Recent Advances in Rheumatology

Recent Advances in Rheumatology

Edited by Travis Reagan

hayle medical
New York

Hayle Medical,
750 Third Avenue, 9th Floor,
New York, NY 10017, USA

Visit us on the World Wide Web at:
www.haylemedical.com

ISBN: 978-1-63241-762-6

Printed in China.

Cataloging-in-Publication Data

Recent advances in rheumatology / edited by Travis Reagan.
p. cm.
Includes bibliographical references and index.
ISBN 978-1-63241-762-6
1. Rheumatology. 2. Rheumatism. I. Reagan, Travis.

RC927 .R47 2019
616.723--dc23

Table of Contents

Preface

Rheumatology is concerned with the diagnosis and therapy of rheumatic diseases. These diseases can be classified into degenerative arthropathies, systemic conditions and connective tissue diseases, inflammatory arthropathies and soft tissue rheumatism. Rheumatoid arthritis, septic arthritis, spondyloarthropathies, etc. are categorized as inflammatory arthropathies. Tennis elbow, low back pain and Golfer's elbow fall within soft tissue rheumatism. The incorporation of biologics such as inhibitors of JAK-STAT signaling pathway, TNF-alpha and certain interleukins are one of the most important developments in this field. Autoimmune diseases are a principal cause of many rheumatic disorders. Therefore, much of research in rheumatology is focused in this direction. Clinical trials of monoclonal antibody therapies for the treatment of arthritic disorders are another emerging focus in rheumatology. This book elucidates the concepts and innovative models around prospective developments with respect to rheumatology. It presents researches and studies performed by experts across the globe. It is meant for students who are looking for an elaborate reference text on rheumatology.

All of the data presented henceforth, was collaborated in the wake of recent advancements in the field. The aim of this book is to present the diversified developments from across the globe in a comprehensible manner. The opinions expressed in each chapter belong solely to the contributing authors. Their interpretations of the topics are the integral part of this book, which I have carefully compiled for a better understanding of the readers.

At the end, I would like to thank all those who dedicated their time and efforts for the successful completion of this book. I also wish to convey my gratitude towards my friends and family who supported me at every step.

Editor

1

Etanercept-Induced Myelopathy in a Pediatric Case of Blau Syndrome

Fabiola Caracseghi,[1] Jaume Izquierdo-Blasco,[2] Angel Sanchez-Montanez,[3] Susana Melendo-Perez,[4] Manuel Roig-Quilis,[2] and Consuelo Modesto[1]

[1] *Pediatric Rheumatology Department, Vall d'Hebron University Hospital, P. Vall d'Hebron 119-129, 08035 Barcelona, Spain*
[2] *Pediatric Neurology Department, Vall d'Hebron University Hospital, P. Vall d'Hebron 119-129, 08035 Barcelona, Spain*
[3] *Pediatric Radiology Department, Vall d'Hebron University Hospital, P. Vall d'Hebron 119-129, 08035 Barcelona, Spain*
[4] *Pediatric Emergency Department, Vall d'Hebron University Hospital, P. Vall d'Hebron 119-129, 08035 Barcelona, Spain*

Correspondence should be addressed to Fabiola Caracseghi, fabiola.caracseghi@gmail.com

Academic Editor: D. Aeberli

Blau syndrome is a rare autoinflammatory disorder within the group of pediatric granulomatous diseases. Mutations in nucleotide-binding oligomerization domain 2 (NOD2/CARD15) are responsible for this condition, which has an autosomal dominant pattern of inheritance and variable expressivity. The clinical picture includes arthritis, uveitis, skin rash, and granulomatous inflammation. Central nervous system involvement is seldom reported, although some isolated cases of seizures, neurosensorial hearing loss, and transient cranial nerve palsy have been described. Treatment consists of nonsteroidal anti-inflammatory drugs, corticosteroids, and immunosuppressive agents, among which anti-tumor-necrosis-factor-alpha (TNF-α) biologic agents, such as etanercept, play an important role. Among the major adverse effects of TNF-α inhibitors, demyelinating disease, multiple sclerosis, and acute transverse myelitis have been reported in adults. We describe a case of pediatric Blau syndrome affected by etanercept-induced myelopathy, manifesting as a clinical syndrome of transverse myelitis. The patient experienced rapid recovery after etanercept was discontinued. To our knowledge, this is the first such case reported in the literature and, possibly, the one with the latest onset, following 8 years of treatment. We discuss the etiopathogenic mechanisms of this reaction and possible explanations for the imaging findings.

1. Introduction

Blau syndrome is a rare autoinflammatory disorder within the group of pediatric granulomatous diseases, together with early-onset sarcoidosis [1, 2]. Mutations in nucleotide-binding oligomerization domain 2 (NOD2/CARD15), a member of the NOD-like receptor family of intracellular proteins, are responsible for the disease, which has an autosomal dominant pattern of inheritance and variable expressivity.

The clinical picture includes arthritis, uveitis, skin rash, and granulomatous inflammation [1, 3]. Central nervous system (CNS) involvement is seldom reported, although isolated cases of seizures, neurosensorial hearing loss and transient cranial nerve palsy have been described [4]. Fever and acute-phase reaction are not always present [2, 3].

Treatment consists of nonsteroidal anti-inflammatory drugs, corticosteroids, and, in refractory cases, immunosuppressive agents, such as methotrexate, azathioprine, mycophenolate mofetil and, recently, interleukin 1 blockers (anakinra), and anti-tumor-necrosis-factor-alpha (TNF-α) biologic agents. Anti-TNF-α drugs, such as etanercept, infliximab, and adalimumab have been on the market since 1998. Etanercept, a soluble recombinant dimer of human TNF receptor proteins fused and bound to human IgG_1, acts competitively to inhibit TNF binding to its cell surface receptor. Infliximab and adalimumab are monoclonal anti-TNF-α antibodies, the first a murine chimeric and the latter a humanized antibody [3].

Anti-TNF-α treatment has been successfully used for several autoimmune and autoinflammatory conditions, such as rheumatoid arthritis, psoriasis with or without arthritis, ankylosing spondylitis, juvenile idiopathic arthritis, and Crohn's disease. Because of the low prevalence of Blau syndrome, there is little information on anti-TNF-α use in pediatric patients with this disease.

The major adverse effects of TNF-α inhibitors include local injection site and systemic reactions after intravenous infusion, infections (particularly opportunistic, due to fungi and mycobacteria), lymphoproliferative diseases, and systemic lupus erythematosus-like syndromes. Demyelinating diseases, multiple sclerosis, and acute transverse myelitis have also been reported in adults [5].

We describe the case of a pediatric patient with Blau syndrome affected by etanercept-induced myelopathy, manifesting as a clinical syndrome of transverse myelitis. To our knowledge, this is the first such case reported in the literature. A distinctive feature was its late onset, 8 years after the start of treatment.

2. Case Presentation

A 13-year-old boy presented to the emergency unit with inability to stand or walk. Eight days previously, he had experienced a mild coccygeal trauma while playing soccer. Seven days later he presented paresthesia of the lower limbs and, less than 24 hours later, bilateral hypoesthesia and paraparesis. He was unable to initiate urination or defecation, but was not incontinent. He denied fever and any infectious episodes over the previous weeks.

The patient had been diagnosed of Blau syndrome at the age of 5. The condition manifested as a generalized papulous rash, recurrent arthritis, and tenosynovitis, which started when he was 2 years old. His mother had been misdiagnosed as having rheumatoid arthritis as a child, after presenting similar symptoms. Genetic study confirmed an autosomal dominant mutation in the NOD2/CARD15 gene. The patient had been treated earlier with corticosteroids and methotrexate and, over the previous 8 years, since the diagnosis, had also received etanercept, with good disease control. He had never presented ocular manifestations.

Physical examination revealed a normal mental status, with no cranial nerve involvement. Funduscopic examination was normal. Muscle tone strength and deep tendon reflexes of the upper limbs were normal. He had hyperreflexia in both lower limbs, an extensor plantar reflex and bilateral exhaustible clonus. Muscle strength in the lower limbs was decreased, graded 2 to 4 out of a maximum of 5 in the different muscle groups, the most highly affected being the psoas and quadriceps. He had tactile and pain hypoesthesia with a sensitive level at T12 and normal thermal and vibratory sensation. Painless camptodactyly and flexion contractures of the proximal interphalangeal joints of the fourth and fifth fingers had already been documented, and there were no inflamed joints. He had no spleen or liver enlargement and no acute skin lesions. The remainder of the examination was normal.

Blood analyses were unremarkable, except for a high erythrocyte sedimentation rate (85 mm/h, normal value <10 mm/h). Cerebrospinal fluid glucose level was normal, protein was slightly elevated (78 mg/dL, normal value 15–45 mg/dL), and IgG level was high (7.4 mg/dL, normal value <3.4 mg/dL), without pleocytosis or oligoclonal bands. Bacterial, viral, and fungal microbiological tests were negative, including mycobacteria.

Cranial magnetic resonance imaging (MRI) study was normal. MRI of the spinal cord revealed bifocal high-intensity white matter lesions on T2-weighted images (T2WI), one extending from the second to the fourth cervical (C_2–C_4) level and another at the conus medullaris (T_{12}-L_1), which enhanced after contrast administration (Figures 1 and 2). Diffusion-weighted imaging (DWI) and apparent diffusion coefficient maps failed to show water movement restriction.

Considering the previous reports of similar adverse reactions with anti-TNF-α [5–12], etanercept was discontinued. The patient received intravenous methylprednisolone pulse therapy (1 g/day) during 5 days, followed by oral prednisone starting at 1 mg/kg, with slow dose tapering for 6 weeks. Clinical improvement was noted 36 hours after the first infusion, and the patient was able to walk without help and regain sphincter control 5 days later. Mild proximal muscle weakness, hyperreflexia, and paresthesia persisted during the next 2 weeks, with progressive amelioration. Four weeks later, his recovery was nearly complete, with slight hyperreflexia in the lower limbs.

Follow-up MRI performed 6 weeks after the first study revealed complete resolution of the cervical cord lesion and an improvement with no enhancement of the conus medullaris lesion (Figure 3).

At his last clinical follow-up visit, 3 months after onset, the patient was completely symptom-free, and the neurological examination was normal. His baseline treatment was switched to corticosteroids and methotrexate. New biological drugs will be reconsidered depending on his disease control, but anti-TNF-α agents are excluded.

3. Discussion

The patient exhibited a clinical syndrome of acute transverse myelitis. The mild coccygeal trauma he had sustained previously may have acted as a triggering event, as has been previously reported [6]. Although etanercept undoubtedly played a role in this patient's myelopathy, the underlying mechanisms are difficult to establish, especially in the absence of pathological studies. It is noteworthy that imaging study revealed 2 lesions at different levels, but the cervical lesion showed no clinical expression on detailed neurological examination and the clinical and MRI manifestations progressively disappeared over a 4- to 6-week period.

The shape of the lesions, the lateral position within the spinal cord, and the enhancement suggest demyelination as the most plausible origin of the patient's MRI findings. MRI studies in cases of anti-TNF-α-associated complications reported to date usually show single or multiple lesions on T2WI, attributed to demyelination [5, 7]. As the cervical lesion completely disappeared 6 weeks after drug withdrawal

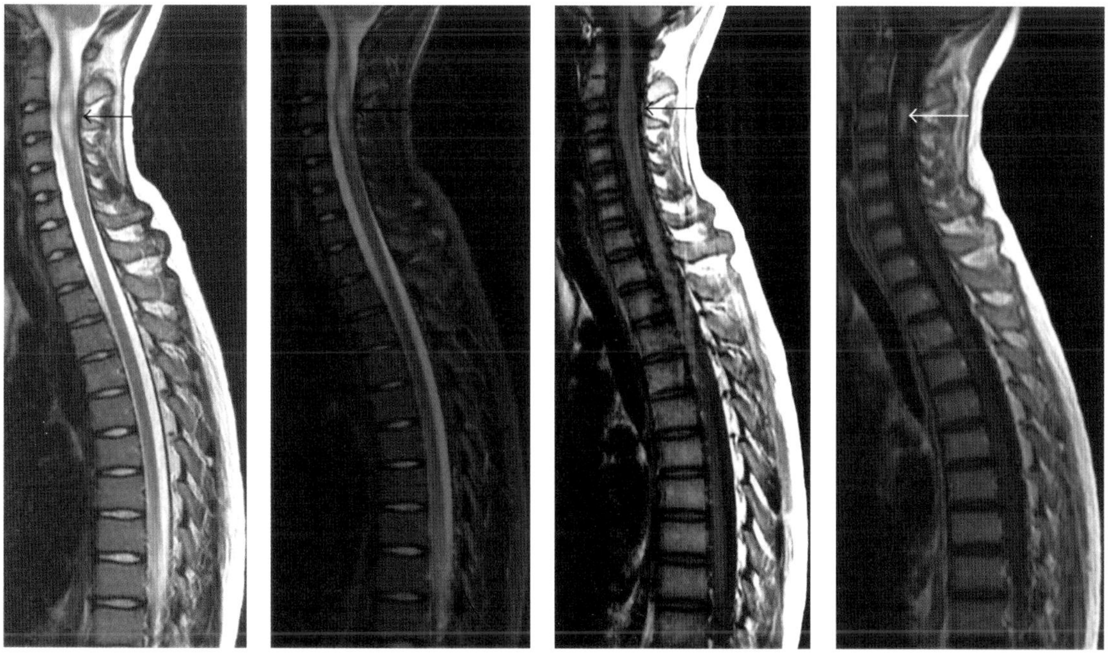

(a) (b) (c) (d)

Figure 1: MR images of the cervicodorsal spinal cord. Sagittal T2WI (a) and STIR-T2WI (b) show a well defined, ovoid-shaped, high-intensity lesion (black arrow) within the cervical cord at C_2–C_4, with mild fusiform expansion of the cord. On sagittal T1WI (c), the lesion is slightly hypointense (black arrow). After gadolinium administration (d), the lesion enhances intensely and homogeneously (white arrow).

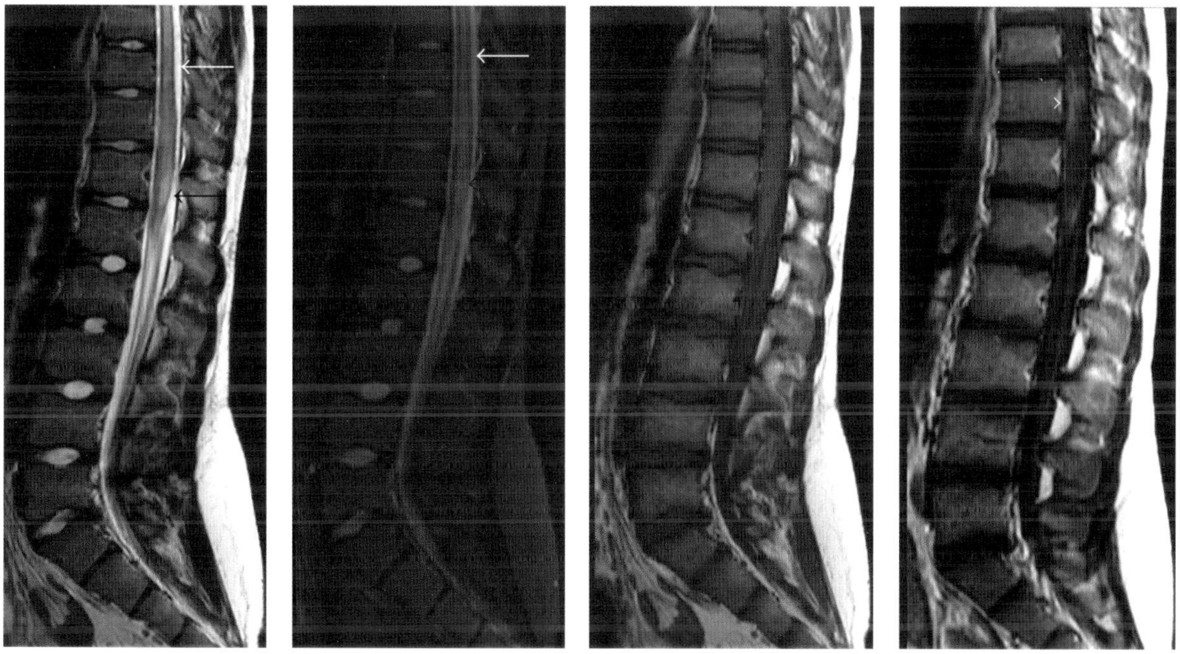

(a) (b) (c) (d)

Figure 2: MR images of the dorsolumbar spinal cord. Sagittal T2WI (a) and STIR-T2WI (b) show patchy hyperintense lesions involving the distal lumbar spinal cord and the conus medullaris (black arrows). Mild spinal cord edema is also present (white arrows). Incidentally, posterior disc bulging is visualized at the level of L_5-S_1 (black arrowhead). The lesions are isointense on T1WI (c). T1WI after intravenous gadolinium injection (d) demonstrates heterogeneous enhancement (white arrowhead).

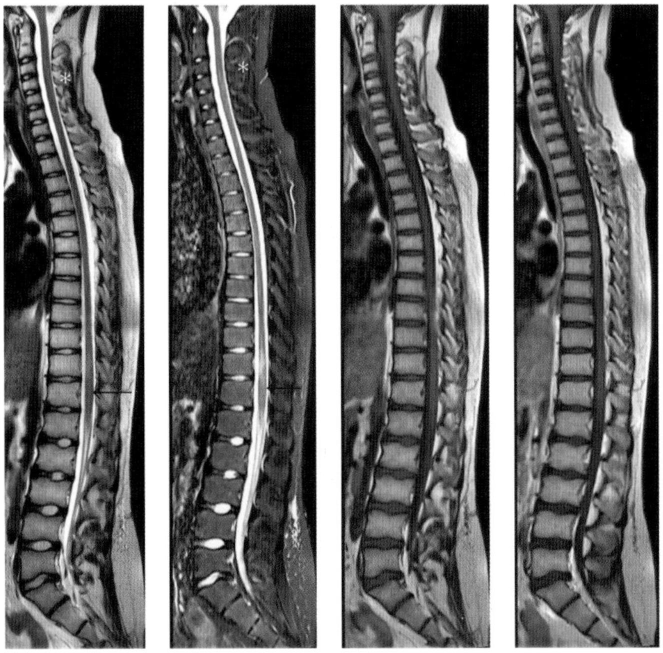

FIGURE 3: Whole cord MR images 6 weeks after the first MRI. Sagittal T2WI (a) and STIR-T2WI (b) show resolution of the cervical lesion (white asterisks), whereas a slight hyperintensity is seen in the lumbar cord (black arrows). There are no abnormalities on sagittal T1WI without (c) and with intravenous gadolinium (d).

and there are no previous reports of histological confirmation, other potential explanations should be considered.

Osmotic demyelination, defined as acute demyelination without inflammation, attributed to osmotic stress or rapid shifts in serum osmolality (classically due to rapid correction of hyponatremia), can produce a similar MRI pattern. The imaging findings may be due to a focal disruption of the brain blood barrier, leading to extravasation and transudation of fluid and macromolecules through arteriolar walls, similarly to what occurs in posterior reversible encephalopathy syndrome. Nonetheless, enhancement following gadolinium administration is not a common feature in these conditions. The imaging characteristics are also consistent with small-vessel lesion due to vasculitis or ischemia. However, although an ischemic etiology cannot be ruled out, the absence of ventral cord predilection and the lack of restriction on DWI make this possibility less likely. Lastly, infectious diseases of the spine can have a similar MRI appearance, but the clinical scenario rules out this possibility.

TNF-expressing macrophages are the effector cells responsible for active demyelination and axonal injury [5]. TNF-α is an important proinflammatory cytokine that is involved in the pathogenesis of inflammatory demyelination in many conditions [5]. It has heterogenic effects in the inflammatory cascade and immune regulation, some of which are not well understood and even antagonistic, depending on the type of receptors involved. For example, although it is an important cytokine implicated in neuronal inflammation, particularly when its type 1 receptor (TNFR1) is involved, TNF-α can also have a protective effect on the CNS and is a key element in remyelination through activation of its type 2 receptor (TNFR2) [5]. The effects of this cytokine on the CNS also depend on the underlying disease. A good example is multiple sclerosis, in which anti-TNF-α treatment worsens the disease, whereas in other conditions, such as chronic dysimmune neuropathies, it is successfully used to treat autoimmune demyelination.

The reported neurological complications related to anti-TNF-α drugs include visual disturbances, confusion, paresthesia, gait disturbances, ataxia, apraxia, dysarthria and even complete Miller-Fisher or Guillain-Barré syndromes, optic neuritis (unilateral or bilateral), pure sensory neuropathy, spasticity, neurogenic bladder, transverse myelitis, and seizures [5, 7, 8]. CNS demyelinating disease and peripheral neuropathy syndromes seem to be the most common [5].

Cerebrospinal fluid can be normal, but low glucose, high protein levels, pleocytosis (mononuclear or polynuclear), increased IgG, and the presence of oligoclonal bands have been reported [5–9].

Symptoms due to etanercept-related demyelination usually develop after a mean of 5 months of therapy [5], with a broad range, from 1 week to several years [5–10]. Our case is among those with the latest reported onset, occurring after 8 years of treatment.

It is difficult to establish an association between anti-TNF therapy and the development of demyelinating disease and peripheral neuropathy. There is, however, a temporal association between the use of these drugs and the development of symptoms, which improve after interrupting treatment and/or reappear after reexposure in most reported cases, as in ours. There are some factors against this association, such as the existence of an underlying condition, which could predispose to myelination defects (this is the case of multiple sclerosis, in which patients are at high risk of demyelination regardless of anti-TNF-α treatment) [5, 7]. Demyelinating lesions are not characteristic of Blau syndrome. Several theories have been put forth to explain this relation [5, 9], such as local immune dysregulation by TNF-α blockage leading to prolonged survival of myelin-specific activated T cells and increased cytokine production, vasculitis-induced ischemia and altered repairing of axonal injuries, and myelin damage by TNRF2 inhibition. But, up to now, long-term clinical studies assessing the safety of anti-TNF-α drugs have failed to show a higher rate of neurological disorders in treated patients than in the general population [5, 9, 11].

There is no specific treatment for this complication, but the immediate withdrawal of the causative drug seems reasonable, together with high-dose courses of corticosteroids, intravenous immunoglobulins (IVIG), or plasmapheresis [5 9]. The use of cyclophosphamide, interferon β-1a, azathioprine, or gabapentin, usually in association with steroids or IVIG, has also been reported, with variable results [5, 9]. In most cases, the prognosis is favorable, with partial or complete resolution of the symptoms (occurring spontaneously in some cases) and, sometimes, with persistent imaging abnormalities [5, 6]. Long-term followup has shown a variable course, suggesting that treatment withdrawal may not be necessary for disease control in individual patients who do not have disabling involvement and for whom there are no other available treatment options [10].

Cerebral demyelination possibly associated with etanercept treatment in children has been reported in the single case of a 5-year-old girl with systemic-onset juvenile idiopathic arthritis, but it was difficult to establish whether it was drug-related [12].

4. Conclusions

Anti TNF therapy should be avoided in patients with a history of predisposing conditions, such as multiple sclerosis or peripheral neuropathy. Clinicians should carefully monitor their patients for new or unusual neurological symptoms appearing during treatment and discontinue therapy if there is a suspected drug related complication. Based on the current experience, in individual cases, in which other treatment options are limited, anti-TNF drugs might be continued at a lower dose, under strict supervision.

Acknowledgments

The authors gratefully acknowledge Dr. Elida Vázquez for her useful comments on the paper and Celine Cavallo for language editing.

References

[1] D. Rigante, "Autoinflammatory syndromes behind the scenes of recurrent fevers in children," *Medical Science Monitor*, vol. 15, no. 8, pp. RA179–RA187, 2009.

[2] J. I. Aróstegui and J. Yagüe, "Hereditary systemic autoinflammatory diseases. Hereditary periodic fever syndromes," *Medicina Clinica*, vol. 129, no. 7, pp. 267–277, 2007.

[3] L. Punzi, A. Furlan, M. Podswiadek et al., "Clinical and genetic aspects of Blau syndrome: a 25-year follow-up of one family and a literature review," *Autoimmunity Reviews*, vol. 8, no. 3, pp. 228–232, 2009.

[4] A. Emaminia, M. Nabavi, M. M. Nasab, and S. Kashef, "Central nervous system involvement in Blau syndrome: a new feature of the syndrome?" *Journal of Rheumatology*, vol. 34, no. 12, pp. 2504–2505, 2007.

[5] A. G. Tristano, "Neurological adverse events associated with anti-tumor necrosis factor alpha treatment," *Journal of Neurology*, vol. 257, no. 9, pp. 1421–1431, 2010.

[6] N. Al Saieg and M. J. Luzar, "Etanercept induced multiple sclerosis and transverse myelitis," *Journal of Rheumatology*, vol. 33, no. 6, pp. 1202–1204, 2006.

[7] N. L. Sicotte and R. R. Voskuhl, "Onset of multiple sclerosis associated with anti-TNF therapy," *Neurology*, vol. 57, no. 10, pp. 1885 1888, 2001.

[8] C. J. van der Laken, W. F. Lems, R. M. van Soesbergen, I. I. van der Sande, and B. A. C. Dijkmans, "Paraplegia in a patient receiving anti-tumor necrosis factor therapy for rheumatoid arthritis: comment on the article by Mohan et al," *Arthritis and Rheumatism*, vol. 48, no. 1, pp. 269–270, 2003.

[9] N. Mohan, E. T. Edwards, T. R. Cupps et al., "Demyelination occurring during anti-tumor necrosis factor α therapy for inflammatory arthritides," *Arthritis and Rheumatism*, vol. 44, no. 12, pp. 2862–2869, 2001.

[10] P. Lozeron, C. Denier, C. Lacroix, and D. Adams, "Long-term course of demyelinating neuropathies occurring during tumor necrosis factor-α-blocker therapy," *Archives of Neurology*, vol. 66, no. 4, pp. 490–497, 2009.

[11] L. Klareskog, M. Gaubitz, V. Rodriguez-Valverde, M. Malaise, M. Dougados, and J. Wajdula, "A long-term, open-label trial of the safety and efficacy of etanercept (Enbrel) in patients with rheumatoid arthritis not treated with other disease-modifying antirheumatic drugs," *Annals of the Rheumatic Diseases*, vol. 65, no. 12, pp. 1578–1584, 2006.

[12] S. Kunzmann, M. Warmuth-Metz, and H. J. Girschick, "Cerebral demyelination in association with TNF-inhibition therapy in a 5-year-old girl with aseptic meningitis as the first symptom of Still's disease," *Scandinavian Journal of Rheumatology*, vol. 34, no. 1, pp. 76–78, 2005.

2

Reduced Quadriceps Motor-Evoked Potentials in an Individual with Unilateral Knee Osteoarthritis

Michael A. Hunt, Jeanie R. Zabukovec, Sue Peters, Courtney L. Pollock, Meghan A. Linsdell, and Lara A. Boyd

Department of Physical Therapy, University of British Columbia, Vancouver, BC, Canada V6T 1Z3

Correspondence should be addressed to Michael A. Hunt, michael.hunt@ubc.ca

Academic Editors: L.-P. Erwig, K. P. Makaritsis, P. E. Prete, and T. Takahashi

One male with unilateral osteoarthritis (OA) of the knee underwent testing of corticospinal (CS) excitability (as quantified from motor-evoked potentials (MEPs) in the rectus femoris (RF) using transcranial magnetic stimulation) and quadriceps muscle strength. Baseline data indicated reduced MEP amplitudes in the RF of the affected limb compared to the unaffected limb. Increases in RF MEP amplitudes from both limbs were observed immediately following a 30-minute exercise session focusing on muscle strengthening. Following an 8-week muscle strengthening intervention, the participant exhibited increased MEP amplitudes and muscle strength in the affected limb. These findings suggest that alterations in peripheral muscle function found in patients with knee OA may have an origin centrally within the motor cortex and that interlimb differences may be evident in those with unilateral disease. These findings also suggest that CS excitability may be improved following a muscle strengthening intervention.

1. Introduction

Osteoarthritis (OA) is a prevalent chronic condition often associated with symptoms of pain and physical dysfunction. Biomechanical studies in this patient population have typically focused on the measurement of knee joint load obtained from three-dimensional gait analysis and/or methods of assessing neuromuscular function. Altered or excessive joint loading is a recognized risk factor for the degradation of articular cartilage [1, 2], and biomechanical studies have identified joint-specific measures of load during movement, that are predictive of disease progression. For example, the magnitude of the external knee adduction moment (KAM) measured during walking—an indirect measure of dynamic load in the medial compartment of the knee joint [3]—has been shown to be a strong predictor of medial compartment tibiofemoral knee OA progression [4].

In addition to producing movement, the muscles of the lower limb are believed to play a role in the dissipation of load away from articular cartilage in the knee joint [5]. However, patients with knee OA often exhibit strength deficiencies [6–8] and altered neuromuscular control [9] compared to those without OA, which may result in suboptimal load dissipation within the knee. Electromyographical studies during walking have also shown increased muscle cocontraction in those with knee OA [10, 11], indicative of altered motor output. Due to these differences in neuromuscular outcomes, many researchers and clinicians have attempted to restore muscle strength and function in those with knee OA using a variety of treatment approaches ranging from simple muscle strengthening programs to complex neuromuscular retraining interventions, all with varying effects on muscle and joint function.

Though the motor output changes resulting from knee OA have been well-studied, the central contribution to muscle activity is less well known. Noninvasive activation of the motor cortex using transcranial magnetic stimulation (TMS) to evoke responses in peripheral muscles (termed motor evoked potentials (MEPs)) provides a reliable and accurate method of assessing corticospinal (CS) excitability and the contribution of central structures to muscle activity [12]. This method has been used for a number of patient populations ranging from those with neurological impairments including stroke [12] to orthopaedic involvement such as those with muscle weakness [13], knee pain [14], or anterior cruciate ligament injury [15]. We are unaware of any studies that have used TMS to study CS excitability and central contributions to muscle activity in patients with knee OA. As a result, the purpose of the present study was to assess CS excitability and quadriceps muscle strength in an individual with unilateral knee OA before and after a muscle strengthening program.

2. Case Presentation

A 67-year-old, right leg dominant male (1.63 m; 61.4 kg) underwent physical assessment pertaining to reports of unilateral left knee pain and muscle weakness. He first experienced moderate left knee pain five months previously when attempting to carry a heavy object up a flight of stairs. There were no reports of previous injuries to the feet, knees, hips, or back that required medical attention. The pain was self-managed using anti-inflammatory medication and glucosamine with chondroitin, however he still reported a moderate (4/10) amount of knee pain on most days. He was able to ambulate unaided, but occasionally used a cane when walking longer distances. Radiographs confirmed the presence of mild OA in the left knee with definite medial joint space narrowing and one small medial tibial osteophyte (Kellgren and Lawrence grade 2 [16]). Radiographs of the right knee were unremarkable. Clinical examination did not reveal any ligamentous laxity or patellofemoral involvement, or any observable difference in knee circumference or thigh muscle girth. In accordance with established and institutional safety guidelines for the use of TMS, the participant was screened for history of seizure, medication use, metal implants in the brain or head, and history of neurological diagnosis prior to inclusion in this study [17, 18].

Assessment of neuromuscular function included measurement of CS excitability (as quantified using MEPs) and isometric muscle strength. CS excitability was assessed using TMS with a 70 mm double cone coil (Magstim Super Rapid, Magstim Company, Ltd.). Surface bipolar Ag-AgCl electrodes (10 mm diameter) were placed 25 mm apart on the belly of the left and right rectus femoris (RF), and a ground electrode was placed on the patella. The skin was shaved, cleaned, and abraded prior to application of the electrodes to reduce electrical impedance. During stimulation, the coil trajectory that elicited the best MEP for the RF for each leg was marked using BrainSight software (Rogue, Montreal) and stored for future reference, and the marker for the RF trajectory was placed on a template MRI brain image. To reduce both intra- and intersession variability in the application of TMS, the same reference brain and RF trajectory marker were used in each TMS mapping time point. Active motor threshold (AMT) was determined while the participant maintained a low level contraction and defined as the lowest stimulator intensity that generated 5 MEPs across 10 trials, each with a peak-to-peak amplitude (Figure 1) of at least 200 μV. MEPs were then elicited from the motor cortex at stimulus intensities of 105%, 115%, 120%, 125%, 130%, 135%, and 145% AMT. A stimulus response (motor recruitment) curve [19] was generated for each limb by calculating the average peak MEP magnitude from ten consecutive stimuli at each intensity, with approximately 1 sec to 4 sec between each stimulus. To account for the possibility of baseline variability, data from each stimulus intensity were normalized to 105% AMT for each stimulation session. Linear regression was then used to compute the slope parameter for the curve, as suggested previously [15, 20]. This procedure was repeated immediately following a 30-minute exercise session, using the same electrode placement and coil trajectory. This exercise session was intended to familiarize the participant with a home-based exercise program and included unilateral (affected limb only) open-kinetic chain knee extension in sitting, knee flexion in standing, and hip abduction in standing and side lying. Closed kinetic chain exercises include half-squats against a wall, forward lunges, and seated leg presses (not part of the home program due to equipment requirements), all involving both limbs. Resistance, when applicable, was provided from cuff weights attached around the ankle and chosen based on the ability to perform 10 repetitions with moderate difficulty.

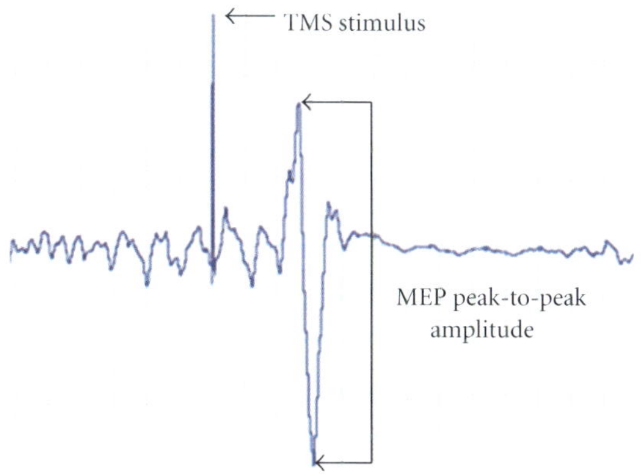

FIGURE 1: MEP magnitude was determined by identifying the peak-to-peak amplitude of the quadriceps EMG trace following each TMS-evoked stimulus.

On a separate visit to the laboratory within the same week as the assessment of CS excitability, maximal isometric muscle strength was measured while the participant was seated in an isokinetic dynamometer (Biodex System 4; Biodex Medical Systems Inc., Shirley, NY). Maximal isometric knee extension torque from each limb was measured with the hip in 90° of flexion and the knee in 30° of flexion. After a warm-up trial for the purposes of equipment familiarization, three isometric trials of five-second duration were completed for each limb. The maximum torque exerted onto the dynamometer from the three trials was identified and normalized to body mass (Nm/kg).

Following baseline muscle strength testing, the participant was prescribed the series of six muscle-strengthening exercises described above and instructed to complete each exercise for 3 sets of 10 repetitions at home on at least four days per week over 8 weeks. Ankle cuff weights were provided for resistance to the seated knee extension, side lying hip abduction, as well as the standing knee flexion, and hip abduction. The participant met with a physiotherapist four times over this period to ensure proper exercise performance and safe progression of resistance, and to perform additional exercises (e.g., seated leg press and standing hip adduction with cable resistance) not possible as part of the home program. CS excitability (using the same electrode placement and coil trajectory from baseline, AMT was determined again) and muscle strength were assessed again at the end of the 8-week muscle strengthening intervention, using the same techniques with the isokinetic dynamometer and outcomes previously described. Finally, overall average knee pain was assessed before and after the strengthening intervention, using an 11-point numerical rating scale with 0 representing "no pain" and 10 representing "worst pain imaginable".

Between-limb differences in MEP amplitude were evident across all stimulus intensities at baseline (Figure 2). In general, RF MEPs were higher in the unaffected limb compared to the affected limb across all stimulus intensities prior to 30 minutes of exercise. Following the 30-minute exercise familiarization session, MEP amplitudes in both limbs increased at all stimulus intensities, with the exception of 120% and 145% AMT in the unaffected limb. Differences between limbs in the postexercise session were small at all stimulus intensities. Following 8 weeks of lower limb muscle strengthening, MEP amplitudes in the affected limb increased, compared to baseline at all stimulus intensities except 115% of AMT (Figure 3). Finally, overall knee pain was reduced from 4/10 to 0/10, and maximal isometric quadriceps torque increased from 1.25 Nm/kg to 1.60 Nm/kg following the 8-week strengthening intervention.

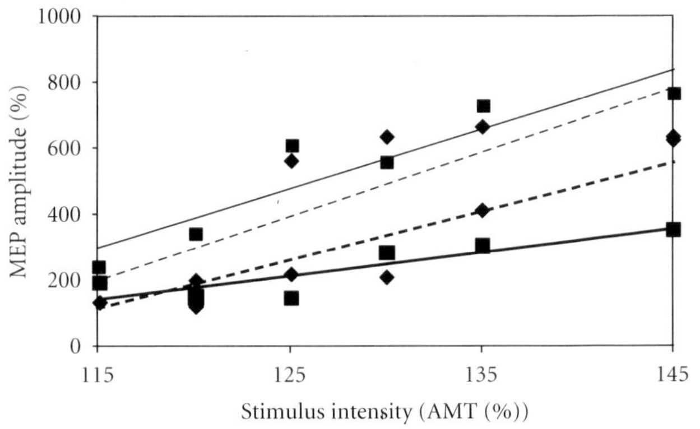

Figure 2: Stimulus response curves at the baseline testing session produced by calculating average MEP magnitudes at TMS stimulus intensities equal to 115%, 120%, 125%, 130%, 135%, and 145% of the active motor threshold (AMT) for each limb. Values are represented as a normalized percentage of the average MEP amplitude calculated at 105% of the AMT for the affected limb (squares and solid lines) and unaffected limb (diamonds and dashed lines). Thick lines correspond to the first baseline testing session (before the initial 30-minute exercise session), while thin lines correspond to the second baseline testing session (immediately following the initial 30-minute exercise session).

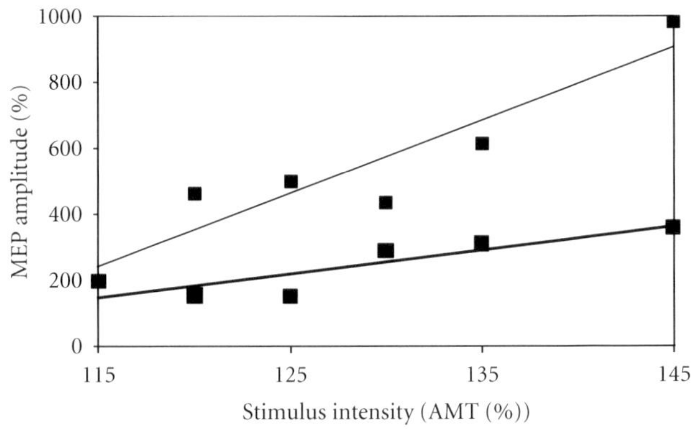

Figure 3: Stimulus response curves for the affected limb from the baseline, preexercise testing session (thick line) and 8-week follow-up testing session (thin line) produced by calculating average MEP amplitudes at TMS stimulus intensities equal to 115%, 120%, 125%, 130%, 135%, and 145% of the active motor threshold (AMT). Values are represented as a normalized percentage of the average MEP magnitude calculated at 105% of the AMT from each testing session.

3. Discussion

Results from this case study show that interlimb differences in CS excitability existed in an individual with unilateral OA of the knee. Specifically, CS excitability was reduced in the RF muscle crossing the knee affected with OA, compared to the contralateral, unaffected limb. Further, increases in CS excitability in the hemisphere controlling the affected limb were evident immediately following a single muscle strengthening exercise session as well as after completing an 8-week intervention focusing on improving muscle strength. Taken together, these findings indicate the likelihood of alterations along the CS tract in individuals with knee OA, as well as the possibility of improving motor function with exercise training.

Though there are no data in the literature reporting cortical excitability in individuals with knee OA, there are previous examinations of patients with other knee pathologies. On et al. [14] reported increases in MEP magnitudes in the vastus medialis obliques and vastus lateralis muscles in a cohort of younger (ages 23 to 37 years) individuals with patellofemoral pain syndrome compared to healthy controls. Héroux and Tremblay [15] identified three unique subgroups of patients with anterior cruciate ligament injures based on their interlimb differences in RF MEP amplitudes. Of the 10 participants, three exhibited steeper stimulus response curves (i.e., higher MEPs across all stimulus intensities) in their injured limb compared to the uninjured; four participants exhibited steeper stimulus response curves in the uninjured limb, while the remaining three participants exhibited symmetry between the two limbs. They postulated that these differences in MEP presentation were the result of impairments in quadriceps activation in some individuals and distinguished between "copers" and "noncopers" known to exist in this patient population that reflect either an ability to exhibit near normal biomechanics and joint function despite the injury, or an increasing risk of reinjury and functional decline [21]. Identification of similar subgroups in individuals with knee OA would have important implications for the management of the disease given that proper muscle function is believed to play an important role in cartilage offloading during movement. Thus, identification of those who exhibit impairments in cortical excitability and motor output would permit more focused rehabilitation and improvements in subsequent joint protection. In contrast, those without cortical and motor impairments may not necessarily require muscle reconditioning approaches and alternate treatment strategies could be provided.

The individual in the current case study exhibited increases in MEP amplitude following 8 weeks of muscle strengthening exercises. Results from previous studies examining the effect of muscle strengthening on MEP amplitudes point to differences in outcomes based on the muscle being examined. Strengthening exercises have not been shown to increase MEP amplitude from the flexor digitorum indices muscle [22, 23] nor the biceps brachii muscle [24], but have been shown to increase MEP amplitudes from the soleus muscle [25]. Modulation of MEPs is also dependent on the functional implication of muscles in the task. Schieppati et al. [26] demonstrated an increase in MEPs in prime movers in precision tasks requiring control compared to power tasks, despite comparable EMG levels. Jensen and colleagues [24] also demonstrated that several weeks of skill training induced CS excitability, whereas strength training induced a decrease. Thus, it may be that the MEP response to exercise is not only dependent on the muscle group, but the biomechanical requirements of the muscles for movement.

The increases in MEP amplitudes from the RF of the affected limb in the present study suggest some form of plasticity in the motor system of the participant that may have occurred due to improved neuromuscular efficiency, cortical changes resulting from decreased pain responses, or both. Importantly, increases in MEP magnitude were evident following a single 30-minute exercise session. This may have been the result of upregulation of central nervous system, a general improvement in activation of the quadriceps with force production compared to the preexercise, sedentary situation, or a reduction in muscle inhibition after exercise due to decreased joint pain. Indeed, the term "arthrogenic muscle inhibition" has been used to describe a diminished ability to contract a muscle following an injury [27], which may reduce the excitability of motor neurons and subsequent motor output [28]. Many authors suggest that these changes are manifested at the cortical level to produce deficits in strength following orthopaedic injuries [29–32], while others suggest that these changes in cortical excitability result from prolonged muscle activation and movement impairments [33, 34]. Regardless, a viscous cycle of pain and movement restrictions—common in those with knee OA—may result in impairments in CS excitability and motor output, causing further movement restrictions and subsequent joint pain. Given the suggested role of muscle in OA pathogenesis [5], identification of methods to enhance neuromuscular efficiency while simultaneously reducing joint pain represents an important clinical and research objective for this patient population. That said, the limited ability to draw firm conclusions of the relationship between OA and cortical excitability and resultant MEPs from a single patient must be acknowledged. Further work in this area is warranted to better understand these relationships, with an aim to improve the clinical management of the disease.

4. Conclusions

These findings show that CS excitability and subsequent RF MEPs are different based on the presence or absence of knee OA within an individual. It was also shown that increases in MEP amplitudes can be achieved with short-term (30-minute) and longer-term (8-week) exercise. Given the continued use of strengthening exercises in clinical management of knee OA as well as the recent focus on the use of neuromuscular retraining programs for knee OA, continued research is needed to determine the optimal methods of restoring neuromuscular function in this patient population. Further, an understanding of the role of reduced CS excitability and MEPs on measures of joint loading during movement a known risk factor for OA progression—is needed to better understand disease pathology and develop effective treatments focusing on improving muscle and joint function.

Acknowledgments

Partial funding for this study was provided from the Canadian Arthritis Network. L. A. Boyd received salary support from the Canada Research Chairs and the Michael Smith Foundation for Health Research.

References

[1] E. L. Radin and I. L. Paul, "Response of joints to impact loading. I. In vitro wear," *Arthritis and Rheumatism*, vol. 14, no. 3, pp. 356–362, 1971.

[2] E. L. Radin, H. G. Parker, J. W. Pugh, R. S. Steinberg, I. L. Paul, and R. M. Rose, "Response of joints to impact loading III. Relationship between trabecular microfractures and cartilage degeneration," *Journal of Biomechanics*, vol. 6, no. 1, pp. 51–57, 1973.

[3] O. D. Schipplein and T. P. Andriacchi, "Interaction between active and passive knee stabilizers during level walking," *Journal of Orthopaedic Research*, vol. 9, no. 1, pp. 113–119, 1991.

[4] T. Miyazaki, M. Wada, H. Kawahara, M. Sato, H. Baba, and S. Shimada, "Dynamic load at baseline can predict radiographic disease progression in medial compartment knee osteoarthritis," *Annals of the Rheumatic Diseases*, vol. 61, no. 7, pp. 617–622, 2002.

[5] K. L. Bennell, M. A. Hunt, T. V. Wrigley, B. W. Lim, and R. S. Hinman, "Role of muscle in the genesis and management of knee osteoarthritis," *Rheumatic Disease Clinics of North America*, vol. 34, no. 3, pp. 731–754, 2008.

[6] R. S. Hinman, M. A. Hunt, M. W. Creaby, T. V. Wrigley, F. J. McManus, and K. L. Bennell, "Hip muscle weakness in

individuals with medial knee osteoarthritis," *Arthritis Care and Research*, vol. 62, no. 8, pp. 1190–1193, 2010.

[7] S. P. Messier, R. F. Loeser, J. L. Hoover, E. L. Semble, and C. M. Wise, "Osteoarthritis of the knee: effects on gait, strength, and flexibility," *Archives of Physical Medicine and Rehabilitation*, vol. 73, no. 1, pp. 29–36, 1992.

[8] C. Slemenda, K. D. Brandt, D. K. Heilman et al., "Quadriceps weakness and osteoarthritis of the knee," *Annals of Internal Medicine*, vol. 127, no. 2, pp. 97–104, 1997.

[9] T. Hortobágyi, J. Garry, D. Holbert, and P. Devita, "Aberrations in the control of quadriceps muscle force in patients with knee osteoarthritis," *Arthritis Care and Research*, vol. 51, no. 4, pp. 562–569, 2004.

[10] J. L. Astephen, K. J. Deluzio, G. E. Caldwell, M. J. Dunbar, and C. L. Hubley-Kozey, "Gait and neuromuscular pattern changes are associated with differences in knee osteoarthritis severity levels," *Journal of Biomechanics*, vol. 41, no. 4, pp. 868–876, 2008.

[11] C. L. Hubley-Kozey, K. J. Deluzio, S. C. Landry, J. S. McNutt, and W. D. Stanish, "Neuromuscular alterations during walking in persons with moderate knee osteoarthritis," *Journal of Electromyography and Kinesiology*, vol. 16, no. 4, pp. 365–378, 2006.

[12] A. Cacchio, M. Paoloni, N. Cimini et al., "Reliability of TMS-related measures of tibialis anterior muscle in patients with chronic stroke and healthy subjects," *Journal of the Neurological Sciences*, vol. 303, no. 1-2, pp. 90–94, 2011.

[13] D. Urbach, A. Berth, and F. Awiszus, "Effect of transcranial magnetic stimulation on voluntary activation in patients with quadriceps weakness," *Muscle and Nerve*, vol. 32, no. 2, pp. 164–169, 2005.

[14] A. Y. On, B. Uludağ, E. Taşkiran, and C. Ertekin, "Differential corticomotor control of a muscle adjacent to a painful joint," *Neurorehabilitation and Neural Repair*, vol. 18, no. 3, pp. 127–133, 2004.

[15] M. E. Héroux and F. Tremblay, "Corticomotor excitability associated with unilateral knee dysfunction secondary to anterior cruciate ligament injury," *Knee Surgery, Sports Traumatology, Arthroscopy*, vol. 14, no. 9, pp. 823–833, 2006.

[16] J. H. Kellgren and J. S. Lawrence, "Radiological assessment of osteo-arthrosis," *Annals of the Rheumatic Diseases*, vol. 16, no. 4, pp. 494–502, 1957.

[17] E. M. Wassermann, "Risk and safety of repetitive transcranial magnetic stimulation: report and suggested guidelines from the International Workshop on the Safety of Repetitive Transcranial Magnetic Stimulation, June 5-7, 1996," *Electroencephalography and Clinical Neurophysiology*, vol. 108, no. 1, pp. 1–16, 1998.

[18] S. Rossi, M. Hallett, P. M. Rossini, and A. Pascual-Leone, "Safety, ethical considerations, and application guidelines for the use of transcranial magnetic stimulation in clinical practice and research," *Clinical Neurophysiology*, vol. 120, no. 12, pp. 2008–2039, 2009.

[19] M. C. Ridding and J. C. Rothwell, "Stimulus/response curves as a method of measuring motor cortical excitability in man," *Electroencephalography and Clinical Neurophysiology*, vol. 105, no. 5, pp. 340–344, 1997.

[20] J. Ray, B. McNamara, and S. Boniface, "Acquisition and expression of proximal and distal upper limb stimulus-response curves to transcranial magnetic stimulation," *Muscle and Nerve*, vol. 25, no. 2, pp. 202–206, 2002.

[21] T. L. Chmielewski, S. Stackhouse, M. J. Axe, and L. Snyder-Mackler, "A prospective analysis of incidence and severity of quadriceps inhibition in a consecutive sample of 100 patients with complete acute anterior cruciate ligament rupture," *Journal of Orthopaedic Research*, vol. 22, no. 5, pp. 925–930, 2004.

[22] D. J. Kidgell and A. J. Pearce, "Corticospinal properties following short-term strength training of an intrinsic hand muscle," *Human Movement Science*, vol. 29, no. 5, pp. 631–641, 2010.

[23] T. J. Carroll, S. Riek, and R. G. Carson, "The sites of neural adaptation induced by resistance training in humans," *Journal of Physiology*, vol. 544, no. 2, pp. 641–652, 2002.

[24] J. L. Jensen, P. C. D. Marstrand, and J. B. Nielsen, "Motor skill training and strength training are associated with different plastic changes in the central nervous system," *Journal of Applied Physiology*, vol. 99, no. 4, pp. 1558–1568, 2005.

[25] S. Beck, W. Taube, M. Gruber, F. Amtage, A. Gollhofer, and M. Schubert, "Task-specific changes in motor evoked potentials of lower limb muscles after different training interventions," *Brain Research*, vol. 1179, no. 1, pp. 51–60, 2007.

[26] M. Schieppati, C. Trompetto, and G. Abbruzzese, "Selective facilitation of responses to cortical stimulation of proximal and distal arm muscles by precision tasks in man," *Journal of Physiology*, vol. 491, no. 2, pp. 551–562, 1996.

[27] J. T. Hopkins and C. D. Ingersoll, "Arthrogenic muscle inhibition: a limiting factor in joint rehabilitation," *Journal of Sport Rehabilitation*, vol. 9, no. 2, pp. 135–159, 2000.

[28] R. M. Palmieri, J. A. Tom, J. E. Edwards et al., "Arthrogenic muscle response induced by an experimental knee joint effusion is mediated by pre- and post-synaptic spinal mechanisms," *Journal of Electromyography and Kinesiology*, vol. 14, no. 6, pp. 631–640, 2004.

[29] L. G. Elmqvist, R. Lorentzon, C. Johansson, and A. R. Fugl-Meyer, "Does a torn anterior cruciate ligament lead to change in the central nervous drive of the knee extensors?" *European Journal of Applied Physiology and Occupational Physiology*, vol. 58, no. 1-2, pp. 203–207, 1988.

[30] H. Gauffin, G. Pettersson, Y. Tegner, and H. Tropp, "Function testing in patients with old rupture of the anterior cruciate ligament," *International Journal of Sports Medicine*, vol. 11, no. 1, pp. 73–77, 1990.

[31] D. Urbach, W. Nebelung, H. T. Weiler, and F. Awiszus, "Bilateral deficit of voluntary quadriceps muscle activation after unilateral ACL tear," *Medicine and Science in Sports and Exercise*, vol. 31, no. 12, pp. 1691–1696, 1999.

[32] E. M. Wojtys and L. J. Huston, "Neuromuscular performance in normal and anterior cruciate ligament- deficient lower extremities," *American Journal of Sports Medicine*, vol. 22, no. 1, pp. 89–104, 1994.

[33] J. Liepert, M. Tegenthoff, and J. P. Malin, "Changes of cortical motor area size during immobilization," *Electroencephalography and Clinical Neurophysiology*, vol. 97, no. 6, pp. 382–386, 1995.

[34] G. Zanette, P. Manganotti, A. Fiaschi, and S. Tamburin, "Modulation of motor cortex excitability after upper limb immobilization," *Clinical Neurophysiology*, vol. 115, no. 6, pp. 1264–1275, 2004.

Granulomatosis with Polyangiitis Presenting as a Choroidal Tumor

Taro Masuda,[1] Yasumori Izumi,[1] Hayato Takeshita,[1] Chieko Kawahara,[1] Yoshika Tsuji,[1] Hirokazu Kurohama,[2] Nozomi Iwanaga,[1] Miwako Inamoto,[3] Keiichi Kase,[4] Masahiro Ito,[2] Atsushi Kawakami,[5] and Kiyosi Migita[1]

[1]*Departments of General Internal Medicine and Rheumatology, Nagasaki Medical Center, Kubara 2-1001-1, Omura, Nagasaki 856-8562, Japan*
[2]*Department of Pathology, Nagasaki Medical Center, Kubara 2-1001-1, Omura, Nagasaki 856-8562, Japan*
[3]*Department of Ophthalmology, Nagasaki Medical Center, Kubara 2-1001-1, Omura, Nagasaki 856-8562, Japan*
[4]*Department of Otolaryngology, Nagasaki Medical Center, Kubara 2-1001-1, Omura, Nagasaki 856-8562, Japan*
[5]*Department of Rheumatology, Nagasaki University Hospital, Sakamoto 1-7-1, Nagasaki 852-8501, Japan*

Correspondence should be addressed to Kiyosi Migita; migita@nagasaki-mc.com

Academic Editor: Gregory J. Tsay

Granulomatosis with polyangiitis (GPA) sometimes involves the eye orbit; however, choroidal involvements in GPA had been rarely reported. We report a rare case presenting with a choroidal mass in an 83-year-old Japanese woman who presented with left eye pain. Diagnostic biopsy revealed necrotizing vasculitis with infiltrates of inflammatory cells. Diagnosis was localized granulomatosis with polyangiitis. Combined treatments with corticosteroid plus azathioprine resolved the choroidal mass region. Although treatment with corticosteroid and immunosuppressive agents improves the prognosis of the disease, ocular morbidity is still well recognized. Clinicians should consider a differential diagnosis of GPA in patients with inflammatory choroidal tumors.

1. Introduction

Granulomatosis with polyangiitis (GPA) is classically characterized as the triad of necrotizing granulomatosis lesions of the upper and lower respiratory tract, focal segmental glomerulonephritis, and necrotizing vasculitis [1]. The vasculitis preferentially affects small-fiber arterial vessels and, to a lesser extent, small and large vessels, causing arteritis [2]. Affected patients usually present with the disease in the upper respiratory tracts, lungs, and kidneys, although it has been reported to involve almost any organ [3]. GPA also can manifest as ophthalmological disease [4], although there have been few reports of choroidal involvement. Anti-neutrophil cytoplasmic antibody- (ANCA-) directed proteinase-3 (RR3-ANCA) is a diagnostic marker for GPA [5]. A definitive diagnosis of GPA, however, requires the presence of a histologically proved granulomatous inflammatory process, vasculitis, and giant cells [6]. We report the unusual clinical course of a patient with a choroidal tumor accompanied by an elevated serum myeloperoxidase- (MPO-) ANCA titer. The final diagnosis was identified as GPA when the pathological evaluation revealed the presence of necrotizing vasculitis and the serum MAO-ANCA assay was positive. We discuss here this unusual choroidal manifestation of GPA.

2. Case Presentation

An 83-year-old Japanese woman was referred to us with an 8-month history of left periorbital and left eye pain associated with headache migrating temporal region. The patient subsequently developed conjunctivitis of the left eye. The medical history included unstable angina 3 months previously that was treated with percutaneous coronary intervention. Upon admission, the patient had a temperature of 37.3°C, pulse 91/min, and blood pressure 90/63 mmHg. Her lungs were clear, and her abdomen was soft without hepatosplenomegaly.

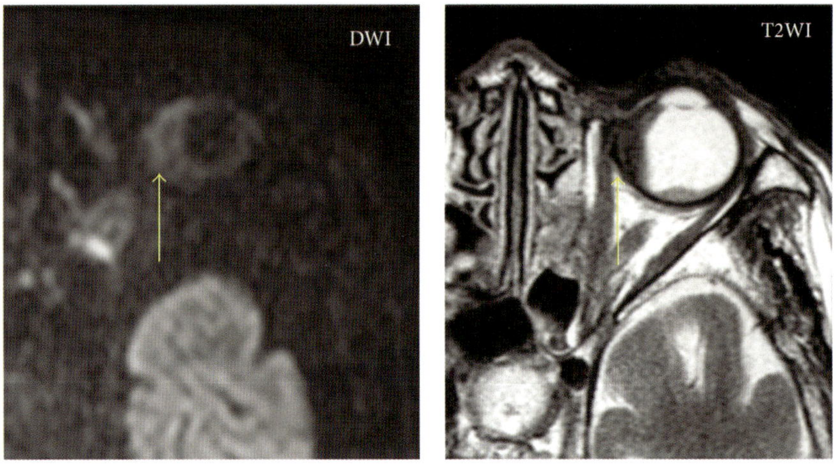

FIGURE 1: MRI images of the choroidal mass. Diffuse-weighted images (DWI) showed high signal intensity in left interior orbital lesion. T2-weighted image (T2WI) showed the choroidal tumor with low intensity of left eye.

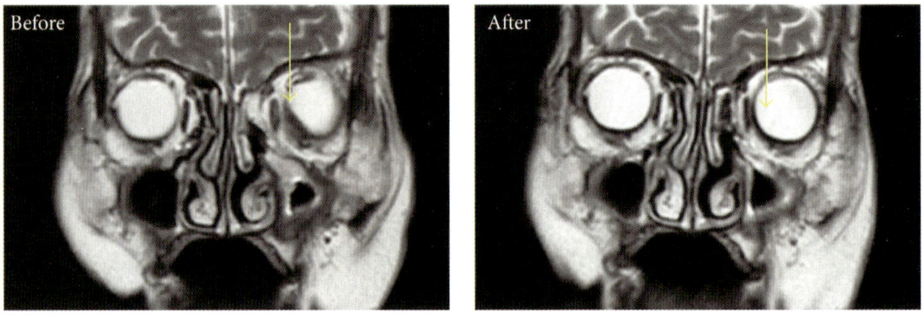

FIGURE 2: Coronal T2-weighted images showing a left choroidal tumor and space-occupying lesions in left paranasal sinus (arrow) before and 3 weeks after steroid treatment.

Neurological examinations revealed no nervous system involvements including cranial nerve palsy or peripheral neuropathy. The patient's pupils were both 3.0 mm, and motility was normal. Confrontational visual-field examinations were normal in both eyes. Intraocular pressures were 16 mmHg on the right and 17 mmHg on the left. Funduscopic examination revealed no abnormalities of the optic nerve or retinal vessels of both eyes.

Laboratory results are shown in Table 1. The patient's erythrocyte sedimentation rate was 86 mm/hr, and her serum C-reactive protein level was 9.73 mg/dL. The peripheral blood white blood cell count was 8400/μL with normal renal function and urinalysis.

Enzyme-linked immunosorbent assays (ELISAs) showed positive results for MPO-ANCA (41.1 IU/mL, normal < 10 IU/mL) and negative results on an anti-proteinase-3-(PR3-) ANCA (3.5 IU/mL, normal < 10 IU/mL). Computed tomography (CT) of the chest and abdomen revealed no abnormal findings (data not shown). In magnetic resonance imaging (MRI) scans of the orbits, diffuse-weighted images (DWI) showed a mass lesion in the interior of left eye. T2-weighted image (T2WI) showed a choroidal tumor with low intensity in left eye (Figure 1). MRI also demonstrated space-occupying lesions in left paranasal sinus (Figure 2). Chest X-ray showed no significant finding and magnetic resonance arteriography (MRA) did not reveal the findings of cerebral vasculitis (Figure 3). There was no pulmonary or renal involvement.

We performed diagnostic biopsy of the choroidal mass. Histopathological evaluation of the specimen revealed granulomatous choroiditis with necrotizing vasculitis with infiltrates of inflammatory cells (Figure 4). Also, surgical biopsy specimens of left paranasal sinus showed vasculitis of small-sized vessels with fibrinoid necrosis (Figure 5). According to the international Chapel Hill Consensus Conference (CHCC) nomenclature for vasculitis syndrome [7], the patient had small-vessel vasculitis and the diagnosis of limited type of GPA was made based on the serological (presence of MPPO-ANCA) and histological evidence of vasculitis and granulators inflammation in choroidal and sinus tissues, without the involvement of respiratory tracts and kidney. Other small-vessel vasculitides, such as microscopic polyangiitis (MPA) or eosinophilic granulomatosis with polyangiitis (EGPA), were ruled out from these clinical findings.

Table 1: Laboratory findings.

Peripheral blood	
Red blood cells	$337 \times 10^4/\mu L$
Hemoglobin	10.4 g/dL
White blood cells	$8400/\mu L$
Neutrophil	83.2%
Monocyte	5.5%
Lymphocyte	10.0%
Eosinophil	0.9%
Basophil	0.5%
Platelet	$30.4 \times 10^4/\mu L$
Blood chemistry	
Total protein	7.6 g/dL
Albumin	2.8 g/dL
Total bilirubin	0.5 mg/dL
Glutamic-oxaloacetic transaminase	19 IU/L (7–33)
Glutamic-pyruvic transaminase	14 IU/L (5–30)
Lactate dehydrogenase	199 IU/L (260–480)
Alkaline phosphatase	261 IU/L (80–250)
Creatinine kinase	39 IU/L (60–160)
Total cholesterol	171 mg/dL
Blood urea nitrogen	15.0 mg/dL
Creatinine	0.4 mg/dL
Na	132 mEq/L
K	4.1 mEq/L
Cl	100 mEq/L
Ca	8.7 mg/dL
Serological tests	
C-reactive protein	9.37 mg/dL (<0.30)
Erythrocyte sedimentation rate	86 mm/hr
IgG	2250 mg/dL (900–2000)
IgA	458 mg/dL
IgM	131 mg/dL
C3	155 mg/dL (86–160)
C4	50 mg/dL (17–45)
Rheumatoid factor	24 (U/mL) (<17)
Antinuclear Ab	< ×40 (Speckled)
PR-3-ANCA	<1.0 U/mL (<3.5)
MPO-ANCA	41.1 U/mL (<3.5)
Anti-CCP Ab	<0.6 U/mL (<4.5)
Virological test	
HCV-Ab	(−)
HBsAg	(−)
Urinalysis	
Protein	(−)
Sugar	(−)
Occult blood	(−)
Sediment	np

HBsAg: hepatitis B surface antigen; Anti-CCP Ab: anti-cyclic citrullinated peptide antibody; HCV: hepatic C virus; MPO-ANCA: myeloperoxidase anti-neutrophil cytoplasmic antibody; PR-3-ANCA: proteinase 3-anti-neutrophil cytoplasmic antibody.

We treated the patient with oral prednisolone (30 mg/day). The symptoms rapidly resolved. MRI findings indicated that the choroidal tumor was also rapidly resolving (Figure 2). Two months later, she was symptom-free with normalized MPO-ANCA levels on orally prednisolone 10 mg daily. However, 3 months later, she experienced a relapse of fever with elevated levels of CRP and MPO-ANCA. She was treated with methylprednisolone pulse therapy (500 mg, 3 successive days) and we increased her prednisolone to 30 mg a day. She was then started with azathioprine (50 mg daily) and her prednisolone was eventually tapered down to 20 mg/day over three months. She continues to be doing well with no further relapse (Figure 6).

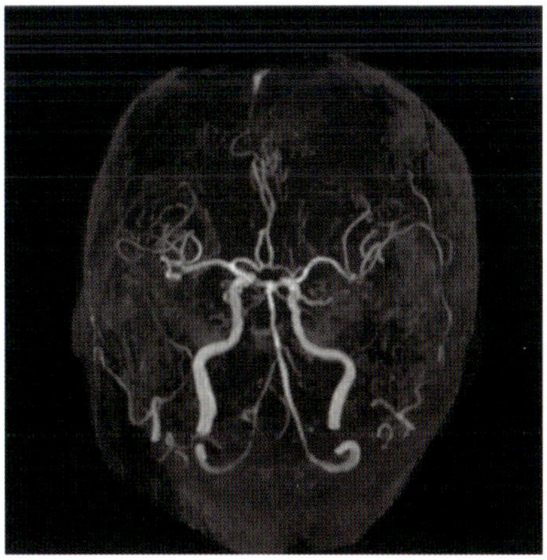

Figure 3: Magnetic resonance arteriography (MRA) before corticosteroid therapy shows no finding of cerebral vasculitis.

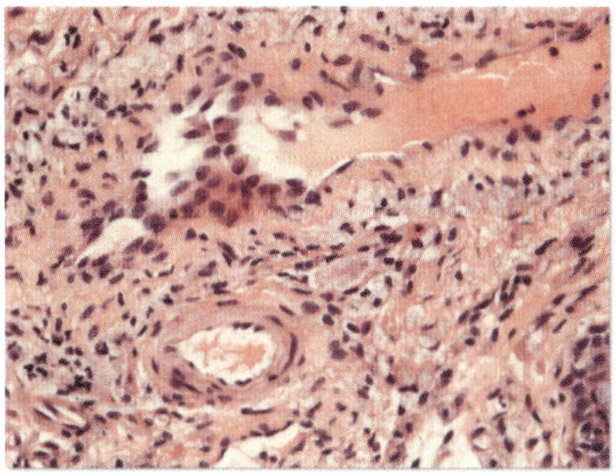

Figure 4: Histology of the left choroidal tumor showing vasculitis of a small-sized artery. Choroidal tumor biopsy specimens showing necrotizing vasculitis with aggregate of inflammatory cells (hematoxylin and eosin staining).

3. Discussion

We report the case of a choroidal tumor in a patient with GPA. Choroidal tumors are not uncommon, but the development of a choroidal tumor caused by GPA is rare. To our knowledge, no choroidal tumor as a direct consequence of GPA has been described, although retrobulbar granuloma is one of the serious complications of GPA [8]. It is often resistant to conventional therapy, and the outcome usually includes visual loss and orbital deformity [9]. Until recently, such patients had undergone surgical resection [9].

In our case, histological examination showed a chronic necrotizing granulomatous inflammation localized in the

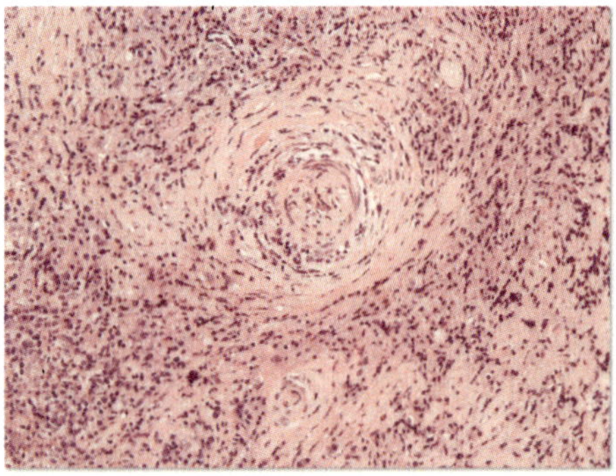

FIGURE 5: Histology of paranasal sinus biopsy specimens. Paranasal sinus biopsy specimens showing vasculitis with fibrinoid necrosis and small-size artery obliterated by concentric inflammatory cells with granulomatous inflammation (hematoxylin and eosin staining).

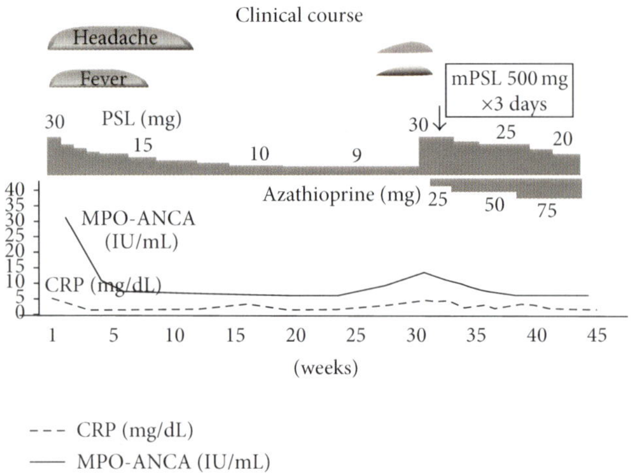

FIGURE 6: Clinical course of the present case.

choroidal tissues, thus creating the picture of a solid choroidal tumor. These clinical and histological findings seem to indicate that choroidal granuloma may be another ocular manifestation of GPA. Although GPA can affect any systemic organ, ophthalmological manifestations occur in 28~77% of GPA patients [10]. The most common manifestation of GPA is orbital disease (15%), followed by scleral, episcleral (3.5%), corneal (8%), and nasolacrimal (7%) abnormalities [11]. The presence of a solid choroidal tumor in patients with GPA is unusual, although choroidal involvement in GPA may manifest as uveitis, retinal vasculitis, choroidal arterial occlusion, or choriocapillaritis. GPA is a systemic inflammatory disease whose histological features often include necrosis, granuloma formation, and vasculitis of small to medium-sized vessels [12]. ANCAs are present in about 80–90% of patients and appear to play a role in the pathogenesis of GPA [5]. RR3-ANCA is a diagnostic marker of GPA [5]. A definitive diagnosis of GPA, however, requires the presence of a histologically proved granulomatous inflammatory process, vasculitis, and the presence of giant cells [6]. GPA was diagnosed in our patient based on the pathological findings. The presence of MPO-ANCA in this patient was somewhat atypical. This finding was similar to that in the GPA case series reported by Chen in which the PR3-ANCA assay was negative and the assay for MPO-ANCA was positive [13]. Therefore, the presence of MPO-ANCA in these patients is not inconsistent with GPA.

The gold standard treatment for GPA combines glucocorticoids (GCs) and cyclophosphamide (CYP) [14]. More severe ocular disease is often not responsive to GCs alone. The use of oral GCs alone achieved good control in a limited number of patients exhibiting serious deterioration [4]. The most dramatic benefits have occurred with the use of GC and CYP. It is therefore believed that the treatment of choice for significant GPA with an ocular component remains the GC-CYP combination [4]. In ANCA-associated vasculitis, glucocorticoid tapering protocol, including the use of less toxic immunosuppressants such as azathioprine in remission-maintenance therapy, has been proposed [15]. The Japanese patients with MPO-ANCA-associated vasculitis (JMAAV) trial revealed the usefulness of severity-based treatment, in which low dose corticosteroid and, if necessary, cyclophosphamide or azathioprine were recommended in patients with mild form [16]. The present case was successfully treated by GCs plus azathioprine against clinical manifestations of GPA. Thus, the less toxic regimens may be considered initially in cases of less aggressive, limited disease, especially in elderly patients with GPA.

In summary, we report a case of choroidal tumor in a patient with granulomatous choroiditis secondary to GPA. GPA is a rare entity that can affect almost any organ system. To our knowledge, no choroidal tumor has been previously described as a direct consequence of GPA. Although ophthalmic involvement is relatively common during the course of the disease, choroidal involvement is rare. It is important, however, to consider GPA in the differential diagnosis of a choroidal tumor. Early diagnosis and an appropriate interdisciplinary approach to management are required to decrease morbidity in patients with GPA-mediated inflammatory ocular disease.

References

[1] C. Comarmond and P. Cacoub, "Granulomatosis with polyangiitis (Wegener): clinical aspects and treatment," *Autoimmunity Reviews*, vol. 13, no. 11, pp. 1121–1125, 2014.

[2] J. C. Jennette, R. J. Falk, P. A. Bacon et al., "2012 Revised International Chapel Hill consensus conference nomenclature of vasculitides," *Arthritis and Rheumatism*, vol. 65, no. 1, pp. 1–11, 2013.

[3] C. G. M. Kallenberg, C. A. Stegeman, W. H. Abdulahad, and P. Heeringa, "Pathogenesis of ANCA-associated vasculitis: new possibilities for intervention," *American Journal of Kidney Diseases*, vol. 62, no. 6, pp. 1176–1187, 2013.

[4] N. Pakrou, D. Selva, and I. Leibovitch, "Wegener's granulomatosis: ophthalmic manifestations and management," *Seminars in Arthritis and Rheumatism*, vol. 35, no. 5, pp. 284–292, 2006.

[5] U. Schönermarck, P. Lamprecht, E. Csernok, and W. L. Gross, "Prevalence and spectrum of rheumatic diseases associated with proteinase 3-antineutrophil cytoplasmic antibodies (ANCA) and myeloperoxidase-ANCA," *Rheumatology (Oxford)*, vol. 40, no. 2, pp. 178–184, 2001.

[6] K. Muller and J. H. Lin, "Orbital granulomatosis with polyangiitis (Wegener granulomatosis): clinical and pathologic findings," *Archives of Pathology & Laboratory Medicine*, vol. 138, no. 8, pp. 1110–1114, 2014.

[7] J. C. Jennette, R. J. Falk, P. A. Bacon et al., "2012 Revised International Chapel Hill consensus conference nomenclature of vasculitides," *Arthritis & Rheumatism*, vol. 65, no. 1, pp. 1–11, 2013.

[8] P. Stavrou, J. Deutsch, C. Rene, D. E. Laws, R. A. Luqmani, and P. I. Murray, "Ocular manifestations of classical and limited Wegener's granulomatosis," *The Quarterly Journal of Medicine*, vol. 86, no. 11, pp. 719–725, 1993.

[9] A. B. Tarabishy, M. Schulte, G. N. Papaliodis, and G. S. Hoffman, "Wegener's granulomatosis: clinical manifestations, differential diagnosis, and management of ocular and systemic disease," *Survey of Ophthalmology*, vol. 55, no. 5, pp. 429–444, 2010.

[10] S. J. Charles, P. A. R. Meyer, and P. G. Watson, "Diagnosis and management of systemic Wegener's granulomatosis presenting with anterior ocular inflammatory disease," *The British Journal of Ophthalmology*, vol. 75, no. 4, pp. 201–207, 1991.

[11] C. L. Bullen, T. J. Liesegang, T. J. McDonald, and R. A. DeRemee, "Ocular complications of Wegener's granulomatosis," *Ophthalmology*, vol. 90, no. 3, pp. 279–290, 1983.

[12] P.-R. Rothschild, C. Pagnoux, R. Seror, A. P. Brézin, E. Delair, and L. Guillevin, "Ophthalmologic manifestations of systemic necrotizing vasculitides at diagnosis: a retrospective study of 1286 patients and review of the literature," *Seminars in Arthritis and Rheumatism*, vol. 42, no. 5, pp. 507–514, 2013.

[13] M. Chen, F. Yu, Y. Zhang, W.-Z. Zou, M.-H. Zhao, and H.-Y. Wang, "Characteristics of Chinese patients with Wegener's granulomatosis with anti-myeloperoxidase autoantibodies," *Kidney International*, vol. 68, no. 5, pp. 2225–2229, 2005.

[14] K. de Groot, N. Rasmussen, P. A. Bacon et al., "Randomized trial of cyclophosphamide versus methotrexate for induction of remission in early systemic antineutrophil cytoplasmic antibody-associated vasculitis," *Arthritis & Rheumatism*, vol. 52, no. 8, pp. 2461–2469, 2005.

[15] C. Mukhtyar, L. Guillevin, M. C. Cid et al., "EULAR recommendations for the management of primary small and medium vessel vasculitis," *Annals of the Rheumatic Diseases*, vol. 68, no. 3, pp. 310–317, 2009.

[16] S. Ozaki, T. Atsumi, T. Hayashi et al., "Severity-based treatment for Japanese patients with MPO-ANCA-associated vasculitis: the JMAAV study," *Modern Rheumatology*, vol. 22, no. 3, pp. 394–404, 2012.

4

Effectiveness of Certolizumab Pegol in Treating Rheumatoid Arthritis Patients with Persistent Inflamed Residual Mono- or Oligosynovitis Resistant to Prior TNF-α Inhibitors

Syuichi Koarada,[1] Masahiko Tsuboi,[2] Mitsunori Komine,[3] Yoshinobu Nakao,[1] Yukiko Tokuda,[1] Yukihide Ono,[1] Satoko Tashiro,[1] Akihito Maruyama,[1] Nobuyuki Ono,[1] Akihide Ohta,[1] and Yoshifumi Tada[1]

[1]*Division of Rheumatology, Faculty of Medicine, Saga University, 5-1-1 Nabeshima, Saga 849-8501, Japan*
[2]*Nagasaki Medical Hospital of Rheumatology, 1-21 Aburaya-machi, Nagasaki 850-0832, Japan*
[3]*Tsuruta Rehabilitation Clinic, 174-8 Ogi-Ushizu, Saga 849-0305, Japan*

Correspondence should be addressed to Syuichi Koarada; koarada@cc.saga-u.ac.jp

Academic Editor: Remzi Cevik

We report four cases of successful treatment with certolizumab pegol (CZP) of rheumatoid arthritis (RA) patients with persistent inflamed residual mono- or oligosynovitis resistant to prior TNF-α inhibitors. Although the patients were in a moderate disease activity, a low activity, or a remission of RA, they sustained inflammatory mono-/oligoarthritis even after treatment with prior TNF inhibitors. They were then all treated with CZP and observed in a serial ultrasonography. In all cases, the positive power Doppler signals in the joint have disappeared promptly and all of the patients were able to retain remission in the long term. The treatment of CZP to the refractory mono-/oligoarthritis of inflammatory synovitis in RA patients has not been previously described. The cases suggest that it may be associated with the feature of CZP, possible effective penetration into the site of inflammation.

1. Introduction

In rheumatoid arthritis (RA), persistent inflamed mono- or oligoarthritis is a frequent clinical problem and is difficult to treat [1, 2]. Even in clinical remission (CR), the prevalence of ultrasound- (US-) detected residual synovitis in patients with RA is frequent [3]. Importantly, residual synovitis is the risk of relapse and structural progression in RA patients with CR by the disease-modifying antirheumatic drugs (DMARDs), including biological therapies [1, 3]. We report four cases of successful treatment with certolizumab pegol (CZP) of RA patients with persistent inflamed residual mono- or oligosynovitis resistant to prior TNF-α inhibitors.

2. Case Presentation

A representative case was a 27-year-old Japanese woman with four-year history of active RA who complained in February 2013 of pain and swelling of the bilateral wrists, shoulders, and foots (case 1). She had been already treated with methotrexate (MTX) 10 mg/week orally. Because she was referred to our clinic with severe polyarthritis, a combination of golimumab administered subcutaneously (SC) and methotrexate (MTX) 10 mg/week orally was medicated. Her symptoms other than the left wrist have quickly disappeared. On clinical examination after a year, although systemic polyarthritis was remarkably improved and she obtained CR in DAS28-CRP (Disease Activity Score 28-CRP), evident monosynovitis of the left wrist had persisted. She complained of restriction of wrist movements for a month. She was referred to a near orthopedic doctor for synovectomy. However, she did not agree on surgical therapy. US imaging showed the persistent left wrist synovitis (PD-positive; grade 2) (baseline). TNF inhibitor was switched to CZP. Her symptom of the left wrist was resolved after 2 weeks and her PD signals in US have disappeared completely after 2 months (PD-negative;

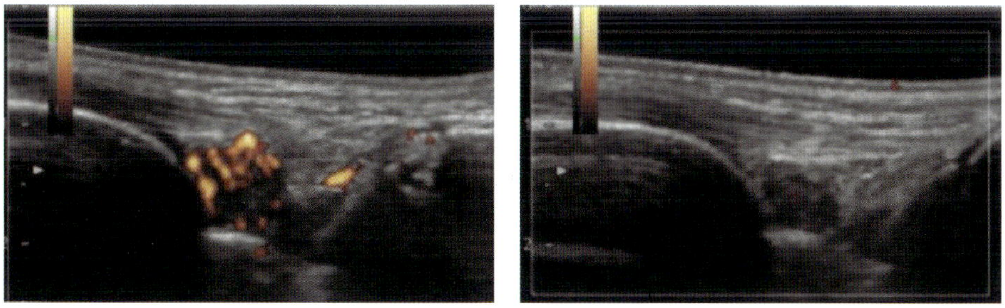

Figure 1: A representative result of US of the wrist of case 3 demonstrated PD-positive synovitis before treatment with CZP. US showed disappearance of PD-positive inflammatory synovitis after treatment with CZP.

grade 0). Since the improvement of clinical symptoms and laboratory data, the administration of MTX was tapered off and CZP was stopped after 8 months. Presently, she achieved drug-free remission for 5 months.

We experienced other three patients with RA who had sustained inflammatory mono- or oligoarthritis even after treatment with prior TNF inhibitors. The patients were all female with a mean (SD) age of 42.3 (14.5) years and a mean (SD) disease duration of 6.0 (4.8) years. A mean (SD) period of treatment with prior TNF inhibitors was 24.8 (16.8) months. In US, all patients had power Doppler- (PD-) positive synovitis. They were then all treated with CZP and observed in a serial US. Each patient had a physical and laboratory evaluation before and after treatment. All patients responded well after the injection of CZP as evaluated by the reduction in the number of swollen and tender joints (Table 1). In all cases, the PD-positive signals in the joints were not detected after treatment (a mean (SD) duration of 1.9 (0.9) months). The effectiveness was associated with the improvement of US findings. The DAS28-CRP score (mean (SD); 2.69 (0.68) $\rightarrow$ 1.55 (0.34)) and PD grade (2 $\rightarrow$ 0) decreased (Figure 1 and Table 1). The effectiveness was associated with the improvement of US findings. No adverse reactions were noted. All of the patients were able to retain remission in the long term with drug off (case 1; 13 months) or with remaining CZP (case 2; 14 months, case 3; 7 months, and case 4; 4 months).

3. Discussion

Persistent mono- or oligoarthritis may be even destructive and necessitate joint replacement surgery in the future. Therefore, surgical synovectomy and intra-articular (IA) steroids, chemical, and tumor necrosis factor-α- (TNF-α-) inhibitors are local therapeutic options in RA resistant to other medical treatments [1, 4]. However, the efficacy of local therapy is not always evident and it may be of short duration [1]. Moreover, injection site reactions [5] and septic arthritis secondary to IA TNF inhibitors [6] have been experienced. IA therapy of TNF inhibitors has not become a mainstay in RA [7]. In this situation, a pharmacological effect of agent at the site of inflammation may be an important factor for the effective treatment of residual arthritis. Most soluble agents are rapidly absorbed from the inflamed joint to systemic circulation and the transience is a major obstacle to attain clinical effect. Modification of drugs is a strategy to prolong the residence time in the joint [7]. PEGylation (conjugation of a PEG (polyethylene glycol) moiety) is a conventional chemical method to increase the bioavailability of drugs and to delay systemic elimination [8]. This approach has also the potential to increase in the drug residence time in inflamed joints. As shown in an animal model, CZP, PEGylated TNF inhibitor, penetrates inflamed joints more effectively than other TNF inhibitors [9]. However, the evidence of these features of CZP in human has not been clinically confirmed.

CZP is efficacious and well tolerated in phase III clinical trials in RA patients with active disease, irrespective of concomitant or previous therapy [10]. Schiff et al. reported that CZP in RA patients who are secondary nonresponders to TNF inhibitors, demonstrating a good response and a safety profile [11]. However, these patients had active disease defined as ≥6 tender and swollen joints of 28-joint count (polyarthritis). There are no published data relating to the treatment with CZP of refractory mono- and oligoarthritis of inflammatory synovitis resistant to prior TNF inhibitors in RA. Our cases suggested the efficacy of CZP in the patients with RA having residual mono- or oligoarthritis. In conclusion, the clinical benefits may be associated with the drug's feature of localized distribution of CZP compared to other TNF inhibitors. Because potentially effective, safe, and long-lasting treatment for persistent and residual mono- or oligoarthritis is greatly required in clinical practice of RA, further examination in a prospective, randomized, controlled, and multicenter comparative effectiveness study of CZP versus other TNF inhibitors is important to draw rational conclusion.

Data Sharing Statement

Additional data and information about the study can be accessed by contacting the corresponding author.

Ethical Approval

Patient consent was obtained and this study was approved by the Ethics Committee of Saga University.

Table 1: Clinical and laboratory changes in patients with RA and mono- or oligoarthritis treated with CZP.

Case	Age/sex	Stage	DD (year)	DMARD	Prior biologics (duration)	NSJ/NTJ prior → before → after	DAS28-CRP prior → before → after	Imaged joint	PD (grade) Before	After	Duration
1	27 F	I	4	MTX	GLM (12 m)	4/3 → 1/1 → 0/0	3.87 → 2.21 → 1.45	Wrist	2	0	2 m
2	41 F	III	2	BUC	GLM (10 m)	1/3 → 1/1 → 0/0	2.34 → 2.02 → 1.11	1st IP	2	0	3 m
3	39 F	III	13	MTX	IFX (15 m), ETN (30 m)	2/4 → 2/2 → 0/1	3.82 → 3.46 → 1.76	Wrist	2	0	1.5 m
4	62 F	II	4	MTX	ETN (32 m)	5/6 → 3/1 → 1/0	4.24 → 3.05 → 1.88	Elbow	2	0	1 m
Mean (SD)	42.3 (14.5)				24.8 m (16.8 m)	3/4 → 1.75/1.25 → 0.25/0.25	3.56 → 2.69 → 1.55 (0.84) (0.68) (0.34)		2	0	1.9 m (0.9 m)

DD: disease duration, NSJ/NTJ: the number of swollen and tender joints, m: month(s), F: female, stage: Steinbrocker classification, MTX: methotrexate, BUC: bucillamine, GLM: golimumab, IFX: infliximab, ETN: etanercept. Prior: DAS28 scores prior to treatment with the 1st TNF-inhibitor.

Authors' Contribution

All authors were responsible for study concept and design, clinical revision, and drafting of the paper for important intellectual content and approved the final version of the paper to be published. Syuichi Koarada, Masahiko Tsuboi, and Mitsunori Komine were responsible for acquisition of data. Yoshinobu Nakao, Yukiko Tokuda, Yukihide Ono, Satoko Tashiro, Akihito Maruyama, and Nobuyuki Ono were responsible for analysis and interpretation of data. Akihide Ohta and Yoshifumi Tada supervised the study.

Acknowledgments

The authors thank K. Eguchi and M. Sugi for their assistance with the research. Syuichi Koarada is supported by Grant-in-Aid for Scientific Research from the Ministry of Education, Science, Sports, and Culture of Japan (no. 26461466).

References

[1] B. A. C. Fisher and A. Keat, "Should we be using intraarticular tumor necrosis factor blockade in inflammatory monoarthritis?" *Journal of Rheumatology*, vol. 33, no. 10, pp. 1934–1935, 2006.

[2] S. N. Nikas, T. I. Temekonidis, A. K. Zikou, M. I. Argyropoulou, S. Efremidis, and A. A. Drosos, "Treatment of resistant rheumatoid arthritis by intra-articular infliximab injections: a pilot study," *Annals of the Rheumatic Diseases*, vol. 63, no. 1, pp. 102–103, 2004.

[3] H. Nguyen, A. Ruyssen-Witrand, F. Gandjbakhch, A. Constantin, V. Foltz, and A. Cantagrel, "Prevalence of ultrasound-detected residual synovitis and risk of relapse and structural progression in rheumatoid arthritis patients in clinical remission: a systematic review and meta-analysis," *Rheumatology*, vol. 53, no. 11, Article ID keu217, pp. 2110–2118, 2014.

[4] U. Fiocco and L. Punzi, ""Are there any evidences for using the intra-articular TNF-α blockade in resistant arthritis?"," *Joint Bone Spine*, vol. 78, no. 4, pp. 331–334, 2011.

[5] E. L. Arnold, D. Khanna, H. Paulus, and M. P. Goodman, "Acute injection site reaction to intraarticular etanercept administration," *Arthritis and Rheumatism*, vol. 48, no. 7, pp. 2078–2079, 2003.

[6] I. Chatzigiannis, G. Kakavouli, G. Sakellariou et al., "Intra articular injection of infliximab in resistant inflamed joints of rheumatoid arthritis and spondyloarthropathies," *Annals of the Rheumatic Diseases*, vol. 63, supplement, p. 418, 2004.

[7] C. H. Evans, V. B. Kraus, and L. A. Setton, "Progress in intra articular therapy," *Nature Reviews Rheumatology*, vol. 10, no. 1, pp. 11–22, 2014.

[8] G. Pasut, "Pegylation of biological molecules and potential benefits: pharmacological properties of certolizumab pegol," *BioDrugs*, vol. 28, no. 1, pp. S15–S23, 2014.

[9] R. Palframan, M. Airey, A. Moore, A. Vugler, and A. Nesbitt, "Use of biofluorescence imaging to compare the distribution of certolizumab pegol, adalimumab, and infliximab in the inflamed paws of mice with collagen-induced arthritis," *Journal of Immunological Methods*, vol. 348, no. 1-2, pp. 36–41, 2009.

[10] M. E. Weinblatt, R. Fleischmann, T. W. J. Huizinga et al., "Efficacy and safety of certolizumab pegol in a broad population of patients with active rheumatoid arthritis: results from the REALISTIC phase IIIb Study," *Rheumatology*, vol. 51, no. 12, Article ID kes150, pp. 2204–2214, 2012.

[11] M. H. Schiff, J. von Kempis, R. Goldblum, J. R. Tesser, and R. B. Mueller, "Rheumatoid arthritis secondary non-responders to TNF can attain an efficacious and safe response by switching to certolizumab pegol: a phase IV, randomised, multicentre, double-blind, 12-week study, followed by a 12-week open-label phase," *Annals of the Rheumatic Diseases*, vol. 73, pp. 2174–2177, 2014.

5

Radiological Followup of the Evolution of Inflammatory Process in Sacroiliac Joint with Magnetic Resonance Imaging: A Case with Pyogenic Sacroiliitis

Muhammet Cinar,[1] Hatice Tugba Sanal,[2] Sedat Yilmaz,[1] Ismail Simsek,[1] Hakan Erdem,[1] Salih Pay,[1] and Ayhan Dinc[1]

[1] *Division of Rheumatology, Gulhane Military Medical Academy School of Medicine, 06018 Etlik, Ankara, Turkey*
[2] *Department of Radiology, Gulhane Military Medical Academy School of Medicine, 06018 Etlik, Ankara, Turkey*

Correspondence should be addressed to Muhammet Cinar, muhcinar@hotmail.com

Academic Editors: U. Gresser and F. Schiavon

Pyogenic sacroiliitis (PS) is an acute form of sacroiliitis that mostly starts with very painful buttock pain. Here in this case, the followup magnetic resonance (MR) images of a 49-year-old male patient with PS is displayed. After his sacroiliitis was documented by MR images, he was treated with the combination of rifampicin plus streptomycin and moxifloxacin. Serial MR investigations were done to disclose acute and subsequent imaging changes concerning sacroiliac joint and surrounding bone structures. Although after treatment all the symptoms were completely resolved, 20 months later changes suggesting active sacroiliitis on MR images were continuing.

1. Introduction

Pyogenic sacroiliitis (PS) is a relatively rare condition, representing only 1-2% of all cases of septic arthritis [1, 2]. Nonspecific initial symptoms and physical examination findings sometimes make it difficult to diagnose, thus delaying appropriate treatment. It is a treatable condition with few long-term complications if appropriate treatment is initiated promptly [3, 4]. Low awareness of the clinical presentation and lack of knowledge of the diagnostic procedure usually lead to delay in diagnosis [2, 4]. Magnetic resonance imaging (MRI) appears to be the most useful imaging technique in evaluating early and subsequent changes involving the joint [5].

It is important to know distinction between infectious and noninfectious sacroiliitis in terms of treatment options. Here, we reported an adult patient who presented with signs, symptoms, and radiologic evidence of unilateral PS that resolved with antibiotic treatment. In this case, we aimed to show the time course of the PS through MR images from the time of first diagnosis to the treatment. In this aspect, this is the first case demonstrating the long-term course of PS with MRI.

2. Case Report

A 49-year-old man without significant medical history was admitted to hospital with a 7-day history of pain in the right hip and buttock, and low-grade fever. He said his pain began acutely one week ago while sleeping. The pain was severe, sharp and progressed over the next several hours. There was no history of trauma. The radiographs showed no abnormalities in the pelvis and hip. The patient was treated with suspected infection in the right hip joint and had been given antibiotics (cefazolin sodium 3 × 500 mg/day plus ciprofloxacin 2 × 500 mg/day) and anti-inflammatory medications on his discharge from the emergency department.

He was admitted to hospital one week after because of worsening buttock pain and associated lower back pain. At the time of admission, he had a mild low-grade fever with a peak temperature of 38°C, and he reported night

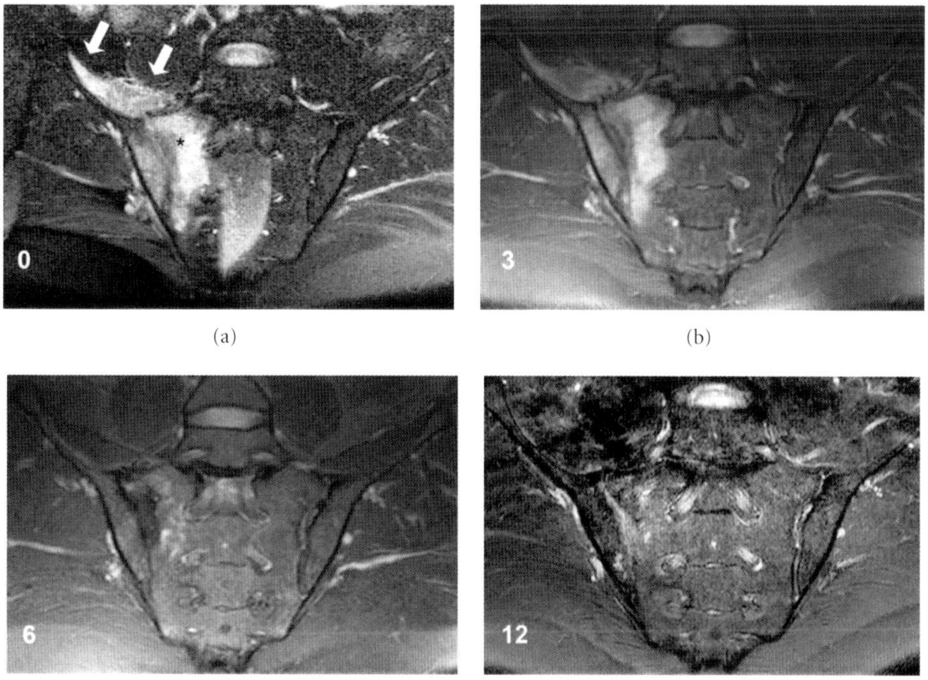

(a) (b) (c) (d)

Figure 1: Fluid sensitive sequence on coronal MR images on the first admission (0), and on followups of 3rd, 6th, and 12th months. Bone marrow edema on the right-sided sacroiliac joint is well seen (*) indicating active inflammation. An accompanying increased signal in the iliopsoas muscle (arrow) is also noticable. Note the diminishing inflammation intensity and distribution in the consecutive months.

sweats. The right sacroiliac joint showed tenderness on pelvic compression. Right hip flexion, internal, and external rotation was very painful and limited. The erythrocyte sedimentation rate (ESR), C-reactive protein (CRP), and white blood cell (WBC) count were 65 mm/h, 228 mg/L, and 8.2×10^9/L, respectively. Bone scan showed an increased uptake in the right sacroiliac joint. A Rose Bengal test for brucellosis was positive and a Wright agglutination test titer was >1/320. HLA-B27 was negative. Blood, urine, and stool cultures were negative.

On MR imaging, mild expansion of the right sacroiliac joint (SIJ) space, along with effusion and bone marrow edema on the joint surfaces indicating active inflammation were detected. An accompanying increased signal in the iliopsoas muscle neighboring right sacroiliac joint was also detected. These findings were yielded to the impression of infective sacroiliitis (Figures 1 and 2).

The patient was diagnosed as pyogenic sacroiliitis due to brusellosis based on imaging, and clinical and laboratory findings, and he was started on antibiotic therapy with moxifloxacin (400 mg daily, for 2.5 months), rifampicin (600 mg daily for 2.5 months), and streptomycin (1 g daily, for 21 days), along with nonsteroidal anti-inflammatory drugs (NSAIDs). Following treatment his symptoms and complaints improved dramatically.

Serial MR images were performed to disclose subsequent changes concerning sacroiliac joint and surrounding structures. Three months following the institution of treatment, he had mild pain in the right gluteal region, but no fever and back pain. Acute phase response was within normal limits. At this time on MR images, the signal intensity of inflammation and contrast enhancement pattern at the subchondral bone and the iliopsoas muscle were detected to be mildly decreased. Six months later, he had only mild pain on right gluteal region. After that time, the patient received NSAIDs on as needed basis. Chronic changes (not shown) including joint surface irregularity, sclerosis, and fatty infiltration were first observed on MRI images obtained at this time. Some active inflammatory changes such as bone marrow edema and contrast enhancement were still observed, yet diminished. Same findings were noticeable on MR images on the twelfth month control as well (Figures 1 and 2). Twenty months following the initial diagnosis, bone marrow edema suggesting acute inflammation around the sacroiliac joint was evident on MR images (not shown). These findings were the same with twelfth month control. The patient's clinical and MRI findings and their changes over time were shown in Table 1.

3. Discussion

Pyogenic sacroiliitis is considered to be an uncommon condition and can be seen in patients of any age. Female patients tend to have a higher incidence than do male patients, especially in the elderly [2]. The diagnosis of PS requires a degree of clinical suspicion and should be confirmed by imaging methods. It has been reported that the varied presentation of symptoms and signs of PS were always remote from the site of infection [3]. Plain radiograms may be normal in early stages of the disease. In one of the

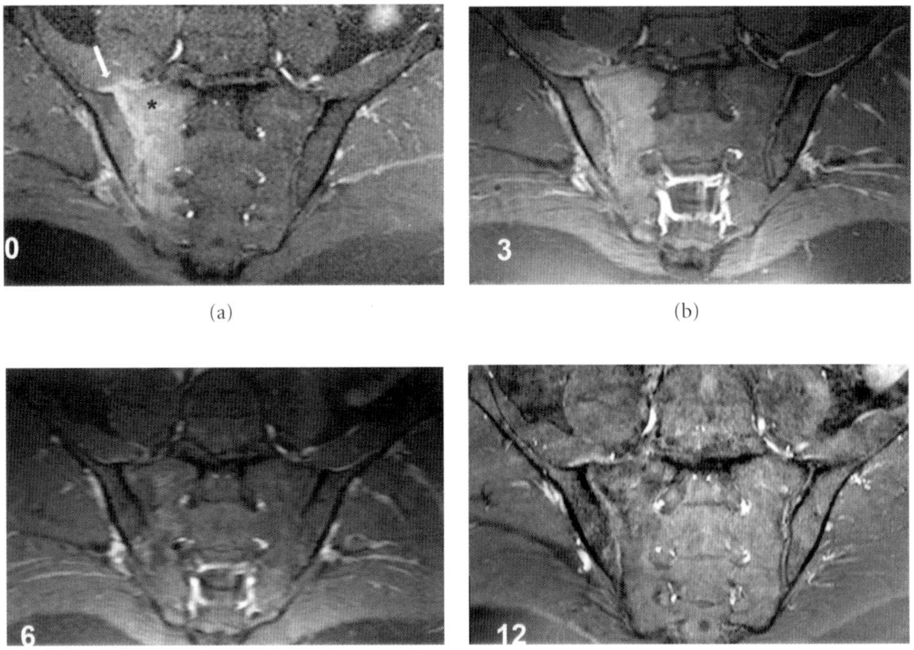

(a) (b) (c) (d)

Figure 2: Contrast enhanced images on coronal MR planes through the sacroiliac joints on the first admission (0), and on follow-ups of 3rd, 6th and 12th months. Note the synovitis (arrow) and contrast enhancement indicating active inflammation in the subchondral bone (∗). Contrast enhancement indicating synovitis has been diminished on the 3rd month and disappeared on the consecutive months as well as the bone marrow edema which is more pronounced in the first 3 months.

Table 1: Clinical course of pyogenic sacroiliitis.

	0 Mo	3 Mo	6 Mo	12 Mo	20 Mo
Clinic findings					
(i) Fever	+	–	–	–	–
(ii) Night sweat	+	–	–	–	–
(iii) Right gluteal pain	Very severe	Moderate	Mild	No pain	No pain
(iv) Pain with sacroiliac stretch	Very severe	Mild	No pain	No pain	No pain
(v) Limitation of spinal mobility measurements	–	–	–	–	–
WBC, $\times 10^9$/L	8.2	5.1	7.5	6.1	6.6
ESR, mm/h	65	4	5	5	5
CRP, mg/L	228	3,32	2.66	<3.4	<3.4
Rose Bengal	Positive	Positive	Negative	Not studied	Not studied
Wright agglutination	>1/320	1/160	<1/80	Not studied	Not studied
MRI findings					
(i) Expansion of the sacroiliac joint space	++	++	+	–	–
(ii) Joint effusion of posteroinferior part of the joint	+	±	–	–	–
(iii) Bone marrow edema on the iliac and sacral surfaces	++++	+++	++	+	+
(iv) Sclerosis and irregularity	–	–	+	+	+
(v) Fatty bone marrow changes	–	–	+	+++	+++
(vi) Edematous changes on neighborhood muscles	+	+	–	–	–
Treatment					
(i) NSAID use	Used	Used	On demand	On demand	Not used
(ii) Antibiotics	Used	Not used	Not used	Not used	Not used

The plus (+) and minus (−) signs were used instead of absent and present meaning. The severity of MRI findings are shown with plus sign. ++++ is defined as very high severity; +++ as high severity; ++ as moderate severity; and + as mild severity.

cohort patients with PS, only 63.6% of the patients presented with the full clinical symptoms typical of PS [2]. Therefore, it is suggested that physicians should keep a high index of suspicion while evaluating adult patients with atypical presentations.

In the previous series, the blood culture yield rate was low. However, local synovial fluid cultures had a high yield rate for pathogens [2]. Synovial fluid aspiration was not universally performed in patients owing to the difficulty in the application of the technique. In our case, we did not perform sacroiliac joint synovial fluid aspiration. Body fluid cultures did not display any bacterial growth. Although the definitive diagnosis requires bacteria isolation from blood or joint fluid cultures, acute onset, one-sided involvement of the joints, and severe gluteal pain accompanied by high fever as in this case were considered as findings supporting PS. Therefore, MR imaging is probably the imaging method of choice to detect PS [6–8]. It provides a detailed evaluation of the joint and surrounding soft tissues [3, 8]. As in our case, together with clinical findings, unilateral involvement, bone marrow edema adjacent to the SIJ surfaces and edema in the neighborhood soft tissues help to diagnose and distinguish infectious from noninfectious sacroiliitis (i.e., some spondyloarthropathies). After a course of intravenous antibiotics, the symptoms completely resolved, thus supporting our diagnosis of infective sacroiliitis.

MR imaging of SIJs has evolved as the most relevant imaging modality for diagnosing early SIJ changes, particularly in patients with ankylosing spondylitis (AS). Active inflammatory lesions such as bone marrow edema (BME)/osteitis, synovitis, enthesitis, and capsulitis can be detected by MRI. Among these, the clear presence of BME/osteitis was considered essential for defining active sacroiliitis. Structural damage lesions such as sclerosis, erosions, fat deposition, and ankylosis can also be detected by MRI, which are accepted as chronic changes [9]. Although the course of MRI changes was comprehensively defined for patients having AS, little is known for patients with infective sacroiliitis.

In this case, consecutive MRIs of a 49-year-old male diagnosed with PS was displayed. We showed that although clinical findings disappear within three months, the MRI findings of suggesting active sacroiliitis did not resolve completely. Even twenty months following the initial diagnosis, bone marrow edema suggesting acute inflammation around the sacroiliac joint was evident on MR images. Interestingly, the patient did not have any complaints at this time (Table 1). We did not perform histologic evaluation to correlate the imaging and clinical findings. Indeed, there is a lack in the literature concerning infective sacoiliitis and its clinical and histologic findings in the time course. Histology-based studies to match the MR imaging findings were conducted mainly in patients with noninfective sacroiliitis [10, 11]. In one of these studies, despite the findings of positive histopathologic results indicating active inflammation, interestingly, it was reported that no MRI findings may be observed [10].

In conclusion, our case demonstrated that in patients with infective sacroiliitis, correlation of the clinical and radiological findings might be far from being perfect. Considering this case, it is obvious that radiological recovery takes longer and it would be more appropriate to rely on clinical and laboratory findings instead of radiological images for the followup of those patients.

Consent

The authors obtained informed consent from the patient.

References

[1] B. F. Hodgson, "Pyogenic sacroiliac joint infection," *Clinical Orthopaedics and Related Research*, no. 246, pp. 146–149, 1989.

[2] M. S. Wu, S. S. Chang, S. H. Lee, and C. C. Lee, "Pyogenic sacroiliitis—a comparison between paediatric and adult patients," *Rheumatology*, vol. 46, no. 11, pp. 1684–1687, 2007.

[3] G. T. Abbott and H. Carty, "Pyogenic sacroiliitis, the missed diagnosis?" *British Journal of Radiology*, vol. 66, no. 782, pp. 120–122, 1993.

[4] M. Doita, S. Yoshiya, Y. Nabeshima et al., "Acute pyogenic sacroiliitis without predisposing conditions," *Spine*, vol. 28, no. 18, pp. E384–E389, 2003.

[5] C. Groves and V. Cassar-Pullicino, "Imaging of bacterial infections of the sacroiliac joint," *Radiologe*, vol. 44, no. 3, pp. 242–253, 2004.

[6] C. E. Althoff, E. Feist, E. Burova et al., "Magnetic resonance imaging of active sacroiliitis: do we really need gadolinium?" *European Journal of Radiology*, vol. 71, no. 2, pp. 232–236, 2009.

[7] X. Baraliakos, K. G. A. Hermann, R. Landewé et al., "Assessment of acute spinal inflammation in patients with ankylosing spondylitis by magnetic resonance imaging: a comparison between contrast enhanced T1 and short tau inversion recovery (STIR) sequences," *Annals of the Rheumatic Diseases*, vol. 64, no. 8, pp. 1141–1144, 2005.

[8] M. A. Klein, C. S. Winalski, M. R. Wax, and D. R. Piwnica-Worms, "MR imaging of septic sacroiliitis," *Journal of Computer Assisted Tomography*, vol. 15, no. 1, pp. 126–132, 1991.

[9] M. Rudwaleit, A. G. Jurik, K. G. A. Hermann et al., "Defining active sacroiliitis on magnetic resonance imaging (MRI) for classification of axial spondyloarthritis: a consensual approach by the ASAS/OMERACT MRI group," *Annals of the Rheumatic Diseases*, vol. 68, no. 10, pp. 1520–1527, 2009.

[10] H. Appel, C. Loddenkemper, Z. Grozdanovic et al., "Correlation of histopathological findings and magnetic resonance imaging in the spine of patients with ankylosing spondylitis," *Arthritis Research and Therapy*, vol. 8, no. 5, article R143, 2006.

[11] R. J. François, D. L. Gardner, E. J. Degrave et al., "Histopathologic evidence that sacroiliitis in ankylosing spondylitis is not merely enthesitis," *Arthritis & Rheumatism*, vol. 43, no. 9, pp. 2011–2024, 2000.

6

Nonbacterial Osteitis of the Clavicle: Longitudinal Imaging Series from Initial Diagnosis to Clinical Improvement

E. Roos,[1] M. Maas,[2] S. J. M. Breugem,[1] G. R. Schaap,[1] and J. A. M. Bramer[1]

[1]*Department of Orthopedic Surgery, Academic Medical Center, P.O. Box 22660, 1100DD Amsterdam, Netherlands*
[2]*Department of Radiology, Academic Medical Center, Amsterdam, Netherlands*

Correspondence should be addressed to E. Roos; eva.roos18@gmail.com

Academic Editor: Jamal Mikdashi

Nonbacterial osteitis is a rare autoinflammatory disease. Often it is mistaken for a tumor or osteomyelitis. We present a case of a twelve-year-old girl referred to our hospital because of a lesion of the right clavicle. The differential diagnoses were sarcoma, osteitis, and Langerhans cell histiocytosis. After biopsy the diagnosis nonbacterial osteitis (NBO) was established. Treatment of choice is a nonsteroidal anti-inflammatory drug. This case report gives a complete follow-up of the disease, showing the pitfalls of the diagnosis.

1. Introduction

Nonbacterial osteitis is a rare condition, most often of the femur or tibia, which occurs in children around the age of eleven [1–4]. We present a case in which the onset of the disease coincided with a trauma the entire process and therefore was depicted in imaging and closely monitored, providing a unique overview of the condition.

2. Case Report

A twelve-year-old girl was presented in our bone tumor meeting because of pain and swelling of the right clavicle. Four months earlier in April she had fallen during exercise. She was presented at the emergency room of a hospital in the periphery with a painful right shoulder. An X-ray was made because of a suspected fractured clavicle (Figure 1): in retrospect a minor swelling of the medial clavicle was observed, with a slight heterogeneous aspect. However this went unnoticed at that time. She was sent home with painkillers.

Four months later in August, the patient had persistent pain and a swelling of the clavicle during physical examination. A new X-ray was made (Figure 2): this showed a large, heterogeneous mass of the medial side, without a soft tissue component. The bony part had a moth eaten aspect. A lamellated periosteal reaction is observed. This was considered to be callus after the trauma in April. The patient was treated conservatively.

After a few weeks though the swelling increased and pain persisted. Blood tests showed a c-reactive protein (CRP) of 22 and a sedimentation rate (ESR) of 81.

In retrospect especially the moth eaten aspect and periosteal reaction of the lesion were suspect. The differential diagnosis is osteitis/osteomyelitis because of the heterogeneous moth eaten aspect and the localization. The lamellated periosteal reaction however could also be apparent in Ewing sarcoma; however a more lytic lesion and more expansion in the soft tissue usually characterize Ewing sarcoma. Osteosarcoma was also thought of but is very rare in the clavicle and is not distinguished by a lamellated periosteal reaction, but by a more spiculated or sunburst periosteal reaction. The image however could fit Langerhans cell histiocytosis; a rare multisystem disease involving clonal proliferation of Langerhans cells. A moth eaten aspect and lamellated periosteal reaction on X-ray also distinguishes the early phases of the condition.

It was decided to make a MRI scan to differentiate between a malign or benign origin. On this MRI made in the end of August, we observe a large bony mass, with

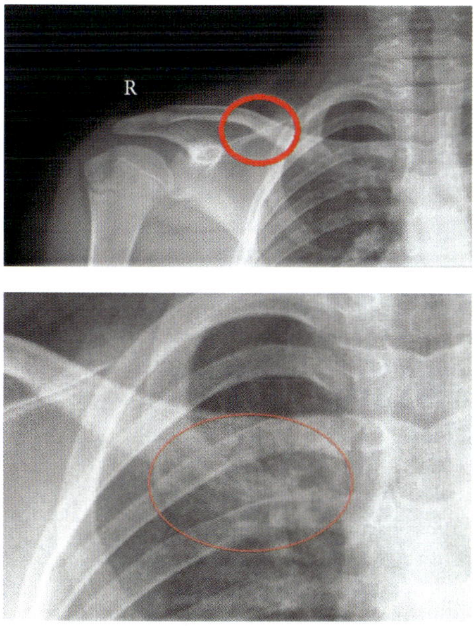

FIGURE 1: A subtle osteitis is seen. The medial site of the clavicle shows an unclear restriction and a heterogeneous aspect.

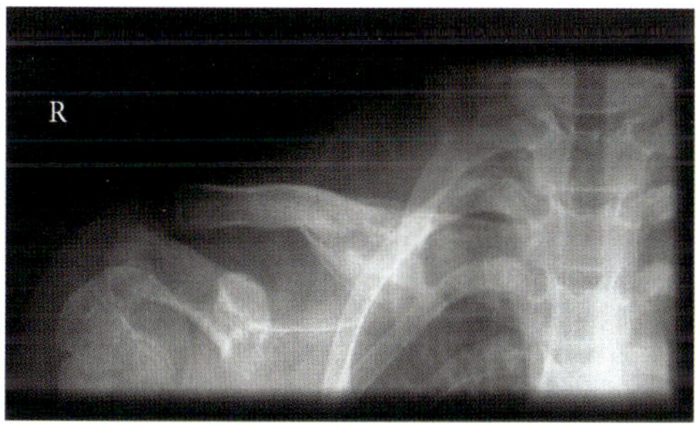

FIGURE 2: A large mass of the medial clavicle, misread as a callus. It has a moth eaten aspect: typical for osteitis.

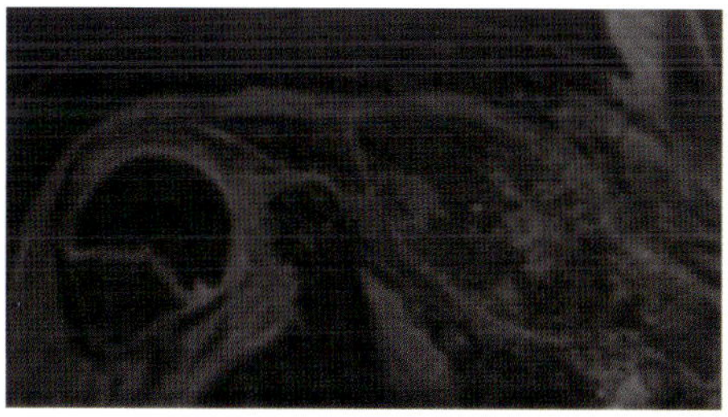

FIGURE 3: A large bony mass with heterogenous aspect and translucent areas.

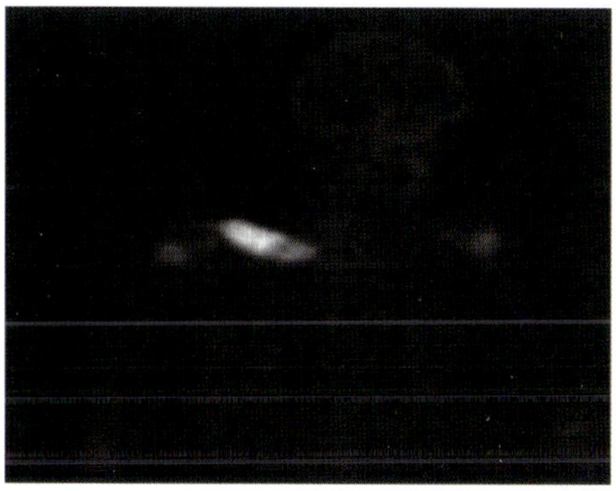

FIGURE 4: A distinctive hot spot of the right clavicle.

a heterogeneous aspect and translucent areas. A lamellated periosteal reaction, especially in the superior part, was seen. There seemed to be no soft tissue involvement. The size of the lesion at that moment was 10 × 5 cm. The lack of soft tissue involvement made Ewing sarcoma and osteosarcoma less likely. The absence of osteolysis and a spiculated periosteal reaction attributed to the possibility of a benign origin. An osteitis seemed to be a plausible cause; although Langerhans cell histiocytosis could not be ruled out (Figure 3).

As osteitis is sometimes multifocal a bone-scintigraphy was made on which a hot spot in the right clavicle was seen. Therefor a multifocal disease was unlikely (Figure 4).

The patient was referred to our musculoskeletal referral center, as it was not clear if the lesion was malign or benign.

After referral, the radiological material was reassessed. In retrospect the lesion was rather suggestive for osteitis, as is described above in the differential diagnosis. It was decided to do an open biopsy, to exclude malignancy or Langerhans cell histiocytosis. Cultures were taken and tissue was sent for pathological evaluation. Pathological investigation showed existing bone with extensive reactive bone formation along the periosteal surface. In both the trabecular and cortical bone osseous transformation was seen, resulting in a more plexiform aspect of the cortex. The stromal spaces and marrow existed of well-vascularized stroma and especially in the trabecular bone chronic and active inflammation was observed (Figure 5). In the adjacent bone a zone with osteoclast activity and more to the periphery osteoblast activity was seen (Figure 6). No Langerhans cells were observed. Cultures and PCR were negative. Nonbacterial osteitis seemed to be the most likely diagnosis.

Because an unknown bacterial pathogen could not be ruled out completely, antibiotics were prescribed pragmatically, first flucloxacillin for six weeks and then because of relapse a switch to clindamycin for three months. There was not much radiological or clinical improvement. Because of the unsuccessful antibiotic treatment, the negative cultures, and the relatively low infection parameters the diagnosis of nonbacterial osteitis was now confirmed.

According to the reports on the topic nonsteroidal anti-inflammatory drugs (NSAIDs) are the preferred treatment for the condition. Therefor NSAIDs were started [1, 2, 4]. The patient's condition improved dramatically. Inflammation values went down and pain diminished. Eighteen months after the first presentation a follow-up X-ray was made (Figure 7). It showed the same tumor-like mass, which was observed before, but now it had calcified. The moth eaten aspect was gone. This is the natural course of nonbacterial osteitis. At the moment our patient has been free of symptoms for two years.

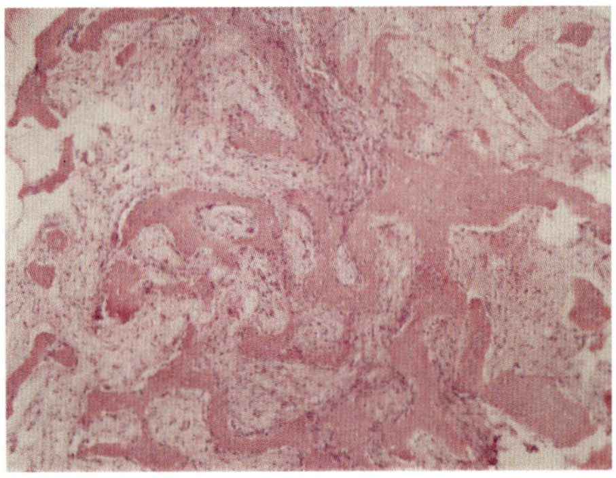

Figure 5

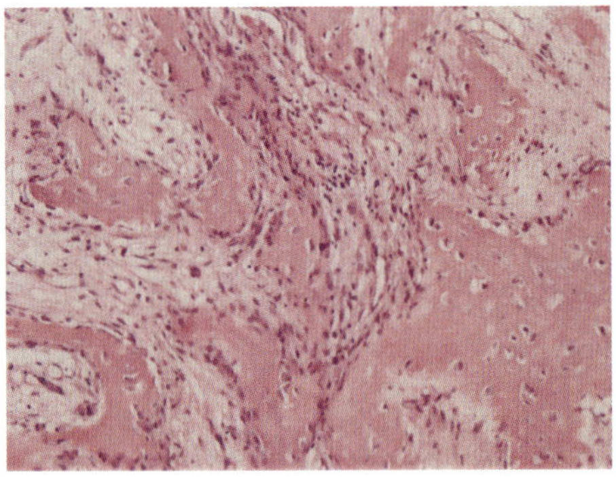

Figure 6

3. Discussion

Nonbacterial osteitis (NBO) is a relatively rare disease [1, 2]. It is a unifocal or multifocal sterile bone lesion, can be acute or recurrent, and is considered to be an autoinflammatory disease [1, 3]. Sometimes it is associated with the SAPHO syndrome (synovitis, acne, pustulosis, hyperostosis, osteitis) and in multifocal and recurrent cases it is called CRMO (chronic recurrent multifocal osteomyelitis) [4, 5]. NBO is considered a diagnosis per exclusionem, because an infectious agent should be ruled out by negative cultures and polymerase chain reaction (PCR) [4, 6].

The median age of presentation is eleven years, with local pain, swelling, and malaise as the leading symptoms [1, 7, 8]. The most common bones affected according to Gikas et al. are the clavicle, femur, and tibia, while Jansson et al. consider the femur, tibia, pelvis, and vertebrae as the most common sites of disease [1, 6, 7, 9, 10].

Imaging shows a characteristic poorly defined, moth eaten, destructive lesion, with expansion, sclerosis, and a solid or multi lamellated periosteal reaction [6, 10]. Sometimes a minor to moderate soft tissue reaction is seen [7]. The absence of an extraosseous mass rules out sarcomas, like Ewing sarcoma and osteosaroma, which are always to be considered in the differential diagnosis [7].

Magnetic resonance imaging (MRI) is regarded as a better diagnostic tool than computer tomography (CT), for it excludes marrow infiltration and soft tissue swelling [7]. Blood tests often show mildly elevated inflammatory markers

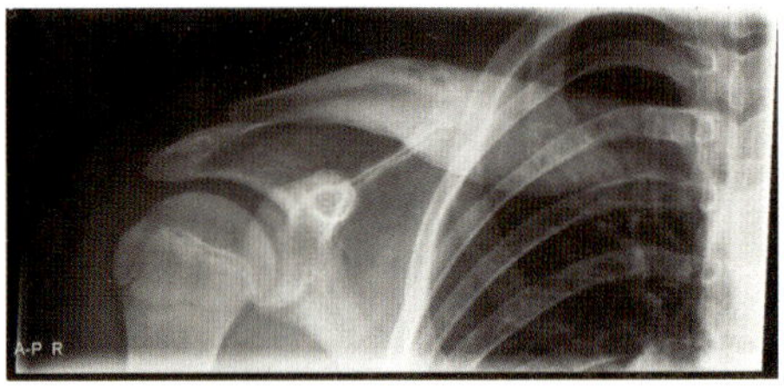

Figure 7: Ossification of the lesion.

[1, 7]. In an early stage NBO might look like a callus formation, misleading the clinician, especially when a trauma has preceded the patient's symptoms.

Gikas et al. argue, based on their experience, that a biopsy is no longer necessary. Imaging, clinical, and biochemical findings are sufficient to diagnose NBO [7].

However we still deem biopsy an important diagnostic tool, especially valuable if other symptoms, for example, those of SAPHO, are not present [1, 4, 7, 10].

It is important to determine between malignant, infectious, and autoinflammatory etiology and so biopsy attributes to the choice of a proper treatment [9, 11].

Traditionally antibiotics were prescribed in NBO, based on the thought that there might be an infectious agent involved that cannot be cultured. Though, as it is considered an autoinflammatory disease without an infectious cause, not antibiotics but NSAIDS are considered the best therapeutic choice [1, 4, 7, 10].

TNF-alpha blockage has been described to be successful for the treatment of relapsing cases of NBO [7, 12], supporting the hypothesis that it is indeed an auto-inflammatory disease. Surgery is advised as a last resort, when patients experience significant morbidity despite adequate medical therapy [7].

Because of a minor trauma, our patient was seen at the first aid department and the early signs of NBO were not detected. In retrospect on the X-ray a subtle osteitis is already exposed. We see how the disease has evolved four months later; now the subtle change has transformed in a clear swelling with bone formation and a moth eaten aspect. To differentiate between a malign or benign origin, a MRI scan is made. As there is now extensive osteolysis or spiculated periosteal reaction a malign origin seems unlikely. The imaging is suspect for osteitis. A bone scintigraphy rules out multifocal osteitis, as there is only one hot spot visible. The biopsy and cultures exclude a malignant or bacterial cause. The further course of treatment confirms the diagnosis of nonbacterial osteitis: antibiotics have no effect; however symptoms subside and the lesion calcifies under treatment with NSAIDs, which is the preferred medication.

As far as we know this is the first case with imaging of nonbacterial osteitis in its earliest stages, showing the pitfalls of this diagnosis as the condition can look like a malignancy or an osteomyelitis. One should be aware though that NBO exists, even without the accompanying symptoms of SAPHO. To exclude a malignant or infectious origin, especially if further symptoms of NBO are not present, biopsy is an important diagnostic tool. NSAIDs are the treatment of choice if NBO seems to be the most likely diagnosis. This case provides a complete follow-up of a patient with nonbacterial osteitis, from a subtle start to active inflammation and to calcification once more.

References

[1] A. Jansson, E. D. Renner, J. Ramser et al., "Classification of non-bacterial osteitis: retrospective study of clinical, immunological and genetic aspects in 89 patients," *Rheumatology*, vol. 46, no. 1, pp. 154–160, 2007.

[2] A. Deutschmann, C. J. Mache, K. Bodo, D. Zebedin, and E. Ring, "Successful treatment of chronic recurrent multifocal osteomyelitis with tumor necrosis factor-α blockage," *Pediatrics*, vol. 116, no. 5, pp. 1231–1233, 2005.

[3] S. R. Hofmann, A. Roesen-Wolff, G. Hahn, and C. M. Hedrich, "Update: cytokine dysregulation in chronic nonbacterial osteomyelitis (CNO)," *International Journal of Rheumatology*, vol. 2012, Article ID 310206, 7 pages, 2012.

[4] H. J. Girschik, P. Raab, S. Surbaum et al., "Chronic non-bacterial osteomyelitis in children," *Annals of the Rheumatic Diseases*, vol. 64, pp. 279–285, 2005.

[5] J. L. Wipff, F. Costantino, I. Lemelle et al., "A large national cohort of french patients with chronic recurrent multifocal osteitis," *Arthritis & Rheumatology*, 2014.

[6] A. F. Jansson, T. H. Müller, L. Gliera et al., "Clinical score for nonbacterial osteitis in children and adults," *Arthritis and Rheumatism*, vol. 60, no. 4, pp. 1152–1159, 2009.

[7] P. D. Gikas, L. Islam, W. Aston et al., "Nonbacterial osteitis: a clinical, histopathological, and imaging study with a proposal for protocol-based management of patients with this diagnosis," *Journal of Orthopaedic Science*, vol. 14, no. 5, pp. 505–516, 2009.

[8] A. Ziobrowska-Bech, B. Fiirgaard, C. Heuck, O. R. Hansen, and T. Herlin, "Ten-year review of Danish children with chronic non-bacterial osteitis," *Clinical and Experimental Rheumatology*, vol. 31, no. 6, pp. 974–979, 2013.

[9] G. Peffers, S. L. J. James, A. Stirling, and P. Jobanputra, "Thoracic spine osteitis: a distinct clinical entity, a variant of SAPHO or late-onset non-bacterial osteitis?" *Rheumatology*, vol. 51, no. 1, pp. 191–193, 2012.

[10] A. Jansson, E. D. Renner, J. Ramser et al., "Classification of non-bacterial osteitis: retrospective study of clinical, immunological and genetic aspects in 89 patients," *Rheumatology*, vol. 46, no. 1, pp. 154–160, 2007.

[11] B. Bjorksten and L. Boquist, "Histopathological aspects of chronic recurrent multifocal osteomyelitis," *Journal of Bone and Joint Surgery. British Volume*, vol. 62, no. 3, pp. 376–380, 1980.

[12] D. Eleftheriou, T. Gerschman, N. Sebire, P. Woo, C. A. Pilkington, and P. A. Brogan, "Biologic therapy in refractory chronic non-bacterial osteomyelitis of childhood," *Rheumatology*, vol. 49, no. 8, pp. 1505–1512, 2010.

7

Fatal Cytomegalovirus Disease after Combination Therapy with Corticosteroids and Rituximab for Granulomatosis with Polyangiitis

Talal Hilal

Department of Internal Medicine, University of Kentucky College of Medicine, Charles T. Wethington Building 304B, 900 South Limestone Street, Lexington, KY 40536, USA

Correspondence should be addressed to Talal Hilal; talal.hilal@uky.edu

Academic Editor: Suleyman Serdar Koca

The association of cytomegalovirus (CMV) with autoimmune disease is poorly understood with suggested causality and reported viral reactivation coinciding with active inflammation. We report a case of a patient who presented with diffuse alveolar hemorrhage and acute renal failure from rapidly progressive glomerulonephritis ultimately diagnosed with granulomatosis with polyangiitis (GPA). She was acutely managed with plasmapheresis to reduce antibody-mediated end-organ damage, hemodialysis for worsening hyperkalemia and acidosis, and high-dose intravenous methylprednisolone. She was transitioned to oral prednisone and started on weekly rituximab with resultant remission induction over a three-week period at which point she developed reactivation of CMV causing severe fatal lung disease and viremia. The case highlights the multiple factors associated with CMV reactivation in cases of severe systemic inflammatory states and the need for further research to help establish practice guidelines regarding antimicrobial prophylaxis in patients with autoimmune diseases on prolonged courses of corticosteroids and biologic agents.

1. Introduction

Granulomatosis with polyangiitis (GPA) is a small-vessel vasculitis characterized by necrotizing granulomatous inflammation in the upper and/or lower respiratory tract and glomeruli. Circulating anti-neutrophil cytoplasmic antibodies (ANCAs) predominantly directed against the neutrophil serine proteinase- (PR-) 3, but also myeloperoxidase (MPO), is seen in 80–94% of affected patients [1]. The cause of this disease and other autoimmune conditions remains unclear with several postulated theories. An association with cytomegalovirus (CMV) has been reported as an etiologic trigger. Furthermore, CMV reactivation is being diagnosed more frequently in active autoimmune disease with resulting deleterious effects. We report a case of a patient who presented with manifestations of severe pulmonary-renal syndrome (PRS) secondary to GPA and who developed fatal CMV disease causing severe pneumonitis and viremia three weeks into her hospital stay and discuss the factors that contribute to CMV reactivation and the potential indications for antimicrobial prophylaxis.

2. Case Report

A 55-year-old female presented to a local emergency department with a 2-week history of progressively worsening shortness of breath and 1 episode of hemoptysis on day of admission. Her past medical history was significant for severe chronic sinusitis for which she took multiple courses of antibiotics over the preceding four-month period. She denied smoking, alcohol, or illicit drug use. Vital signs revealed tachycardia and tachypnea, with a temperature of 36.7°C, heart rate of 120/min, blood pressure of 130/75 mmHg, respiratory rate of 26 breaths/min, and oxygen saturation of 92% on ambient air. Physical examination revealed an obese female in mild respiratory distress. Examination of the chest revealed bilateral inspiratory and expiratory crackles. Cardiovascular exam revealed normal heart sounds without

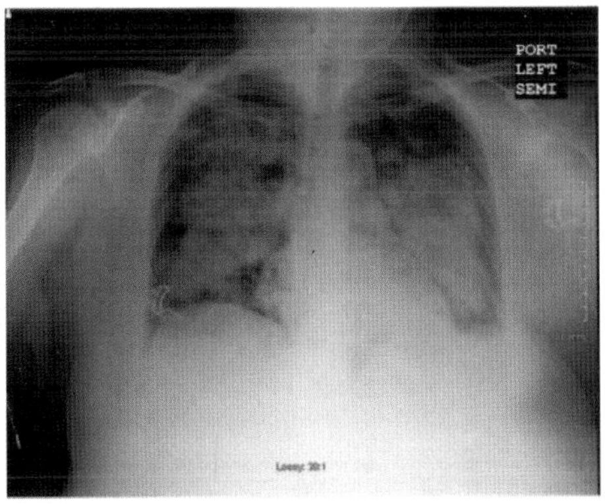

(a)

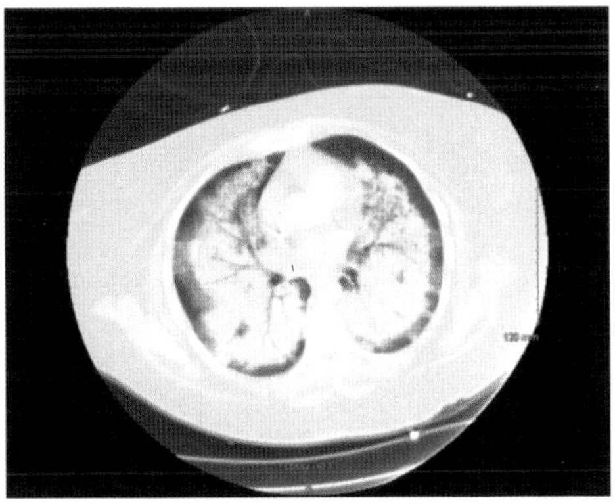

(b)

FIGURE 1: (a) Chest X-ray showing bilateral pulmonary infiltrates in an airspace pattern. (b) Computed tomography of the chest without contrast showing airspace opacities bilaterally sparing the periphery.

murmurs and moderate to severe lower extremity edema extending to the thighs without overlying chronic skin changes. Abdominal exam was unremarkable.

Initial laboratory evaluation revealed a leukocyte count of 16 k/μL, hemoglobin of 6.8 g/dL, platelet count of 318 k/μL, creatinine of 5.2 mg/dL, blood urea nitrogen of 68 mg/dL, and a potassium of 7 mmol/L. Chest X-ray revealed diffuse ground glass opacities bilaterally (Figure 1(a)). Computed tomography (CT) of the chest without contrast revealed diffuse airspace disease bilaterally across upper and lower lung fields sparing the periphery (Figure 1(b)). The patient's presentation of acute respiratory failure and kidney injury was worrisome for autoimmune PRS. The differential diagnosis included GPA, microscopic polyangiitis (MPA), and Goodpasture's syndrome. Her history of chronic sinusitis made GPA the most likely diagnosis. Autoimmune work-up, including ANCAs, PR3, MPO, anti-glomerular basement membrane antibody, and antinuclear antibody, was requested.

The patient was started on pulse-dose steroids with 1 gram of intravenous methylprednisolone daily for 3 days followed by 1 mg/kg of oral prednisone and emergently received renal replacement therapy in the form of hemodialysis for worsening metabolic acidosis and hyperkalemia. She was then transferred to our institution where she was intubated and placed on mechanical ventilation upon arrival for worsening respiratory failure. She was started on plasmapheresis with fresh frozen plasma (FFP) replacement to decrease the level of circulating immunoglobulins mediating neutrophil activation and vascular inflammation. Diagnostic bronchoscopy revealed DAH. Autoimmune work-up revealed positive c-ANCA, and the PR3 level was 1351 (normal 0–19 AU/mL) confirming the diagnosis of GPA. Treatment with intravenous rituximab was initiated in addition to steroids and plasmapheresis. Based on anecdotal experience, the patient was started on trimethoprim-sulfamethoxazole (TMP-SMX) and fluconazole for prophylaxis against *Pneumocystis jirovecii* and fungal disease, respectively.

On Day 10 of hospital stay, CT of the chest revealed marked improvement in airspace disease (Figure 2(a)). The patient at that point was extubated. She had received three days of IV methylprednisolone with transition to oral prednisone, five treatments of plasmapheresis, and two doses of rituximab. On Day 20 of hospital stay, she had received two additional plasmapheresis treatments and a third dose of rituximab. Her PR3 level had decreased from 1351 on admission to 767 on Day 10 and 383 on Day 20. The patient was requiring intermittent hemodialysis but was recovering lung function.

On Day 25 of hospital stay, the patient developed acute respiratory decompensation and required reintubation and mechanical ventilation. It was thought that she had developed fluid overload and was in need of further ultrafiltration. However, the patient's gas exchange did not show improvement after three days of hemodialysis with a net negative fluid balance. She received her fourth and final dose of rituximab afterwards and was weaned off the ventilator and extubated on Day 30. To rule out the possibility of a pulmonary embolus, a repeat CT of the chest with contrast was obtained and revealed worsening airspace and interstitial lung disease bilaterally (Figure 2(b)).

Following extubation, the patient was having high oxygen requirements and complaining of severe shortness of breath on minimal exertion. A repeat PR3 level was lower at 310 on Day 30, indicating that symptoms were unlikely to be related directly to active GPA. A repeat diagnostic bronchoscopy with bronchial washings and lung biopsy was positive for CMV on BAL and tissue culture. Polymerase chain reaction (PCR) testing in plasma for quantification of CMV DNA was positive with a value of 188,000 International Units/mL. The patient was initiated on ganciclovir and IV CMV immunoglobulin for CMV pneumonitis and viremia. Her respiratory status continued to deteriorate and she required reintubation a week after starting antiviral therapy.

On Day 40, her PR3 level had decreased further to 150, but repeat CT scan of the chest without contrast revealed worsening airspace and interstitial disease (Figure 2(c)). At that point, the family decided to withdraw aggressive measures in favor of comfort care. Antivirals, steroids, and dialysis were

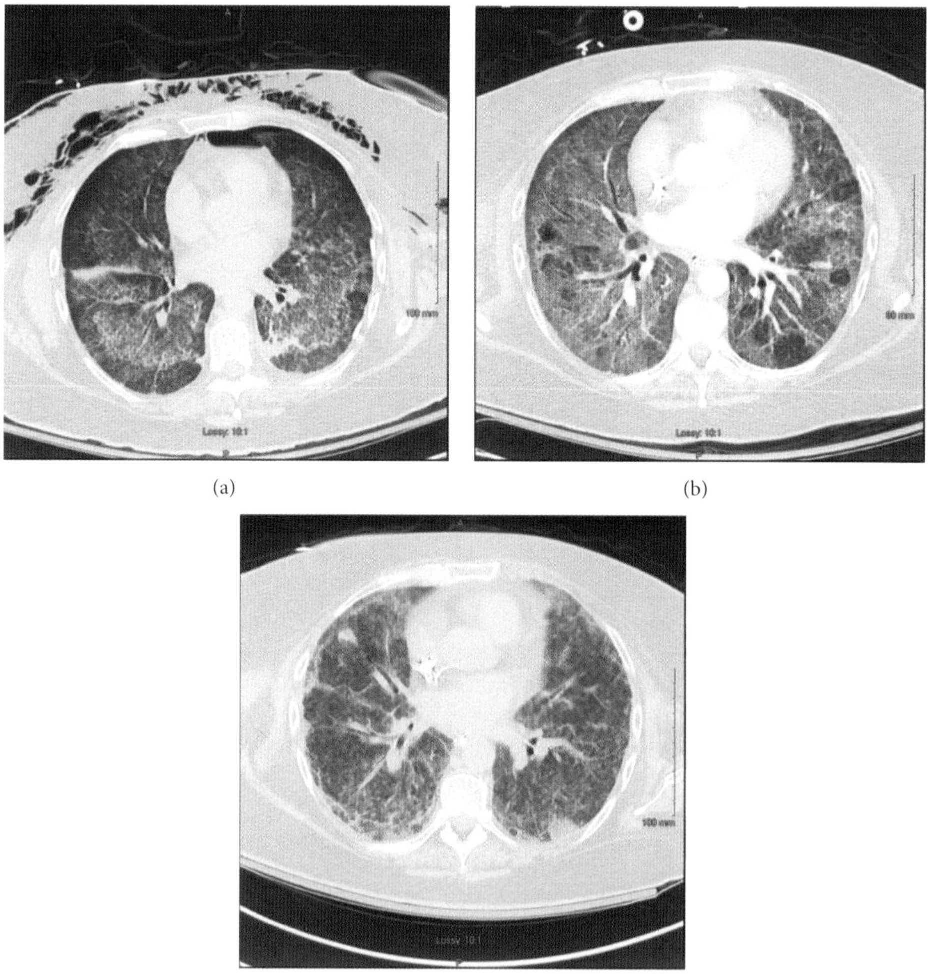

(a) (b) (c)

FIGURE 2: (a) CT of the chest without contrast on Day 10 showing marked improvement in airspace opacities, (b) Day 30 showing increase in diffuse ground glass opacities with associated reticular abnormality, (c) and Day 40 showing further increase in ground glass opacities with evidence of interstitial fibrosis.

stopped and the patient expired within a week. An autopsy was denied.

3. Discussion

Cytomegalovirus (CMV) is a ubiquitous virus belonging to the Herpesviridae family, which includes herpes simplex viruses (HSV) types 1 and 2, varicella zoster virus (VZV), and Epstein-Barr virus (EBV) [2]. The prevalence of CMV seropositivity in the United States increases with age from 36.3% in 6–11-year-olds to 90.8% in those aged >80 years [3]. The virus is typically acquired early in life from contact with bodily fluids and manifests in the two main forms of disease—primary infection, which is usually subclinical in immunocompetent hosts, and endogenous infection in CMV-seropositive individuals who experience reactivation from latency [2].

Endogenous infection from reactivation is always a concern with immunosuppression as seen in patients with hematologic malignancies or solid tumors who are receiving immunosuppressive chemotherapy and particularly transplant recipients. As a result, guidelines were developed for antimicrobial prophylaxis in neutropenic patients and transplant recipients. The two approaches in preventing CMV disease in those particular patient populations who are CMV seropositive are universal prophylaxis and preemptive therapy. With the prophylactic approach, patients receive antiviral therapy for a defined period of time, while, with the preemptive approach, CMV DNA monitoring is carried out every 1 to 2 weeks and patients are treated when viral DNA is detected or is on the rise on repeat testing [4–7].

The association of CMV with autoimmune disease has been described in two nonmutually exclusive ways: as a causal relationship wherein CMV triggers the pathogenesis autoimmune disease and as a complication of autoimmune disease wherein active inflammation causes endogenous CMV infection from reactivation. The evidence for the latter comes from immunocompetent patients with critical illness admitted to the intensive care unit and highlights the systemic inflammatory state as a possible trigger [8].

Table 1: Time course of illness with corresponding PR3 level, treatment regimen, and reactivation of CMV disease.

	Day 5	Day 10	Day 20	Day 25	Day 30	Day 40
PR3 level	1351	767	383		310	150
Corticosteroid	Prednisone 80 mg	Prednisone 80 mg	Prednisone 80 mg	Prednisone 70 mg	Prednisone 70 mg	Prednisone 70 mg
Rituximab		Second dose	Third dose		Fourth dose	
Symptoms and signs of CMV disease				Hypoxia, fever	Worsening pulmonary infiltrates	Persistent viremia

Approximately a third of these patients with latent infection develop reactivation of CMV [9]. This has been linked to impaired natural killer (NK) cell activity [10] and high levels of circulating tumor necrosis factor- (TNF-) α-producing T helper 1 cells [11, 12]. Along the same thought process, the septic stimuli that cause a systemic inflammatory response are also as seen in autoimmune diseases, acute graft rejection, and graft versus host disease (GVHD), all of which have a higher incidence of CMV reactivation.

In cases of ANCA-associated vasculitides, such as GPA, CMV infection seems to be related to the onset of inflammatory disease or to the initiation of immunosuppressive therapy [13–16], as seen in the present case. The distinction between the two is a difficult one to make. In examining the present case, the immunosuppressive effect was probably related to prednisone use rather than rituximab. Initial pulsed dosing of methylprednisolone was unlikely to have contributed as described in a study by Chibane et al. [17], which examined the tolerance profile associated with the three-day use of high-dose intravenous pulse methylprednisolone. A total of 146 patients were followed prospectively for 6 months. The majority (88.4%) developed complications, mostly neuropsychiatric (e.g., insomnia), but also cardiac (e.g., hypertension, bradycardia), and metabolic (e.g., hyperglycemia, hyperkalemia). There were no reports of infections even with such high doses. The immunosuppressive effect of corticosteroids seems to be related to the duration and not the quantity. The present patient was on high doses of oral prednisone for three weeks prior to onset of new symptoms.

Rituximab, the anti-CD20 monoclonal antibody, is becoming more widely utilized as a treatment option for GPA. Studies examining CMV reactivation rates in patients receiving rituximab are conflicting. Patel et al. [18] examined the incidence of CMV in 55 patients who received rituximab in the postrenal transplant setting and failed to show a difference between rituximab- and non-rituximab-treated patients. The rituximab-treated group did, however, have an increased incidence of other viral and fungal infections. Aksoy et al. [19] examined 64 case reports of patients with B-cell non-Hodgkin's lymphoma who developed serious viral infections after receiving rituximab and found that CMV was the second most common encountered infection, after hepatitis B. Case reports seem to be confounded by multiple associated risk factors that would predispose patients to CMV reactivation in addition to rituximab, including hematologic malignancies and transplantation [20, 21].

The exact mechanism of CMV reactivation in the present case points towards a multifactorial process. The use of prednisone very likely played a role, but the duration of treatment prior to reactivation is less than what would be expected in cases of reactivation in the posttransplant setting. Rituximab-induced CMV reactivation is a possibility with the aforementioned growing body of evidence in support of herpes viral reactivation, but the temporal relation and onset of viral illness remain unclear. Although the disease was under control when symptoms of CMV disease appeared, as evident by a stable PR3 level, the initial severe inflammatory state the patient presented with strongly supports it as an etiologic factor that mediated initial reactivation of CMV disease (see Table 1). Other factors that must not be overlooked include the underlying viral load [9] and the location of inflammation (i.e., lungs) [22].

Antimicrobial prophylaxis that includes TMP-SMX, fluconazole, and acyclovir/ganciclovir is currently used in patients with critical illness due to autoimmune disease based on anecdotal evidence, as seen in the present case. This highlights the need for research that seeks to determine the incidence of these opportunistic infections in patients with severe manifestations of autoimmune disease and those on prolonged corticosteroid therapy and biologic agents. Ultimately, structured practice guidelines need to be instituted to aid the physician in deciding whether to use antimicrobial prophylaxis in a somewhat overlooked patient population.

4. Conclusion

Endogenous infection from CMV reactivation is mediated by several factors in the setting of severe illness and inflammatory states. Guidelines currently do not exist for antimicrobial prophylaxis in patients with autoimmune diseases receiving prolonged courses of corticosteroids or biologic agents. The need to revisit the issue is essential, and larger studies need to be undertaken to examine the incidence of CMV disease in this particular population. The use of antiviral prophylaxis or establishing a preemptive therapy approach may prove to be an effective measure that prevents morbidity and mortality.

References

[1] J. D. Finkielman, A. S. Lee, A. M. Hummel et al., "ANCA are detectable in nearly all patients with active severe Wegener's granulomatosis," *The American Journal of Medicine*, vol. 120, no. 7, pp. 643.e9–643.e14, 2007.

[2] S. Varani and M. Landini, "Cytomegalovirus-induced immunopathology and its clinical consequences," *Herpesviridae*, vol. 2, no. 1, article 6, 2011.

[3] S. A. S. Staras, S. C. Dollard, K. W. Radford, W. D. Flanders, R. F. Pass, and M. J. Cannon, "Seroprevalence of cytomegalovirus infection in the United States, 1988–1994," *Clinical Infectious Diseases*, vol. 43, no. 9, pp. 1143–1151, 2006.

[4] M. Wadhawan, S. Gupta, N. Goyal et al., "Cytomegalovirus infection: its incidence and management in cytomegalovirus-seropositive living related liver transplant recipients: a single-center experience," *Liver Transplantation*, vol. 18, no. 12, pp. 1448–1455, 2012.

[5] M. Sandherr II, H. Einsele, H. Hebart et al., "Antiviral prophylaxis in patients with haematological malignancies and solid tumours: guidelines of the infectious diseases working party (AGIHO) of the German society for hematology and oncology (DGHO)," *Annals of Oncology*, vol. 17, no. 7, pp. 1051–1059, 2006.

[6] M. Slifkin, S. Doron, and D. R. Snydman, "Viral prophylaxis in organ transplant patients," *Drugs*, vol. 64, no. 24, pp. 2763–2792, 2004.

[7] E. Meijer, G. J. Boland, and L. F. Verdonck, "Prevention of cytomegalovirus disease in recipients of allogeneic stem cell transplants," *Clinical Microbiology Reviews*, vol. 16, no. 4, pp. 647–657, 2003.

[8] F. G. Frantzeskaki, E.-S. Karampi, C. Kottaridi et al., "Cytomegalovirus reactivation in a general, nonimmunosuppressed intensive care unit population: incidence, risk factors, associations with organ dysfunction, and inflammatory biomarkers," *Journal of Critical Care*, 2014.

[9] C. H. Cook, "Cytomegalovirus reactivation in 'immunocompetent' patients: a call for scientific prophylaxis," *The Journal of Infectious Diseases*, vol. 196, no. 9, pp. 1273–1275, 2007.

[10] C. A. Biron, K. S. Byron, and J. L. Sullivan, "Severe herpesvirus infections in an adolescent without natural killer cells," *The New England Journal of Medicine*, vol. 320, no. 26, pp. 1731–1735, 1989.

[11] W. D. Döcke, S. Prösch, E. Fietze et al., "Cytomegalovirus reactivation and tumour necrosis factor," *The Lancet*, vol. 343, no. 8892, pp. 268–269, 1994.

[12] C. Söderberg-Nauclér, "HCMV microinfections in inflammatory diseases and cancer," *Journal of Clinical Virology*, vol. 41, no. 3, pp. 218–223, 2008.

[13] M. F. Meyer, B. Hellmich, S. Kotterba, and H. Schatz, "Cytomegalovirus infection in systemic necrotizing vasculitis: causative agent or opportunistic infection?" *Rheumatology International*, vol. 20, no. 1, pp. 35–38, 2000.

[14] T. Mori, H. Kameda, H. Ogawa et al., "Incidence of cytomegalovirus reactivation in patients with inflammatory connective tissue diseases who are under immunosuppressive therapy," *Journal of Rheumatology*, vol. 31, no. 7, pp. 1349–1351, 2004.

[15] Y. Kabata, G. Takahashi, and H. Tsuneoka, "Cytomegalovirus retinitis treated with valganciclovir in Wegener's granulomatosis," *Clinical Ophthalmology*, vol. 6, no. 1, pp. 521–523, 2012.

[16] S. Varani, A. Mastroianni, G. Frascaroli et al., "Generalized Wegener's granulomatosis in an immunocompetent adult after cytomegalovirus mononucleosis and bacterial urinary tract infection," *Arthritis and Rheumatism*, vol. 60, no. 5, pp. 1558–1562, 2009.

[17] S. Chibane, S. Feldman-Billard, I. Rossignol, R. Kassaei, F. Mihoubi-Mantout, and E. Héron, "Short-term tolerance of three days pulse methyprednisolone therapy: a prospective study in 146 patients," *Revue de Medecine Interne*, vol. 26, no. 1, pp. 20–26, 2005.

[18] S. J. Patel, J. M. Devos, R. J. Knight et al., "Effects of rituximab on the development of viral and fungal infections in renal transplant recipients," *ISRN Transplantation*, vol. 2013, Article ID 819025, 8 pages, 2013.

[19] S. Aksoy, H. Harputluoglu, S. Kilickap et al., "Rituximab-related viral infections in lymphoma patients," *Leukemia and Lymphoma*, vol. 48, no. 7, pp. 1307–1312, 2007.

[20] M. Sharma, J. Moore, V. Nguyen, and K. van Besien, "Fatal CMV pneumonitis in a lymphoma patient treated with rituximab," *American Journal of Hematology*, vol. 84, no. 9, pp. 614–616, 2009.

[21] M.-Y. Lee, T.-J. Chiou, L.-T. Hsiao et al., "Rituximab therapy increased post-transplant cytomegalovirus complications in Non-Hodgkin's lymphoma patients receiving autologous hematopoietic stem cell transplantation," *Annals of Hematology*, vol. 87, no. 4, pp. 285–289, 2008.

[22] M. Balthesen, M. Messerle, and M. J. Reddehase, "Lungs are a major organ site of cytomegalovirus latency and recurrence," *Journal of Virology*, vol. 67, no. 9, pp. 5360–5366, 1993.

8

A Case of Rheumatoid Arthritis and Limited Systemic Sclerosis Overlap Successfully Treated with Tocilizumab for Arthritis and Concomitant Generalized Lymphadenopathy and Primary Biliary Cirrhosis

Eiko Saito,[1] Shinji Sato,[1] Shinichi Nogi,[1] Noriko Sasaki,[1] Naofumi Chinen,[1] Kiri Honda,[1] Takayuki Wakabayashi,[1] Chiho Yamada,[1] Naoya Nakamura,[2] and Yasuo Suzuki[1]

[1] *Division of Rheumatology, Department of Internal Medicine, Tokai University School of Medicine, 142 Shimokasuya, Isehara 160-8582, Japan*

[2] *Department of Pathology, Tokai University School of Medicine, 142 Shimokasuya, Isehara 160-8582, Japan*

Correspondence should be addressed to Shinji Sato; shinsjam@tokai-u.jp

Academic Editor: Masataka Kuwana

A 57-year-old woman with rheumatoid arthritis (RA) and limited systemic sclerosis (lSSc) was suspected to have lymphadenopathy and primary biliary cirrhosis (PBC). Lymph node biopsy showed reactive follicular lymphadenopathy with intrafollicular plasmacyte infiltration that was interleukin-6 positive by immunohistostaining. Because of gradually worsening arthritis, tocilizumab was administered and arthritis improved markedly. Interestingly, lymphadenopathy and PBC improved simultaneously. This suggested that interleukin-6 might play an important role in reactive lymphadenopathy and PBC associated with RA/lSSc.

1. Introduction

More than 50% of patients with rheumatoid arthritis (RA) exhibit lymphadenopathy [1], and reactive follicular hyperplasia is one of most distinctive histological characteristics of it [2]. There are 3 main causes of lymphadenopathy complicated with RA. These are due to extra-articular manifestation of RA itself, complication of Sjögren syndrome [3], and treatment with immunosuppressive agents including methotrexate (MTX) or tumor necrosis factor-α (TNF-α) blockers [4–9].

If a patient develops lymphadenopathy during treatment with MTX, the possibility of MTX associated lymphoproliferative disease (LPD) arises and MTX should be discontinued promptly [8]. Here we report a case of RA overlapping with limited systemic sclerosis (lSSc) with refractory arthritis, generalized lymphadenopathy, and primary biliary cirrhosis (PBC). In this case, treatment with tocilizumab (TCZ) was successful in management of these concurrent conditions.

2. Case Report

A 57-year-old woman with RA was referred to Tokai University Hospital for further evaluation and treatment. She was initially treated with 200 mg daily of Bucillamine without improvement. Therefore, 6 mg weekly of MTX was started and then increased to 8 mg weekly and continued for another 8 weeks. At that time, her joint symptoms were still active and she had polyarthritis. Although she had Raynaud's phenomenon and sclerodactyly, she had no keratoconjunctivitis sicca and xerostomia, and parotid gland swelling was not observed. Therefore, she was diagnosed with lSSc but did not fulfill the criteria of Sjögren syndrome. Laboratory findings revealed an erythrocyte sedimentation rate (ESR) of 89 mm/hr, C-reactive protein (CRP) of 3.85 mg/dL. Anti-CCP antibody and RF were positive. Anti-nuclear antibody (centromere pattern) and anti-centromere antibody were also positive. She had 6 tender joints (TNJ) and 8 swollen joints (SWJ). DAS28-ESR was 5.83 which indicated that she had still high disease activity. Therefore, she was admitted to

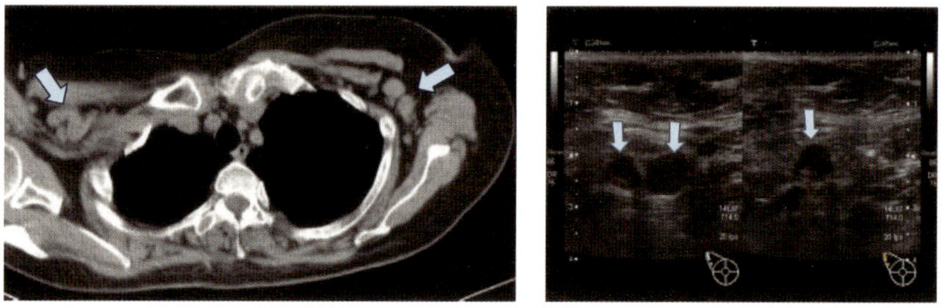

(a) (b)

Figure 1: Lymphadenopathy at first admission. Lymphadenopathy was seen in both axial lymph nodes at first admission (a). Malignant lymphoma was suspected because lymph nodes echogram showed elliptical shape and reticular or hypoechoic pattern with deviation of lymph node hilum (b).

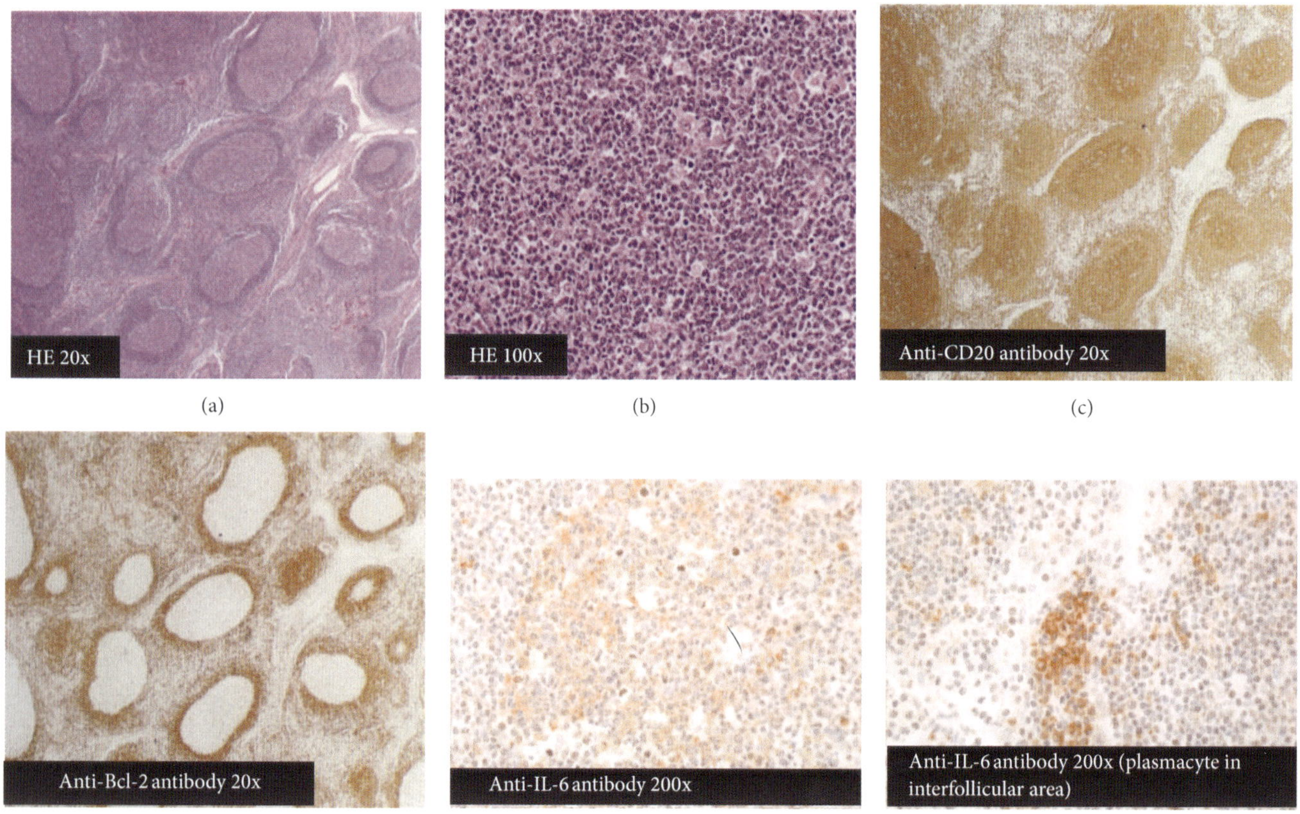

(a) (b) (c) (d) (e) (f)

Figure 2: Histopathological and histoimmunochemical features of lymph node biopsy. Lymph node biopsy showed follicular hyperplasia and germinal center proliferation with narrowed mantle-zone ((a): HE stain, ×20). No dysplasia was seen in germinal center and hemophagocytic cells are scattered in this area ((b): HE stain, ×100). The lymphocytes forming in the germinal center were CD20 positive (c), BCL-2 negative (d), and IL-6 positive (e). Plasmacytes in interfollicular area were also IL-6 positive (f).

our hospital to introduce infliximab (IFX) therapy. Prior to starting the combination therapy with IFX and MTX, computed tomography (CT) was performed to rule out active tuberculosis infection. CT revealed that she had generalized lymphadenopathy (Figure 1(a)) and she was suspected to have malignant lymphoma (ML) based on the results of ultrasound sonography (Figure 1(b)). Treatment with IFX and MTX was discontinued in case generalized lymphadenopathy was due to MTX. A lymph node biopsy was immediately performed from the swollen right neck lymph node. Histology showed follicular hyperplasia throughout the lymph node and germinal center proliferation with a narrowed mantle-zone (Figure 2(a)). Germinal centers consisted of mainly centroblasts and centrocytes with tingible body macrophages, indicating reactive follicular hyperplasia (Figure 2(b)). These centroblasts and centrocytes showed CD20 positive, BCL-2 negative and IL-6 positive immunohistochemically (Figures 2(c)–2(e)). In interfollicular area, many

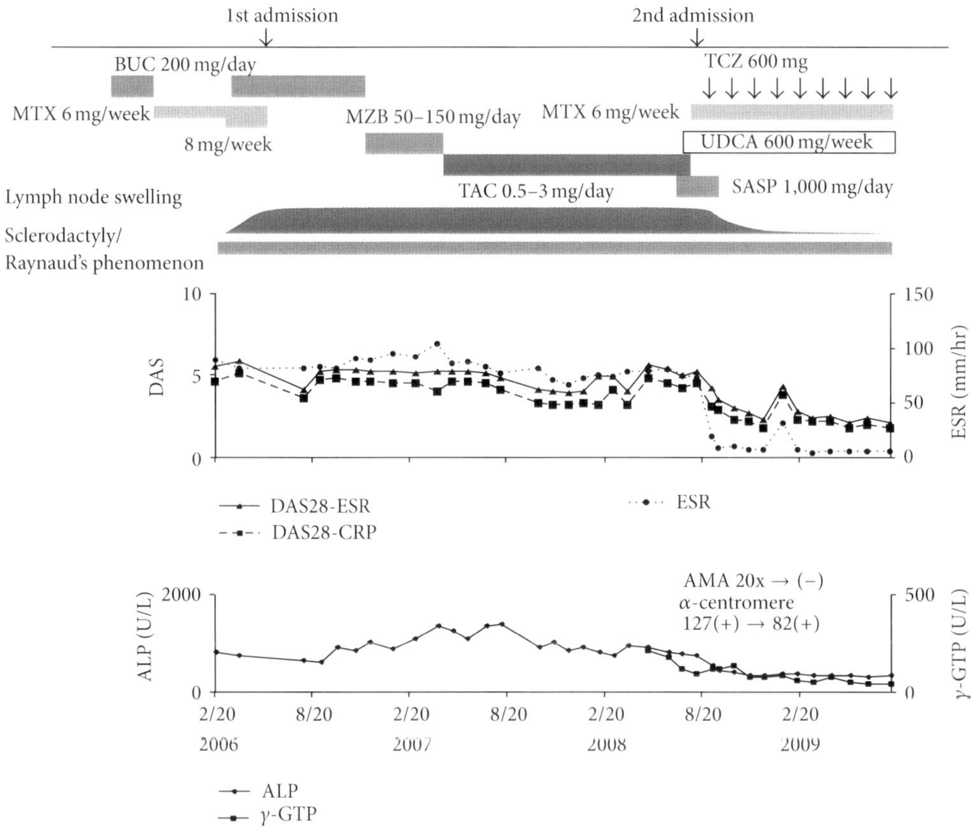

FIGURE 3: Clinical course and changes in articular manifestations, lymph node swelling, and serum ALP, γ-GTP concentration. The improvements of articular manifestations, lymph node swelling, and serum ALP, γ-GTP concentration were closely linked to TCZ therapy.

mature plasma cells are infiltrated and these also showed IL-6 positive (Figure 2(f)). Epstein-Bar virus in situ hybridization was negative (not shown). At the same time, alkaline phosphatase (ALP) and gamma glutamyl transpeptidase (γ-GTP) gradually increased. Blood test revealed positive anti-mitochondrial antibody (AMA) and otherwise unexplained high ALP and γ-GTP concentrations that lead to the diagnosis of PBC. Thus, treatment with ursodeoxycholic acid was initiated. In spite of discontinuation of MTX, lymphadenopathy did not improve, contrary to expectations. Because her joint symptoms worsened rapidly during the same period, mizoribine, tacrolimus, and sulfasalazine were used to relief her articular inflammation in turn; however, none of them were effective. Her lymphadenopathy persisted and the size of lymph nodes remained the same during the clinical course. Because her arthritis worsened gradually, she was again hospitalized to receive combination therapy with tocilizumab (TCZ), a humanized monoclonal antibody against interleukin-6 (IL-6) receptor, and MTX. On the second admission, TNJ count was 3 and SWJ count was 5. Generalized lymph node swelling was still observed. Laboratory data indicated an ESR of 75 mm/hr, CRP of 4.21 mg/dL, and matrix metalloproteinase-3 of 739 ng/mL. DAS28-ESR score of 5.39 showed she still had high disease activity. ALP and γ-GTP were elevated to 787 U/L and 117 U/L, respectively. Treatment with 600 mg of TCZ monthly plus 6 mg of MTX weekly was initiated (Figure 3). After introduction of TCZ, her polyarthritis improved markedly.

Nine months after the introduction of the TCZ, her DAS28-ESR score was 1.53 (her TNJ count was 1 and SWJ count was 2) showing clinical improvement. Interestingly, the generalized lymphadenopathy regressed rapidly (Figure 4) and serum ALP and γ-GTP concentration as well as AMA titer also decreased to within normal range in parallel with the improvement of polyarthritis. However, sclerodactyly and Raynaud's phenomenon did not improve apparently even after the initiation of TCZ therapy. Her arthritis has been well controlled for more than 2 years and she continues to take TCZ and MTX with no adverse events or complications.

3. Discussion

Here we reported a patient with overlapping RA and lSSc who was successfully treated with TCZ for polyarthritis as well as generalized lymphadenopathy and PBC. The predominant feature of present case is the efficacy of TCZ for generalized lymphadenopathy and PBC.

Lymphadenopathy is one of the extra-articular manifestations of RA and increasing relative risk of ML in RA and Sjögren syndrome is also well known [3]. Besides, it has been reported that MTX and TNF-α blockers

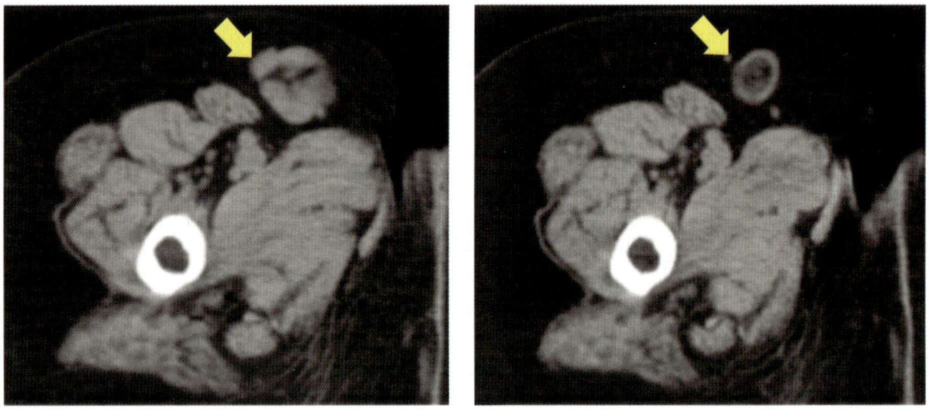

(a) (b)

Figure 4: Change in lymph node size by TCZ therapy. Generalized lymphadenopathy was observed before TCZ therapy (left panel, right inguinal area) but it regressed rapidly with central necrosis after TCZ therapy (right panel, right inguinal area).

induce lymphadenopathy in RA that are known as "iatrogenic immunodeficiency-associated lymphoproliferative disorders" [10]. Histopathological patterns of lymphadenopathy associated with RA are diverse. According to Kojima et al. [11], LPDs in RA are classified as benign, atypical, and malignant types. Histopathological finding of lymphadenopathy that is frequently seen in RA is reactive follicular hyperplasia with interfollicular plasmacytosis, which is classified as benign [2].

As the pathological manifestation of the present case showed reactive follicular hyperplasia and appeared to be benign, we suspected that a generalized lymphadenopathy was due to MTX associated LPD because it was discovered during MTX therapy. Therefore, we discontinued the administration of MTX immediately. However, lymphadenopathy did not improve in spite of MTX discontinuation. TNF-α blockers should be avoided in such a condition because Food and Drug Administration has issued warning that there is an increased risk of malignancy in patients treated with TNF-α blockers [1]. Numata et al. reported an RA patient with lymphadenopathy that showed follicular hyperplasia with increased expression of IL-6 in germinal centers that was identical to the pathologic characteristics of Castleman disease and the lymphocytes from this lymph node produced IL-6 in in vitro culture [12]. This patient showed the same histopathological features and also exhibited the increased expression of IL-6 in the germinal centers and interfollicular area. These results might indicate that one of histopathological characteristics of RA-associated lymphadenopathy are the same as those of Castleman disease. Therefore, TCZ is a possible candidate to treat RA patients with these conditions.

In addition, this case was complicated with PBC and showed high serum ALP and γ-GTP levels. However, these values decreased after injection of TCZ and AMA also became negative in parallel with the normalization of serum ALP and γ-GTP level after 9 months of TCZ treatment. These findings suggest that increased serum IL-6 concentration might play a role in PBC. However, as far as we know, there are few reports of the association of PBC with increased serum IL-6 level. Yamashiki et al. reported that sera from PBC patients showed a higher percentage of IL-6 receptor positive T lymphocytes by PHA activation compared with healthy controls [13]. They also reported that there is a significant correlation between the percentage of IL-6 positive T lymphocytes and AMA titer [13]. These results suggest that IL-6 might play an important role in pathogenesis of PBC. Improvement of PBC in this case might support this hypothesis. However, this is only a single case and further study of similar patients should help draw a more rigorous conclusion.

Currently, TCZ, monoclonal anti-IL-6 receptor antibody, has been approved for treatment of RA, Castleman disease, and juvenile idiopathic arthritis in Japan. Moreover, TCZ is expected to be potentially useful in the treatment of other IL-6 associated diseases such as Crohn's disease. In this context the present case might suggest that the potential use for the treatment of LPD and PBC associated with RA/lSSc overlap. Although Shima et al. reported that sclerosis of skin was improved by TCZ [14], sclerodactyly and Raynaud's phenomenon did not improve obviously in this patient. As the stage of her skin thickening was late phase and involved in only the fingers, it might be difficult to evaluate the improvement of skin thickening.

In summary, we reported a case of refractory RA/lSSc overlapping with generalized lymphadenopathy and PBC successfully treated with TCZ. This case suggested that increased serum IL-6 concentration might play an important role in lymphadenopathy and PBC associated with RA/lSSc. TCZ might be effective for these conditions as well as for treatment of the articular manifestation in RA.

References

[1] M. D. Robertson, F. D. Hart, W. F. White, G. Nuki, and P. L. Boardman, "Rheumatoid lymphadenopathy," *Annals of the Rheumatic Diseases*, vol. 27, no. 3, pp. 253–260, 1968.

[2] M. Kojima, Y. Hosomura, H. Itoh et al., "Reactive proliferative lesions in lymph nodes from rheumatoid arthritis patients: a clinicopathological and immunohistological study," *Acta Pathologica Japonica*, vol. 40, no. 4, pp. 249–254, 1990.

[3] E. Theander, R. Manthorpe, and L. T. H. Jacobsson, "Mortality and causes of death in primary Sjögren's syndrome: a prospective cohort study," *Arthritis and Rheumatism*, vol. 50, no. 4, pp. 1262–1269, 2004.

[4] L. Georgescu, G. C. Quinn, S. Schwartzman, and S. A. Paget, "Lymphoma in patients with rheumatoid arthritis: association with the disease state or methotrexate treatment," *Seminars in Arthritis and Rheumatism*, vol. 26, no. 6, pp. 794–804, 1997.

[5] A. C. Moseley, H. B. Lindsley, B. S. Skikne, and O. Tawfik, "Reversible methotrexate associated lymphoproliferative disease evolving into Hodgkin's disease," *Journal of Rheumatology*, vol. 27, no. 3, pp. 810–813, 2000.

[6] J. Askling, C. M. Fored, E. Baecklund et al., "Haematopoietic malignancies in rheumatoid arthritis: lymphoma risk and characteristics after exposure to tumour necrosis factor antagonists," *Annals of the Rheumatic Diseases*, vol. 64, no. 10, pp. 1414–1420, 2005.

[7] F. Wolfe and K. Michaud, "The effect of methotrexate and antitumor necrosis factor therapy on the risk of lymphoma in rheumatoid arthritis in 19,562 patients during 89,710 person-years of observation," *Arthritis and Rheumatism*, vol. 56, no. 5, pp. 1433–1439, 2007.

[8] R. Rizzi, P. Curci, M. Delia et al., "Spontaneous remission of "methotrexate-associated lymphoproliferative disorders" after discontinuation of immunosuppressive treatment for autoimmune disease. Review of the literature," *Medical Oncology*, vol. 26, no. 1, pp. 1–9, 2009.

[9] A. K. Wong, S. Kerkoutian, J. Said, H. Rashidi, and S. T. Pullarkat, "Risk of lymphoma in patients receiving antitumor necrosis factor therapy: a meta-analysis of published randomized controlled studies," *Clinical Rheumatology*, vol. 31, no. 4, pp. 631–636, 2012.

[10] P. Gaulard, S. H. Swerdlow, N. L. Harris, E. S. Jaffe, and C. Sundstrom, "Other iatrogenic immunodeficiency-associated lymphoproliferative disorders," in *World Health Organization Classification of Tumours. Pathology and Genetics: Tumours of Haematopoietic and Lymphoid Tissues*, S. H. Swerdlow, E. Campo, N. L. Harris et al., Eds., pp. 350–351, IARC Press, Lyon, France, 4th edition, 2008.

[11] M. Kojima, T. Motoori, and S. Nakamura, "Benign, atypical and malignant lymphoproliferative disorders in rheumatoid arthritis patients," *Biomedicine and Pharmacotherapy*, vol. 60, no. 10, pp. 663–672, 2006.

[12] Y. Numata, Y. Matsuura, S. Onishi et al., "Case report: interleukin-6 positive follicular hyperplasia in the lymph node of a patient with rheumatoid arthritis," *The American Journal of Hematology*, vol. 36, no. 4, pp. 282–284, 1991.

[13] M. Yamashiki, Y. Kosaka, J. Nishioka et al., "Flow cytometric analysis of IL-6 Receptors on peripheral lymphocytes in patients with primary billiary cirrhosis," *Journal of Clinical Laboratory Analysis*, vol. 12, pp. 83–87, 1998.

[14] Y. Shima, Y. Kuwahara, H. Murota et al., "The skin of patients with systemic sclerosis softened during the treatment with anti-IL-6 receptor antibody tocilizumab," *Rheumatology*, vol. 49, no. 12, Article ID keq275, pp. 2408–2412, 2010.

9

Acute Fibrinous and Organizing Pneumonia and Undifferentiated Connective Tissue Disease

Valéria Valim, Roberta Hora Rocha, Roberta Barcelos Couto, Thaysa Simões Paixão, and Érica Vieira Serrano

Department of Internal Medicine, Universidade Federal do Espirito Santo, Marechal Campos Avenue 1355, 29040-715 Vitoria, ES, Brazil

Correspondence should be addressed to Valéria Valim, val.valim@gmail.com

Academic Editors: T. C. Hsu and M. Salazar-Paramo

Acute fibrinous and organizing pneumonia (AFOP), recently described, is a histologic pattern characterized by the presence of fibrin "balls" within alveolar spaces. The term undifferentiated connective tissue disease (UCTD) is used to identify autoimmune systemic diseases that do not fulfill the criteria to be classified as a definitive connective tissue disease. The AFOP has never been reported in association with UCTD. The present reported case is a 39-year-old Caucasian, female with dry cough and progressive dyspnea. Eight months later, she was diagnosed with "organizing pneumonia" based on clinical history and radiologic images. She manifested Raynaud's Phenomenon, sicca syndrome, boot and gloves neuropathic pain, and previous hypothyroidism. Antinuclear antibody, rheumatoid factor, and specific autoantibodies were negative. Salivary gland biopsy and electroneuromyiography were normal. The capillaroscopy showed a "scleroderma" pattern with capillary deletion and ectasia. She experienced clinical and radiologic worsening. Despite being submitted to cyclophosphamide pulse, she developed hemorrhage and then died. Thoracotomy pulmonary specimen showed histological pattern of AFOP. This paper shows a rare association of AFOP with UCTD.

1. Introduction

Acute fibrinous and organizing pneumonia (AFOP) is an unusual type of lung injury characterized by a typical histological pattern recently described whose main features are the presence of intra-alveolar fibrin in the form of "balls" and organizing pneumonia with patchy distribution, which does not meet the classic histologic criteria for bronchiolitis obliterans with organizing pneumonia (BOOP), eosinophilic pneumonia (EP), or diffuse alveolar damage (DAD) [1–3].

This entity described in 2002 by Beasley et al. presents clinically as a lung injury. There seem to be two distinct patterns of disease progression and outcome: an acute, with fulminant course and rapid progression to death, and subacute, with chances of survival and recovery [1].

Acute fibrinous and organizing pneumonia (AFOP) may be idiopathic in nature or associated with many factors, such as autoimmune rheumatic diseases, occupational exposure (exotic animals, coal and tungsten mines, and hairspray [1, 4]), altered immune status (long-term steroids use, poorly controlled diabetes, alcoholism, lymphoma, acute myeloid leukemia and allogeneic hematopoietic stem cell transplantation, HIV infection, and *Pneumocystis jiroveci* pneumonia [1, 5, 6]), infectious causes (*Haemophilus influenzae, Acinetobacter baumannii,* and coronavirus [1, 3]), and exposure to drugs (abacavir, decitabine, and amiodarone) [1, 7–9].

The term undifferentiated connective tissue disease (UCTD) is used to identify autoimmune systemic diseases that do not fulfill the criteria to be classified as a definitive connective tissue disease (CTD) such as systemic lupus erythematosus, Sjögren's syndrome, systemic sclerosis, mixed connective tissue disease, rheumatoid arthritis, systemic vasculitis, and polymyositis/dermatomyositis. Some studies observed that this condition could progress into some of these diseases. The onset of UCTD is similar to most CTDs, peaking in the middle years of life [10, 11].

The natural history of these rare entities is variable: a high percentage of patients with UCTD maintain an undifferentiated clinical course and do not evolve to a distinct CTD, whereas some patients can evolve over time [11].

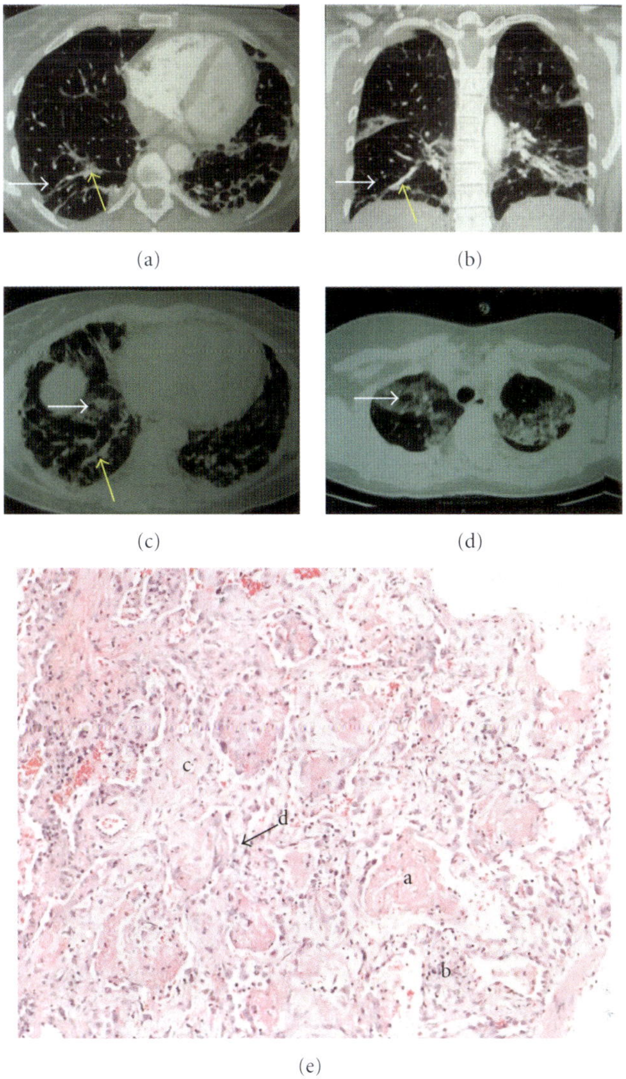

Figure 1: (a) and (b) CT findings of "focal areas of lung parenchymal infiltrates with ground-glass opacities, associated (white arrow) with septal thickening (yellow arrow), with peripheral distribution." (c) and (d) CT findings of interstitial infiltrate, with diffuse ground glass opacity with foci of parenchymal densification (yellow arrow) and some air bronchograms (white arrow). (e) Histhopatological examination showing (1) intra-alveolar accumulation of fibrin in the form of solid blocks; (2) acute inflammatory infiltrate in the interstitium; (3) alveolar septal edema and congestion; (4) *xantomatososum* macrophages accumulation.

Lung involvement as the first clinical manifestation of UCTD is rarely reported and usually appears as a complication in established UCTD [11].

There are only six cases of AFOP associated with rheumatic disease described.

There is no previously published case of AFOP and UCTD.

2. Case Report

A 39-year-old female Caucasian psychologist sought medical attention complaining of cough. Chest radiography showed changes that were attributed to pneumonia, treated with cefuroxime at the time. After eight months, progressive dyspnea was associated.

Initial diagnosis by pulmonologist was "organizing pneumonia," based on clinical history and computed tomographic (CT) findings, described as "focal areas of lung parenchymal infiltrates with ground-glass opacities, associated with septal thickening, with peripheral distribution, predominating in the lower lobes" (Figures 1(a) and 1(b)). Transbronchial biopsy was performed, which showed "scant fragments of bronchial wall and adjacent alveolar collapse exhibiting a minimum focus of interstitial inflammatory infiltrate." It was prescribed treatment with prednisone 20 mg/day.

After twelve months of evolution since the onset of symptoms, she went to a rheumatologist for differential diagnosis evaluation. On this occasion, the pulmonologist had already searched and excluded tuberculosis and she had dyspnea on minimal exertion. Diffuse pain in arms and legs, burning in

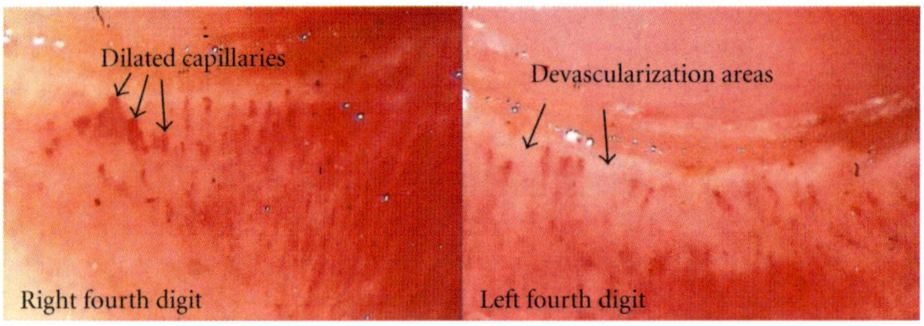

Figure 2: Panoramic nailfold capillaroscopy of the left and right fourth digits showing a scleroderma standard microangiopathy: dilated capillaries and devascularization areas.

the fingertips, fatigue, sleep disorder, Raynaud's phenomenon (RP), xerostomia, and xerophthalmia were present at the symptomatology interrogation and physical examination. She had positive personal and family history of Hashimoto's thyroiditis. On physical examination there was no skin thickening or arthritis, oroscopy was normal, blood pressure was 90 × 60 mmHg, and heart frequency was 96 beats per minute. Upon respiratory system examination basal crackles bilaterally and 20 breaths per minute were observed. There were no changes in cardiovascular and abdominal examination.

Tests were requested for the investigation of rheumatic diseases including systemic sclerosis, Sjögren's syndrome, and vasculitis. On this occasion, the prednisone dose was increased to 1 mg/kg/day.

Inflammatory activity tests and serologic and antibodies tests are demonstrated in Table 2.

In the evaluation of lung function a pattern compatible with incipient restrictive ventilatory disorder was observed. As evidence of inflammatory activity, CRP was always negative and ESR was increased. Autoantibodies were negative (antinuclear antibodies-ANA, rheumatoid factor, anti-SCL 70, anti-Jo-1, anti-RNP, anti-SS-A, anti-SS-B, and c-ANCA), except a 1 : 20 p-ANCA reagent. The patient presented a normocytic normochromic anemia, and the hemoglobin value ranged from 9.8 to 13.3 mg/dL and the hematocrit range was 30.3 to 41.7%, probably due to the underlying disease. In two occasions, the patient presented lymphopenia that could indicate disease activity or could be related to steroid therapy. Chlamydia pneumonia IgG serology was reagent 1 : 512 and IgM was negative. Mycoplasma pneumonia serology was negative. The exams allowed excluding Sjögren's syndrome (negative anti-SS-A and anti-SS-B and normal salivary biopsy). Renal, liver, and hormonal functions were normal.

A panoramic nailfold capillaroscopy showed the presence of moderate capillary ectasia and mild devascularization of focal distribution, described as "well-defined scleroderma (SD) standard microangiopathy, consistent with systemic sclerosis, dermatomyositis or overlap syndrome with scleroderma component" (Figure 2).

Given the results of capillaroscopy and the presence of RP she was diagnosed with systemic sclerosis in the early stages. Then it was proposed to start cyclophosphamide pulse 1 g.

However, after three weeks of diagnosis, the patient developed high fever (39 degrees) and dyspnea at rest, requiring hospitalization. On admission, her respiratory frequency was 40 incursions per minute, the arterial oxygen tension was 48.4 mmHg, and oxygen saturation was 88.5% and she had basal crackles bilaterally. On the third day she developed respiratory failure, requiring ventilatory support and intensive care. The chest CT showed interstitial infiltrate, with diffuse ground-glass opacity in both lungs, associated with foci of parenchymal densification, predominantly peripheral, some air bronchograms and mild pleural thickening marginally, more evident in right lung basis and apex. Small calcified nodules of residual aspect, scattered in both lungs, without pleural effusion (Figures 1(c) and 1(d)), were observed. An echocardiogram was done to exclude pulmonary hypertension. The pulmonary arterial pressure was 31 mmHg.

Hemoculture and urine culture were negative. Virus B and C serologies were negative. The CRP increased from 42 to 147 mg/dL.

At that moment the pulmonologist considered three possible diagnosis: nonspecific interstitial pneumonia, pneumonia caused by *Pneumocystis carinii*, or pneumonia caused by virus (CMV, adenovirus, herpes 1 and 2).

On the fourth day, she underwent an open biopsy (microthoracotomy), which consisted of pulmonary segmentectomy of right middle and lower lobes. Some part of the material was sent to investigate fungus, mycobacteria, and general culture, all of them presented negative results. The biopsy revealed that there were no infectious process and no granulomas. Histopathological examination showed "a parenchymal diffuse involvement, intra-alveolar fibrin accumulation in the form of solid blocks, pneumocytes hyperplasia, interstitial mild acute inflammatory infiltrate, alveolar septal edema and congestion, intra-alveolar fibroblastic Masson bodies and *xantomatososum* accumulation of macrophages, a typical pattern of acute Fibrinous and Organizing Pneumonia (AFOP)" (Figure 1(e)).

After excluding any infection etiology including bacteria, virus, mycobacteria, and fungus, she received pulse therapy with cyclophosphamide 1 g and methylprednisolone 1 g for three days. Despite treatment, the patient developed respiratory failure by pulmonary hemorrhage.

3. Discussion

We reported the case of a female patient of 39 years with diagnosis of undifferentiated connective tissue disease (UCTD)

Table 1: Described cases of acute fibrinous organizing pneumonia, 2002–2011.

Rheumatologic disease	Age	Sex	Treatment	Time	Outcome evolution	Author, year
Ankylosing spondylitis	55	M	Corticoid	—	Survived	Beasley et al., 2002, [1]
Polymyositis	78	F	Corticoid	—	Death	Beasley et al., 2002, [1]
Fibromyalgia	58	F	Antibiotic	—	Survived	Beasley et al., 2002, [1]
Juvenile dermatomyositis	14	F	Azithromycin, immunoglobulin, cyclophosphamide, methylprednisolone, and cyclosporine	2 months	Death	Prahalad et al., 2005, [12]
Stigma of rheumatic disease	47	M	Prednisone	3 months	Survived	Balduin et al., 2007, [13]
SLE and APS	16	M	Prednisone, cyclophosphamide, anticoagulants	2,5 months	Survived	Hariri et al., 2010, [14]

SLE: systemic erythematosus lupus; APS: antiphospholipid syndrome.

Table 2: Inflammatory activity tests and serologic and autoantibodies tests.

	09/12/2007	10/30/2007	03/06/2008	07/02/2008
ESR (mm/h) RV: <20	67	54		55
CRP (mg/dL) RV: <0,5	<0,5	<0,5		<0,5
Total protein (g/dL) RV: 6–8		72		
ANA RV: nonreactive	Nonreactive	Nonreactive	Nonreactive	
RF (UI/mL) RV: <40	<40	<40	<40	
P-ANCA RV: negative			1 : 20	
Anti-TPO (UI/mL) RV: <35			842	
Anti-TBG (UI/mL) RV: <40			141	
Negative autoantibodies: anti-Scl70, anti-Jo1, c-ANCA, anti-RNP, anti-SS-A, anti-SS-B, anti-CCP, antinative DNA, and anticentromere.				
Mycoplasma pneumoniae, *Chlamydia pneumoniae*, HBV and HCV negative serologic tests.				

ESR: erythrocyte sedimentation rate; CRP: C-reactive protein; ANA: antinuclear antibodies; RF: rheumatoid factor; P-ANCA: perinuclear antineutrophil cytoplasmic antibodies; anti-TPO: antithyroid peroxidase; anti-TGB: antithyroxine binding globulin; anti-Scl 70: antitopoisomerase antibodies; anti-Jo 1: antisynthetase antibodies; c-ANCA: cytoplasmic antineutrophil cytoplasmic antibodies; anti-RNP: antiribonucleoproteins antitopoisomerase antibodies; anti-SS-A: anti Sjogren's Syndrome antigen A; anti SS B: anti Sjogren's syndrome antigen B; anti CCP: anticitrulline containing peptide; HBV: hepatitis B virus; HCV: hepatitis C virus; RV: reference value.

and manifestations suggestive of systemic sclerosis (SSc) as Raynaud's phenomenon (RP) and capillaroscopic pattern SD associated with acute fibrinous and organizing pneumonia (AFOP).

There were some difficulties to complete the diagnosis in relation to both pulmonary and systemic aspects.

A detailed assessment by a rheumatologist specialist noted the presence of RP, which is a symptom guide to SSc diagnosis [15, 16]. Raynaud's phenomenon is one of the most common symptoms in SSc (90–95%) but also can be find in other rheumatic diseases like lupus, rheumatoid arthritis, Sjögren's syndrome, myositis, and overlap diseases. It often precedes rheumatic disease manifestations by a variable period of time [15, 17]. At the present time capillaroscopy is recommended as mandatory exam to investigate RP for the diagnosis of early SSc [16, 18, 19]. In patients with RP, the presence of capillaroscopy abnormalities that characterize the scleroderma pattern indicates a high specificity and a positive predictive value for the diagnosis of SSc and related disorders, more than a positive antinuclear antibodies test [16].

The manifestations strongly suggested the SSc, but it was not possible to give the diagnosis based on the American College of Rheumatology criteria [20]. Also the patient did not have skin or characteristic pulmonary manifestation. Then, we concluded with the diagnosis of UCTD.

Acute fibrinous and organizing pneumonia (AFOP) is a histological pattern characterized by intra-alveolar fibrin accumulation associated with organizing pneumonia consisting of intraluminal loose connective tissue within the alveolar bronchioles and ducts associated with the fibrin [1, 2]. In this case, the histopathological study of the patient showed a lung parenchymal diffuse involvement, intra-alveolar fibrin in the form of solid blocks, pneumocytes hyperplasia, mild acute inflammatory infiltrate in the interstitium, alveolar septal edema and congestion and intra-alveolar fibroblastic Masson bodies, also reported by Beasley et al. [1].

Beasley et al. noted that the period between the onset of symptoms and the biopsy performance did not exceed two months, and, among patients who died, the average number of days between onset of symptoms and death was 29 days [1]. In this patient, 15 months have passed from the onset of initial symptoms until the biopsy and death. The need for mechanical ventilation (MV) was the only significant parameter that correlated with prognosis in cases studied by Beasley et al., and all patients who required mechanical ventilation died [1]. The same was observed in the patient of this case.

Steroids and antibiotics, associated or not, diuretics and mechanical ventilation were used in the treatment of AFOP by Beasley et al., and therapeutic modality used did not correlate with the outcome background [1]. It was not found yet an ideal treatment for AFOP, but there are reports in the literature of successful treatments with mycophenolate mofetil and methylprednisolone [21] and prednisone and cyclophosphamide [22]. The patient in this study received cyclophosphamide and methylprednisolone pulse therapy in the intensive critical unit but progressed to respiratory failure by pulmonary hemorrhage.

We believe that early therapy institution could have resulted in a more favorable outcome in this case, although further studies are still needed on this new entity to support this understanding.

Clinically, the diagnosis of AFOP is undistinguishable from the others lung injuries diagnosis. Adding the radiologic aspects there is a range of differential diagnoses as atypical pneumonia, pulmonary edema, and interstitial pneumoniae [1]. In the presented current case, initially pneumonia was diagnosed. Then, according to the clinical and radiographic aspects she was diagnosed with organizing pneumonia (OP). However, the result of the histopathological examination showed, posteriorly, the AFOP standard. The diagnosis of AFOP is essentially histological. In the series studied by Beasley et al., cases of patients who had only transbronchial biopsy were excluded from the study [1] since, due to the localized nature of the injury, this kind of biopsy may fail on histologic diagnosis [1, 2]. Acute fibrinous and organizing pneumonia (AFOP) diagnosis should only be made on large biopsy specimen when it is quite certain that there are not otherwise diagnostic features of diffuse alveolar damage (DAD), eosinophilic pneumonia (EP) or OP, histological patterns that make differential diagnosis with AFOP [2]. No hyaline membranes were seen as in DAD, and despite the presence of eosinophils in some specimens, they were never predominant as in EP [22]. Although fibrin deposits have been described in both the DAD and OP patterns, they do not comprise a major component of the process [1].

Regarding the association with autoimmune rheumatic diseases and AFOP, Beasley et al. noted in their series an association with ankylosing spondylitis and polymyositis [1]. Association with rheumatic diseases as systemic lupus erythematosus and juvenile dermatomyositis was already described in literature [12–14] (Table 1).

There are no previous reports in the literature about the association of UCTD and AFOP and this is the first reported case. It is a rare association that may be increasingly reported in the literature as this new terminology is best known and most biopsies are early performed with proper technique.

4. Conclusion

In this paper it was presented a rare combination of acute fibrinous and organizing pneumonia (AFOP) with an undifferentiated connective tissue disease (UCTD).

References

[1] M. B. Beasley, T. J. Franks, J. R. Galvin, B. Gochuico, and W. D. Travis, "Acute fibrinous and organizing pneumonia: a histologic pattern of lung injury and possible variant of diffuse alveolar damage," *Archives of Pathology and Laboratory Medicine*, vol. 126, no. 9, pp. 1064–1070, 2002.

[2] M. B. Beasley, "The pathologist's approach to acute lung injury," *Archives of Pathology and Laboratory Medicine*, vol. 134, no. 5, pp. 719–727, 2010.

[3] C. R. Cordeiro, "Airway involvement in interstitial lung disease," *Current Opinion in Pulmonary Medicine*, vol. 12, no. 5, pp. 337–341, 2006.

[4] C. Santos, F. Fradinho, and A. Catarino, "Acute fibrinous and organizing pneumonia," *Revista Portuguesa de Pneumologia*, vol. 16, no. 4, pp. 607–616, 2010.

[5] S. M. Lee, J. J. Park, H. S. Sun et al., "Acute fibrinous and organizing pneumonia following hematopoietic stem cell transplantation," *Korean Journal of Internal Medicine*, vol. 24, no. 2, pp. 156–159, 2009.

[6] J. Y. Heo, J. Y. Song, J. Y. Noh, H. S. Yong, H. J. Cheong, and W. J. Kim, "Acute fibrinous and organizing pneumonia in a patient with HIV infection and Pneumocystis jiroveci pneumonia," *Respirology*, vol. 15, no. 8, pp. 1259–1261, 2010.

[7] N. Yokogawa and D. V. Alcid, "Acute fibrinous and organizing pneumonia as a rare presentation of abacavir hypersensitivity reaction," *AIDS*, vol. 21, no. 15, pp. 2116–2117, 2007.

[8] T. S. Vasu, R. Cavallazzi, A. Hirani, and P. E. Marik, "A 64-year-old male with fever and persistent lung infiltrate," *Respiratory Care*, vol. 54, no. 9, pp. 1263–1265, 2009.

[9] S. A. Papiris, C. Triantafillidou, L. Kolilekas, D. Markoulaki, and E. D. Manali, "Amiodarone: review of pulmonary effects and toxicity," *Drug Safety*, vol. 33, no. 7, pp. 539–558, 2010.

[10] L. F. Guerrero, J. C. Rueda, R. Arciniegas, and J. M. Rueda, "Undifferentiated connective tissue disease in a rheumatology center in Cali, Colombia: clinical features of 94 patients followed for a year," *Rheumatology International*. In press.

[11] F. Lunardi, E. Balestro, B. Nordio et al., "Undifferentiated connective tissue disease presenting with prevalent interstitial lung disease: case report and review of literature," *Diagnostic Pathology*, vol. 6, no. 1, article 50, 2011.

[12] S. Prahalad, J. F. Bohnsack, C. G. Maloney, and K. O. Leslie, "Fatal acute fibrinous and organizing pneumonia in a child with juvenile dermatomyositis," *Journal of Pediatrics*, vol. 146, no. 2, pp. 289–292, 2005.

[13] R. Balduin, C. Giacometti, L. Saccarola et al., "Acute fibrinous and organizing pneumonia in a patient with collagen vascular disease 'stigma'," *Sarcoidosis Vasculitis and Diffuse Lung Diseases*, vol. 24, no. 1, pp. 78–80, 2007.

[14] L. P. Hariri, S. Unizony, J. Stone et al., "Acute fibrinous and organizing pneumonia in systemic lupus erythematosus: a case report and review of the literature," *Pathology International*, vol. 60, no. 11, pp. 755–759, 2010.

[15] S. P. Toya and G. E. Tzelepis, "The many faces of scleroderma sine scleroderma: a literature review focusing on cardiopulmonary complications," *Rheumatology International*, vol. 29, no. 8, pp. 861–868, 2009.

[16] R. De Angelis, W. Grassi, and M. Cutolo, "A growing need for capillaroscopy in rheumatology," *Arthritis Care and Research*, vol. 61, no. 3, pp. 405–410, 2009.

[17] S. N. Lambova and U. Müller-Ladner, "The role of capillaroscopy in differentiation of primary and secondary Raynaud's phenomenon in rheumatic diseases: a review of the literature and two case reports," *Rheumatology International*, vol. 29, no. 11, pp. 1263–1271, 2009.

[18] M. Matucci-Cerinic, V. Steen, P. Nash, and E. Hachulla, "The complexity of managing systemic sclerosis: screening and diagnosis," *Rheumatology*, vol. 48, pp. 8–13, 2009.

[19] M. Cutolo, C. Pizzorni, M. E. Secchi, and A. Sulli, "Capillaroscopy," *Best Practice and Research: Clinical Rheumatology*, vol. 22, no. 6, pp. 1093–1108, 2008.

[20] A. T. Masi, G. P. Rodnan, and T. A. Medsger, "Preliminary criteria for the classification of systemic sclerosis (scleroderma)," *Arthritis and Rheumatism*, vol. 23, no. 5, pp. 581–590, 1980.

[21] S. Bhatti, A. Hakeem, J. Torrealba, J. P. McMahon, and K. C. Meyer, "Severe acute fibrinous and organizing pneumonia (AFOP) causing ventilatory failure: successful treatment with mycophenolate mofetil and corticosteroids," *Respiratory Medicine*, vol. 103, no. 11, pp. 1764–1767, 2009.

[22] C. Damas, A. Morais, C. S. Moura, and J. A. Marques, "Acute fibrinous and organizing pneumonia," *Revista Portuguesa de Pneumologia*, vol. 12, no. 5, pp. 615–620, 2006.

10

Gouty Panniculitis with Ulcerations in a Patient with Multiple Organ Dysfunctions

Lu Wang,[1] Crystal Rose,[2] Paul Mellen,[2] George Branam,[2] and Maria M. Picken[1]

[1] *Department of Pathology and Laboratory Medicine, Loyola University Medical Center, 2160 S 1st Avenue, Maywood, IL 60153, USA*
[2] *Department of Pathology, Ball Memorial Hospital, Indiana University Health, 2401 W University Avenue, Muncie, IN 47303, USA*

Correspondence should be addressed to Maria M. Picken; mmpicken@aol.com

Academic Editor: Shoichiro Ikuyama

Gouty panniculitis is a rare manifestation of gout. Clinically, it is characterized by indurated subcutaneous nodules in nonjoint areas. Pathologically, typical characteristic gouty tophi can be seen in subcutaneous tissue. It is postulated that gouty panniculitis develops as a consequence of uric acid accumulation in the body and localized inflammatory changes in subcutaneous tissue. We report a case of a 46-year-old man with 20-year history of gout, who developed multiple subcutaneous nodules over the abdomen and right groin/thigh area over a 2-year period. After a recent episode of congestive heart failure and acute renal failure, the nodules increased in size and the overlying skin became erythematous and ulcerated. Pathologic examination demonstrated typical tophi in the dermis and subcutaneous tissue. A review of the literature yielded fifteen similar cases that had been previously reported. We conclude that gouty panniculitis may be a manifestation of undertreated gout and may be exacerbated by the deterioration of other systemic functions.

1. Introduction

Gouty panniculitis is a rare manifestation of gout. It is characterized clinically by indurated, erythematous, or ulcerated subcutaneous nodules. Histologic confirmation is achieved by identification of tophaceous crystal deposition in the lobular subcutaneous tissue [1, 2]. The clinical presence of indurated subcutaneous plaques may precede, or appear subsequently to the articular clinical expression of tophaceous gout [1]. We report a case of gouty panniculitis manifesting as multiple subcutaneous nodules in different locations with and without ulceration. The recent literature related to this disease entity is also reviewed.

2. Case Report

A 46-year-old male with a 20-year history of gout presented with nontender nodules in the subcutaneous tissue of the abdomen, groin, and right thigh. The nodules had been present for two years; however, over the past three weeks, some of the nodules became erythematous and eventually ulcerated. In addition, the patient had recently been admitted for congestive heart failure and acute renal failure 3.5 weeks prior to presentation. His gout had never been treated. Furthermore, the patient's medical history was complicated by type II diabetes and morbid obesity with a BMI of 40.6.

Physical examination revealed multiple, whitish subcutaneous nodules and 4 skin ulcers in the lower half of the abdomen, right groin, and right thigh. All ulcers measured between 1 and 3 cm; fibrinous, necrotic, and chalky whitish material covered poorly formed granulation tissue. The nonulcerated pale, white nodules with focal erythema could be palpated subcutaneously and averaged from 1.0 to 1.5 cm in diameter (Figure 1(a)). Clinically, there was also significant swelling of the right elbow and the MCP joints on the patient's right hand.

Results of laboratory tests from the patient's most recent admission revealed the following: uric acid 14.3 mg/dL (reference range 4–7 mg/dL), blood glucose 255 mg/dL (reference range 70–99 mg/dL), BUN 47 mg/dL (reference range

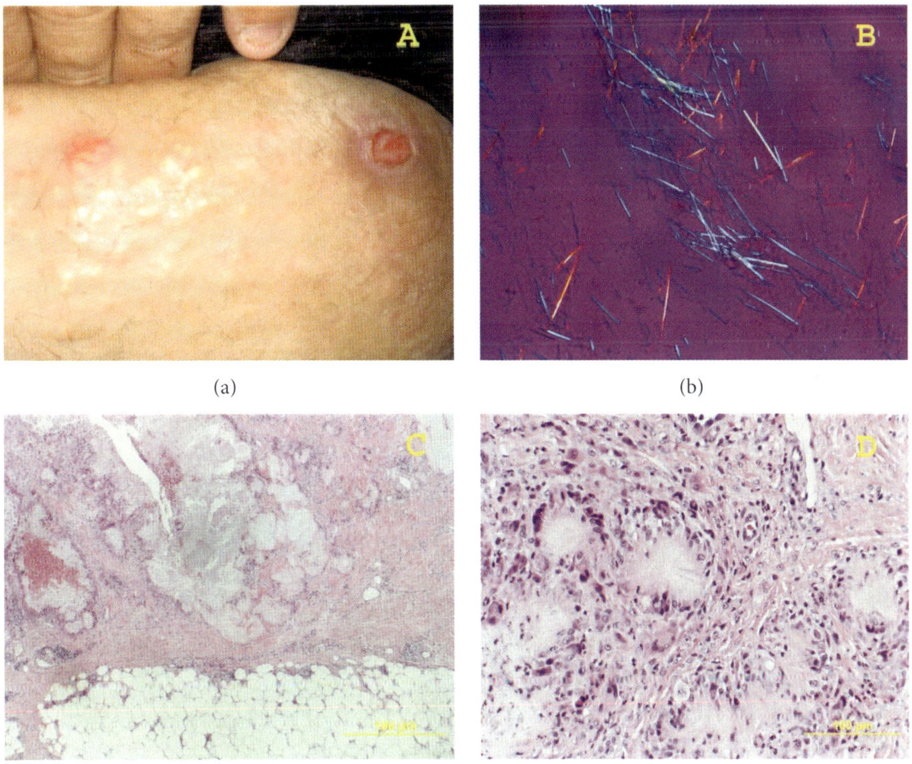

(a) (b)

(c) (d)

FIGURE 1: Skin and subcutaneous lesion. (a) Ulcer and erythematous nodule in right groin area, 1 to 1.5 cm; (b) negative birefringence of urate crystal on fresh tissue touch imprint slide (400x); (c) and (d) subcutaneous lesion: low power picture shows subcutaneous tissue erosion with pools of pale staining or slightly eosinophilic amorphous/feathery material surrounded by collagen fibers and chronic inflammatory cells (c, 40x); high power picture shows feathery eosinophilic crystalline material converging in the center and surrounded by palisading histiocytes and multinucleated giant cells (d, 200x).

5–20 mg/dL), creatinine 1.61 mg/dL (reference range 0.8–1.4 mg/dL), and estimated GFR 46 mL/min/1.73 m^2 (reference range ≥59). His uric acid levels were 10.8 mg/dL and 11.2 mg/dL at the time of surgical removal of the ulcerated nodules, 3 and 4 weeks later. At that time also, his renal function and blood glucose levels were still abnormal: BUN 38 mg/dL, creatinine 1.65 mg/dL, GFR 45 mL/min/1.73 m^2, and blood glucose 147 mg/dL.

The patient underwent 3 excisional biopsies, including 2 from an abdominal skin lesion and 1 from the right thigh. All 3 specimens were submitted separately, over a 3 week period, for histological evaluation. Sectioning of the specimens revealed multifocal areas filled with white, chalky material. Touch imprint slides were prepared before tissue fixation. Microscopic examination under polarized light showed multiple needle-shaped crystals displaying negative birefringence (Figure 1(b)). Permanent histology slides showed pools of pale and slightly eosinophilic amorphous as well as feathery material in the dermis and subcutaneous tissue (Figures 1(c) and 1(d)). The lesions demonstrated different stages of development. The smaller lesions had a central area of feathery crystalline material surrounded by palisading histiocytes and multinucleated giant cells. The larger lesions consisted of disorganized, laminated material surrounded by collagen fibers and chronic inflammation. The lesions eroded outward to the skin surface leading to ulceration. Based on the clinical, laboratory, and histologic findings, a diagnosis of multifocal gouty tophi was made.

3. Discussion

Gout has become increasingly common in the Western world, such that the lifetime risk of acquisition is now approximately 1-2% [3, 4]. Tophi are a common clinical manifestation of gout. They contain collections of monosodium urate crystals and are commonly located in the vicinity of joints of the elbows, hands, and feet. They lead to joint destruction and chronic (long-term and continuous) joint pain and stiffness. Gouty panniculitis is characterized by inflammation of the subcutaneous fat and manifests itself clinically as nodular (lumpy) lesions on the legs and trunk, which ulcerate and ooze fluid containing monosodium urate crystals [5]. In contrast to tophi, panniculitis has been reported, thus far, only in a very small percentage of patients with gout. Thus, Webershock [2] reported one case in 2010 and reviewed 8 prior reported cases from 1977 to 2007 [2, 6–9]. Recently, however, Ochoa et al. [1] reported an additional 6 cases from a single institution and concluded that panniculitis should be considered as one of the principal clinical manifestations of gout. These authors also raised the question of whether this particular manifestation has hitherto been under reported.

The pathogenesis of gouty panniculitis is currently not well understood. Some predisposing factors may enhance the deposition of monosodium urate crystals in the subcutaneous tissue. As expected, hyperuricemia is present in the vast majority of patients diagnosed with this condition [7]. A high metabolic rate, leading to increased production of uric acid, may lead to an oversaturation of monosodium urate with joint deposition and deposition in the lobular subcutaneous tissue [1]. In addition, preexisting subcutaneous tissue damage is known to increase the risk of subcutaneous panniculitis. Additional factors may include venous stasis, varicosities, or chronic edema related to cardiac failure and elevated serum amylase or lipase [2, 7]. Elevated serum amylase and lipase, in patients with renal failure and end stage renal disease, may be due to decreased renal clearance of these enzymes [10, 11]. Hence, chronic renal insufficiency associated with hypertensive nephropathy or other medical conditions represents a potential risk factor for gouty panniculitis [1].

Ochoa et al. postulated that gouty panniculitis could be caused by localized inflammatory changes in the lobular subcutaneous tissue. This inflammation may be triggered or perpetuated by blood supply disruption caused by monosodium urate crystals, consequently resulting in microtrauma to the terminal capillary walls and adipose tissues. This hypoxia then renders the subcutaneous tissues vulnerable to further injury [1].

More recently, uric acid has been shown to activate the NLRP3 (NOD (nucleotide-binding oligomerization domain) like receptors, pyrin domain 3) inflammasome, which plays a key role in innate immunity. In lipopolysaccharide (LPS) stimulated mice, monosodium urate (as well as calcium pyrophosphate dihydrate) crystals have been shown to cause an increase in caspase-1 activation and the secretion of IL-1β. However, mice deficient for inflammasome components were defective in crystal-induced IL-1β secretion [12]. Moreover, in a peritoneal murine model of gout, monosodium urate crystal-recruited monocytes differentiate into proinflammatory M1-like macrophages producing more IL-1 along with other cytokines and chemokines [13]. These experimental findings support the concept that the innate immune system may play a critical role in the triggering of crystal-induced acute inflammation. Consonant with these findings, IL-1 inhibitors appear to be beneficial in the treatment of gout.

Our patient had a long history of untreated gout. Over two years, he progressively developed subcutaneous nodules over his abdomen, groin, and right thigh area. His blood uric acid levels ranged between 10.8 mg/dL and 14.3 mg/dL during his recent hospitalization. The subcutaneous nodules became erythematous and ulcerated soon after the development of congestive heart failure and acute renal failure. His renal failure was a likely consequence of his cardiac insufficiency, the latter providing low blood perfusion of the kidney. In addition, this patient was diabetic and may have had underlying diabetic nephropathy. This in turn could have made the kidney more susceptible to impaired perfusion due to the acute onset of heart failure. The deterioration of kidney function and the use of the loop diuretic furosemide may have accelerated the accumulation of uric acid in the patient's body [14], ultimately exacerbating his gouty panniculitis. Furthermore, the severe hyperuricemia might have led to further deterioration of renal function. Histologically, the newly developed small lesions, which were surrounded by palisading histiocytes, may be indicative of the active phase of his panniculitis. The patient's other medical conditions, which contributed to gout development, included type II diabetes [15] and morbid obesity [16].

The differential diagnosis of gouty panniculitis encompasses a wide range of disorders including sclerema neonatorum, subcutaneous fat necrosis, pancreatic panniculitis, poststeroid panniculitis, factitial panniculitis, hemorrhagic panniculitis, and many others [1, 2, 7]. Although gouty panniculitis can often demonstrate a granulomatous reaction, the detection of feathery crystalline material, although rare, is helpful. Since monosodium urate crystals can be dissolved during paraffin fixation and routine hematoxylin and eosin (H&E) staining, the feathery structures seen on permanent histology slides actually represent empty spaces previously occupied by the needle-shaped crystals of monosodium urate. Thus, the direct detection of crystals using polarized light requires either touch imprint slides prepared from fresh tissue or the use of ethanol fixation during tissue processing.

All gouty panniculitis cases (18 in total, including the current case) are reviewed. The average age of onset is 47.2 years old. In general, gouty panniculitis is a late clinical manifestation of chronic gout (average 17 years). However, the skin lesions may also be manifested before the onset of classic gout [1]. Gouty panniculitis appears more likely to develop in male patients, with a male to female ratio of 7 : 1. Hyperuricemia (mean 9.8 mg/dL) plays an important role in the development gouty panniculitis. Some patients, who have a normal uric acid level at diagnosis, may have experienced long-term hyperuricemia at an earlier time. Among all 18 cases, abnormal renal function was noted in 12 (66.7%) patients [1, 6, 8, 9, 17, 18]. Due to the lack of complete metabolic panel (CMP) data, renal function in the remaining 6 cases could not be assessed [2, 7, 19]. Also, elevation of erythrocyte sedimentation rate and C-reactive protein have been noted in some cases [2, 7, 8].

With regard to gouty panniculitis, although no specific treatment for this condition is currently available, systemic anti-inflammatory therapy, including corticosteroids, can often rapidly ameliorate the symptoms [2, 7]. The nonhealing ulcerated lesions can also be surgically resected. Our patient was treated with NSAIDs (naproxen) and prednisone with a fair response.

4. Conclusion

Although gouty panniculitis is an uncommon symptom of gout, the development of nodules in subcutaneous tissue should alert the clinician to the need for a more careful monitoring of the patient. Uncontrolled hyperuricemia can lead to devastating dermatopathologic consequences. Skin manifestations can be an indicator of undertreated or untreated gout, as well as the decompensation of other systemic conditions such as renal dysfunction. Further systemic workup or close clinical monitoring should be considered in such patients.

References

[1] C. D. Ochoa, V. Valderrama, J. Mejia et al., "Panniculitis: another clinical expression of gout," *Rheumatology International*, vol. 31, no. 6, pp. 831–835, 2011.

[2] T. Weberschock, P. Gholam, W. Hartschuh, and M. Hartmann, "Gouty panniculitis in a 68-year-old man: case report and review of the literature," *International Journal of Dermatology*, vol. 49, no. 4, pp. 410–413, 2010.

[3] L. X. Chen and H. R. Schumacher, "Gout: an evidence-based review," *Journal of Clinical Rheumatology*, vol. 14, supplement 5, pp. S55–S62, 2008.

[4] P. Richette and T. Bardin, "Gout," *The Lancet*, vol. 375, no. 9711, pp. 318–328, 2010.

[5] G. F. Falasca, "Metabolic diseases: gout," *Clinics in Dermatology*, vol. 24, no. 6, pp. 498–508, 2006.

[6] K. M. Niemi, "Panniculitis of the legs with urate crystal deposition," *Archives of Dermatology*, vol. 113, no. 5, pp. 655–656, 1977.

[7] A. Dahiya, J. Leach, and H. Levy, "Gouty panniculitis in a healthy male," *Journal of the American Academy of Dermatology*, vol. 57, supplement 2, pp. S52–S54, 2007.

[8] A. A. Snider and S. Barsky, "Gouty panniculitis: a case report and review of the literature," *Cutis*, vol. 76, no. 1, pp. 54–56, 2005.

[9] P. E. LeBoit and S. Schneider, "Gout presenting as lobular panniculitis," *American Journal of Dermatopathology*, vol. 9, no. 4, pp. 334–338, 1987.

[10] N. D. Vaziri, D. Chang, A. Malekpour, and S. Radaht, "Pancreatic enzymes in patients with end-stage renal disease maintained on hemodialysis," *The American Journal of Gastroenterology*, vol. 83, no. 4, pp. 410–412, 1988.

[11] C. F. Jiang, K. W. Ng, S. W. Tan et al., "Serum level of amylase and lipase in various stages of chronic renal insufficiency," *Zhonghua Yi Xue Za Zhi*, vol. 65, no. 2, pp. 49–54, 2002.

[12] F. Martinon, V. Petrilli, A. Mayor, A. Tardivel, and J. Tschopp, "Gout-associated uric acid crystals activate the NALP3 inflammasome," *Nature*, vol. 440, no. 7081, pp. 237–241, 2006.

[13] W. J. Martin, O. Shaw, X. Liu, S. Steiger, and J. L. Harper, "Monosodium urate monohydrate crystal-recruited noninflammatory monocytes differentiate into M1-like proinflammatory macrophages in a peritoneal murine model of gout," *Arthritis & Rheumatism*, vol. 63, no. 5, pp. 1322–1332, 2011.

[14] W. F. Boron, *Medical Physiology: A Cellular and Molecular Approach*, W.B. Saunders, Philadelphia, Pa, USA, 2003.

[15] N. Schlesinger, "Diagnosing and treating gout: a review to aid primary care physicians," *Postgraduate Medicine*, vol. 122, no. 2, pp. 157–161, 2010.

[16] A. L. Weaver, "Epidemiology of gout," *Cleveland Clinic Journal of Medicine*, vol. 75, supplement 5, pp. S9–S12, 2008.

[17] A. Iglesias, J. Londono, D. L. Saaibi, M. Pena, H. Lizarazo, and E. B. Gonzalez, "Gout nodulosis: widespread subcutaneous deposits without gout," *Arthritis Care & Research*, vol. 9, no. 1, pp. 74–77, 1996.

[18] C. M. Choi, B. L. Lew, S. Y. Lee, and W. Y. Sim, "Gouty panniculitis also involving the bone marrow," *Acta Dermato-Venereologica*, vol. 93, no. 2, pp. 189–190, 2013.

[19] E. Peñaranda-Parada, N. S. Bejarano, J. Mejía et al., "Gouty arthritis and panniculitis: extensive involvement of the dermis and severe joint damage," *Journal of Clinical Rheumatology*, vol. 18, no. 3, pp. 142–143, 2012.

11

Cranial Nerve Palsies: Sarcoidosis to Systemic Lupus Erythematosus

Fawad Aslam,[1,2] Firas Bannout,[2,3] and Elizabeth B. Russell[1,2]

[1] *Division of Rheumatology, Department of Internal Medicine, University of Arkansas for Medical Sciences, Little Rock, AR 72205, USA*

[2] *Division of Rheumatology, Department of Internal Medicine, John L. McClellan Memorial Veterans Hospital, Little Rock, AR 72205, USA*

[3] *Department of Neurology, University of Arkansas for Medical Sciences, Little Rock, AR 72205, USA*

Correspondence should be addressed to Fawad Aslam; fawadaslam2@gmail.com

Academic Editors: G. S. Alarcon and L.-P. Erwig

Cranial palsies are a very rare feature of SLE. Similarly, peripheral sensory-motor axonal neuropathy is very uncommon in SLE. The combination of the two as the presenting symptoms of SLE is a diagnostic challenge particularly in an elderly male patient with a known diagnosis of sarcoidosis. This case serves to highlight the diagnostic considerations in such a patient. The lack of response to standard therapy and the presence of subtle clues like anemia, proteinuria, and mild serositis should prompt the physician to look for alternate diagnoses. The potential association of SLE and sarcoidosis is also discussed. SLE can be present in elderly male patients with cranial and peripheral neuropathy.

1. Introduction

Central nervous system (CNS) involvement in systemic lupus erythematosus (SLE) is approximated at 50% and ranges from 14 to 75% [1]. Cranial palsies are an unusual central nervous system manifestation of SLE and account for 0.5–1.0% of neuropsychiatric manifestations [2]. Most frequent cranial neuropathies involve the eighth nerve followed by the oculomotor set (third, fourth, and sixth), and then the fifth and seventh nerves [3]. In sarcoidosis, 10% patients develop CNS involvement with 50–75% of cases having cranial involvement, most commonly the facial nerve [4]. Of anecdotal interest, SLE is the most frequent connective tissue disease associated with sarcoidosis [5] and the two share some underlying pathophysiological mechanisms [6]. We report a case of multiple cranial nerve palsies and subacute progressive, symmetric peripheral neuropathy simulating Guillain-Barre syndrome (GBS) in a patient with sarcoidosis who was eventually diagnosed with SLE.

2. Case Report

A 61-year-old African-American male presented to the emergency room with a few days history of double vision, left eyelid droop, and numbness and tingling in both hands and feet. He also endorsed one month history of profound fatigue and a progressive weakness with overhead movements and climbing stairs. Now to the point he was unable to ambulate and a recent fall triggered his visit.

He had a history of biopsy proven sarcoidosis in 1970. He was treated with steroids for one year. He had gout, dyspepsia, and mild obstructive pulmonary disease. His medications included an albuterol inhaler, allopurinol, and omeprazole. He reported a weight loss of 30 pounds in the preceding six months. He had a chronic dry cough.

Physical examination revealed a thin man with normal vital signs. Pertinent findings on exam were a significant ptosis of the left eye with only 1 mm aperture, an inability to fully adduct the left eye and inability to abduct the left

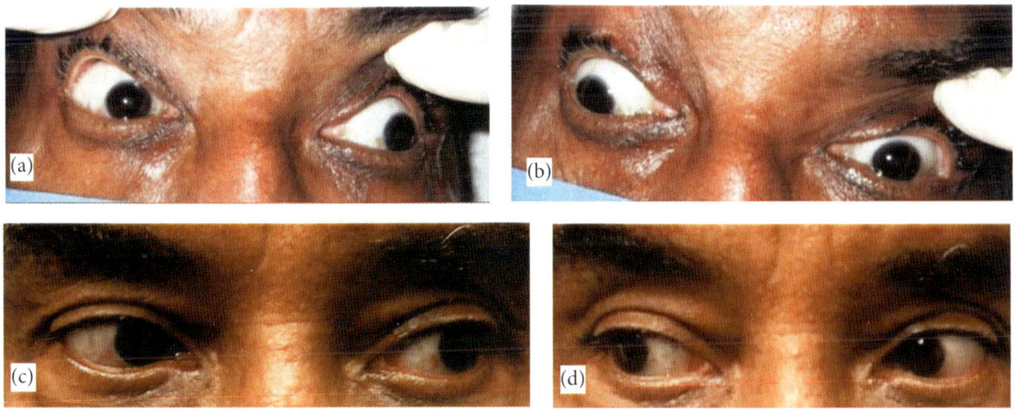

FIGURE 1: Pre-treatment leftward gaze (a), pre-treatment rightward gaze (b), post-treatment leftward gaze (c), post-treatment rightward gaze (d).

eye (Figure 1), and an inability to achieve upward gaze in either eye. This was interpreted as partial right III and VI and almost complete left III and VI cranial neuropathies. There was subtle bilateral facial weakness and mild decrease of left facial sensation to pinprick test. He had proximal muscular atrophy and proximal weakness of both upper and lower extremities with 4/5 upper extremity strength and 3/5 lower extremities. Distal strength was preserved. He reported minimal tenderness on muscle palpation. Reflexes were decreased to absent bilaterally and sensation was somewhat decreased in the distal legs. His abdominal exam revealed slight tenderness with palpation of the entire abdomen. Joint examination was normal.

Admission labs revealed hemoglobin of 10.9 g/dL. Studies including calcium, electrolytes, creatinine, human immunodeficiency virus antibodies, vitamin B12, folate, creatinine protein kinase, aldolase, rapid plasma reagin, thyroid stimulating hormone, hepatitis screen, amylase, and lipase were normal except for mildly elevated AST and total bilirubin. His erythrocyte sedimentation rate (ESR) was elevated at 66 mm/hr (normal 0–40) while his C-reactive-protein (CRP) was normal. His urinalysis showed 3+ proteinuria that was normal 6 months ago. A computed tomography (CT) scan of the head was normal. Based on the initial impression of progressive symmetrical sensorimotor polyneuropathy and multiple cranial neuropathies, simulating GBS-like picture or a Miller-Fisher variant, the patient was treated with inpatient five days of IVIG. A working diagnosis of neurosarcoidosis, paraneoplastic syndrome, and vasculitic neuropathy was entertained.

A CT of the chest confirmed multiple calcified nodules with some increase in size and a small new right lower lobe infiltrate. Magnetic resonance imaging (MRI) and magnetic resonance angiogram (MRA) of the brain (including MRI orbit with and without gadolinium injection) were normal except for a small incidental aneurysm of distal right MCA branch. An electromyographic (EMG) and nerve conductive study (NCS) revealed a diffuse, predominantly axonal sensory-motor length-dependent polyneuropathy and myopathy with some suggestion of a mononeuritis multiplex undergoing generalized transformation. MRI of the lumbosacral spine showed multilevel degenerative changes. A spinal tap including cytology was negative except for elevated protein at 105 mg/dL (albumin-cytologic dissociation).

Workup was done for a paraneoplastic etiology. CT abdomen was normal except a small amount of free fluid in the pelvis. Prostate-specific antigen colonoscopy was normal. A fine needle aspiration biopsy of the lung infiltrate revealed an inflammatory infiltrate with increased plasma cells but no granulomas and all cultures were negative. A muscle biopsy revealed moderately severe inflammatory myopathy with muscle fiber atrophy, regenerating fibers, and few ragged red fibers with no evidence of vasculitis. Endomysial fibrosis was also seen. A Sural nerve biopsy was negative for any acute abnormality but revealed evidence of possible old vasculitis.

Lack of response to five doses of IVIG and a positive antinuclear antibody (ANA) (>1 : 640) prompted a rheumatology consultation on day 7 of his admission. Anti-SSA was strongly positive (>8.0) but other antibodies were negative. Complements were normal. Anticardiolipin, beta-2 glycoprotein-1-antibodies, lupus anticoagulant, and antineutrophil cytoplasmic antibodies were negative. Anti-Hu, anti-Ri, anti-YO, MUSK, antivoltage-gated calcium channel, acetylcholine receptor antibodies, Gq1b, angiotensin converting enzyme, lyme antibodies were negative. A 24 hour urine showed 1.1 gram protein. Serum protein electrophoresis showed slightly increased polyclonal immunoglobulin G (IgG). An echocardiogram revealed small pericardial effusion. On day 12 of admission, patient's Hb dropped to 7 g/dL without any triggering etiology. Serum haptoglobin was decreased and direct/indirect Coombs were positive. He was treated with pulse steroids for 5 days and then oral prednisone thereafter with improvement in his anemia but unchanged neurological status.

Based on the presence of autoantibodies, Coombs positive hemolytic anemia, proteinuria, myositis, serositis as manifested by mild abdominal pain, pelvic free fluid, and small pericardial effusion, symmetrical progressive sensorimotor polyneuropathy simulating GBS and multiple cranial neuropathies, he was diagnosed with SLE. He was begun on IV cyclophosphamide (CYC) approximately 3 weeks after presentation and had very significant improvement in both motor strength and extraocular movement within 4 weeks (Figure 1). He has presently received six infusions of cyclophosphamide and is off the prednisone and doing well on methotrexate. He is undergoing rehabilitation and has had complete resolution of his diplopia and anemia. His serositis and proteinuria also resolved.

3. Discussion

This patient's presentation with cranial neuropathies and axonal peripheral neuropathies were initially felt to be a primary neurologic syndrome and sarcoidosis was the initial concern given his past history. However, the absence of active sarcoidosis on lung, muscle, and nerve biopsy, lack of any leptomeningeal enhancement or white matter lesions on brain MRI suggestive of sarcoidosis, and lack of response to steroids argued against sarcoidosis. Moreover presence of autoantibodies, autoimmune hemolytic anemia, proteinuria, serositis, and evidence of old vasculitis were suggestive of SLE. No occult cancer was identified although this was a major concern. The response to CYC was further convincing of the autoimmune diagnosis.

Ocular manifestations in SLE are fairly common and estimated to occur in up to 60% of patients [7]. However, ocular motor abnormalities are infrequent. Most reported ocular motor abnormalities in SLE are isolated findings but, as in our case, multiple oculomotor cranial neuropathies have been described [8].

Peripheral neuropathy in SLE is predominantly of the sensory variety however, in one study of 1533 SLE patients, 13.5% had some peripheral neuropathic involvement of which only 18.8% were of the sensory-motor type [9]. Usually peripheral neuropathy appears in the established SLE cases, and rarely as the initial presentation. Polyneuropathy in itself is an uncommon presentation of SLE and is responsible for only 2.0-3.0% of all neuropsychiatric SLE cases [2].

The pathogenic mechanism of cranial neuropathies in the setting of SLE is often difficult to verify. Vasculitis is often suspected because the patient has evidence of vasculitis elsewhere. In our patient, there was some evidence of healed vasculitis. Pathologic antibodies have been demonstrated to cause neurotoxicty or demyelination [10]. Another postulated mechanism is damage by local production of inflammatory cytokines [11]. Lastly, antiphospholipid antibodies have been associated with central nervous system disease [12] and the mechanism is assumed to be due to neural ischemia from microangiopathic thrombi. As a general rule, focal symptoms may be attributed to a thrombotic state in the right clinical settings while more generalized symptoms may be due to antibody or inflammatory etiologies [2].

Treatment of cranial nerve palsies in the setting of lupus involves immunosuppression. In cranial SLE, CYC, and intravenous methylprednisone are recommended by published guidelines [3]. An open-label study with rituximab has shown good results in 10 SLE patients with refractory neuropsychiatric lupus [13]. There are reports of the use of IVIG, azathioprine, and plasmapaharesis.

Coexistence of sarcoidosis and SLE has been described in the literature. In one study of biopsy proven sarcoidosis patients, about 29% were positive for ANA [14]. Both diseases share certain features like B and T cell abnormalities and hypergammaglobulinemia, [5, 6]. The exact relationship between the two, if any, remains to be elucidated. Our case was also unique because most cases of co-existent SLE and sarcoidosis have been reported in females [5, 15].

In conclusion, we present a patient with cranial and peripheral neuropathies with a history of sarcoidosis who was eventually diagnosed with SLE and responded well to CYC treatment. SLE should be retained as a differential for cranial neuropathy in patients with known sarcoidosis.

Disclosure

This paper has not been concurrently submitted to any other journal. There is no funding source or conflict of interests pertaining to this paper. The case was presented as a poster presentation at the 34th Scandinavian congress of Rheumatology held in Copenhagen, September 3–5, 2012.

References

[1] A. Bruns and O. Meyer, "Neuropsychiatric manifestations of systemic lupus erythematosus," *Joint Bone Spine*, vol. 73, no. 6, pp. 639–645, 2006.

[2] G. K. Bertsias and D. T. Boumpas, "Pathogenesis, diagnosis and management of neuropsychiatric SLE manifestations," *Nature Reviews Rheumatology*, vol. 6, no. 6, pp. 358–367, 2010.

[3] G. K. Bertsias, J. P. A. Ioannidis, M. Aringer et al., "EULAR recommendations for the management of systemic lupus erythematosus with neuropsychiatric manifestations: report of a task force of the EULAR standing committee for clinical affairs," *Annals of the Rheumatic Diseases*, vol. 69, no. 12, pp. 2074–2082, 2010.

[4] F. G. Joseph and N. J. Scolding, "Sarcoidosis of the nervous system," *Practical Neurology*, vol. 7, no. 4, pp. 234–244, 2007.

[5] R. J. Enzenauer and S. G. West, "Sarcoidosis in autoimmune disease," *Seminars in Arthritis and Rheumatism*, vol. 22, no. 1, pp. 1–17, 1992.

[6] N. K. Veien, F. Hardt, G. Bendixen et al., "Immunological studies in sarcoidosis: a comparison of disease activity and various immunological parameters," *Annals of the New York Academy of Sciences*, vol. 278, pp. 47–51, 1976.

[7] J. B. Davies and P. K. Rao, "Ocular manifestations of systemic lupus erythematosus," *Current Opinion in Ophthalmology*, vol. 19, no. 6, pp. 512–518, 2008.

[8] J. R. Keane, "Eye movement abnormalities in systemic lupus erythematosus," *Archives of Neurology*, vol. 52, no. 12, pp. 1145–1149, 1995.

[9] B. Florica, E. Aghdassi, J. Su, D. D. Gladman, M. B. Urowitz, and P. R. Fortin, "Peripheral neuropathy in patients with systemic lupus erythematosus," *Seminars in Arthritis and Rheumatism*, vol. 41, pp. 203–211, 2011.

[10] R. Omdal, K. Brokstad, K. Waterloo, W. Koldingsnes, R. Jonsson, and S. I. Mellgren, "Neuropsychiatric disturbances in SLE are associated with antibodies against NMDA receptors," *European Journal of Neurology*, vol. 12, no. 5, pp. 392–398, 2005.

[11] R. Dellalibera-Joviliano, M. L. Dos Reis, F. D. Queiroz Cunha, and E. A. Donadi, "Kinins and cytokines in plasma and cerebrospinal fluid of patients with neuropsychiatric lupus," *Journal of Rheumatology*, vol. 30, no. 3, pp. 485–492, 2003.

[12] P. L. Meroni, A. Tincani, N. Sepp et al., "Endothelium and the brain in CNS lupus," *Lupus*, vol. 12, no. 12, pp. 919–928, 2003.

[13] M. Tokunaga, K. Saito, D. Kawabata et al., "Efficacy of rituximab (anti-CD20) for refractory systemic lupus erythematosus involving the central nervous system," *Annals of the Rheumatic Diseases*, vol. 66, no. 4, pp. 470–475, 2007.

[14] I. Weinberg, L. Vasiliev, and I. Gotsman, "Anti-dsDNA antibodies in sarcoidosis," *Seminars in Arthritis and Rheumatism*, vol. 29, no. 5, pp. 328–331, 2000.

[15] S. Begum, C. Li, L. R. Wedderburn, V. Blackwell, and D. A. Isenberg, "Concurrence of sarcoidosis and systemic lupus erythematosus in three patients," *Clinical and Experimental Rheumatology*, vol. 20, no. 4, pp. 549–552, 2002.

12

Diagnosis and Assessment of Disease Activity in Takayasu Arteritis: A Childhood Case Illustrating the Challenge

L. Watson,[1] P. Brogan,[2] I. Peart,[3] C. Landes,[4] N. Barnes,[4] and G. Cleary[5]

[1] *Department of Paediatric Nephrology, Institute of Child Health, Alder Hey Children's NHS Foundation Trust Hospital, Eaton Road, Liverpool L12 2AP, UK*
[2] *Department of Paediatric Rheumatology, Great Ormond Street NHS Hospital, London WC1N 3JH, UK*
[3] *Department of Paediatric Cardiology, Alder Hey Children's NHS Foundation Trust Hospital, Eaton Road, Liverpool L12 2AP, UK*
[4] *Department of Paediatric Radiology, Alder Hey Children's NHS Foundation Trust Hospital, Eaton Road, Liverpool L12 2AP, UK*
[5] *Department of Paediatric Rheumatology, Alder Hey Children's NHS Foundation Trust Hospital, Eaton Road, Liverpool L12 2AP, UK*

Correspondence should be addressed to L. Watson; louise.watson@liverpool.ac.uk

Academic Editors: S. Ikuyama, A. Mak, C. Saadeh, and G. J. Tsay

Takayasu Arteritis (TA) is a rare, debilitating large vessel vasculitis occurring in patients of all ages, including infants, but the disease most commonly presents in the third decade. Diagnosis is often delayed and consequently TA is associated with significant morbidity and mortality. Accurate methods of monitoring disease activity or damage are lacking and currently rely on a combination of clinical features, blood inflammatory markers, and imaging modalities. In this report we describe a case of a 14-year-old boy with childhood-onset TA who, despite extensive negative investigations, did indeed have on-going active large vessel vasculitis with fatal outcome. Postmortem analysis demonstrated more extensive and active disease than originally identified. This report illustrates and discusses the limitations of current modalities for the detection and monitoring of disease activity and damage in large vessel vasculitis. Clinicians must be aware of these limitations and challenges if we are to strive for better outcomes in TA.

1. Introduction

Takayasu Arteritis (TA) is a large vessel vasculitis of unknown aetiology that affects the aorta and its branches. The cause is unknown, but genetic contribution to disease susceptibility is increasingly recognised [1], whilst suggested links with tuberculosis infection remain unproven [2]. Diagnosis is often considerably delayed: in a recent paediatric classification criteria exercise, the mean time from symptom onset to diagnosis was 1.3 years (SD ± 1.6 years) [3]. Even when the diagnosis is secured, challenges occur in distinguishing between the acute or "active" phase of the illness and the chronic, stenotic phase when symptoms or signs are the result of tissue ischaemia from progressive arterial narrowing [4]. It is important to identify active disease since this requires immunosuppressive treatment, but it is unclear whether immunosuppression is effective in the late stage of the disease when a risk-benefit balance must be made [5]. Revascularisation procedures, such as angioplasty and/or stenting, or more invasive surgical interventions such as aortic bypass grafting are commonly required to provide relief from symptomatic ischaemia but are associated with significant life threatening risks and morbidity and are not completely effective in all cases [6, 7]. Moreover the risk of restenosis is high, particularly if the disease is active at the time of surgery [8–11]. We present a case that highlights the difficulties clinicians face in relation to the diagnosis and monitoring of large vessel vasculitis.

2. Case Presentation

Absence of retinal vessel pulsation was noted in a twelve-year-old boy during a routine ophthalmology assessment. He had presented with bilateral congenital glaucoma as an infant requiring surgical correction and hence long-term ophthalmology screening. At the age of eighteen months he had a right seventh nerve palsy that lasted 4 months and subsequently resolved; at the age of two years he developed acute, unexplained cardiac failure with evidence of dilated cardiomyopathy. He was commenced on digoxin, captopril, and frusemide and his cardiac contractility gradually recovered. The underlying cause of cardiomyopathy was never determined.

Between the ages of four and ten years he attended school full time. He had reduced stamina and a long history of calf claudication with a claudication distance of 200 m. He reported recurrent episodes of chest and left arm pain but no unexplained fevers and no cutaneous lesions. His growth parameters were normal (weight and height 50th centile for his age and sex). On examination, he had absent femoral, popliteal, dorsalis pedis, posterior tibialis, and brachial and radial pulses bilaterally. Centrally located abdominal and renal flank bruits were noted. Routine laboratory markers of inflammation (white cell count, erythrocyte sedimentation rate, C reactive protein) were normal, as were routine haematological and biochemistry panels. Antinuclear and antineutrophil cytoplasmic antibodies were negative. Peripheral blood cytokine analysis (TNF alpha, IL-6, and IL10) was normal; in addition he had a normal circulating endothelial cell (CEC) count of 20 cells per mL of whole blood [12]. It was noted however that he had a reversed CD4 : CD8 ratio (32% : 40%, resp.).

Multiple radiological investigations were undertaken to assess for on-going active large vessel vasculitis and/or late stenotic sequelae. Radiological investigations collectively revealed widespread arterial disease with occlusion of the subclavian, common iliac, and proximal tibial and peroneal arteries (Figures 1, 2, and 3). On computer tomography (CT) angiography, and conventional catheter digital subtraction arteriography the descending abdominal aorta was irregular and tapered distal to the renal arteries with severe proximal bilateral renal artery stenosis (Figure 4). The abdominal aorta was thread-like up to the level of the common iliac arteries with some irregular calcific plaque demonstrated on the CT scan (Figures 2 and 4). He had an extensive collateral circulation throughout his arterial tree supplying his limbs.

A half body PET-CT (positron emitting tomography, PET) was performed using fludeoxyglucose (FDG) that showed no uptake of FDG in the large vessels. Echocardiogram showed slight left ventricular impairment with a normal aortic arch, confirmed on angiography, and the coronary arteries appeared normal although selective coronary arteriography was not undertaken.

The clinical history, symptoms, absence of acute phase response, and imaging appearances were compatible with a large vessel vasculitis, currently inactive and in the late stenotic phase of the disease. The exact time of disease onset was unknown. The only positive investigation was a reversed T cell (CD4 : CD8) ratio, and with no FDG uptake on PET-CT, the presence of extensive arterial stenotic lesions, absence of acute phase response including normal peripheral blood cytokines, normal CECs, and aortic intramural calcification, we considered the disease to be in the late fibrotic/stenotic stage. It was therefore felt that immunosuppression was unlikely to confer any benefit. Since there was no obvious angioplasty/revascularisation target; management consisted of a careful and graded return to activity and lifestyle advice to minimise conventional cardiovascular risk factors in the future.

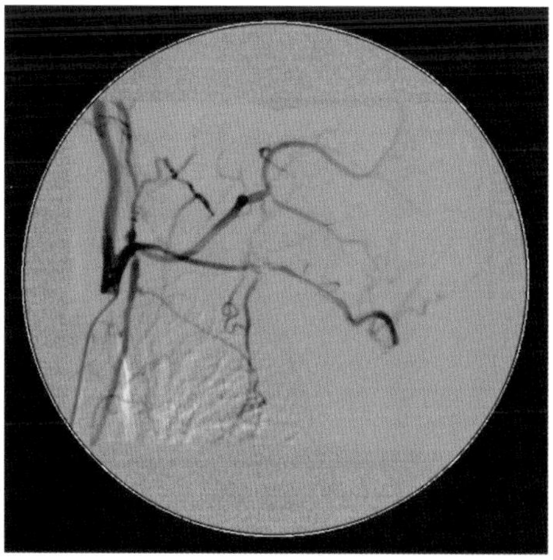

Figure 1: Angiography demonstrating severe stenosis of the aortic branches and complete occlusion below the level of the mesenteric artery.

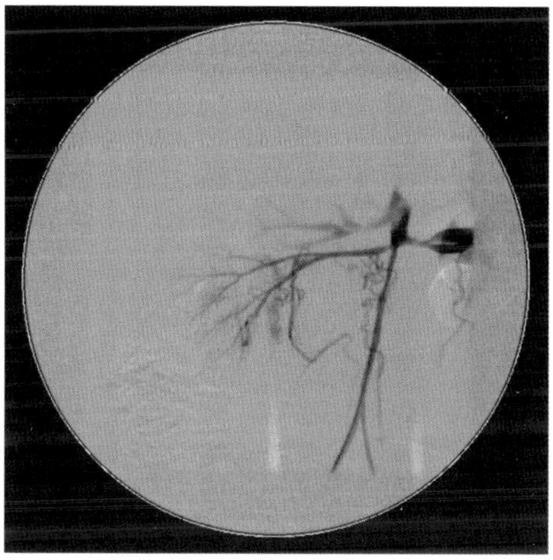

Figure 2: Angiography demonstrating the thread-like aorta up to the level of the common iliac arteries.

At the age of 14 years he collapsed suddenly; resuscitation attempts were unsuccessful. Postmortem examination revealed severe left ventricular hypertrophy and 70% occlusion of the coronary arteries. The abdominal aorta was narrowed with a patchy and sparse chronic inflammatory cell infiltrate and evidence of active inflammation within the vasa vasorum of the distal aorta. There was marked intimal fibrosis with calcification and collateral vessels, as noted on previous imaging.

3. Discussion

Diagnosing TA relies on clinical presentation, characteristic structural arterial abnormalities, and evidence of inflammatory vasculopathy on imaging or histology. A classification of childhood TA exists (Table 1); however the major clinical challenge when considering the disease is distinguishing

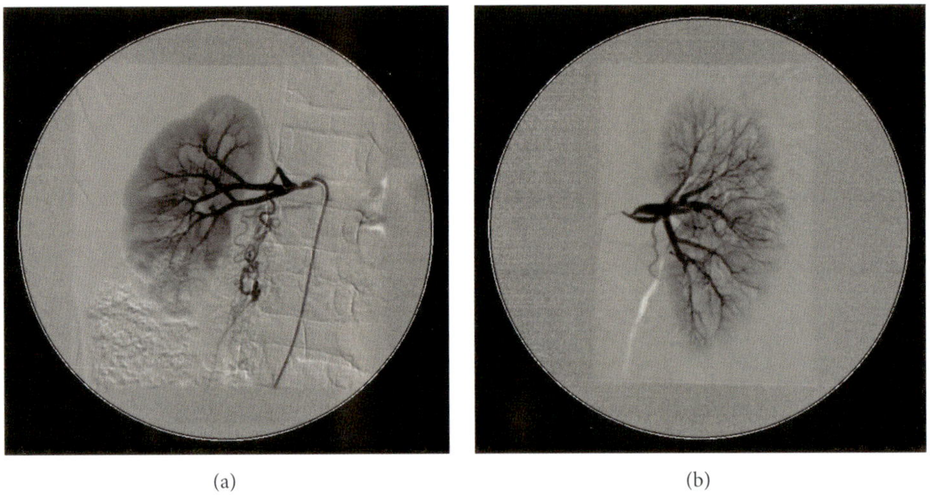

FIGURE 3: Angiography demonstrating severe renal artery stenosis and multiple intrarenal vessel narrowing and collateral blood vessels branching away from the renal artery.

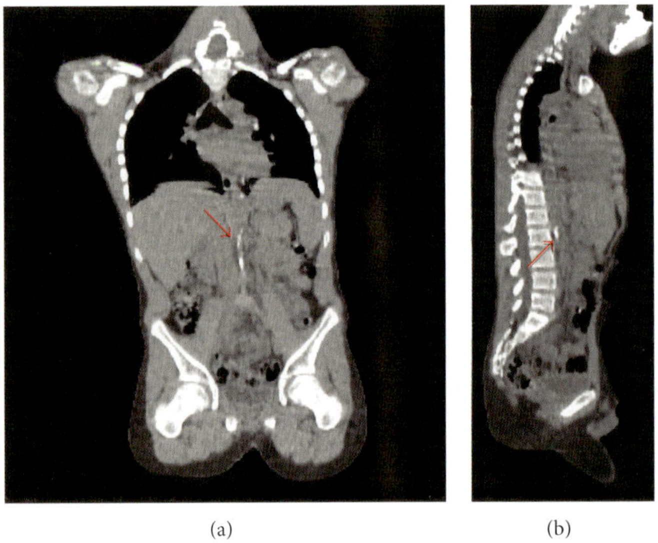

FIGURE 4: An unenhanced computerized tomography (CT) image (coronal and sagittal reformatted) showing aortic calcification (arrow).

this inflammatory large vessel vasculitis from other noninflammatory vasculopathies, since the differential diagnosis is broad (Table 2). This issue is particularly difficult when the disease is in the late stenotic phase, where acute vasculitic disease activity may be minimal or absent.

Since clinical features may be very nonspecific or even absent, delay in the diagnosis of TA is unfortunately very common, sometimes of several years [13]. In this case the onset of inflammatory arteritis may have been present for some time, as collateral vessels take several years to develop, and our patient had an extensive collateral vascular system.

Once the diagnosis of TA is secured, there is currently no gold standard investigation that can be used for monitoring disease activity. A previous study involving 10 Indian patients with TA demonstrated that postmortem analysis identified more active disease than what was detectable clinically [14]. Meticulous monitoring of this condition is therefore essential but poses significant challenges. Clinicians currently combine clinical features with acute phase reactants such as the erythrocyte sedimentation rate and/or C reactive protein; imaging techniques such as PET-CT [15, 16], contrast enhanced MR [17], and CT angiography [18, 19]; and formal digital subtraction arteriography, perceived by most to be the gold standard for defining lumenography to monitor for disease activity and for stenotic sequelae.

Routinely used acute phase reactants may be elevated in the early or active phases of the disease; however their sensitivity and specificity remain poor. In a study by Dagna et al., receiver operating characteristic curves showed an area under the curve value of 0.75 and 0.68 for ESR and CRP, respectively, demonstrating that they were inferior to a novel biomarker, pentraxin-3 [20, 21]. Pentraxin-3 is a protein rapidly produced by many cells, particularly endothelial cells, in response to inflammatory signals [22] and is believed to

Table 1: EULAR/PRINTO/PRES criteria and classification definition of Takayasu Arteritis.

Mandatory criteria	
Angiographic abnormality	Angiography (conventional, CT, and MRI) of the aorta, its main branches or pulmonary arteries showing aneurysm/dilatation, narrowing, occlusion, or thickened arterial wall, not due to any other causes
Additional criteria (need one of the five)	
(1) Pulse deficit or claudication	Lost/decreased/unequal peripheral artery pulse Symptoms of claudication: focal muscle pain induced by physical activity
(2) Blood pressure discrepancy	Discrepancy of four-limb systolic blood pressure >10 mmhg in any limb
(3) Bruits	Audible murmurs or palpable thrills over large arteries
(4) Hypertension	Systolic/diastolic blood pressure >95th centile for height
(5) Acute phase reactant	Erythrocyte sedimentation rate (ESR) >20 mm per hour or C reactive protein (CRP) above normal

Table 2: Differential diagnosis of Takayasu Arteritis.

Classification	Subtype
Primary inflammatory vasculitides	Giant cell arteritis
	Kawasaki disease
	Polyarteritis nodosa
	Wegener's granulomatosis disease
Secondary inflammatory vasculitides	Rheumatic fever
	Sarcoidosis
	SLE
	Behcet's disease
	Spondyloarthropathies
Noninflammatory vascular disease	Fibromuscular dysplasia
	Congenital aortic abnormalities
	Inherited connective tissue disorders
	Neurofibromatosis
Other	Sepsis
	Malignancy
	Human immunodeficiency virus
	Syphilis
	Tuberculosis
	Radiation fibrosis

be an early marker of inflammatory activity in the vessels. Reversal of T cell CD4 : CD8 balance with an increase in the number of CD8 cells has been demonstrated to be a useful marker of disease activity in this condition, as seen in our patient [23]. Whilst emerging data support the use of circulating endothelial cells in small and medium vessel vasculitides [24, 25], their role as potential biomarkers in large vessel vasculitides remains unknown. Large studies assessing the role of anti-CEC antibodies in TA are also lacking [24].

The uptake of 18F-fluorodeoxyglucose on PET imaging is reported as a potentially highly sensitive and accurate method for assessing disease activity in patients with TA. In studies of adult patients with TA (the largest study involving 39 participants) the sensitivity and specificity of 18FDG-PET scanning was shown to be 73–100% and 83–92%, respectively [26–28]. Contrast-enhanced MRI with late gadolinium administration may detect increased arterial wall thickness with evidence of late gadolinium enhancement, suggestive of active large vessel vasculitis [17, 29]. CT angiography is able to detect vessel wall alterations and define luminal changes and may be useful during diagnosis and subsequent monitoring, although this lacks an ability to define active vasculitis [17, 29–31]. In our case, absence of FDG uptake on PET-CT leads us to conclude that contrast induced MRA was unlikely to add further information, and hence this test was not undertaken.

Digital subtraction catheter arteriography is regarded by most as a gold standard for defining lumenography, of particular importance in the assessment of patients potentially requiring revascularisation procedures [32]. Surgical techniques such as angioplasty and bypass are reserved for symptomatic use to restore circulation but do not alter the underlying disease process and are associated with a higher morbidity and even mortality if performed during active disease [33, 34]. This latter point emphasises the importance of accurately defining disease activity if considering a revascularisation process.

In summary, TA can present in childhood and the diagnosis is often significantly delayed despite advances in laboratory biomarkers and imaging to detect vascular inflammation and anatomy. We present a paediatric case with fatal outcome where postmortem studies revealed the true extent of ongoing vasculitic disease activity, and extent of arterial injury, particularly in relation to coronary arterial involvement. We suggest that one of the main reasons the prognosis for TA in the paediatric population remains (arguably) unacceptably poor is through diagnostic delay. If we are to influence this, clinicians must consider the diagnosis earlier and be aware of the limitations of the current technologies for the detection of active large vessel vasculitis. A concerted, international effort of clinical data collection in disease registries and challenging treatments using clinical trials is needed to improve the evidence base for the diagnosis and management of large vessel vasculitis in young patients.

Acknowledgment

Special thanks goes to the family who has kindly given permission and consent for this report.

References

[1] K. A. Morishita, K. Rosendahl, and P. A. Brogan, "Familial Takayasu arteritis—a pediatric case and a review of the literature," *Pediatric Rheumatology*, vol. 9, article 6, 2011.

[2] L. Arnaud, E. Cambau, I. Brocheriou et al., "Absence of Mycobacterium tuberculosis in arterial lesions from patients with Takayasu's arteritis," *Journal of Rheumatology*, vol. 36, no. 8, pp. 1682–1685, 2009.

[3] N. Ruperto, S. Ozen, A. Pistorio et al., "EULAR/PRINTO/PRES criteria for Henoch-Schönlein purpura, childhood polyarteritis nodosa, childhood Wegener granulomatosis and childhood Takayasu arteritis: Ankara 2008. Part I: overall methodology and clinical characterisation," *Annals of the Rheumatic Diseases*, vol. 69, no. 5, pp. 790–797, 2010.

[4] K. Maksimowicz-McKinnon, T. M. Clark, and G. S. Hoffman, "Limitations of therapy and a guarded prognosis in an American cohort of Takayasu arteritis patients," *Arthritis and Rheumatism*, vol. 56, no. 3, pp. 1000–1009, 2007.

[5] C. Mukhtyar, L. Guillevin, M. C. Cid et al., "EULAR recommendations for the management of large vessel vasculitis," *Annals of the Rheumatic Diseases*, vol. 68, no. 3, pp. 318–323, 2009.

[6] S. A. Rao, K. R. Mandalam, V. R. Rao et al., "Takayasu arteritis: initial and long-term follow-up in 16 patients after percutaneous transluminal angioplasty of the descending thoracic and abdominal aorta," *Radiology*, vol. 189, no. 1, pp. 173–179, 1993.

[7] H. J. Kim, C.-S. Lee, J. S. Kim et al., "Outcomes after endovascular treatment of symptomatic patients with Takayasu's arteritis," *Interventional Neuroradiology*, vol. 17, no. 2, pp. 252–260, 2011.

[8] G. S. Kerr, C. W. Hallahan, J. Giordano et al., "Takayasu arteritis," *Annals of Internal Medicine*, vol. 120, no. 11, pp. 919–929, 1994.

[9] J. W. Son, K. K. Koh, Q. Dang, I. S. Choi, and E. K. Shin, "Recurrent restenosis following stent and rotational atherectomy of coronary artery stenosis in Takayasu's arteritis," *International Journal of Cardiology*, vol. 65, no. 3, pp. 295–300, 1998.

[10] J. Amano and A. Suzuki, "Coronary artery involvement in Takayasu's arteritis: collective review and guideline for surgical treatment," *Journal of Thoracic and Cardiovascular Surgery*, vol. 102, no. 4, pp. 554–560, 1991.

[11] R. Pajari, P. Hekali, and P.-T. Harjola, "Treatment of Takayasu's arteritis: an analysis of 29 operated patients," *Thoracic and Cardiovascular Surgeon*, vol. 34, no. 3, pp. 176–181, 1986.

[12] L. A. Clarke, Y. Hong, D. Eleftheriou et al., "Endothelial injury and repair in systemic vasculitis of the young," *Arthritis and Rheumatism*, vol. 62, no. 6, pp. 1770–1780, 2010.

[13] R. Watts, A. Al-Taiar, J. Mooney, D. Scott, and A. MacGregor, "The epidemiology of Takayasu arteritis in the UK," *Rheumatology*, vol. 48, no. 8, pp. 1008–1011, 2009.

[14] B. K. Sharma, S. Jain, and B. D. Radotra, "An autopsy study of Takayasu arteritis in India," *International Journal of Cardiology*, vol. 66, supplement 1, pp. S85–S91, 1998.

[15] S. Sager, S. Yilmaz, M. Ozhan et al., "F-18 Fdg PET/CT findings of a patient with Takayasu arteritis before and after therapy," *Molecular Imaging and Radionuclide Therapy*, vol. 21, pp. 32–34, 2012.

[16] Y. Cheng, N. Lv, Z. Wang, B. Chen, and A. Dang, "18-FDG-PET in assessing disease activity in Takayasu arteritis: a meta-analysis," *Clinical and Experimental Rheumatology*, vol. 31, no. 1, supplement 75, pp. S22–S27, 2013.

[17] M. Papa, F. De Cobelli, E. Baldissera et al., "Takayasu arteritis: intravascular contrast medium for MR angiography in the evaluation of disease activity," *American Journal of Roentgenology*, vol. 198, no. 3, pp. W279–W284, 2012.

[18] W. A. Schmidt, "Imaging in vasculitis," *Best Practice & Research Clinical Rheumatology*, vol. 27, pp. 107–118, 2013.

[19] F. P. Zhu, S. Luo, Z. J. Wang, Z. Y. Jin, L. J. Zhang, and G. M. Lu, "Takayasu arteritis: imaging spectrum at multidetector CT angiography," *British Journal of Radiology*, vol. 85, pp. e1282–e1292, 2012.

[20] R. Moriwaki and F. Numano, "Takayasu arteritis: follow-up studies for 20 years," *Heart and Vessels*, vol. 7, no. 1, supplement, pp. 138–145, 1992.

[21] L. Dagna, F. Salvo, M. Tiraboschi et al., "Pentraxin-3 as a marker of disease activity in takayasu arteritis," *Annals of Internal Medicine*, vol. 155, no. 7, pp. 425–433, 2011.

[22] P. Cieślik and A. Hrycek, "Long pentraxin 3 (PTX3) in the light of its structure, mechanism of action and clinical implications," *Autoimmunity*, vol. 45, no. 2, pp. 119–128, 2012.

[23] S. S. Uppal and S. Verma, "Analysis of the clinical profile, autoimmune phenomena and T cell subsets (CD4 and CD8) in Takayasu's arteritis: a hospital-based study," *Clinical and Experimental Rheumatology*, vol. 21, no. 6, supplement 32, pp. S112–S116, 2003.

[24] J. Eichhorn, D. Sima, B. Thiele et al., "Anti-endothelial cell antibodies in Takayasu arteritis," *Circulation*, vol. 94, no. 10, pp. 2396–2401, 1996.

[25] H. Wang, J. Ma, Q. Wu, X. Luo, Z. Chen, and L. Kou, "Circulating B lymphocytes producing autoantibodies to endothelial cells play a role in the pathogenesis of Takayasu arteritis," *Journal of Vascular Surgery*, vol. 53, no. 1, pp. 174–180, 2011.

[26] I. Karapolat, M. Kalfa, G. Keser et al., "Comparison of F18 FDG PET/CT findings with current clinical disease status in patients with Takayasu's arteritis," *Clinical and Experimental Rheumatology*, vol. 31, no. 1, supplement 75, pp. 15–21, 2012.

[27] D. Tezuka, G. Haraguchi, T. Ishihara et al., "Role of FDG PET-CT in Takayasu arteritis: sensitive detection of recurrences," *JACC: Cardiovascular Imaging*, vol. 5, no. 4, pp. 422–429, 2012.

[28] M. Fuchs, M. Briel, T. Daikeler et al., "The impact of18F-FDG PET on the management of patients with suspected large vessel vasculitis," *European Journal of Nuclear Medicine and Molecular Imaging*, vol. 39, no. 2, pp. 344–353, 2012.

[29] C. Schneeweis, B. Schnackenburg, M. Stuber et al., "Delayed contrast-enhanced MRI of the coronary artery wall in takayasu arteritis," *PLoS One*, vol. 7, Article ID e50655, 2012.

[30] Y. Eshet, R. Pauzner, O. Goitein et al., "The limited role of MRI in long-term follow-up of patients with Takayasu's arteritis," *Autoimmunity Reviews*, vol. 11, pp. 132–136, 2011.

[31] M. K. Yadav, "Takayasu arteritis: clinical and CT—angiography profile of 25 patients and a brief review of literature," *Indian Heart Journal*, vol. 59, no. 6, pp. 468–474, 2007.

[32] N. Khandelwal, N. Kalra, M. K. Garg et al., "Multidetector CT angiography in Takayasu arteritis," *European Journal of Radiology*, vol. 77, no. 2, pp. 369–374, 2011.

[33] J. Hu, H. Huang, X. Zhang et al., "Stent placement for treatment of long segment (>/=80mm) carotid artery stenosis in patients with takayasu disease," *Journal of Vascular and Interventional Radiology*, vol. 23, pp. 1473–1477, 2012.

[34] D. Saadoun, M. Lambert, T. Mirault et al., "Retrospective analysis of surgery versus endovascular intervention in Takayasu arteritis a multicenter experience," *Circulation*, vol. 125, no. 6, pp. 813–819, 2012.

13

A Rare Case of Kikuchi Fujimoto's Disease with Subsequent Development of Systemic Lupus Erythematosus

Yu Zuo, Michelle Foshat, You-wen Qian, Brent Kelly, Brock Harper, and Bernard Karnath

Department of Internal Medicine, University of Texas Medical Branch, 301 University Boulevard, Galveston, TX 77555, USA

Correspondence should be addressed to Yu Zuo, yuzuo@utmb.edu

Academic Editors: D. R. Alpert, M. Salazar-Paramo, and A. Zoli

Kikuchi Fujimoto's disease (KFD) is a rare, immune-mediated, self-limiting disorder with unique histopathological features. KFD is usually seen in young Asian females; however, cases have been reported throughout the world and in all ethnicities. It has been recognized that there is a rare association between Systemic Lupus Erythematosus (SLE) and KFD via sporadic case reports. The exact pathophysiological relationship between these two diseases is still unclear. We report a case of a young Asian female who presented with persistent fever and lymphadenopathy and was diagnosed with Kikuchi Fujimoto's disease based on lymph node biopsy; although an SLE workup was done, she did not meet the American Rheumatology Association (ARA) diagnostic criteria for lupus, and the lymph node biopsy did not show features of SLE. She improved clinically with a short course of steroid therapy. Two months later, the patient presented with central facial rash and arthralgia. SLE workup was repeated, a skin biopsy was done, and the results at this time supported a diagnosis of SLE.

1. Introduction

Kikuchi Fujimoto's disease (KFD) is a rare, immune-mediated, typically self-limiting disease first described in Japan in 1972 [1, 2]. It has been seen in all ethnic groups around the world; however, most cases are reported in Asia and the Far East. Between 1991 and 2005, there were a total of 330 cases of KFD reported in Medline database around the world, and only 22 cases were reported in the US [3]. Clinically, patients present with persistent fever and lymphadenopathy which may be painful; cervical lymph nodes are most commonly involved. Other symptoms such as fatigue, night sweats, nausea and vomiting, weight loss, arthralgias, and a variety of cutaneous lesions are also reported. Laboratory findings are nonspecific including elevated Erythrocyte Sedimentation Rate (ESR), neutropenia, lymphocytosis, mildly elevated transaminase, and elevated Lactate Dehydrogenase (LDH) [3–5]. Diagnosis is made via lymph node biopsy with a histopathological finding characterized by a histiocytic necrotizing lymphadenitis without granulocytic infiltrate [3]. In most cases, KFD is a self-limiting disease; only supportive treatment is required. However, case reports suggest that a short course of corticosteroids can expedite remission. The association of Systemic Lupus Erythematosus (SLE) and KFD is even rarer; out of 330 cases reported between 1991 and 2005, only 28 patients with KFD were also diagnosed with SLE [3]. By Medline search, between 2005 and 2012, there were only 9 more additional SLE-associated KFD cases reported around the world [6–14].

2. Case Presentation

A 23-year-old Asian previously healthy woman presented with persistent fever and cervical, supraclavicular, and axillary lymphadenopathy. She denied chest pain, SOB, nausea, vomiting, weight loss, dizziness, diarrhea, urinary symptoms, rash, joint pain, headache, or vaginal discharge. She denied sick contacts, recent travel, exposure to pets/animals, bug bites, new medications, and herbal supplements. Prior to admission, the patient was evaluated at a community urgent care center where she had negative monospot test, Epstein-Barr Virus (EBV) PCR, and Cytomegalovirus (CMV) IgG. Upon admission, pt had a fever of 102.7, tachycardia at 115, and BP 109/74. Physical exam showed diffuse, rubbery, mobile, and tender lymphadenopathy of bilateral anterior cervical lymph nodes, bilateral axillary lymph nodes, and left supraclavicular lymph nodes. No rash was seen on her skin. There was no joint tenderness, warmness, erythema, or swelling. Cardiovascular and respiratory exams were otherwise unremarkable. CT scan showed enlarged axillary lymph nodes with partially necrotic appearing centers (Figure 1), partially visualized supraclavicular lymphadenopathy, and borderline to mildly enlarged mediastinal lymph nodes. Labs revealed WBC 3700, Antinuclear Antibody (ANA) positive with a titer of 1 : 80, Rheumatoid Factor low positive at 21 IU/mL (normal at 20 IU/mL), anti-dsDNA at 118 u/mL at equivocal range, ESR elevated to 110 mm/hr, elevated C-reactive protein (CRP), Toxoplasma IgG and IgM negative, Parvovirus IgM negative, SSA and SSB negative, and PPD negative. Core lymph node biopsy showed no increased neutrophils, eosinophils, or plasma cells. No typical microscopic signs of vasculitis or Hematoxylin bodies were noted. AFB for mycobacteria, GMS for fungi, and Warthin-Starry for Cat-Scratch disease were all negative. Overall features were consistent with histiocytic necrotizing lymphadenitis. Based on the previous pathological finding, a diagnosis of Kikuchi Fujimoto's disease was made. The patient was given prednisone 40 mg daily; after the first dose, her fever resolved and symptoms improved. She received two doses of prednisone in the hospital and was discharged with an additional 5 days of prednisone 40 mg daily. The patient developed a central facial erythematous patch with scaling (Figure 2) one month after discharge. She denied joint pain or swelling, fever, and fatigue; lymphadenopathy had significantly reduced in size. She was referred to dermatology and was diagnosed with seborrheic dermatitis and discharged home with desonide 0.05% cream and ketoconazole cream 2%. She was also evaluated by a rheumatologist; at that time she did not have the complete picture of SLE. Two months after discharge, she was seen again at the Rheumatology clinic with mild elbow swelling and pain. Physical exam showed small effusion with inability to fully extend her elbows bilaterally. The patient was also seen in the dermatology clinic that same day, with some improvement of her facial rash but with new erythematous patches with scaling on her scalp. A punch skin biopsy was obtained at that time. Labs at that time revealed that CBC, CRP, and CMP were unremarkable. Urinalysis did not show proteinuria, pyuria, or bacteria. ANA was positive with significant IFA titer of 1 : 320, complement C3 and C4 were decreased, and SSA positive, SSB negative, anti-ds DNA positive at 233.6 u/mL, anti-Smith positive at 79.5 units, and anti-ribonucleic protein (RNP) antibodies positive at 113.9 units were evident. These labs were consistent with SLE. The skin punch biopsy showed hyperkeratosis, follicular plugging, interface dermatitis, patchy perivascular, and periadnexal lymphocytic infiltrate with a focal area of increased dermal mucin consistent with discoid lupus erythematosus (Figure 4). She was diagnosed with SLE and placed on hydroxychloroquine.

3. Discussion

KFD is a rare, benign, self-limiting, immune-mediated disorder that usually resolves spontaneously after 1–4 months

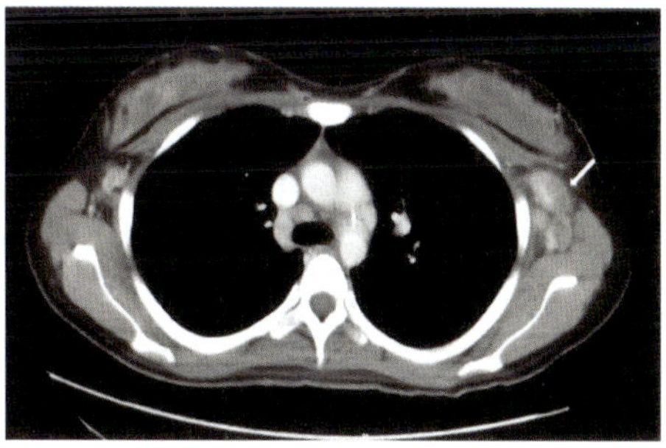

Figure 1: Axillary lymphadenopathy on CT thorax with contrast.

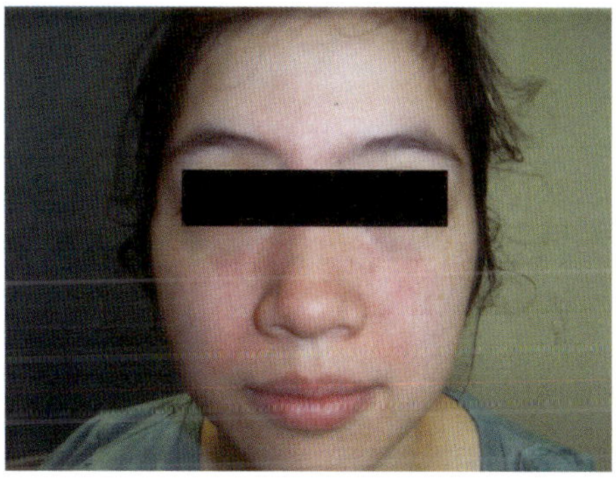

Figure 2: Patient presents with central facial rash 2 months after the diagnosis of KFD.

[15]. It occurs more frequently among young Asian females; however, cases had been reported in all continents and among all ethnic groups [16]. Based on a study done by Kucukardali et al., in 2007, 330 cases of KFD were reported in the Medline database; among those, 77% were females with a mean age of 25, and 70% of patients were under age of 30. Asia had the most reported cases followed by Europe and America. The most common symptoms were persistent fever and lymphadenopathy. High sedimentation rate is observed in a majority of patients, and positive ANA has also been reported in KFD patients. Moreover, 64% of patients improved without any treatment, 16% of patients received steroid treatment and the rest had various other treatments [3, 17]. Sporadic SLE-associated KFD cases have been reported, and the exact clinical and pathophysiological relationships between these two diseases are not known. SLE-associated KFD cases are more common in Asian countries. Among those cases, SLE has been seen to either coincide, proceed, or follow a diagnosis of KFD [16]. Kucukardali et al. reported 28 cases of SLE-associated KDF that meet the diagnostic criteria for SLE. Eighteen patients were diagnosed with KFD and SLE simultaneously, four had a previous diagnosis of SLE, and six were diagnosed with SLE after they were diagnosed with KFD [3]. Santana et al., in 2005, reported a total of 35 cases SLE-associated KFD all over the world based on Medline and LILACS databases. Seven patients were diagnosed with SLE prior to KFD diagnosis, fourteen patients were diagnosed with KFD and SLE simultaneously, and fourteen patients were diagnosed with SLE after

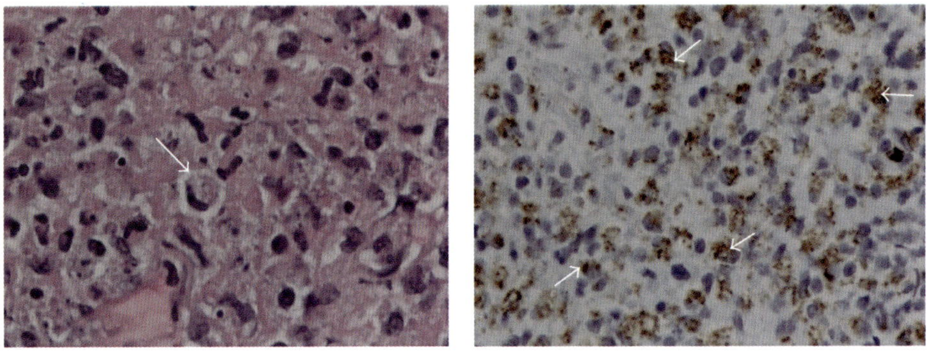

(a) (b)

Figure 3: (a) Crescent histiocyte (arrow) in a background of karyorrhectic debris and histiocyte proliferation, 1000x. (b) Numerous histiocytes show cytoplasmic staining for MPO, 500x.

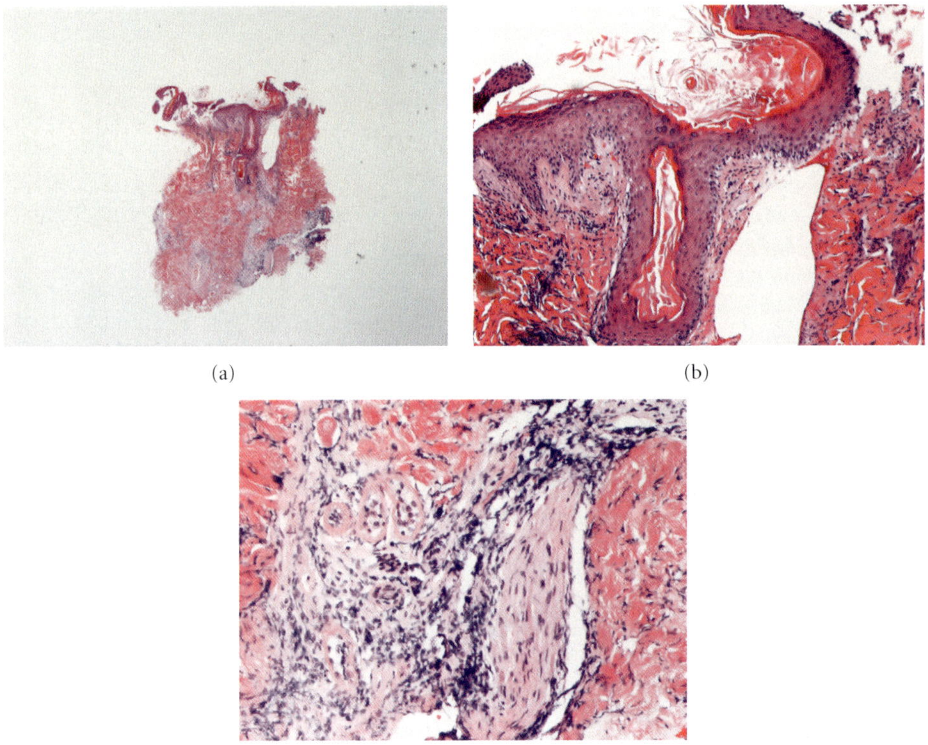

(a) (b)

(c)

Figure 4: (a), (b), and (c) The skin punch biopsy showed hyperkeratosis, follicular plugging, interface dermatitis, and patchy perivascular and periadnexal lymphocytic infiltrate with a focal area of increased dermal mucin consistent with discoid lupus erythematosus.

a diagnosis of KFD [15]. Clinical features of SLE and KFD can be very similar; fever, lymphadenopathy, fatigue, and joint pain can be seen in both diseases. Definite discrimination between those two diseases is based on histopathological findings; the presence of hematoxylin, plasma cells, and deposition of DNA is seen in SLE patients but not in KFD patients. Kim et al. had found that SLE-associated KFD patients tend to have high incidence of skin manifestations [16].

Our patient fits into the epidemiological traits of KFD and has a typical KFD clinical presentation. She is a young, Asian, previously healthy female who presented with persistent fever and lymphadenopathy. No joint pain or skin manifestation was present initially. Infectious disease workup has all been negative. ESR was elevated. She did have a positive ANA but with a low titer. Anti-dsDNA was in the equivocal range. SSA and SSB were negative. Lymph node biopsy shows partially preserved lymphoid architecture with rare lymphoid follicles and extensive coagulative necrosis. The necrotic areas contain abundant karyorrhectic debris. The necrosis is often surrounded by and intermingled with many histiocytes that occasionally contain engulfed nuclear debris with the nuclei pushed to the periphery giving the nuclei crescent appearances (Figure 3(a)). The histiocytes, highlighted by CD68, demonstrate myeloperoxidase (MPO) positivity (Figure 3(b)). Noted in the cellular area are some large cells with prominent nucleoli and amphophilic cytoplasm, morphologically mostly consistent with plasmacytoid dendritic cells. Many small CD3 positive T-lymphocytes are scattered in the necrotic areas with CD8 positive T-cells outnumbering CD4 positive T-cells. CD20 shows few residual lymphoid follicles. The overall findings are that of a Kikuchi Hashimoto lymphadenopathy [18–20]. The CD20 and CD3 staining results do not support a diagnosis of B- or T-cell lymphoma. Due to the fact that there are no increased neutrophils, eosinophils, or plasma cells, and vasculitis and hematoxylin bodies are not noted in the biopsy, a diagnosis of lupus lymphadenitis is not suggested pathologically.

She did not meet the diagnosis criteria for SLE upon admission. History, clinical, laboratory, and biopsy findings all support a diagnosis of KFD. Two months later, the patient presented with malar rash, joint pain, positive ANA at high titer, increased anti-ds DNA, and positive anti-RNP antibodies; at that point, the patient met the American Rheumatology Association diagnostic criteria for SLE. Her skin core biopsy finding is consistent with discoid lupus erythematosus which further confirms a diagnosis of SLE.

In conclusion, although KFD is a rare and self-limiting condition, it is important to recognize this condition in a patient who fits the epidemiological background with typical clinical features to avoid burdensome investigative workup and adding unnecessary anxiety to patients. In addition, when managing patient with KFD, it is crucial to recognize the relationship between SLE and KFD and carry out careful clinical surveillance to identify potential coexistence of SLE and to monitor for future development of SLE.

References

[1] M. Kikuchi, "Lymphadenitis showing focal reticulum cell hyperplasia with nuclear debris and phagocytes," *Acta haematologica Japonica*, vol. 35, pp. 379–380, 1972.

[2] Y. Fujimoto, Y. Kojima, and K. Yamaguchi, "Cervical Subacute necrotizing lymphadenitis," *Naika*, vol. 20, pp. 920–927, 1972.

[3] Y. Kucukardali, E. Solmazgul, E. Kunter, O. Oncul, S. Yildirim, and M. Kaplan, "Kikuchi-fujimoto disease: analysis of 244 cases," *Clinical Rheumatology*, vol. 26, no. 1, pp. 50–54, 2007.

[4] A. Hrycek, P. Cieślik, W. Szkróbka, and J. Pajak, "Kikuchi-Fujimoto disease: a case report," *RRheumatology International*, vol. 26, no. 2, pp. 179–181, 2005.

[5] E. M. Bailey, N. C. Klein, and B. A. Cunha, "Kikuchi's disease with liver dysfunction presenting as fever of unknown origin," *The Lancet*, vol. 2, no. 8669, p. 986, 1989.

[6] P. Pace-Asciak, M. A. Black, R. P. Michel, and K. Kost, "Case series: raising awareness about kikuchi-fujimoto disease among otolaryngologists: is it linked to systemic lupus erythematosus?" *Journal of Otolaryngology*, vol. 37, no. 6, pp. 782–787, 2008.

[7] P. Singhania, R. Paul, S. Maitra, A. Banerjee, and M. Hashmi, "Kikuchi-fujimoto disease from eastern India," *Journal of Global Infectious Diseases*, vol. 2, no. 3, pp. 305–306, 2010.

[8] D. Khanna, A. Shrivastava, P. R. Malur, and R. Kangle, "Necrotizing lymphadenitis in systemic lupus erythematosus: is it kikuchi-fujimoto disease?" *Journal of Clinical Rheumatology*, vol. 16, no. 3, pp. 123–124, 2010.

[9] V. A. Londhey, A. S. Buche, S. H. Kini, and G. C. Rajadhyaksha, "Kikuchi fujimoto disease and systemic lupus erythematosus—a rare association," *Journal of Association of Physicians of India*, vol. 58, no. 10, pp. 642–643, 2010.

[10] M. Abraham, I. Lazareth, G. Bonardel et al., "Kikuchi disease and lupus: case report, literature review and FDG PET/CT interest," *Journal des Maladies Vasculaires*, vol. 36, no. 4, pp. 274–279, 2011.

[11] D. Khanna, A. Shrivastava, P. R. Malur, and R. Kangle, "Necrotizing lymphadenitis in systemic lupus erythematosus: is it kikuchi-fujimoto disease?" *Journal of Clinical Rheumatology*, vol. 16, no. 3, pp. 123–124, 2010.

[12] S. C. Murthy, S. M. Dandin, A. Dandin, and M. Y. Patwardan, "Kikuchi's disease associated with systemic lupus erythematosus," *Indian Journal of Dermatology, Venereology and Leprology*, vol. 71, no. 5, pp. 338–341, 2005.

[13] H. C. Chen, J. H. Lai, G. S. Huang et al., "Systemic lupus erythematosus with simultaneous onset of Kikuchi-Fujimoto's disease complicated with antiphospholipid antibody syndrome: a case report and review of the literature," *Rheumatology International*, vol. 25, no. 4, pp. 303–306, 2005.

[14] T. Kampitak, "Fatal Kikuchi-Fujimoto disease associated with SLE and hemophagocytic syndrome: a case report," *Clinical Rheumatology*, vol. 27, no. 8, pp. 1073–1075, 2008.

[15] A. Santana, B. Lessa, L. Galrão, I. Lima, and M. Santiago, "Kikuchi-Fujimoto's disease associated with systemic lupus erythematosus: case report and review of the literature," *Clinical Rheumatology*, vol. 24, no. 1, pp. 60–63, 2005.

[16] S. K. Kim, M. S. Kang, B. Y. Yoon et al., "Histiocytic necrotizing lymphadenitis in the context of systemic lupus erythematosus (SLE): is histiocytic necrotizing lymphadenitis in SLE associated with skin lesions?" *Lupus*, vol. 20, no. 8, pp. 809–819, 2011.

[17] J. Iba Ba, J. R. Nzenze, L. Missounga et al., "Kikuchi-Fujimoto disease in Gabon. Description of first 2 cases in Gabon," *Médecine Tropicale*, vol. 70, no. 2, pp. 175–176, 2010.

[18] C. B. Hutchinson and E. Wang, "Kikuchi-Fujimoto disease," *Archives of Pathology & Laboratory Medicine*, vol. 134, no. 2, pp. 289–293, 2010.

[19] B. Sopeña, A. Rivera, C. Vázquez-Triñanes et al., "Autoimmune manifestations of Kikuchi disease," *Seminars in Arthritis and Rheumatism*, vol. 41, no. 6, pp. 900–906, 2012.

[20] M. Kojima, T. Motoori, S. Asano, and S. Nakamura, "Histological diversity of reactive and atypical proliferative lymph node lesions in systemic lupus erythematosus patients," *Pathology Research and Practice*, vol. 203, no. 6, pp. 423–431, 2007.

14

Disseminated Tuberculosis Mimicking Ankylosing Spondylitis

Valérie Huyge,[1] Serge Goldman,[1] and Muhammad S. Soyfoo[2]

[1] *Department of Nuclear Medicine, Hôpital Erasme, Université Libre de Bruxelles (ULB), 1070 Brussels, Belgium*
[2] *Department of Rheumatology, Hôpital Erasme, Université Libre de Bruxelles (ULB), 1070 Brussels, Belgium*

Correspondence should be addressed to Valérie Huyge, vhuyge@ulb.ac.be

Academic Editors: D. Aeberli, R. Cevik, and F. Maillot

Ankylosing spondylitis is a chronic inflammatory disorder affecting mainly the axial skeleton. Here we report a case of a man with a clinical suspicion of ankylosing spondylitis but with a persistence of increased inflammatory markers. In this case, ^{18}F-FDG-PET/CT revealed multiple hypermetabolic lesions in axial skeleton, lymph nodes, and the lung, suggestive of either disseminated tuberculosis or lymphoma. Histological analysis of the pulmonary lesion revealed mycobacterium tuberculosis. This case highlights, firstly, the importance of excluding other diagnoses in the presence of clinical picture of ankylosing spondylitis and high inflammatory markers and, secondly, the determining role of PET/CT.

1. Introduction

Ankylosing spondylitis (AS) is a chronic inflammatory disorder affecting mainly the axial skeleton, the peripheral joints, and the entheses. The prevalence of AS is reported to be between 0.1 and 0.8% with more males being affected than females, in a 3 to 1 ratio [1]. AS is often diagnosed between the age of 20 and 40 years. The clinical spectrum of AS ranges from low back pain to systemic features including uveitis and renal failure [1]. More frequently, the symptoms of AS encompass inflammatory back pain, joint stiffness, and loss of spinal mobility. The diagnosis of AS is made according to the new ASAS criteria which include clinical, biological, and imaging features [2]. As such, patients suffering from AS might have increased inflammatory markers such as elevated C-reactive protein (CRP) levels and erythrocyte sedimentation rate (ESR) [3]. However, in patients with very high CRP and ESR, other causes should be searched for such as inflammatory bowel diseases [4]. Disseminated tuberculosis (DT) with insidious clinical presentation can mimic several clinical syndromes [5]. Bone involvement in DT is protean harvesting Pott's disease and Poncet's arthritis. Sacroiliac joint involvement in DT is rare (less than 10%) and reported as mainly unilateral [6, 7]. We hereby report the case of a young man with typical clinical features of AS, marked inflammatory syndrome, and bilateral sacroiliitis revealing DT.

2. Case Presentation

A 30-year-old man, of East African origin, was admitted to our hospital for a constrictive chest pain. The patient's history included acute methanol intoxication with bilateral permanent blindness, due to necrosis in bilateral putamen demonstrated on magnetic resonance imaging (MRI). The patient was followed in the rheumatology outpatient clinic for AS. There was no history of smoking or illicit drug consumption but the patient admitted drinking alcohol occasionally. The patient reported low inflammatory back pain for more than one year, good response to nonsteroid anti-inflammatory drugs (NSAIDs) and computer tomography imaging (CT) of bilateral sacroiliitis (grade 2), leading to the diagnosis of AS according to the ASAS criteria (Figure 1).

The initial physical examination revealed a satisfactory general condition, no fever, normal vital signs, and synovitis of the knees. The cardiopulmonary examination was normal. Initial blood examination showed increased ESR at 80 mm/h ($N < 20$ mm/h) and CRP 5.8 mg/dL ($N < 0.5$ mg/dL), moderate hepatic cytolysis (<2X Normal values), and anicteric cholestasis. Total bilirubin, hematological tests, and renal function were normal. Troponin level was initially increased to 0.091 mg/dL; it decreased after 3 hours to 0.023 mg/dL. Chest radiography revealed no abnormalities. An electrocardiogram revealed widespread concave S-T elevation and a P-R depression (D2 D3). Cardiac echography was normal.

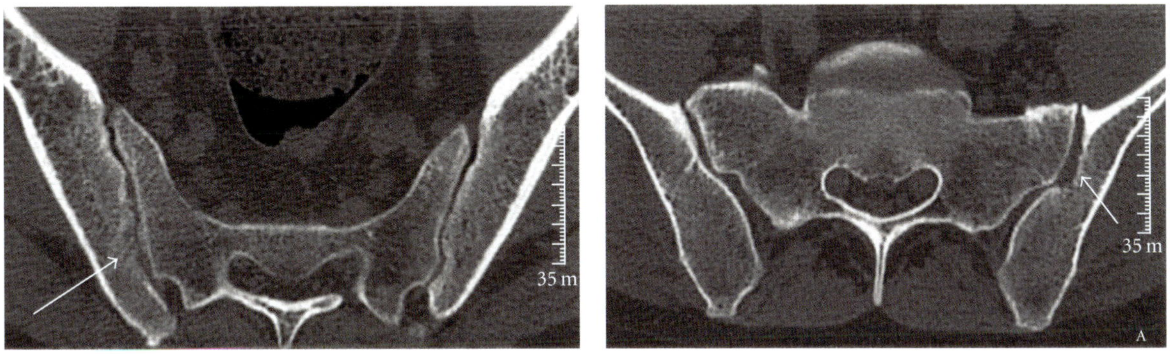

(a) (b)

Figure 1: (a) CT scan demonstrates erosions on the right SIJ (*arrow*). (b) CT scan demonstrates erosions on the left SIJ (*arrow*).

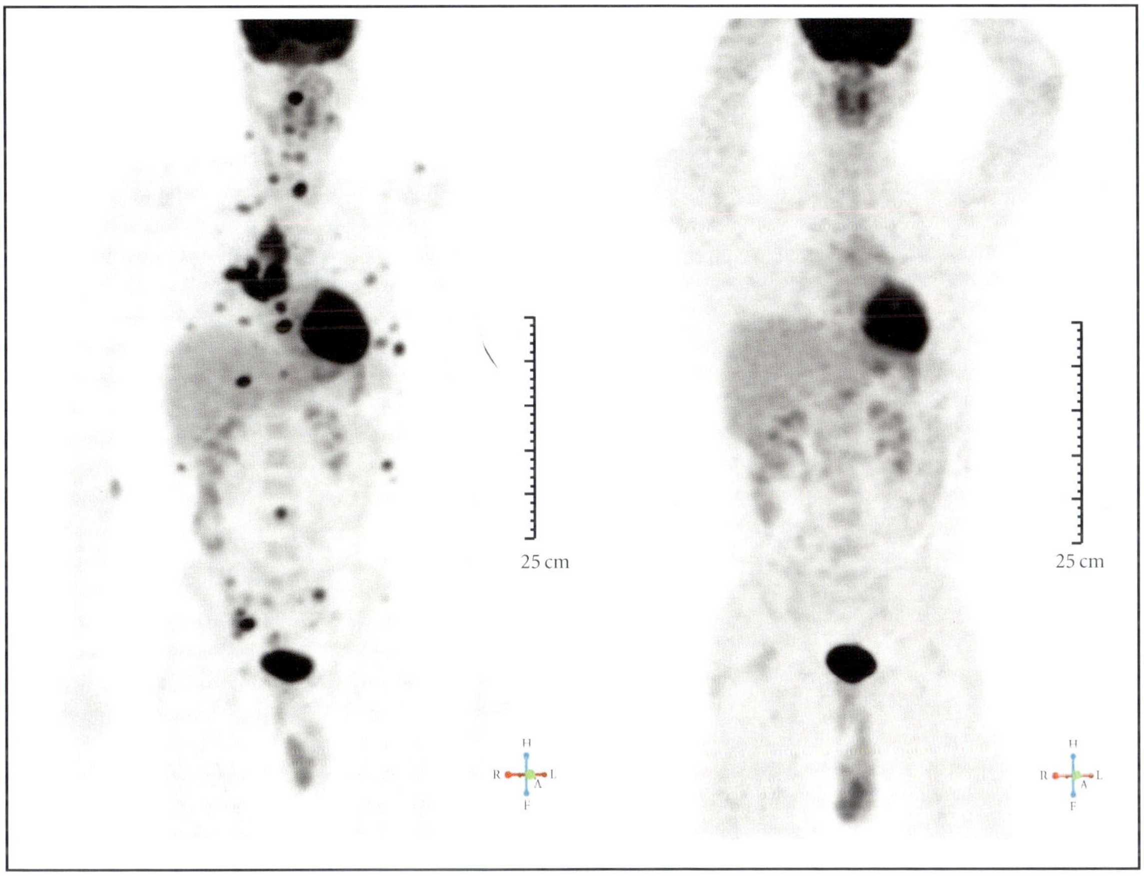

(a) (b)

Figure 2: (a) represents ^{18}F-FDG-PET/CT imaging showing multifocal hypermetabolic lesions of the sacroiliac joints, lungs and axillary, cervical, supraclavicular lymphadenopathy suggestive of systemic disease. (b) represents ^{18}F-FDG PET/CT imaging one year after anti-tuberculosis treatment. All hypermetabolic lesions have been cleared, confirming efficient therapy of tuberculosis.

Myocardial infarction was ruled out, and the patient was treated with NSAIDs with good clinical response.

Because of the persistence of increased inflammatory markers and negative biological infectious investigations and first imaging studies (chest X-Ray and abdominal ultrasound), a whole-body positron emission tomography combined with a computed tomography (PET/CT) using F18-fluorodeoxyglucose as radiotracer (^{18}F-FDG) was performed to detect any occult infectious or inflammatory sites. The ^{18}F-FDG-PET/CT revealed mediastinal, hilar pulmonary, supraclavicular and cervical bilateral hypermetabolic lymph nodes, hypermetabolic condensation in the right lung, multiple hypermetabolic lesions of axial skeleton (Figure 2(a)), in particular the thoracic spine, rib cage, and bilateral sacroiliac joints (Figure 3). This was suggestive of either DT or lymphoma. A tuberculin skin test was done and was highly

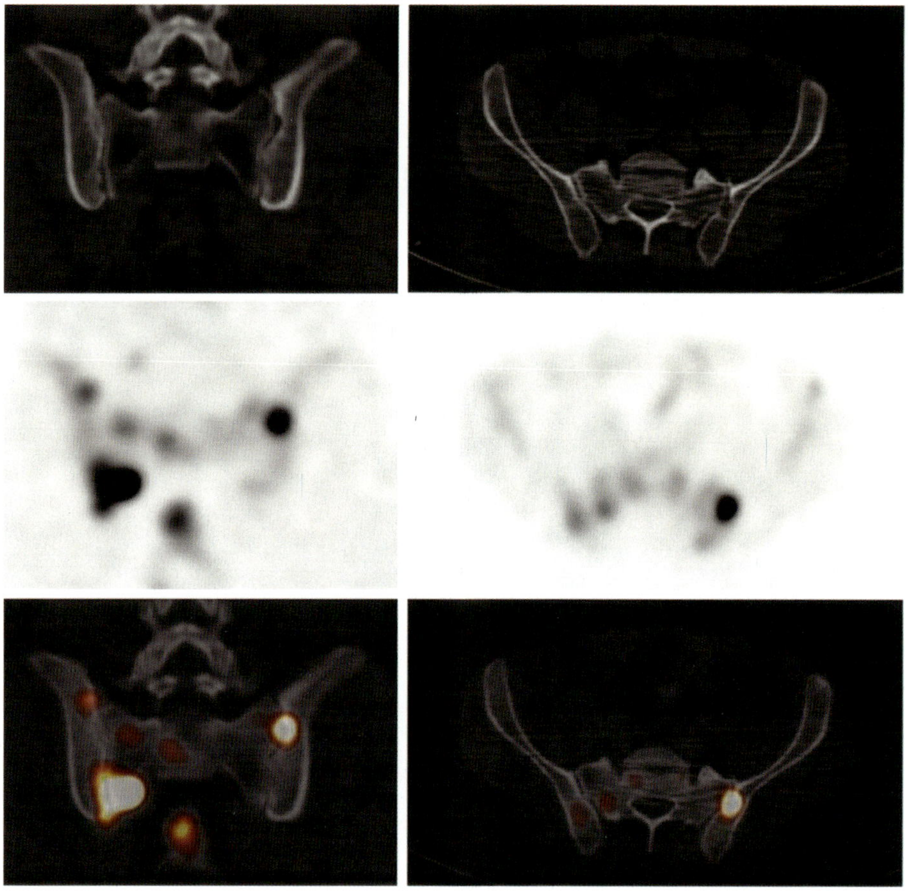

Figure 3: The figure shows sacroiliac joint involvement as hypermetabolic lesions as seen on ^{18}F-FDG-PET/CT. Left row: coronal CT, PET, and fused PET/CT slices. Right row: transverse CT, PET, and fused PET/CT slices.

positive (22 × 27 mm), whereas analysis for TB was negative in the sputum and urine. Bronchoscopy with biopsy of the right pulmonary lesion was performed. Histological analysis of the lesions showed the presence of necrotic granuloma, and microbiological examination revealed mycobacterium tuberculosis. The diagnosis of DT with axial skeleton, lung, and lymph node involvement was retained, and the patient was treated with Isoniazid 300 mg/d, Rifampicin 300 mg bid, Pyrazinamide 500 mg/d, and Ethambutol 400 mg qid. ^{18}FDG-PET/CT was repeated after 1 year of treatment and showed total disappearance of the aforementioned lesions (Figure 2(b)).

3. Discussion

Skeletal lesions are present in 2% of all cases of tuberculosis, and sacroiliac joint (SIJ) involvement has been reported in up to 9.7% of patients with skeletal tuberculosis [5]. We here report the case of a patient presenting with clinical features of AS revealing multifocal skeletal tuberculosis with bilateral SIJ involvement. Pouchot and colleagues reported 11 cases of SIJ tuberculosis, but none of them had bilateral involvement [6]. Ramlakan and Govender reported 17 patients of SIJ tuberculosis, with only one case with bilateral involvement [7]. Multifocal skeletal tuberculosis is often difficult to diagnose because of the insidious presentation and the paucity of systemic symptoms such as fever, weight lost, and night sweat. Hong and colleagues also reported a case of multifocal skeletal tuberculosis, which was misdiagnosed as AS and did not respond to antirheumatic drugs [8]. Our patient was also initially diagnosed as AS because of clinical and bilateral sacroiliitis CT scan features but persisting inflammatory markers in our patient prompted further investigations. Indeed, patients with AS might present with increased inflammatory markers but those generally are normalized with NSAIDs [3]. Moreover, many patients with axial involvement have normal or slightly elevated values of ESR and CRP, in comparison to patients with predominant involvement of the peripheral joints, IBD, or rheumatoid arthritis [4]. A bone scan or an MRI of SIJ was not being performed because CT scan of SIJ already demonstrated bilateral sacroiliitis. Conventional imaging investigations were negative. A CT thorax and CT abdomen were not performed because of the high-dose irradiation of this examination and the possibility of access to a whole-body FDG-PET/CT low dose. This hybrid imaging technique is well accepted for routine assessment of oncology disorders [9] but it is also increasingly used for the assessment and monitoring of infectious and inflammatory processes [10–12]. Indeed, ^{18}F-FDG accumulates not only in malignant tissues but also at the sites of infection and inflammation. Moreover, ^{18}F-FDG-PET/CT is a whole-body procedure allowing delineation of both the localization and the number of foci, even at sites that are clinically silent. In the present case, polyarticular pain with bilateral sacroiliitis was the most salient clinical features inveigling the diagnosis of AS. Value of ^{18}F-FDG-PET/CT in the diagnosis and assessment of multisystemic diseases is illustrated in this case with the detection of a lung lesion, lymphadenopathies, and bone lesions, including lesions of sacroiliac joints. As here shown, ^{18}F-FDG-PET/CT also permits to guide biopsy procedures for pathological and bacteriological diagnosis, and it helps in the monitoring of response to therapy.

This case highlights the importance of excluding other diagnoses in the presence of clinical picture of AS and high inflammatory markers. As such, ^{18}FDG-PET/CT might be a valuable tool in the detection of inflammatory and infectious processes.

Acknowledgments

The authors would like to thank Drs. Vandergheynst and Herpain for their assistance in the management of the clinical case.

References

[1] J. Braun and J. Sieper, "Ankylosing spondylitis," *The Lancet*, vol. 369, no. 9570, pp. 1379–1390, 2007.

[2] M. Rudwaleit, D. van der Heijde, R. Landewé et al., "The development of Assessment of SpondyloArthritis international Society classification criteria for axial spondyloarthritis (part II): validation and final selection," *Annals of the Rheumatic Diseases*, vol. 68, no. 6, pp. 777–783, 2009.

[3] M. Benhamou, L. Gossec, and M. Dougados, "Clinical relevance of C-reactive protein in ankylosing spondylitis and evaluation of the NSAIDs/coxibs' treatment effect on C-reactive protein," *Rheumatology*, vol. 49, no. 3, pp. 536–541, 2010.

[4] A. Spoorenberg, D. van der Heijde, E. de Klerk et al., "Relative value of erythrocyte sedimentation rate and C-reactive protein in assessment of disease activity in ankylosing spondylitis," *Journal of Rheumatology*, vol. 26, no. 4, pp. 980–984, 1999.

[5] J. H. Kim, A. A. Langston, and H. A. Gallis, "Miliary tuberculosis: epidemiology, clinical manifestations, diagnosis, and outcome," *Reviews of Infectious Diseases*, vol. 12, no. 4, pp. 583–590, 1990.

[6] J. Pouchot, P. Vinceneux, J. Barge et al., "Tuberculosis of the sacroiliac joint: clinical features, outcome, and evaluation of closed needle biopsy in 11 consecutive cases," *The American Journal of Medicine*, vol. 84, no. 3, part 2, pp. 622–628, 1988.

[7] R. J. Ramlakan and S. Govender, "Sacroiliac joint tuberculosis," *International Orthopaedics*, vol. 31, no. 1, pp. 121–124, 2007.

[8] L. Hong, J. G. Wu, J. G. Ding et al., "Multifocal skeletal tuberculosis: experience in diagnosis and treatment," *Medecine et Maladies Infectieuses*, vol. 40, no. 1, pp. 6–11, 2010.

[9] I. Ak, M. P. Stokkel, and E. K. Pauwels, "Positron emission tomography with 2-[18F] fluoro-2-deoxy-D-glucose in oncology. Part II. The clinical value in detecting and staging primary tumours," *Journal of Cancer Research and Clinical Oncology*, vol. 126, no. 10, pp. 560–574, 2000.

[10] R. Kumar, S. Basu, D. Torigian, V. Anand, H. Zhuang, and A. Alavi, "Role of modern imaging techniques for diagnosis of infection in the era of 18F-fluorodeoxyglucose positron emission tomography," *Clinical Microbiology Reviews*, vol. 21, no. 1, pp. 209–224, 2008.

[11] H. Zhuang and A. Alavi, "18-fluorodeoxyglucose positron emission tomographic imaging in the detection and monitoring of infection and inflammation," *Seminars in Nuclear Medicine*, vol. 32, no. 1, pp. 47–59, 2002.

[12] K. Strobel and K. D. Stumpe, "PET/CT in musculoskeletal infection," *Seminars in Musculoskeletal Radiology*, vol. 11, no. 4, pp. 353–364, 2007.

15

The Coexistence of Systemic Lupus Erythematosus and Thyrotoxicosis: The Diagnostic Value of Antihistone Antibodies

Marta Baleva,[1] Krasimir Nikolov,[2] Emil Manov,[3] Anastas Stoikov,[3] Rebhat Shabani,[3] Lyubomir Dourmishev,[4] and Milena Nikolova[5]

[1] *Department of Clinical Immunology, University Hospital Alexandrovska, Sofia, Bulgaria*
[2] *Department of Dermatology and Venereology, Medical University, 9002 Varna, Bulgaria*
[3] *Department of Internal Medicine II, University Hospital Alexandrovska, Sofia, Bulgaria*
[4] *Department of Dermatology and Venereology, University Hospital Alexandrovska, Sofia, Bulgaria*
[5] *Department of Nephrology, University Hospital Alexandrovska, Sofia, Bulgaria*

Correspondence should be addressed to Marta Baleva, marta_baleva@yahoo.com

Academic Editors: D. Aeberli, A. Giusti, and J. Mikdashi

We report four female patients with Graves' disease with positive ANA antibodies and possibility for development of systemic lupus erythematosus. All four patients have been treated with antithyroid drugs. SLE symptoms have appeared from 4 to 12 months after the beginning of therapy with methysol in two of them. The third patient had no symptoms for SLE, but her ANA, anti-DNA, and antihistone antibodies had been positive at the time of the onset of thyrotoxicosis. The fourth patient had alopecia areata with positive ANA and antihistone antibodies.

1. Introduction

The association between Hashimoto's thyroiditis and systemic lupus erythematosus (SLE) has been described by a number of authors [1, 2], but in contrast Mulhern et al. [3] report that there is not clear association between these two diseases. The coexistence of SLE and thyrotoxicosis was less known till now. In some cases thyrotoxicosis preceded the manifestation of SLE, in other ones the signs of SLE appeared firstly, and in some patients both diseases began simultaneously [4].

We describe four patients with Graves' disease with positive antinuclear antibodies (ANAs) and a possibility for development of SLE.

ANAs were determined by an indirect immunofluorescent method on HEp-2 cells, anti-ds DNA, anti-Sm, anni-RNP, and antihistone antibodies, as well as T_3, T_4, and TTH—by an ELISA technique.

2. Case Report

Patient 1. A 39-year-old female patient had suffered from weakness, weight loss, tachyarrhythmia, tremor, exophthalmos, moist skin, and goiter during the last year. For four months she was treated with propylthiouracil (PTU) with no effect, but one month ago she had edema on the legs, pleural effusion, and dyspnea. At the time of hospitalization in the intensive care department, she had exophthalmus, tachyarrhythmia (140 bpm), and anasarca with no effect of treatment with PTU 60 mg daily. Leading clinical manifestations were signs and symptoms for cardiac decompensation with cardiomegaly, absolute tachyarrhythmia with atrial flutter, T_3 gallop rhythm, positive venous pulse of the jugular veins, hypotension, and anasarca. Her skin and mucus were icteric; she had xanthelasmas on the upper eyelids and goiter (III-IV grade) with an auscultatory thrill, and the pleural effusion and the hepatomegaly persisted. Laboratory tests showed normal values of ESR,

RBC, WBC, and platelet counts and of serum creatinine, urea, and ASAT and ALAT levels, bilirubinemia (total—48, 3 μmol/L, direct—17, 3 μmol/L), elevated levels of cholestatic enzymes (alkaline phosphatase 168 Units, gamma-GTP 62 Units), negative ANA, DNA, Sm, and RNP, but positive antihistone antibodies, T_3-3, T_4-124, and TTH-0, 1 pmol/L. 12-lead ECG: absolute tachyarrhythmia and atrial flutter, P-pulmonale, diffuse changes in repolarisation showing positive results after therapy. Echocardiography: left ventricle sizes and volumes are within the normal range, and moderate enlargement of the left atrium exists. Elevated pulmonary artery pressure (systolic: 60 mm Hg, median 38 mm Hg) and overburdened right ventricle with relative tricuspidal regurgitation II degree and enlargement of the right atrium were detected. EF was 44%, and FS was 22%. She was treated with methylprednisolone 30 mg daily and furosemide 40 mg daily and showed improvement.

Patient 2. The case is a 44-year-old female patient, who had suffered from tachycardia, moist skin, and goiter in the last years. She had pericardial effusionseveral months ago. At that time the values of T_3 and T_4 were 8 and 115 pmol/L, respectively. The patient was treated with methysol (6 tablets daily, later 4 tablets daily). Since last summer she had had photosensitivity, arthralgia, alopecia areata, and malar rush. ANAs were positive (1:640), and DNA and Sm antibodies were positive as well, but antihistone antibodies were negative. All blood tests, including ESR, erythrocytes, leukocytes, thrombocytes, ASAT, ALAT, creatinine, and urea, were normal. The levels of thyroid hormones were as followes: FT_3 = 5.3 pg/mL (normal 2.3–4.2 pg/mL); FT_4 = 9.3 μg/dL (normal 0.8–1.8 ng/L), TSH-below 0.15 μIU/mL (normal 0.5–4.70 μIU/mL). Arthralgia, photosensitivity, alopecia, and malar rash persist till now. In addition this patient had WPW syndrome and allergy to antibiotics.

The patient was treated with methysol, but because of an elevation of the serum transaminases levels during the course of treatment (ASAT-37, ALAT-64 U) and hyperbilirubinemia, the treatment with methysol was stopped and PTU (3 tablets daily) was given. Additionally she took syllimarine (6 tablets daily) and chloroquine (1 tablet).

Patient 3. A 29-year-old female patient was admitted to the hospital because of tachycardia (100 bpm), tremor, weakness, edema on the upper eyelids and legs, skin itching, and enlarged goiter. Tc 99 m thyroid scan revealed increased uptake and uneven distribution of radioactivity. EST, hemoglobin, erythrocytes, leukocytes, thrombocytes, creatinine, and urea were normal, and the following results were obtained: ASAT = 55 IU/L, ALAT = 58 IU/L, alkaline phosphatase = 138 IU/L, FT_3 = 11, FT_4 = 60, anti-DNA and antihistone antibodies-positive, Sm, RNP-negative. The patient was treated with methysol 2 tablets 3 times daily, propranolol 60 mg daily, and Hismanal.

Patient 4. A 29-year-old female patient had suffered from thyrotoxicosis for the last 15 years. The first symptoms were weakness, tremor, tachycardia, diffuse goiter, exophthalmus, and alopecia areata. She had been treated with thymidazol, propranolol, and medazepam for the following 3 years. Alopecia disappeared, and symptoms for thyrotoxicosis showed an improvement. Ten years ago she had alopecia areata again. The treatment with low doses of prednisolone (20 mg daily) and laser therapy was followed by episodical disappearance of the alopecia. At the admission to hospital, her T_3 was 6 mmol/L, T_4-9, 5 mmol/L and the clinical symptoms for thyrotoxicosis were negative, but she had reticular alopecia areata. ANAs were positive (1:160), while Sm, RNP, and DNA antibodies were negative, but antihistone antibodies were positive.

All clinical and laboratory data are summarized in Table 1.

3. Discussion

Graves' disease and SLE are multisystemic autoimmune disorders. It is well known that many patients with SLE have positive thyroglobulin and microsome autoantibodies [1, 5, 6], and they have higher frequency of thyroid disorders [4, 7, 8]. Some authors suggest that the existence of Graves' disease induced SLE. For example Searles et al. [9], Amrhein et al. [10], Sato-Matsumura et al. [11], and Horton et al. [12] discuss the existence of PTU-induced lupus-like syndrome. The coexistence of thyrotoxicosis and SLE has been described by others [4, 13, 14]. According to Rodrigue et al. [4], the onset of hyperthyroidism preceded by 6 months to five years the onset of lupus manifestations in 3 from 6 patients; in 2 patients both diseases began simultaneously, and in the last patient the diagnosis of SLE preceded that of thyrotoxicosis.

In 2 of four patients described in this paper the SLE signs and symptoms follow those of thyrotoxicosis for a period of 4 and 12 months (patient 1 and patient 2, resp.). In the third patient, positive ANA appeared simultaneously with the signs and symptoms of thyrotoxicosis. The fourth patient had alopecia areata at the onset of thyrotoxicosis, but her ANAs were not determined at the beginning of the disease. At the time of observation, she had alopecia areata and positive ANA and antihistone antibodies. All four patients have been treated with PTU, methysol, and thymidazol for a typical Graves' disease: goiter, exophthalmas, tremor, tachycardia, and changes in thyroid function. Two of them had some symptoms characteristic for SLE: polyserositis and antihistone antibodies (N 1) and arthralgia, alopecia, photosensitivity, malar rush, and positive ANA, DNA, and Sm antibodies (N 2). The third patient had positive ANA, anti-DNA and antihistone antibodies, and no clinical data for SLE. The fourth one had only alopecia areata and photosensitivity as symptoms of SLE; ANA titer was elevated, and antihistone antibodies were positive.

In 1992 Loviselli et al. [15] reported that 13% of the patients with Graves' disease are positive for ds-DNA antibodies, determined by RIA, 11% for ss-DNA antibodies (ELISA), 2% for antihistone antibodies (ELISA), and 7% for ANA (immunofluorescence). Park et al. [6] do not find any significant differences in the concentration of anti-DNA antibodies in SLE patients with normal thyroid function,

Table 1: Clinical symptoms and laboratory data in four patients with thyrotoxicosis.

N	Clinical symptoms for thyrotoxicosis	T_3/FT_3	T_4/FT_4	Clinical symptoms for SLE	ANA	Sm Ab*	RNP Ab	ds DNA Ab	histone Ab
1	Diffuse goiter, exophthalmus, tachycardia, moist skin, weight loss	6.8	183	Polyserositis	—	–	–	–	+
2	Diffuse goiter, tachycardia, moist skin	8	115	Pericarditis, photosensitivity, arthralgia, alopecia areata, malar rash	1 : 640	+	–	+	–
3	Tachycardia, tremor, diffuse goiter, weakness	11	60	No	1 : 160	–	–	+	+
4	Weakness, tachycardia, diffuse goiter, tremor, exophthalmus	6	9.5	Alopecia areata, photosensitivity	1 : 160	–	–	–	+

*Ab: antibodies.

Graves' disease, Hashimoto's thyroiditis, and euthyroid sick syndrome. All 6 patients with coexistence of SLE and thyrotoxicosis, described by Rodrigue et al. [4] are ANA positive and 4 of them anti-DNA antibodies positive. Krausz et al. [16] report a patient in whom SLE has preceded Graves' disease for several years, and after treatment with methimazole, an exacerbation of SLE activity has been observed as well as an elevation of ANA titer.

Recently there are at least 4 opinions about the relations between SLE and thyrotoxicosis:

(1) the coexistence of SLE and thyrotoxicosis [4, 17];

(2) the possibility of drug-induced SLE after treatment with antithyroid drugs [10, 12];

(3) the presence of autoimmune thyroid disorders in SLE patients [5, 8, 18];

(4) the possibility of drug-induced serological changes after treatment with propylthiouracil (positive ANA of different type without presence of SLE) [19, 20].

The four patients examined by us have different antinuclear antibodies (Table 1), but only one of them (N 2) fulfills the ARA criteria for SLE. All four patients have been treated with antithyroid drugs, but 3 of them have positive antihistone antibodies. SLE symptoms have appeared 12 months after the beginning of methysol therapy in the second patient and the polyserositis in the first patient 4 months after the beginning of therapy with PTU.

We share the opinion of Rodrigue et al. [4] that the early differential diagnosis between SLE and thyrotoxicosis is very difficult. The reasons for this are some similar clinical manifestations of both diseases. Another explanation is the possibility of drug-induced SLE in some patients, treated with antithyroid drugs. The determination of ANA, including antihistone antibodies, could be of great interest in these cases.

Acknowledgment

This manuscript was supported by Grant no. DOO2/125 from the Ministry of Education, Bulgaria.

References

[1] A. P. Weetman and M. J. Walport, "The association of autoimmune thyroiditis with Systemic Lupus Erythematosus," *British Journal of Rheumatology*, vol. 26, no. 5, pp. 359–361, 1987.

[2] J. J. Garber, J. W. Worthington, R. V. Randall, and R. R. Kierland, "Lupus erythematosus and Hashimoto's thyroiditis," *Postgraduate Medicine*, vol. 46, no. 4, pp. 100–105, 1969.

[3] L. M. Mulhern, A. T. Masi, and L. E. Shulman, "Hashimoto's disease: a search for associated disorders in 170 clinically detected cases," *The Lancet*, vol. 2, no. 7462, pp. 508–511, 1966.

[4] S. Rodrigue, H. Laborde, and P. M. Catoggio, "SLE and thyrotoxicosis: a hitherto little recognized association," *Annals of the Rheumatic Diseases*, vol. 48, no. 5, pp. 424–427, 1989.

[5] M. L. Boey, P. H. Fong, J. S. C. Lee, W. Y. Ng, and A. C. Thai, "Autoimmune thyroid disorders in SLE in Singapore," *Lupus*, vol. 2, no. 1, pp. 51–54, 1993.

[6] D. J. Park, C. S. Cho, S. H. Lee et al., "Thyreoid disorders in korean patients with Systemic Lupus Erythematosus," *Scandinavian Journal of Rheumatology*, vol. 24, pp. 13–17, 1995.

[7] F. W. Miller, G. F. Moore, B. D. Weintranb, and A. D. Steinberg, "Prevalence of thyroid disease and abnormal thyroid function test results in patients with Systemic Lupus Erythematosus," *Arthritis & Rheumatism*, vol. 30, no. 10, pp. 10124–10131, 1987.

[8] K. L. Goh and F. Wang, "Thyroid disorders in SLE," *Annals of the Rheumatic Diseases*, vol. 45, pp. 579–583, 1986.

[9] R. P. Searles, S. R. Plymate, and G. M. Troup, "Familial thioamide-induced lupus syndrome in thyrotoxicosis," *Journal of Rheumatology*, vol. 8, no. 3, pp. 498–500, 1981.

[10] J. A. Amrhein, F. M. Kenny, and D. Ross, "Granulocytopenia, lupus-like syndrome, and other complications of propylthiouracil therapy," *The Journal of Pediatrics*, vol. 76, no. 1, pp. 54–63, 1970.

[11] K. C. Sato-Matsumura, H. Koizumi, T. Tatsumura et al., "Lupus erythematosus-like syndrome induced by thiamasole and propylthiouracil," *The Journal of Dermatology*, vol. 21, pp. 501–507, 1994.

[12] R. C. Horton, M. C. Sheppard, and P. Emery, "Propylthiouracil-induced Systemic Lupus Erythematosus," *The Lancet*, vol. 2, no. 8662, p. 568, 1989.

[13] C. Papadopoulos, R. Jiji, and E. Maher, "Lupus erythematosus and hyperthyroidism," *American Journal of Diseases of Children*, vol. 118, no. 4, pp. 621–625, 1969.

[14] M. E. Oren and M. S. Cohen, "Immune thrombocytopenia, red cell aplasia, lupus, and hyperthyroidism," *Southern Medical Journal*, vol. 71, no. 12, pp. 1577–1578, 1978.

[15] A. Loviselli, F. Velluzzi, R. Pala et al., "Circulating antibodies to DNA-related antigens in patients with autoimmune thyroid disorders," *Autoimmunity*, vol. 14, no. 1, pp. 33–36, 1992.

[16] Y. Krausz, A. Blum, and A. Rubinow, "Hyperthyroidism and Systemic Lupus Erythematosus: chance or genetic predisposition?" *Clinical and Experimental Rheumatology*, vol. 9, no. 4, pp. 438–439, 1991.

[17] Z. Abraham, M. Rozenbaum, E. J. Feuerman, A. Kinarty, and N. Lahat, "Adolescent Systemic Lupus Erythematosus and Graves' disease," *Clinical and Experimental Rheumatology*, vol. 12, no. 1, pp. 90–91, 1994.

[18] J. Kosmo,, N. Naito, K. Saito et al., "Anti-thyroid peroxidase antibody activity in sera of patients with Systemic Lupus Erythematosus," *Clinical and Experimental Immunology*, vol. 75, no. 2, pp. 217–221, 1989.

[19] S. S. Wing and I. G. Fantus, "Adverse immunologic effects of antithyroid drugs," *Canadian Medical Association Journal*, vol. 136, no. 2, pp. 121–127, 1987.

[20] M. N. G. Dukes and L. Beeley, Eds., *Side Effects of Drugs Annual 14*, Elsevier, Amsterdam, The Netherlands, 1990.

16

Multicentric Reticulohistiocytosis Presenting with Papulonodular Skin Lesions and Arthritis Mutilans

Raya Saba, Shawn G. Kwatra, Bishwas Upadhyay, Aibek E. Mirrakhimov, and Farah N. Khan

Department of Internal Medicine, Saint Joseph Hospital, 2900 N. Lake Shore, Chicago, IL 60657, USA

Correspondence should be addressed to Aibek E. Mirrakhimov; amirrakhimov1@gmail.com

Academic Editors: T. C. Hsu and M. A. Hunt

Multicentric reticulohistiocytosis is a rare multisystem disorder of unknown etiology that is characterized by erosive polyarthritis and papulonodular lesions on the skin, mucous membranes, and internal organs. We report the case of a 54-year-old female who was misdiagnosed as having rheumatoid arthritis and underwent numerous joint replacement surgeries for progressively destructive arthritis in her hands, shoulders, hips, and knees. The patient finally received a diagnosis of multicentric reticulohistiocytosis after histopathological examination of the patient's left knee arthroplasty which revealed a diffuse histiocytic infiltrate, multinucleated giant cells, and finely granulated eosinophilic cytoplasm with a ground-glass appearance.

1. Introduction

Multicentric reticulohistiocytosis (MRH) is a rare multisystem disorder of unknown etiology, characterized by erosive polyarthritis and papulonodular lesions on the skin, mucous membranes, and internal organs. MRH is the most destructive chronic inflammatory arthritis, manifesting more aggressively than either rheumatoid arthritis (RA) or psoriatic arthritis [1], and progressing to arthritis mutilans in 45% of cases [2]. The onset of the disease is usually in the forth decade of life, affecting females two to three times more often than males [3, 4], and presenting insidiously with joint symptoms preceding skin manifestations in the majority of patients. Herein, we describe the case of a patient found to have multicentric reticulohistiocytosis who was previously misdiagnosed as having rheumatoid arthritis for several years.

2. Description of Case

A 54-year-old African-American female with a history of multiple joint replacements presented to clinic complaining of severe diffuse arthritis. She reported progressive morning stiffness and arthralgias in her knees that first started 10 years prior, followed shortly by the development of skin nodules on the dorsum of both hands. Since this time, multiple other joints became affected including her bilateral hands, hips, and shoulders.

She was initially seen by a rheumatologist 10 years ago and diagnosed with RA. Over the course of her disease, she tried numerous therapies including ibuprofen, prednisone, etanercept, methotrexate, and adalimumab. However, she had a poor response to these medications, and her arthritis continued to worsen. She eventually underwent bilateral hip and knee replacement surgeries to improve her deteriorating functional ability.

On physical exam, the patient had multiple nonpruritic reddish-brown papulonodular lesions on the dorsum of the hands that were present for the past 8 years (Figure 1). The skin rash started approximately 2 years after the onset of symptoms. She also had eyelid xanthelasmas along with arthritic deformities involving the metacarpophalangeal (MCP), proximal interphalangeal (PIP), and distal interphalangeal (DIP) joints. Other features observed included telescoping of the digits bilaterally, ulnar deviation of the wrists, and limited abduction and flexion of the shoulders.

Extensive laboratory workup was significant for a microcytic hypochromic anemia, elevated erythrocyte sedimentation rate (ESR) and C-reactive protein (CRP), and an

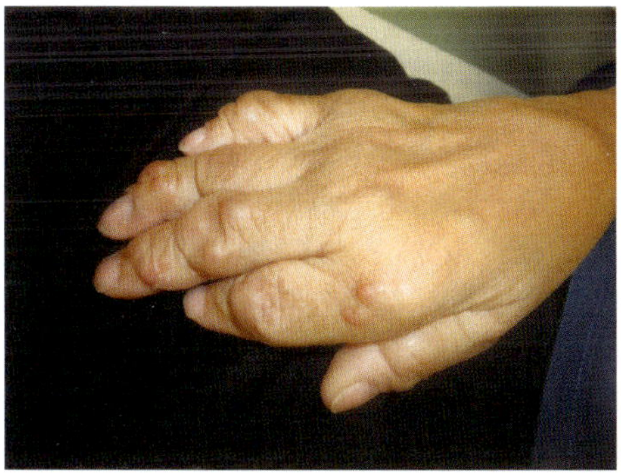

FIGURE 1: Reddish-brown papulonodular lesions on the dorsum of the hand.

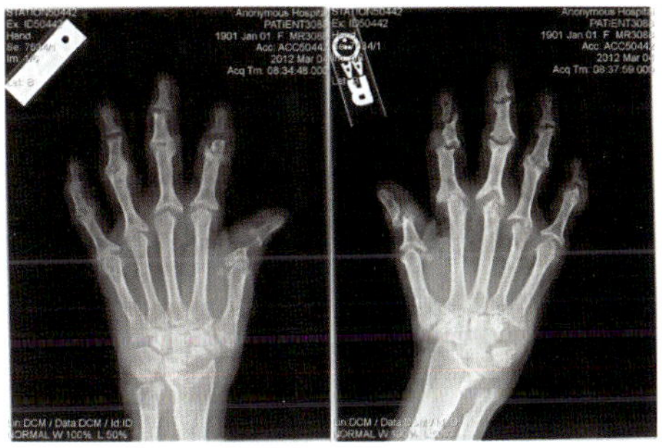

FIGURE 2: X-ray of the hand showing the "pencil-in-cup" phenomenon and narrowing of the joint spaces.

abnormal lipid panel. The following tests were within normal limits: antinuclear antibodies, rheumatoid factor, anticyclic citrullinated protein antibody, liver function tests, and thyroid studies.

X-ray of the hand showed severe diffuse destruction of the carpometacarpal, metacarpophalangeal, and interphalangeal joints with widening of joint spaces and expanded bases of proximal and middle phalanges giving the appearance of a pencil-in-cup deformity (Figure 2). Shortening and complete resorption of certain phalanges was also seen along with interphalangeal joint fusion and subluxation. There was also significant periarticular osteoporosis, narrowing of the joint spaces, and new bone formation. X-ray of the shoulder revealed destructive changes and multiple erosions of the acetabulum, humeral head, and acromioclavicular articulation, without any associated fracture or dislocation (Figure 3). These findings were consistent with arthritis mutilans.

Finally, histopathological examination of the patient's left knee arthroplasty reported marked histiocytic infiltration with multinucleated giant cells (Figure 4). Other features noted include a finely granulated eosinophilic cytoplasm with a ground-glass appearance, vesicular nuclei, hyperplastic synovial tissue, and chronic inflammation with fibrin deposition. Histiocytes and histiocytic giant cells contained periodic acid Schiff (PAS) reactive material (Figure 5(a)) and stained positive for CD68 (Figure 5(b)).

The patient's combination of clinical presentation, laboratory testing, imaging, and histopathology was consistent with a diagnosis of multicentric reticulohistiocytosis. Due to poor compliance, the patient failed to undergo screening for an associated malignancy.

Treatment regimens have been adjusted frequently. She failed a combination of adalimumab and methotrexate as well as a trial of azathioprine. Her current regimen consists of etanercept, methotrexate, and prednisone, which provides symptomatic relief including decreased stiffness, edema, and pain. This treatment regimen has unfortunately failed to resolve her irreversible arthritic deformities.

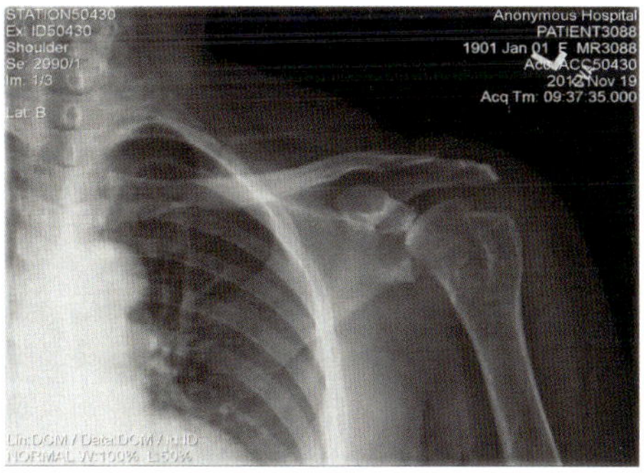

FIGURE 3: X-ray of the shoulder displaying multiple erosions of the acetabulum, humeral head, and acromioclavicular articulation.

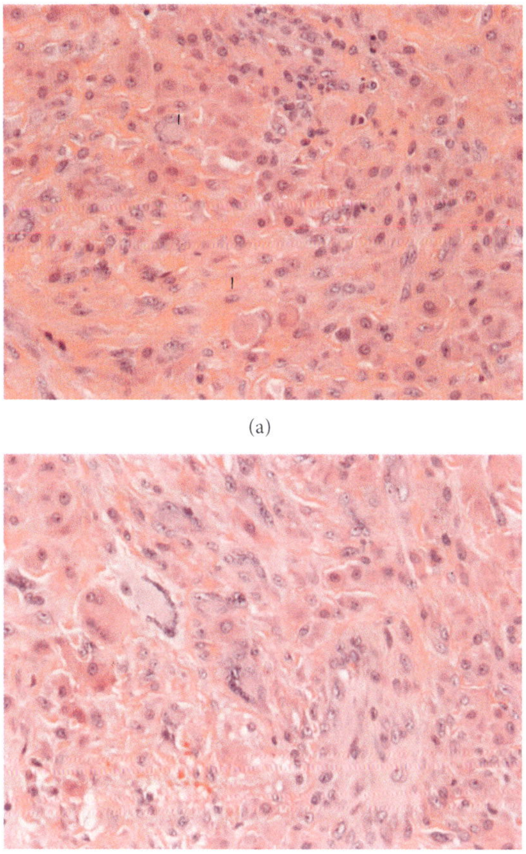

(a)

(b)

FIGURE 4: Histiocytic infiltration with multinucleated giant cells.

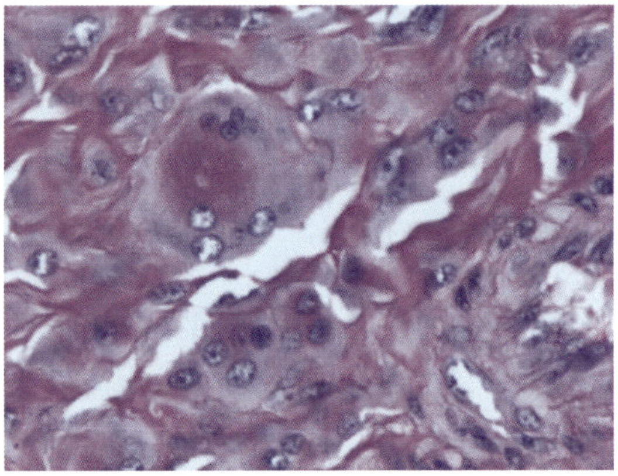

(a)

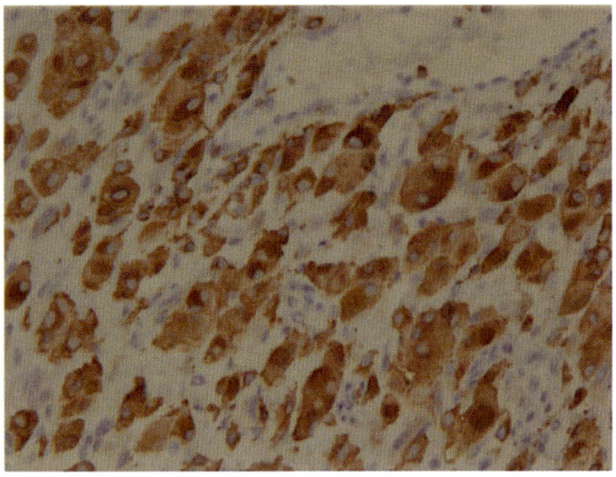

(b)

Figure 5: (a) Histiocytes with PAS material; (b) histiocytes staining positive for CD68.

3. Discussion

MRH is a rarely diagnosed rheumatologic condition. While only approximately 250 cases have been reported worldwide, this is likely to be a significant underrepresentation of the disease. Owing to its rarity, the diagnosis can be challenging, and many patients are misdiagnosed with more common causes of erosive polyarthritis, such as RA. Hence, increased awareness plays a crucial role, and a high index of suspicion is warranted by clinicians in patients presenting with erosive polyarthritis. Helpful clues (which were all present in our case) include the development of characteristic skin lesions, X-ray findings including involvement of the distal interphalangeal joints (DIP), rapid progression to arthritis mutilans, and confirmatory histopathology findings.

Arthritis associated with MRH is inflammatory in nature and tends to be symmetrical. There is maximal involvement of the interphalangeal joints of the hands that can lead to the disabling "accordion" or "opera glass" hand [3]. Involvement of the distal interphalangeal (DIP) joints is present in 75% of patients, representing an important diagnostic clue in distinguishing MRH from other types of erosive arthritis, mainly rheumatoid arthritis [5].

Skin involvement is a characteristic of MRH and involves multiple flesh-colored to reddish-brown nonpruritic firm papules and nodules, ranging in size from a few millimeters to 2 cm in size. Most of these lesions are commonly located over the dorsal aspects of the hands, the elbows, and on the head. Systemic complaints have also been observed and most often affect the pulmonary, cardiac, and muscular systems.

MRH has been described in association with various conditions: hyperlipidemia (30–58%), a positive skin tuberculin test (12–50%), and many autoimmune diseases (5–20%) including RA, Sjogren's syndrome [6], primary biliary cirrhosis [7], and systemic vasculitis [8]. A higher association with underlying internal malignancy has been reported in up to 25% of MRH patients with hematological, breast, and stomach carcinomas being the most common [9, 10]. It has, thus, been classified by several authors as a paraneoplastic syndrome, occurring in close proximity to the onset of a new neoplasm or the recurrence of a previously diagnosed one, and regressing upon treatment of the primary tumor [11]. A thorough investigation to exclude malignancy is highly recommended in patients with newly diagnosed MRH.

Laboratory investigations lack specificity and diagnostic relevance. These investigations may reveal a microcytic anemia, elevated ESR, elevated CRP, and hyperlipidemia. Imaging, on the other hand, plays a key diagnostic role. Radiologic findings include well-circumscribed marginal erosions, widening of joint spaces, loss of cartilage, and resorption of subchondral bone. In contrast to other types of inflammatory arthritis, periarticular osteopenia and heterotrophic new bone formation are rarely reported [1, 12].

The diagnosis is confirmed histologically, with a skin or synovial tissue biopsy demonstrating pleomorphic mononuclear histiocytes, multinucleated giant cells, and eosinophilic ground-glass cytoplasm that is PAS positive [3].

These cells have also been shown to stain positively with the osteoclast markers tartrate-resistant acid phosphatase (TRAP) and Cathepsin K. This finding, along with good response to treatment with bisphosphonates, provides support for the notion of MRH being a systemic osteoclastic disease [13].

Although symptoms associated with MRH may spontaneously remit within 5–10 years of diagnosis, aggressive treatment is recommended to avoid irreversible sequelae of the active inflammation period. Due to the limited number of cases, treatment continues to be experimental. Remission has been achieved in patients with MRH with methotrexate, chlorambucil, and cyclophosphamide. These drugs have been used in various combinations with adjuvant nonsteroidal anti-inflammatory agents, hydroxychloroquine, and corticosteroids [14]. MRH has also shown a successful response to azathioprine [15] and leflunomide [16]. More recent data show excellent results achieved with antitumor necrosis factor (TNFα) therapy including etanercept [17], infliximab [18], and adalimumab [19]. Finally, improvement has also been noted with bisphosphonates, including alendronate [20] and zoledronic acid [13].

4. Conclusion

Clinicians should have a high index of suspicion for MRH in patients presenting with erosive polyarthritis and papulonodular skin lesions. Helpful clues for diagnosis include involvement of the DIP, rapid progression to arthritis mutilans, and characteristic histopathological findings including a diffuse histiocytic infiltrate, multinucleated giant cells, and finely granulated eosinophilic cytoplasm with a ground-glass appearance.

Acknowledgment

The authors would like to thank Drs. Yongsuk Lertratanakul, Teresita Zdunek, and Harry Brown for providing important clinical, pathologic, and radiographic insight into the case.

References

[1] D. A. Campbell and N. L. Edwards, "Multicentric reticulohistiocytosis: systemic macrophage disorder," *Bailliere's Clinical Rheumatology*, vol. 5, no. 2, pp. 301–319, 1991.

[2] J. D. Gorman, C. Danning, H. R. Schumacher, J. H. Klippel, and J. C. Davis Jr., "Multicentric reticulohistiocytosis: case report with immunohistochemical analysis and literature review," *Arthritis & Rheumatism*, vol. 43, no. 4, pp. 930–938, 2000.

[3] M. V. Barrow and K. Holubar, "Multicentric reticulohistiocytosis. A review of 33 patients," *Medicine*, vol. 48, no. 4, pp. 287–305, 1969.

[4] F. B. Luz, A. P. Gaspar, N. Kalil-Gaspar, and M. Ramos-E-Silva, "Multicentric reticulohistiocytosis," *Journal of the European Academy of Dermatology and Venereology*, vol. 15, no. 6, pp. 524–531, 2001.

[5] D. Santilli, A. Lo Monaco, P. L. Cavazzini, and F. Trotta, "Multicentric reticulohistiocytosis: a rare cause of erosive arthropathy of the distal interphalangeal finger joints," *Annals of the Rheumatic Diseases*, vol. 61, no. 6, pp. 485–487, 2002.

[6] K. Ben Abdelghani, I. Mahmoud, E. Chatelus, C. Sordet, J. E. Gottenberg, and J. Sibilia, "Multicentric reticulohistiocytosis: an autoimmune systemic disease? Case report of an association with erosive rheumatoid arthritis and systemic Sjogren syndrome," *Joint Bone Spine*, vol. 77, no. 3, pp. 274–276, 2010.

[7] M. Doherty, M. F. R. Martin, and P. A. Dieppe, "Multicentric reticulohistiocytosis associated with primary biliary cirrhosis: successful treatment with cytotoxic agents," *Arthritis & Rheumatism*, vol. 27, no. 3, pp. 344–348, 1984.

[8] G. F. Oliver, I. Umbert, R. K. Winkelmann, and S. A. Muller, "Reticulohistiocytoma cutis—review of 15 cases and an association with systemic vasculitis in two cases," *Clinical and Experimental Dermatology*, vol. 15, no. 1, pp. 1–6, 1990.

[9] J. L. Snow and S. A. Muller, "Malignancy-associated multicentric reticulohistiocytosis: a clinical, histological and immunophenotypic study," *British Journal of Dermatology*, vol. 133, no. 1, pp. 71–76, 1995.

[10] L. Han, Q. Huang, K. H. Liao et al., "Multicentric reticulohisti ocytosis associated with liver carcinoma: report of a case," *Case Reports in Dermatology*, vol. 4, no. 2, pp. 163–169, 2012.

[11] B. El-Haddad, D. Hammoud, T. Shaver, and S. Shahouri, "Malignancy-associated multicentric reticulohistiocytosis," *Rheumatology International*, vol. 31, no. 9, pp. 1235–1238, 2011.

[12] D. Resnick, "Lipidoses, histiocytoses, and hyperlipoproteinemias," in *Diagnosis of Bone and Joint Disorders*, D. Resnick, Ed., pp. 2206–2214, WB Saunders, Philadelphia, Pa, USA, 3rd edition, 1995.

[13] K. A. Codriansky, T. M. Rünger, J. Bhawan, A. Kantarci, and E. Y. Kissin, "Multicentric reticulohistiocytosis: a systemic osteoclastic disease?" *Arthritis Care and Research*, vol. 59, no. 3, pp. 444–448, 2008.

[14] G. C. Liang and A. S. Granston, "Complete remission of multicentric reticulohistiocytosis with combination therapy of steroid, cyclophosphamide, and low-dose pulse methotrexate," *Arthritis & Rheumatism*, vol. 39, no. 1, pp. 171–174, 1996.

[15] A. Rudd, C. Dolianitis, G. Varigos, and A. Howard, "A case of multicentric reticulohistiocytosis responsive to azathioprine in a patient with no underlying malignancy," *Australas Journal of Dermatology*, vol. 52, no. 4, pp. 292–294, 2011.

[16] A. A. Lonsdale-Eccles, A. E. Haworth, F. C. McCrae, and S. A. Young-Min, "Successful treatment of multicentric reticulohistiocytosis with leflunomide," *The British Journal of Dermatology*, vol. 161, no. 2, pp. 470–472, 2009.

[17] B. T. Kovach, K. T. Calamia, J. S. Walsh, and W. W. Ginsburg, "Treatment of multicentric reticulohistiocytosis with etanercept," *Archives of Dermatology*, vol. 140, no. 8, pp. 919–921, 2004.

[18] A. H. Kalajian and J. P. Callen, "Multicentric reticulohistiocytosis successfully treated with infliximab: an illustrative case and evaluation of cytokine expression supporting anti-tumor necrosis factor therapy," *Archives of Dermatology*, vol. 144, no. 10, pp. 1360–1366, 2008.

[19] S. E. Shannon, H. R. Schumacher, S. Self, and A. N. Brown, "Multicentric reticulohistiocytosis responding to tumor necrosis factor-α inhibition in a renal transplant patient," *Journal of Rheumatology*, vol. 32, no. 3, pp. 565–567, 2005.

[20] H. Goto, M. Inaba, K. Kobayashi et al., "Successful treatment of multicentric reticulohistiocytosis with alendronate: evidence for a direct effect of bisphosphonate on histiocytes," *Arthritis & Rheumatism*, vol. 48, no. 12, pp. 3538–3541, 2003.

17

Early-Onset Neutropenia Induced by Rituximab in a Patient with Lupus Nephritis and Hemolytic Anemia

Mariangelí Arroyo-Ávila, Ruth M. Fred-Jiménez, and Luis M. Vilá

Division of Rheumatology, Department of Medicine, University of Puerto Rico, Medical Sciences Campus, San Juan, PR 00936, USA

Correspondence should be addressed to Luis M. Vilá; luis.vila2@upr.edu

Academic Editor: Graciela S. Alarcon

Rituximab is an anti-CD20 monoclonal antibody that has been used to treat several complications of systemic lupus erythematosus (SLE) including nephritis, cerebritis, and hematological disorders. Neutropenia is among the adverse events associated with rituximab; this usually occurs several weeks after therapy. However, early-onset neutropenia has been reported only in a few cases. Herein, we describe a 36-year-old Hispanic SLE woman who developed severe early-onset neutropenia (0.3×10^9/L) after the second weekly rituximab infusion (375 mg/m^2 weekly $\times$ 4) given for nephritis and hemolytic anemia. She also had early-onset thrombocytopenia after rituximab therapy. Both hematological disorders resolved 12 days after the fourth and final dose. This case, together with few others, suggests that early-onset neutropenia may occur during rituximab therapy. Even though rituximab-induced neutropenia seems to be transient, it may predispose SLE patients to severe complications such as infections.

1. Introduction

Rituximab is a chimeric monoclonal antibody directed against CD20 positive B cells. It was initially approved for the treatment of non-Hodgkin's lymphoma and later indicated for autoimmune rheumatic diseases such as rheumatoid arthritis and antineutrophil cytoplasmic antibody-associated vasculitis [1–3]. Furthermore, rituximab has been used as a second-line treatment for systemic lupus erythematosus (SLE), especially in refractory nephritis, cerebritis, and hematological disorders [1, 4–6]. In general, rituximab has a favorable safety profile; however, several adverse events have been described. Among the most commonly reported are infusion reactions, infections, and late-onset neutropenia [3–5, 7, 8]. The latter occurs after 4 weeks of rituximab treatment, with a median time to development reported between 14 and 23 weeks in patients with rheumatic disorders [7, 9]. Early-onset neutropenia during rituximab infusion is rare [8–11]. Herein, we report an SLE patient who developed severe early-onset neutropenia during treatment with rituximab given for lupus nephritis and hemolytic anemia.

2. Case Presentation

A 36-year-old Puerto Rican woman was hospitalized to our institution in March 2010 because of nephrotic syndrome and hemolytic anemia. Seven years before admission, she was diagnosed with SLE manifested by constitutional symptoms, malar rash, photosensitivity, oral ulcers, alopecia, Raynaud's phenomenon, arthritis, myalgias, lymphadenopathy, lymphopenia, anemia, positive antinuclear antibodies (ANA), elevated anti-dsDNA antibodies, and hypocomplementemia (C3 and C4). Early during the course of disease, she developed autoimmune pancreatitis, serositis, and membranous glomerulonephritis. Initially, she was treated with corticosteroids (including intravenous [IV] methylprednisolone therapy), hydroxychloroquine, IV pulse cyclophosphamide, and azathioprine. However, she had either partial clinical response or adverse events to these drugs for which she was started on mycophenolate mofetil in 2007. She achieved good clinical response with this therapy.

One month before admission, mycophenolate mofetil was discontinued due to severe diarrhea resulting in a severe

SLE exacerbation. Upon admission she had oral ulcers, an erythematous maculopapular rash on her face, neck, and upper extremities, and anasarca. Initial laboratories showed a white blood cell (WBC) count of 6.6×10^9/L, neutrophil count of 6.3×10^9/L, lymphocyte count of 1.3×10^9/L, platelet count of 100×10^9/L, and hemoglobin of 8.7 g/dL. The peripheral blood smear revealed slight hypochromasia, anisocytosis, and poikilocytosis and the presence of reticulocytes. No schistocytes were seen. The reticulocyte count was elevated at 2.6% and the haptoglobin was decreased at 5.8 mg/dL. She had a serum creatinine of 1.53 mg/dL that rapidly worsened to 2.29 mg/dL after 48 hours. Serum albumin was decreased at 1.8 g/dL. The urinalysis showed >50 red blood cells (RBC)/high power field (hpf), 0–4 leukocytes/hpf, 3+ protein, and 0–2 granular casts/hpf. The urine protein-to-creatinine ratio was 2.1 which worsened to 8.6 eleven days later. The Westergren sedimentation rate was elevated at 48 mm/hr. Complement C3 and C4 were decreased at 14.6 mg/dL (90–180 mg/dL) and 2.0 mg/dL (10–40 mg/dL), respectively. Anti-dsDNA antibodies were not elevated.

The patient was treated with methylprednisolone 250 mg IV every six hours for 3 days, followed by methylprednisolone 1-2 mg/kg/day. Mycophenolate mofetil was restarted. During her hospital course she developed several complications including seizures, oliguria requiring transient hemodialysis, hypertensive crisis, and ascites. Rituximab 675 mg (375 mg/m^2) IV weekly was started. Fifteen days after the first rituximab dose (7 days after the second infusion), the WBC count decreased to 2.8×10^9/L, neutrophil count to 2.0×10^9/L, and lymphocyte count to 0.6×10^9/L (Figure 1). The next day, platelets decreased to 52×10^9/L. Cell counts continued to decrease with a nadir of 0.8×10^9/L for leukocytes, 0.3×10^9/L for neutrophils, and 28×10^9/L for platelets, 19 days after the first rituximab dose. Conversely, hemoglobin levels increased during this time. Thirty-nine days after the first rituximab dose (12 days after the fourth and final infusion), WBC and platelet counts returned to normal limits.

She responded favorably to rituximab therapy. Renal function improved and proteinuria significantly decreased. Upon discharge she had a WBC count of 4.6×10^9/L, neutrophil count of 3.3×10^9/L, platelet count of 122×10^9/L, hemoglobin of 11.4 g/dL, and serum creatinine of 0.9 mg/dL. She was discharged on prednisone 60 mg daily, hydroxychloroquine 200 mg twice daily, and mycophenolate mofetil 500 mg twice daily. Prednisone dose was gradually decreased until discontinued. After 4 years of follow-up the patient remained in clinical remission with normal WBC and platelet counts and renal function.

3. Discussion

We describe a patient with SLE manifested by nephritis and hemolytic anemia who developed early-onset neutropenia after the second weekly infusion of rituximab. Early-onset neutropenia, occurring earlier than 4 weeks after initiation of rituximab therapy, has been rarely reported in SLE. To our knowledge, three additional cases have been described (Table 1) [8, 11]. Enríquez et al. reported a 48-year-old woman with SLE and diffuse proliferative glomerulonephritis refractory to cyclophosphamide and high-dose corticosteroids who developed severe neutropenia 5 days after the second dose of rituximab [11]. Additionally, Gottenberg et al. described 2 patients with resistant SLE treated with rituximab after failing several immunosuppressive therapies including cyclophosphamide [8]. Both patients developed severe neutropenia in less than 15 days after the first rituximab infusion. One of these 2 patients, as well as our case, was concomitantly taking mycophenolate mofetil. In the LUNAR trial, Rovin et al. reported that patients receiving rituximab concurrently with mycophenolate mofetil (1.5 gm/day–3 gm/day) for lupus nephritis had a higher frequency of neutropenia compared with those taking mycophenolate mofetil alone (2.7% versus 1.4%). The severity or degree of neutropenia was not reported [4].

The differential diagnosis of transient neutropenia in our patient includes lupus itself, infections, and other drugs besides rituximab, but these possibilities seem unlikely. The patient had mild leukopenia in the past. However, the lowest leukocyte count was 3.0×10^9/L which was documented 3 months prior to current hospitalization. She did not present clinical findings of viral or bacterial infection and had negative blood cultures during the period of rituximab treatment. Other than rituximab, she did not receive drugs that could potentially induce neutropenia.

In addition to neutropenia, early-onset thrombocytopenia may occur following rituximab therapy [10, 12, 13]. Our patient developed transient thrombocytopenia after the second rituximab infusion. Likewise, Larrar et al. reported a two-year-old boy with resistant autoimmune hemolytic anemia who developed uncomplicated transient thrombocytopenia 1 week after the third dose of rituximab [10]. He had spontaneous recovery of platelet count 7 days later. Similar abnormalities have been reported in patients with hairy cell leukemia and mantle cell lymphoma [12, 13]. To our knowledge, no cases of early-onset thrombocytopenia, aside from ours, have been reported in SLE patients receiving rituximab treatment.

Rituximab-induced cytopenias, either early or late, appear to be transient and self-limited [7–11]. While some authors report successful therapy with granulocyte-colony stimulating factor [10, 11], others note recovery of cell counts after discontinuation of rituximab alone [7–9]. Rituximab-induced neutropenia may cause neutropenic fever, infections, and sepsis [5, 7–9, 11]. Our patient had complete resolution of hematological abnormalities after rituximab discontinuation and she did not develop any complications related to neutropenia. Interestingly, our patient had an increase of neutrophil and platelet counts between rituximab doses 3 and 4. This rebound was probably related to the effect of corticosteroid therapy. As described before, during this period the patient was receiving high-dose intravenous methylprednisolone but this was increased from 80 mg daily to 120 mg daily 1 day prior to the rebound.

The pathophysiology of rituximab-induced cytopenia remains unclear as neutrophils and platelets do not express CD20. Using direct immunofluorescence testing, Voog et al. described anti-neutrophil IgG antibodies bound to the

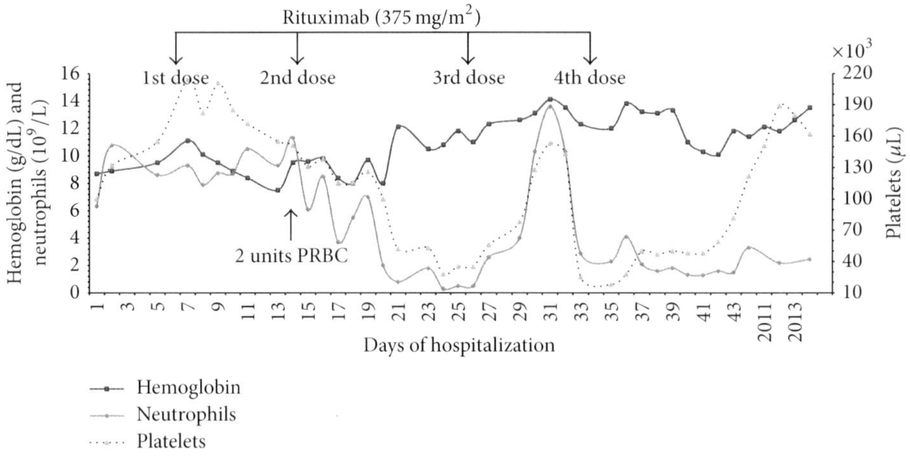

Figure 1: Hemoglobin, neutrophil count, and platelet count during hospitalization. Marked decreases in neutrophils and platelets are observed after seven days of the second rituximab infusion. Hemoglobin levels increased eight days after the second rituximab infusion and remained stable throughout hospitalization. Cell count returned to normal levels twelve days after the final rituximab dose. After four years of follow-up, hemoglobin, neutrophil count, and platelet count remained normal.

Table 1: Adult SLE patients presenting with early-onset neutropenia associated with rituximab therapy.

Author/year	Gender/age (years)/ethnicity	Active clinical manifestations	Prior immunosuppressive therapy	Concomitant immunosuppressive treatment	Number of weekly rituximab infusions/dose	Time to neutropenia after 1st dose of rituximab (days)
Gottenberg et al./2005 [8]	F/30/NA	Pleuropericarditis	NA	None	1/375 mg/m^2	10
Gottenberg et al./2005 [8]	F/22/NA	Articular	Cyclophosphamide	Mycophenolate mofetil	4/375 mg/m^2	15
Enríquez et al./2007 [11]	F/48/Caucasian	Polyarthritis, nonnephrotic range proteinuria	Cyclophosphamide	None	2/375 mg/m^2	15
Current report/2014	F/32/Hispanic	Oral ulcers, rash, hemolytic anemia, and nephrotic syndrome	Cyclophosphamide	Mycophenolate mofetil	4/375 mg/m^2	15

SLE: systemic lupus erythematosus; NA: not available.

surface of neutrophils in two lymphoma patients treated with rituximab who developed neutropenia. However, serum anti-neutrophil IgG antibodies were not detected in these patients [14]. Weissmann-Brenner et al. found that plasma from a lymphoma patient who developed neutropenia after rituximab completely inhibited granulocyte growth of a healthy bone marrow [15]. Nevertheless, most proposed mechanisms attempt to explain the development of late-onset neutropenia, which is more commonly seen. Early-onset neutropenia following rituximab administration may occur through different mechanisms that have yet to be elucidated.

In summary, we report a Hispanic woman with SLE who presented with early-onset neutropenia after the second weekly infusion of rituximab. She also had transient thrombocytopenia. Although cytopenias are common in SLE, in our patient they do not seem to be related with active disease given that other activity parameters such as anemia, proteinuria, and renal insufficiency were resolving. Hemoglobin levels began to increase 16 days after the first rituximab infusion (coinciding with neutrophil decrease) and remained stable thereafter. In addition, there was a sequential association between rituximab administration and the development of cytopenias. Although early-onset cytopenias have been rarely reported, they may be underestimated since follow-up blood cell counts are not routinely performed after rituximab infusions. While rituximab-induced cytopenias seem to be transient they may predispose SLE patients to more severe complications such as infections and sepsis. Clinicians should be aware of the possibility of early-onset neutropenia and thrombocytopenia following rituximab treatment. Repeated clinical assessments to evaluate cytopenia-related complications are reasonable and may be used to guide therapy.

Acknowledgment

Grant support was provided in part by an unrestricted educational grant from Abbvie.

References

[1] I. Danés, A. Agustí, A. Vallano et al., "Available evidence and outcome of off-label use of rituximab in clinical practice," *European Journal of Clinical Pharmacology*, vol. 69, no. 9, pp. 1689–1699, 2013.

[2] J. A. Gómez-Puerta, L. F. Quintana, J. H. Stone, M. Ramos-Casals, and X. Bosch, "B-cell depleting agents for ANCA vasculitides: a new therapeutic approach," *Autoimmunity Reviews*, vol. 11, no. 9, pp. 646–652, 2012.

[3] M. Sebastiani, M. G. Anelli, F. Atzeni et al., "Efficacy and safety of rituximab with and without methotrexate in the treatment of rheumatoid arthritis patients: results from the GISEA register," *Joint Bone Spine*, vol. 81, no. 6, pp. 508–512, 2014.

[4] B. H. Rovin, R. Furie, K. Latinis et al., "Efficacy and safety of rituximab in patients with active proliferative lupus nephritis: the Lupus Nephritis Assessment with Rituximab Study.," *Arthritis and rheumatism*, vol. 64, no. 4, pp. 1215–1226, 2012.

[5] B. Terrier, Z. Amoura, P. Ravaud et al., "Safety and efficacy of rituximab in systemic lupus erythematosus: results from 136 patients from the French autoimmunity and rituximab registry," *Arthritis and Rheumatism*, vol. 62, no. 8, pp. 2458–2466, 2010.

[6] M. Ramos-Casals, M. J. Soto, M. J. Cuadrado, and M. A. Khamashta, "Rituximab in systemic lupus erythematosus A systematic review of off-label use in 188 cases," *Lupus*, vol. 18, no. 9, pp. 767–776, 2009.

[7] D. Tesfa, S. Ajeganova, H. Hägglund et al., "Late-onset neutropenia following rituximab therapy in rheumatic diseases: association with B lymphocyte depletion and infections," *Arthritis & Rheumatism*, vol. 63, no. 8, pp. 2209–2214, 2011.

[8] J.-E. Gottenberg, L. Guillevin, O. Lambotte et al., "Tolerance and short term efficacy of rituximab in 43 patients with systemic autoimmune diseases," *Annals of the Rheumatic Diseases*, vol. 64, no. 6, pp. 913–920, 2005.

[9] E. Besada, W. Koldingsnes, and J. Nossent, "Characteristics of late onset neutropenia in rheumatologic patients treated with rituximab: a case review analysis from a single center," *QJM*, vol. 105, no. 6, pp. 545–550, 2012.

[10] S. Larrar, C. Guitton, M. Willems, and B. Bader-Meunier, "Severe hematological side effects following Rituximab therapy in children," *Haematologica*, vol. 91, no. 8, supplement, p. ECR36, 2006.

[11] E. Enríquez, J. Borrás-Blasco, A. E. Sirvent, M. Masía, and F. Amorós, "Early onset neutropenia after rituximab in lupus nephritis," *Clinical and Experimental Rheumatology*, vol. 25, no. 2, p. 345, 2007.

[12] Z. K. Otrock, R. A. R. Mahfouzd, G. O. Oghlakian, Z. M. Salem, and A. Bazarbachi, "Rituximab-induced acute thrombocytopenia: a report of two cases," *Haematologica*, vol. 90, supplement, Article ID ECR23, 2005.

[13] R. Ram, L. Bonstein, A. Gafter-Gvili, I. Ben-Bassat, O. Shpilberg, and P. Raanani, "Rituximab-associated acute thrombocytopenia: an under-diagnosed phenomenon," *The American Journal of Hematology*, vol. 84, no. 4, pp. 247–250, 2009.

[14] E. Voog, F. Morschhauser, P. Solal-Céligny, M. C. Benyunes, P. S. Multani, and A. Saunders, "Neutropenia in patients treated with rituximab," *The New England Journal of Medicine*, vol. 348, no. 26, pp. 2691–2694, 2003.

[15] A. Weissmann-Brenner, B. Brenner, I. Belyaeva, M. Lahav, and E. Rabizadeh, "Rituximab associated neutropenia: description of three cases and an insight into the underlying pathogenesis," *Medical Science Monitor*, vol. 17, no. 11, pp. CS133–CS137, 2011.

18

Tongue Necrosis as an Initial Manifestation of Giant Cell Arteritis

Jose R. Zaragoza, Natalia Vernon, and Gisoo Ghaffari

Division of Allergy & Immunology, Penn State Hershey Allergy, Asthma & Immunology, 500 University Drive, UPC II, Suite 1300, Hershey, PA 17033, USA

Correspondence should be addressed to Gisoo Ghaffari; gghaffari@hmc.psu.edu

Academic Editor: Suleyman Serdar Koca

Giant cell arteritis (GCA) is a systemic vasculitis of medium and large arteries that mainly affects the external carotid artery. It is a diagnosis of the elderly that typically presents as low-grade fever, temporal tenderness, claudication of the jaw, and in some patients vision loss. In cases where GCA presents with atypical manifestations, the diagnosis may be more difficult, causing a delay in both diagnosis and treatment and ultimately leading to irreversible complications. In this paper, we present an atypical presentation of GCA with symptoms of neck swelling and lingual pain in an elderly female. These symptoms progressed to bilateral necrosis and eventual dislodgement of the tongue. Lingual necrosis is a severe potential complication in GCA. In patients presenting with lingual swelling, pain, and discoloration, GCA should be suspected and prompt therapy should be initiated to avoid irreversible complications.

1. Introduction

Giant cell arteritis is a chronic vasculitis of large and medium sized vessels that commonly affects those above the age of 50 years. It has an estimated incidence of 20 cases per 100,000 individuals and a prevalence of 1 in 500 individuals [1]. Scandinavian and North American females are most commonly affected. Clinical presentation is usually fever, claudication of the jaw, and temporal headache. Less common presenting symptoms include dysphagia, cough, hearing loss, and necrosis of the tongue [2].

The diagnosis of GCA is clinicopathological for which the American College of Rheumatology (ACR) has established classification criteria. To meet the diagnosis criteria, patients should present at least 3 out of 5 positive findings. The ACR diagnostic tool does not include any lingual symptomatology amongst its criteria [3, 4] (Table 1).

Lingual necrosis is a known complication of GCA that commonly affects one side of the tongue [5–8]. In a few cases bilateral necrosis has been described and is considered extremely rare due to the rich lingual vascular supply [2, 5, 9–11]. This paper presents a case of lingual pain and bilateral tongue necrosis secondary to GCA along with a literature review of this rare complication.

2. Case Report

A 68-year-old female patient was initially evaluated by her primary care physician for a nonspecific moderate headache and swelling of the neck for four weeks. She was treated with a course of antibiotics and nonsteroidal anti-inflammatory medications for ten days. After completing this therapy, the patient presented to the Emergency Department for acute onset of severe pain and progressive swelling of the tongue that was compromising her speech and deglutition. She was admitted to the hospital and treated with empiric antibiotic therapy and intermittent doses of systemic glucocorticoids for suspected sialadenitis. Progressive swelling of the tongue compromised feeding so the patient was then transferred to a tertiary care institution for further treatment and consulted with the allergy service for evaluation of angioedema as possible culprit on swelling.

Patient denied symptoms of fever, malaise, or weight loss. She did not have vision loss, jaw claudication, or temporal

Table 1: Three out of five criteria are required to make the diagnosis of GCA.

American College of Rheumatology diagnostic criteria
(1) Age older than 50 years at onset of disease.
(2) New onset of localized headache.
(3) Abnormal temporal artery with tenderness or decreased pulse.
(4) Erythrocyte sedimentation rate higher than 50 mm/hr.
(5) A biopsy of the artery showing necrotizing arteritis with predominant mononuclear cell infiltrate or granulomatous process with multinucleated giant cells.

Table 2: Differential diagnosis in lingual necrosis.

Differential diagnosis in lingual necrosis
(1) Malignancy: (carcinoma, lymphoma, and sarcoma)
(2) Drugs: (vasopressin, chemotherapy, and ergotamine)
(3) Radiation therapy
(4) Cardiovascular: (hemorrhage, embolism, and cardiac arrest)
(5) Infection: (syphilis, tuberculosis)
(6) Systemic vasculitis: (giant cell arteritis, ANCA positive vasculitis)

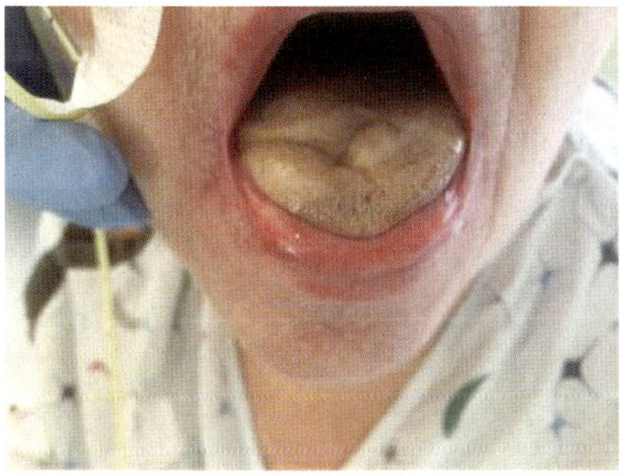

Figure 1: Discoloration and swelling of the anterior half of the tongue upon initial evaluation.

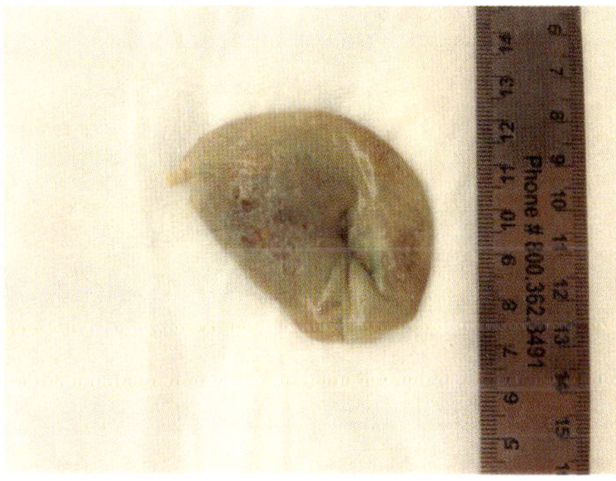

Figure 2: Necrotic appearance of the tongue posterior to dislodgement.

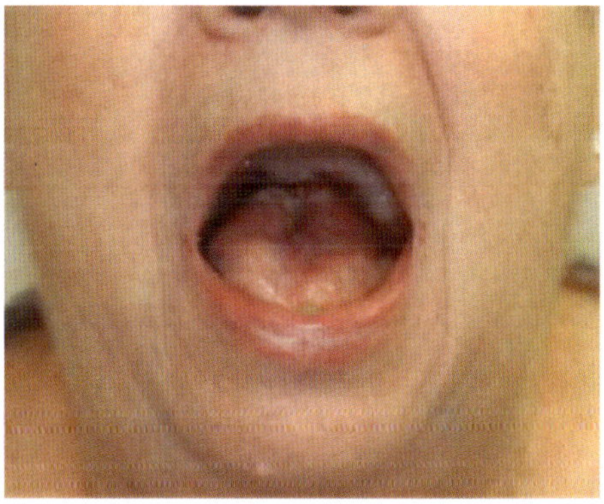

Figure 3: Appearance of the healed tongue.

tenderness. Past medical history was negative for vasoconstrictor use, radiation therapy, cardiac arrest, or embolization. Vital signs were within normal limits with no evidence of cardiac or pulmonary abnormalities. Edema and discoloration involving the anterior half of the tongue with movement limitation were the main findings on physical examination. No temporal artery tenderness was noted (Figure 1).

Hematologic testing revealed mild leukocytosis, anemia and thrombocytosis (WBC: 13.8 ku/L, Hgb: 12.4 g/dL, Hct: 37.8%, Plt: 414 ku/L), and mild neutrophilia on differential. The comprehensive metabolic panel was unremarkable.

Elevation in both C-reactive protein (CRP) and erythrocyte sedimentation (ESR) (1.3 mg/dL and 55 mm/hr, resp.) was concordant with an acute inflammatory process. Antineutrophil cytoplasmic antibody was negative. Even though her presentation was atypical for angioedema, serum C4 levels and C1 esterase inhibitor and function were measured and found to be normal.

A tongue biopsy was performed and showed coagulative necrosis, and no malignant cells or amyloid deposits were identified. Imaging studies including a CT-angiography showed luminal irregularity of right cervical internal carotid artery described to have a "beaded appearance," suggesting arterial involvement and segmental luminal narrowing. A soft tissue defect of the anterior part of the tongue, consistent with avascular necrosis of the tongue, was noted.

GCA was confirmed with bilateral biopsies of the temporal arteries, which showed mixed inflammatory infiltrate composed of lymphocyte, histiocyte, and multinucleated giant cells with focal destruction of internal elastic lamina and marked intimal thickening significantly decreasing the lumen of both arteries, consistent with GCA vasculitis. Our patient met 3 of the 5 ACR criteria: age older than 50, elevated ESR, and histology consistent with GCA on both temporal arteries. Treatment with high dose corticosteroids was initiated at 1 mg/kg. Unfortunately, the patient had extensive necrosis of the tongue that progressed to self-amputation of the anterior half of the tongue (Figures 2 and 3). No other organ system was involved.

TABLE 3: Literature review of bilateral necrosis of the tongue in giant cell arteritis.

Reference	Patient age	Previous symptoms	Presentation	Studies	ACR criteria	Treatment
Oliver et al. [2]	79	An episode of collapse, decreased vision on left eye, and abdominal pain with segmental small bowel necrosis	New-onset, spontaneous bilateral necrosis of the tongue	Erythrocyte sedimentation rate (ESR): 78 Ultrasound of temporal artery: thickened artery with halo	Yes	Prednisolone and azathioprine 100 mg/d each
Zadik et al. [5]	78	Pain of the right head, neck, and shoulder. Fatigue, visual blurring, and weight loss for last 2 mo	Sore tongue, bilateral swelling and pain	Erythrocyte sedimentation rate (ESR): 69 Ultrasound of left temporal artery revealed occlusion	Yes	Prednisone 60 mg/d
Schurr et al. [9]	66	Slurred speech, dysphagia for 2 weeks	Swelling of the tongue with a greyish-purple color	Erythrocyte sedimentation rate (ESR): 120 CT angio.: 3 cm long stenosis with 50% at left common carotid artery	No	Prednisone 500 mg/d × 3 d, then 100 mg/d
Sainuddin and Saeed [10]	82		Acute abdominal pain, fever, and intestinal infarction	Autopsy confirmed giant cell arteritis affecting intestine and temporal artery	Yes	
Patterson et al. [11]	88	Generalized weakness. Painful, swollen, and discolored tongue for 10 days	Ischemic tongue, tender to palpation, and decreased movement		Yes	Prednisone 40 mg daily

3. Literature Review

A PubMed based search was conducted combining the terms "giant cell arteritis and bilateral tongue necrosis," "lingual necrosis," and "ischemia." It included articles published in English and Spanish. We found that bilateral tongue necrosis in GCA has been previously reported in 5 patients. A history of atypical symptoms like dysphagia, lingual pain, and swelling was present in all the cases described. Typical symptoms were only seen in one patient described by Zadic et al., who presented with pain on right side of the head, visual blurring, and fatigue before evaluation (Table 3).

4. Discussion

In general, necrosis of the tongue is rare and may be caused by a wide array of different pathologies ranging from lingual malignancy, use of vasoconstrictor, and radiation therapy [12–17] (Table 2). This paper presents a case of bilateral tongue necrosis and eventual self-amputation of the tongue as a rare complication of GCA. Our case and the literature review of patients with this rare complication reveal that these patients often present with lingual pain and the absence of the typical symptoms of GCA ultimately delaying diagnosis and treatment. Patients with lingual pain or swelling nonresponsive to treatment for infection or angioedema should raise a high index of suspicion for a vasculitic process such as GCA, especially in patients above the age of 50. Physicians should be familiarized with this presentation since lingual swelling may prompt a consultation for evaluation for suspected angioedema, as was the case in our patient.

Acknowledgments

Thanks are due to Timothy Craig D.O. for his guidance and support and Thomas Samson MD for his contribution.

References

[1] J. M. Evans, W. M. O'Fallon, and G. G. Hunder, "Increased incidence of aortic aneurysm and dissection in giant cell (temporal) arteritis: a population-based study," *Annals of Internal Medicine*, vol. 122, no. 7, pp. 502–507, 1995.

[2] M. Oliver, B. Hugl, L. Posch et al., "Subtotal tongue necrosis in delayed diagnosed giant-cell arteritis: a case report," *The American Journal of Otolaryngology—Head and Neck Medicine and Surgery*, vol. 25, no. 6, pp. 438–441, 2004.

[3] G. G. Hunder, D. A. Bloch, B. A. Michel et al., "The American College of Rheumatology 1990 criteria for the classification of giant cell arteritis," *Arthritis and Rheumatism*, vol. 33, no. 8, pp. 1122–1128, 1990.

[4] B. Dasgupta, M. A. Cimmino, H. M. Kremers et al., "2012 Provisional classification criteria for polymyalgia rheumatic: a European League Against Rheumatism/American College of Rheumatology collaborative initiative," *Arthritis & Rheumatism*, vol. 64, no. 4, pp. 943–954, 2012.

[5] Y. Zadik, M. Findler, A. Maly, H. Rushinek, and R. Czerninski, "A 78-year-old woman with bilateral tongue necrosis," *Oral Surgery, Oral Medicine, Oral Pathology, Oral Radiology and Endodontology*, vol. 111, no. 1, pp. 15–19, 2011.

[6] M. Goicochea, J. Correale, L. Bonamico et al., "Tongue necrosis in temporal arteritis," *Headache*, vol. 47, no. 8, pp. 1213–1215, 2007.

[7] S. L. Pendás, J. C. de Vicente Rodríguez, M. G. García, L. M. J. Gutierrez, and J. S. L. Arranz, "Tongue necrosis as a complication of temporal arteritis," *Oral Surgery, Oral Medicine, Oral Pathology*, vol. 78, no. 4, pp. 448–451, 1994.

[8] O. Marcos, A. I. Cebrecos, A. Prieto, and M. Sancho De Salas, "Tongue necrosis in a patient with temporal arteritis," *Journal of Oral and Maxillofacial Surgery*, vol. 56, no. 10, pp. 1203–1206, 1998.

[9] C. Schurr, A. Berthele, M. Burghartz, and J. Kiefer, "Spontaneous bilateral necrosis of the tongue: a manifestation of giant cell arteritis?" *European Archives of Oto-Rhino-Laryngology*, vol. 265, no. 8, pp. 993–998, 2008.

[10] S. Sainuddin and N. R. Saeed, "Acute bilateral tongue necrosis—a case report," *British Journal of Oral and Maxillofacial Surgery*, vol. 46, no. 8, pp. 671–672, 2008.

[11] A. Patterson, C. Scully, N. Barnard, M. J. Griffiths, J. W. Eveson, and M. Novelli, "Necrosis of the tongue in a patient with intestinal infarction," *Oral Surgery Oral Medicine and Oral Pathology*, vol. 74, no. 5, pp. 582–586, 1992.

[12] X. Leroy, A. Delobelle, J. L. Lefebvre, V. Cabaret, F. Bloget, and M. O. Vilain, "Epithelioid sarcoma of the tongue," *Journal of Clinical Pathology*, vol. 50, no. 10, pp. 869–870, 1997.

[13] A. Pollett, B. Perez-Ordonez, R. C. K. Jordan, and M. J. Davidson, "High-grade papillary cystadenocarcinoma of the tongue," *Histopathology*, vol. 31, no. 2, pp. 185–188, 1997.

[14] A. L. Weber, A. Rahemtullah, and J. A. Ferry, "Hodgkin and non-Hodgkin lymphoma of the head and neck: clinical, pathologic, and imaging evaluation," *Neuroimaging Clinics of North America*, vol. 13, no. 3, pp. 371–392, 2003.

[15] J. Bondeson, U. B. Ericsson, P. Falke et al., "Tongue necrosis in temporal arteritis provoked by ergotamine," *Journal of Internal Medicine*, vol. 232, no. 6, pp. 541–544, 1992.

[16] J. M. David, E. Paty, J. M. Bachaud, and J. R. Vignaud, "Lingual necrosis after radiotherapy: radiation arteritis?" *Revue de Stomatologie et de Chirurgie Maxillo-Faciale*, vol. 90, no. 5, pp. 334–336, 1989.

[17] P. Libersa, C. Loison-Blanchard, L. Nawrocki, and S. Duquesnoy, "Bilateral necrosis of the tongue consecutive to cardiac arrest," *Journal of Oral and Maxillofacial Surgery*, vol. 60, no. 3, pp. 322–323, 2002.

19

IgG4-Related Disease without Overexpression of IgG4: Pathogenesis Implications

Naoshi Nishina,[1] Yuko Kaneko,[1] Masataka Kuwana,[1] Hironari Hanaoka,[1] Hideto Kameda,[1] Shuji Mikami,[2] and Tsutomu Takeuchi[1]

[1] *Division of Rheumatology, Department of Internal Medicine, School of Medicine, Keio University, 35 Shinanomachi Shinjuku-ku, Tokyo 160-8582, Japan*
[2] *Division of Diagnostic Pathology, Keio University Hospital, Tokyo 160-8582, Japan*

Correspondence should be addressed to Yuko Kaneko, ykaneko@z6.keio.jp

Academic Editors: L.-P. Erwig, M. Salazar-Paramo, and G. J. Tsay

IgG4-related disease is a new disease group that affects multiple organs. It is characterized by high serum IgG4 and abundant infiltration of IgG4-bearing plasma cells in the affected organ. Here, we describe an intriguing case that suggested that IgG4-related disease might present without IgG4 overexpression or infiltration, at least during a relapse. A 47-year-old man had been diagnosed with systemic lupus erythematosus 15 years. He was admitted due to a pituitary mass, systemic lymphadenopathy, and multiple nodules in the lungs and kidneys. The serum IgG4 level was normal and histopathological examination of the pituitary mass showed abundant lymphocyte and plasma cell infiltration with very few IgG4-positive cells. When we examined specimens preserved from 15 years ago, we found high serum IgG4 levels and IgG4-bearing plasma cell infiltration. This resulted in a diagnosis of IgG4-related disease, and we considered the current episode to be a relapse without IgG4 overexpression. This case indicated that, to clarify the pathogenesis of IgG4-related disease, current cases should repeat specimen evaluations over the course of IgG4-related disease to define diagnostic markers.

1. Introduction

IgG4-related disease, first described in 2001 [1], is a new disease group that affects multiple organs. It is characterized by high serum IgG4 and infiltration of the affected organ with lymphoplasmacytes, IgG4-bearing plasma cells, and fibrosis [2–4]. Because high serum IgG4 and abundant infiltration of IgG4-bearing plasma cells are prominent characteristics, it was suggested that these findings could define the diagnosis of IgG4-related disease [5]. However, the pathogenesis of IgG4 overexpression remains unclear [6], and it is unknown whether IgG4 is related to the cause of the disease.

Here, we described a case of IgG4-related disease that had been exacerbated after 15 years of remission. At the time of the relapse, the patient exhibited several masses in various organs, including pituitary, lung, kidney, and lymph nodes. However, the serum IgG4 level was within normal limits. A histopathological examination of pituitary gland and lung masses showed infiltration of numerous plasma cells, but very few IgG4-bearing cells. This intriguing finding indicated that IgG4-related disease could present without abundant IgG4-bearing plasma cell infiltration, at least at the time of a relapse.

2. Case Presentation

In 2010, a 47-year-old Japanese man was admitted to Keio University Hospital due to a vision abnormality.

In 1994, he had visited our hospital with lymphadenopathy. At that time, he had high serum IgG (6098 mg/dL), and a lymph node specimen from the left inguinal area revealed nonspecific lymphoid hyperplasia, which did not define a diagnosis. In 1995, the suspected diagnosis was systemic lupus erythematosus (SLE), based on observations of polyarthritis, low white blood cell count (1600/μL), positivity for antinuclear antibody, and slightly elevated anti-DNA antibody (12.2 IU/mL by radioimmunoassay; normal range

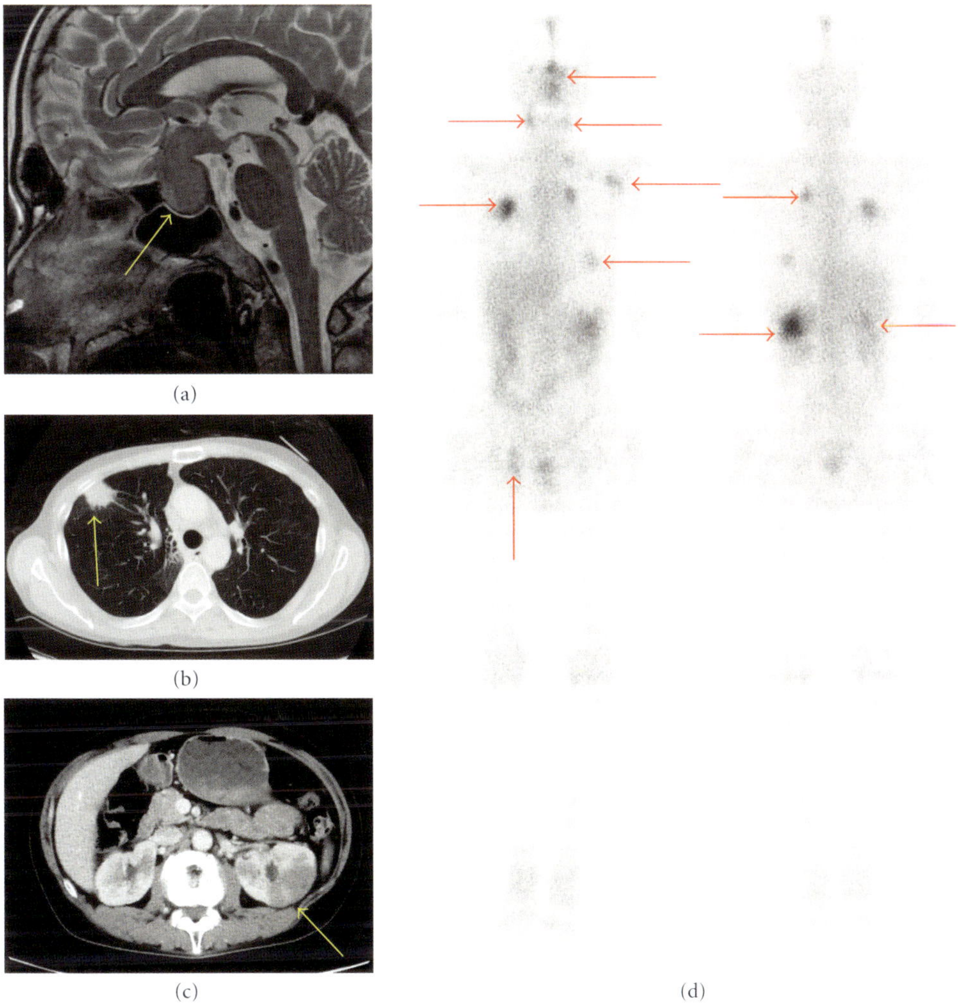

FIGURE 1: Lesions in a patient with IgG4-related disease. (a) Head MRI on a T2-weighted image, sagittal section. A pituitary mass of 30 mm was detected (arrow). (b) Chest CT shows a nodule in the right lung (arrow). (c) Abdominal CT shows that part of the left kidney was not enhanced with contrast media (arrow). (d) ^{67}Gallium accumulated abnormally in the pituitary gland, both sides of the neck, both lungs, both kidneys, and the left inguinal area (arrows).

<6 IU/mL). He was treated with 20 mg daily prednisolone (PSL) and the symptoms disappeared rapidly. Subsequently, the PSL was gradually tapered down. From 2008, he had been taking 2 mg daily PSL and remained in stable condition until he experienced abnormal vision in 2010.

In the 2010 admission, a physical examination showed multiple swollen lymph nodes (1.5 cm maximum diameter) in the neck and inguinal area. A visual field examination revealed bilateral hemianopsia. Laboratory blood tests showed normal results for the blood count, serum electrolytes, serum creatinine, liver enzymes, and lactate dehydrogenase. The C-reactive protein level was slightly elevated to 0.86 mg/dL. The total serum IgG was 3189 mg/dL, with 1550 mg/dL IgG1 (normal range, 320–748), 1100 mg/dL IgG2 (normal range, 208–754), 444 mg/dL IgG3 (normal range, 6.6–88.3), and 94.9 mg/dL IgG4 (normal range, 4.8–105). Magnetic resonance imaging (MRI) of the head revealed a pituitary mass of 30 mm (Figure 1(a)), which was considered the cause of bilateral hemianopsia. A computed tomography (CT) scan showed nodules in both lungs and a lesion in the left kidney that was devoid of contrast enhancement (Figures 1(b) and 1(c)). ^{67}Gallium scintigraphy showed abnormal accumulation in the pituitary gland, both sides of the neck, lungs, kidneys, and the right inguinal area (Figure 1(d)). Biopsies were taken of the pituitary and lung (transbronchial). Both showed similar pathological findings, including mild fibrosis with abundant infiltration of plasma cells and lymphocytes. Nevertheless, immunohistochemical staining for IgG4 was positive for only about 10% of all IgG-positive plasma cells (Figures 2(a) and 2(b)). Although the IgG4 level was normal and IgG4-bearing cells were sparse, we strongly suspected that the patient had IgG4-related disease, due to the appearance and distribution of the lesions. We reevaluated the preserved lymph node biopsy that was acquired in 1994 and the serum that was acquired in 1995. The lymph node showed lymphoid hyperplasia with lymphocytes and plasma cells. Immunohistochemical staining revealed that over half the plasma cells were positive for IgG4 (Figures 2(c), and 2(d)). Moreover, the serum IgG4 was high (317 mg/dL). Taking these findings together,

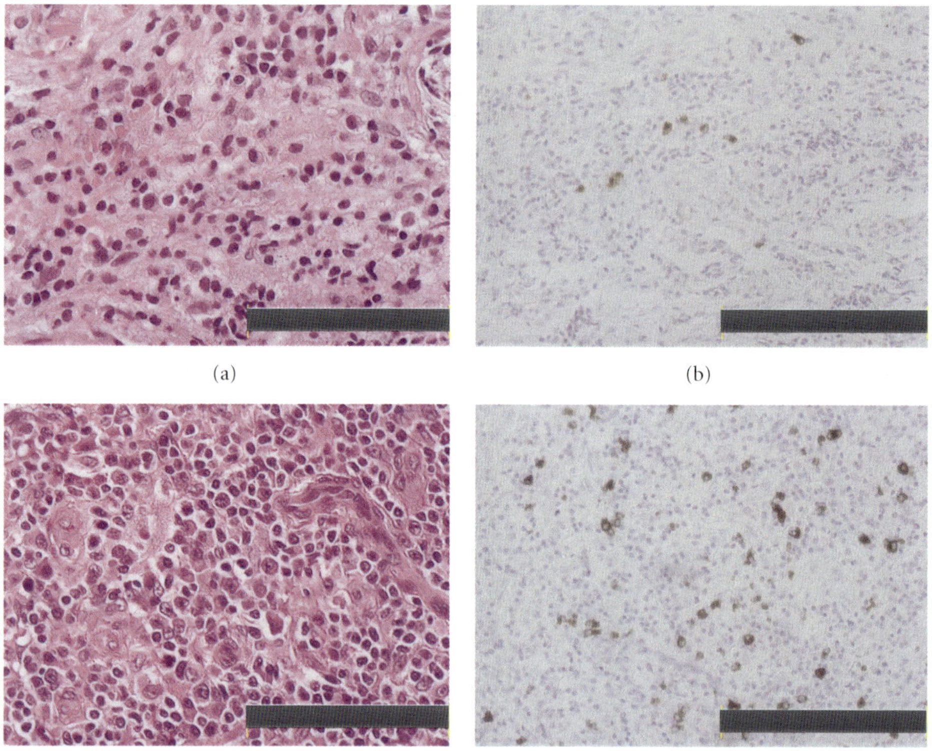

(a) (b) (c) (d)

Figure 2: Histopathology of the pituitary gland and lymph node in a patient with IgG4-related disease. (a) Hematoxylin and eosin staining of the pituitary gland (2010). Bar 100 μm. The gland structure was unclear, and numerous lymphocytes and plasma cells had infiltrated the fibrous tissue. (b) Immunohistochemical staining of the pituitary gland for IgG4 showed that IgG4-positive cells were sparse; they comprised about 10% of all IgG-positive cells. Bar 200 μm. (c) Hematoxylin and eosin staining of the lymph node (1994). Bar 100 μm. Plasma cell infiltration was abundant. (d) Immunohistochemical staining of the lymph node for IgG4 showed abundant IgG4-bearing plasma cells; they comprised over 50% of all IgG-positive cells. Bar 200 μm.

we diagnosed that the patient had had IgG4-related disease from 1994, and that the current complaint was due to a relapse. The patient was given 50 mg (1 mg/kg) PSL daily, and the visual field abnormality and lymph node swelling improved rapidly. After 4 months of treatment, serum IgG levels declined to within the normal range and the abnormal ^{67}Ga accumulation had disappeared. In October 2011, he was taking 5 mg PSL daily, and he has shown no signs of relapse.

3. Discussion

IgG4-related disease is a recently identified lymphoproliferative disorder characterized by hyper-IgG4-γ-globulinemia and IgG4-bearing plasma cell expansion in affected organs with fibrotic or sclerotic changes [5]. The disease frequently progresses in a variable pattern to involve one or multiple characteristic organs; however, the cause of this disease remains poorly understood.

In MRIs, IgG4-related disease can be characterized by hypophysitis in pituitary gland lesions [7], lymphadenopathy in the lymph node [8], inflammatory pseudotumors in the lungs [9], and multiple nodules in the kidney that lack contrast enhancement [10]. Two pathologic features characterize IgG4-related disease. First, hematoxylin and eosin staining shows lymphoplasmacytic infiltration, irregular fibrosis, occasional eosinophilic infiltration, and obliterative vasculitis, regardless of the affected organ [2]. Second, immunostaining shows a greater than 30% proportion of IgG4-positive to IgG-positive plasma cells [2]. In this study, at the current admission, the patient showed normal serum IgG4 concentrations and scarce IgG4-bearing cells in the affected tissues. However, taken together with the CT and MRI images, histopathological features of lymph nodes acquired at the onset showed greater than 50% infiltrations of IgG4-bearing plasma cells, which was consistent with a diagnosis of IgG4-related disease. Moreover, the serum from 15 years ago revealed high IgG4 levels (317 mg/dL). This led us to diagnose this case as IgG4-related disease, according to the criteria proposed by Masaki et al. as follows: (1) Characteristic diffuse/localized swelling or masses in single or multiple organs. (2) Serum IgG4 > 135 mg/dL. (3) Histopathological features that included lymphocyte and IgG4+ plasma cell infiltration (i.e., the proportion of IgG4+ plasma cells to IgG+ plasma cells > 40% and >10 IgG4+plasma cells/HPF), with typical tissue fibrosis [11].

Although the role of IgG4 in IgG4-related disease remains unknown, IgG4 has become a definitive marker; thus, we could discriminate IgG4-related disease from other inflammatory pseudotumors. In this regard, autoimmune pancreatitis is now classified into two distinct subsets, (type 1 and type 2), according to the presence or absence of infiltrating IgG4-positive plasma cells [12, 13]. However, interestingly, in this case, IgG4-positive plasma cells were abundant at the time of onset, but scarce at the time of relapse. It is unclear why IgG4-bearing plasma cell infiltration was scarce at the time of relapse; it may have been the result of long-term PSL treatment. However, the PSL dose was only 2 mg/day for over two years; this is likely to be too insubstantial to abolish infiltration.

When patients diagnosed with IgG4-related disease are admitted during a relapse, a reevaluation of the histology tends to be omitted when the clinical presentation is typical of IgG4-related disease. The present study indicated that histological evaluations of specimens should be obtained from affected organs during the course of the IgG4-related disease; these specimens may provide important information on the pathogenesis of IgG4-related disease.

References

[1] H. Hamano, S. Kawa, A. Horiuchi et al., "High serum IgG4 concentrations in patients with sclerosing pancreatitis," *New England Journal of Medicine*, vol. 344, no. 10, pp. 732–738, 2001.

[2] Y. Zen and Y. Nakanuma, "IgG4-related disease: a cross-sectional study of 114 cases," *American Journal of Surgical Pathology*, vol. 34, no. 12, pp. 1812–1819, 2010.

[3] T. Tabata, T. Kamisawa, K. Takuma et al., "Serum IgG4 concentrations and IgG4-related sclerosing disease," *Clinica Chimica Acta*, vol. 408, no. 1-2, pp. 25–28, 2009.

[4] A. Khosroshahi and J. H. Stone, "A clinical overview of IgG4-related systemic disease," *Current Opinion in Rheumatology*, vol. 23, no. 1, pp. 57–66, 2011.

[5] Y. Masaki, N. Kurose, and H. Umehara, "IgG4-related disease: a novel lymphoproliferative disorder discovered and established in Japan in the 21st century," *Journal of Clinical and Experimental Hematopathology*, vol. 51, no. 1, pp. 13–20, 2011.

[6] H. Takahashi and M. Zeniya, "Acute presentation of autoimmune hepatitis: does it exist? A published work review," *Hepatology Research*, vol. 41, no. 6, pp. 498–504, 2011.

[7] P. Leporati, M. A. Landek-Salgado, I. Lupi, L. Chiovato, and P. Caturegli, "IgG4-related hypophysitis: a new addition to the hypophysitis spectrum," *Journal of Clinical Endocrinology and Metabolism*, vol. 96, no. 7, pp. 1971–1980, 2011.

[8] W. Cheuk, H. K. L. Yuen, S. Y. Y. Chu, E. K. W. Chiu, L. K. Lam, and J. K. C. Chan, "Lymphadenopathy of IgG4-related sclerosing disease," *American Journal of Surgical Pathology*, vol. 32, no. 5, pp. 671–681, 2008.

[9] Y. Zen, S. Kitagawa, H. Minato et al., "IgG4-positive plasma cells in inflammatory pseudotumor (plasma cell granuloma) of the lung," *Human Pathology*, vol. 36, no. 7, pp. 710–717, 2005.

[10] C. Triantopoulou, G. Malachias, P. Maniatis, J. Anastopoulos, I. Siafas, and J. Papailiou, "Renal lesions associated with autoimmune pancreatitis: CT findings," *Acta Radiologica*, vol. 51, no. 6, pp. 702–707, 2010.

[11] H. Umehara, K. Okazaki, Y. Masaki et al., "Comprehensive diagnostic criteria for IgG4 related disease (IgG4-RD), 2011," *Modern Rheumatology*, vol. 22, no. 1, pp. 21–30, 2012.

[12] A. Sugumar, G. Klöppel, and S. T. Chari, "Autoimmune pancreatitis: pathologic subtypes and their implications for its diagnosis," *American Journal of Gastroenterology*, vol. 104, no. 9, pp. 2308–2310, 2009.

[13] D. H. Park, M. H. Kim, and S. T. Chari, "Recent advances in autoimmune pancreatitis," *Gut*, vol. 58, no. 12, pp. 1680–1689, 2009.

20

Three Cases of Previous Smokers with Rheumatoid Arthritis Who Did Not Respond to Tumor Necrosis Factor Inhibitors Were Treated Successfully with an Anti-Interleukin-6 Receptor Antibody

Yasuo Iwata

Iwata Orthopedics and Rheumatology Clinic, No. 13-5, 1A Nakasuji 8-Chome, Takarazuka, Hyogo 665-9874, Japan

Correspondence should be addressed to Yasuo Iwata; iwataseikei@yahoo.co.jp

Academic Editor: Suleyman Serdar Koca

We report three cases of previous smokers who did not respond to TNF inhibitors but who responded successfully to an anti-interleukin-6 receptor antibody (tocilizumab (TCZ)). Case 1 is a 63-year-old woman whose smoking index was 200 and had been complaining of polyarthralgia since 1996. She started treatment with etanercept due to high disease activity, but her DAS28-CRP was 4.2. She was therefore switched to TCZ, which dramatically improved her symptoms; her DAS28-CRP had decreased to 2.1. Case 2 is a 64-year-old man whose smoking index was 1600 and had been complaining of polyarthralgia since 2006. Because his DAS28-CRP score increased over time to 5.9, etanercept and adalimumab were added sequentially, but he showed no response over the course of two years. The patient was therefore switched to TCZ, which dramatically improved his symptoms: his DAS28-CRP decreased to 2.7. Case 3 is a 48-year-old woman whose smoking index was 560 and had been complaining of pain in both knee joints since 2001. She was treated with adalimumab due to high disease activity but showed no response over the course of 1.5 years. The patient was therefore switched to TCZ, and her DAS28-CRP decreased to 1.8. An IL-6 blockade might be suitable for treating these 3 cases of previous smokers.

1. Introduction

Tumor necrosis factor (TNF) inhibitors represent an important advance in therapy for rheumatoid arthritis (RA). RA patients who smoke, however, are reported to be less likely to respond to treatment with TNF inhibitors [1–4]. This report presents three cases of smokers who did not respond to TNF inhibitors but who responded successfully to an anti-interleukin-6 receptor antibody (tocilizumab [TCZ]).

2. A Case Report

Case 1 is a 63-year-old woman whose smoking index was 200 (10 cigarettes/day × 20 years) (Table 1) and had been complaining of polyarthralgia since 1996. She could not take methotrexate due to the adverse effects of liver dysfunction and hair loss. During treatment for RA, she was able to quit smoking as per our instructions. Two years after her first visit, the lateral tibial condyle of her right knee joint collapsed. As a result, she underwent total knee arthroplasty. She started treatment with the TNF inhibitor etanercept due to high disease activity (Disease Activity Score assessing 28 joints with C-reactive protein [DAS28-CRP] was 4) 1.5 years after cessation of smoking but showed no response. Two years after starting this medication, her DAS28-CRP was 4.2 and her MMP-3 was 405 ng/mL. The patient was therefore switched to TCZ (8 mg/kg monthly), which dramatically improved her symptoms. Six months after switching to TCZ, her DAS28-CRP had decreased to less than 2.3 and her MMP-3 had decreased from 405 to less than 59.7 ng/mL (Figure 1). She has satisfied the Boolean-based definition for over 10 months after the cessation of the TCZ therapy. Recent radiograms of the involved joints show nonprogression.

Case 2 is a 64-year-old man whose smoking index was 1600 (40 cigarettes/day × 40 years) (Table 1) and had been complaining of polyarthralgia since 2006. He did not respond

Table 1: Characteristics of patients.

	Case 1	Case 2	Case 3
Sex	Female	Male	Female
Age (years)	63	64	48
Disease duration (years)	12	6	8
Smoking index	200 (10 cigarettes/day × 20 years)	1600 (40 cigarettes/day × 40 years)	560 (20 cigarettes/day × 28 years)
2010 ACR/EULAR classification criteria	Satisfied	Satisfied	Satisfied
Laboratory results	RF 73.8 U/mL ACPA 4.4 U/mL CRP 2.9 mg/dL WBC 11500/μL MMP-3 698.7 ng/mL Platelet $37.1 \times 10^4/\mu$L	RF 60.0 U/mL ACPA 150.0 U/mL CRP 1.5 mg/dL WBC 8600/μL MMP-3 148.1 ng/mL Platelet $35.0 \times 10^4/\mu$L	RF 26.0 U/mL ACPA 128.6 U/mL CRP 0.07 mg/dL WBC 12400/μL MMP-3 179.5 ng/mL Platelet $42.1 \times 10^4/\mu$L
Steinbrocker's roentgenographic classification	Stage IV	Stage III	Stage III
Functional status according to Steinbrocker's revised criteria	Class II	Class II	Class II
Previous treatment: type and dosage (duration in months)	Etanercept 50 mg/week (26) Prednisolone 3 mg/day (62) Bucillamine 200 mg/day (52)	Etanercept 25–50 mg/week (13) Adalimumab 40 mg/2 weeks (4) Methotrexate 8 mg/week (72) Prednisolone 5 mg/day (36) Bucillamine 200 mg/day (48) Gold sodium thiomalate 10 mg/week (24) Mizoribine 150 mg/day (18)	Adalimumab 40 mg/2 weeks (4) Methotrexate 6 mg/week (72) Prednisolone 9 mg/day (36) Salazosulfapyridine 1000 mg/day (6) Mizoribine 200 mg/day (18)
Time (months) to remission of arthritis (DAS28-CRP <2.3)	11	16	1

RF: rheumatoid factor; ACPA: anti-cyclic citrullinated peptide antibody; CRP: C-reactive protein; WBC: white blood cell count; MMP-3: matrix metalloproteinase-3.

to a combination of methotrexate (8 mg/week), prednisolone (10 mg/day), bucillamine (200 mg/day), and intramuscular injections of gold sodium thiomalate (10 mg/week). During treatment for RA, because his DAS28-CRP score increased over time to 5.9 and because he developed active synovitis of the cervical vertebra, etanercept (50 mg/week) was added to his medications one month after he quit smoking as per our instructions, but the patient showed no response over the course of one year. The etanercept was then replaced with adalimumab (40 mg/2 weeks), but the patient still had no response. Four months after adalimumab was started, his DAS28-CRP was 5.7 and his MMP-3 was 251.9 ng/mL. The patient was therefore switched to TCZ (8 mg/kg monthly), which dramatically improved his symptoms. After switching to TCZ, his DAS28-CRP decreased to less than 2.3 and his MMP-3 decreased to 85.9 ng/mL, but his global assessment ranged from 4 to 5 cm (Figure 2). Recent radiograms of the involved joints show no erosive progression.

Case 3 is a 48-year-old woman whose smoking index was 560 (20 cigarettes/day × 28 years) (Table 1) and had been complaining of pain in both knee joints since 2001. She was initially treated with a combination of prednisolone (10 mg/day) and methotrexate (8 mg/week) but did not respond to these medications despite the fact that she was simultaneously undergoing smoking cessation treatment. She was then switched to treatment with adalimumab (40 mg/2 weeks) due to high disease activity 2 months after she quit smoking but showed no response to the new medication over the course of 1.5 years. At the end of this period, her DAS28-CRP was 3.2 and her MMP-3 was 88.2 ng/mL. The patient was therefore switched to TCZ (8 mg/kg monthly), which dramatically improved her symptoms. After a single drip infusion of TCZ, her DAS28-CRP decreased to 1.8 and her MMP-3 decreased to 59.5 ng/mL (Figure 3). She has since satisfied the Boolean-based definition for 5 months. The latest radiographic examination of the involved joints showed no progression of bone erosion.

3. Discussion

Papadopoulos defined a previous smoker as a person who had stopped smoking for at least one year [5]. Cases 2 and 3 were treated with biologics in less than 3 months after smoking cessation; these two cases could therefore be considered current smokers. For case 1 who had smoked for 20 years, the influence of smoking was assumed to exist although etanercept was initiated 1.5 years after quitting smoking. It is said that even if quitting smoking can be achieved, it takes

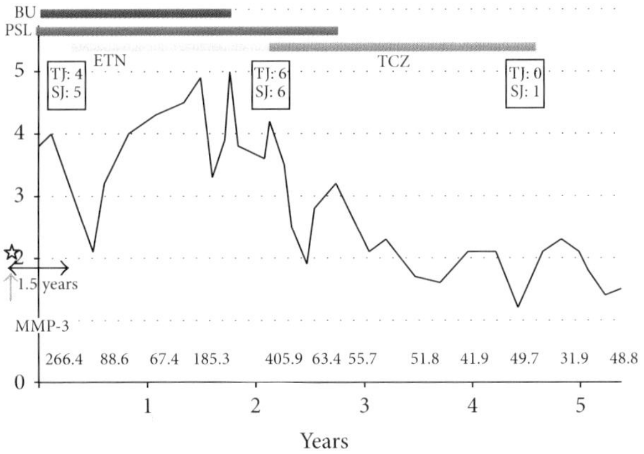

FIGURE 1: Summary of the clinical course of case 1. DAS28-CRP Disease Activity Score assessing 28 joints with C-reactive protein. SASP: salazosulfapyridine, PSL: prednisolone, ETN: etanercept, TCZ: tocilizumab, and MMP-3: matrix metalloproteinase-3. TJ means tender joint counts and SJ means swollen joints counts for the assessment of DAS 28-CRP. The asterisk shows the cessation of smoking. Etanercept was initiated 1.5 years after the cessation of smoking.

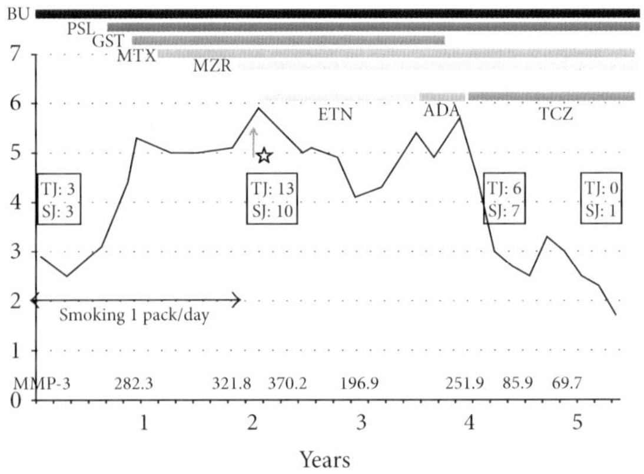

FIGURE 2: Summary of the clinical course of case 2. DAS28-CRP Disease Activity Score assessing 28 joints with C-reactive protein. BU: bucillamine, PSL: prednisolone, GST: gold sodium thiomalate, MTX: methotrexate, MZR: mizoribine, ETN: etanercept, ADA: adalimumab, TCZ: tocilizumab, and MMP-3: matrix metalloproteinase-3. The asterisk shows the cessation of smoking. TJ means tender joint counts and SJ means swollen joints counts for the assessment of DAS 28-CRP.

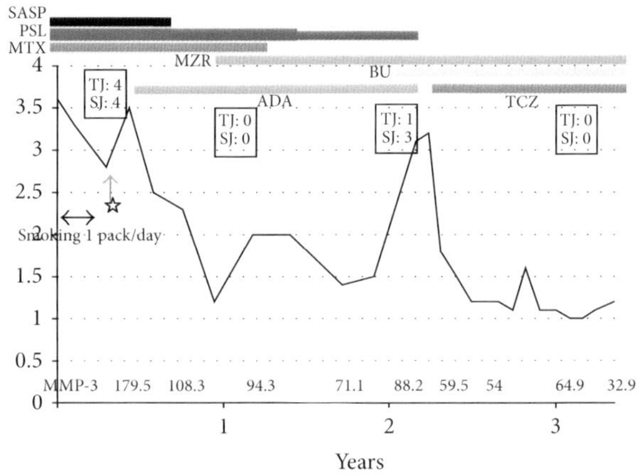

FIGURE 3: Summary of the clinical course of case 3. DAS28-CRP Disease Activity Score assessing 28 joints with C-reactive protein. SASP: salazosulfapyridine, PSL: prednisolone, MTX: methotrexate, MZR: mizoribine, BU: bucillamine, ADA: adalimumab, TCZ: tocilizumab, and MMP-3: matrix metalloproteinase-3. The asterisk shows the cessation of smoking. TJ means tender joint counts and SJ means swollen joints counts for the assessment of DAS 28-CRP.

at least 10 years until the influence of smoking disappears from the body [6]. Karlson et al. reported that duration of smoking was associated with a significantly increased risk of developing RA but that smoking intensity (number of cigarettes/day) was unrelated to risk of RA [7].

In case 3, DAS 28-CRP might get better with the use of mizoribine, but the clinical course showed a relapse of arthritis with the use of mizoribine and, after a single drip infusion of TCZ, her DAS28-CRP decreased to 1.8. It is reasonable to assume that TCZ was effective for her RA.

Anti-TNF-alpha agents were reported to have been less effective for the treatment of RA in current and previous smokers [1–4]. The three cases presented herein were also refractory to anti-TNF agents, although the patients had stopped smoking before the administration of anti-TNF agents. The SAMURAI study demonstrated efficacy in patients with RA treated with TCZ monotherapy [8]. Patients with multidrug refractory adult onset Still's disease (AOSD) were successfully treated with TCZ [9–13].

The relationship between cigarette smoking and the improved response to TCZ probably likely has several explanations. In terms of the relation between smoking and periodontitis, smoking is a major risk factor for periodontitis [14–16]. Sites from refractory patient with periodontitis produced significantly more IL-6 [17]. Fibroblasts from periodontal lesions in vitro produce greater amounts of IL-6 and IL-8 constitutively than healthy controls [18]. In periodontitis stroma, increased citrullinated protein presence (80%) was observed compared with control stroma (33%). Western blotting with monoclonal (F95) antibody to citrullinated proteins revealed the presence of similar citrullinated proteins in both periodontitis and RA-affected synovial tissue [19]. These three cases did not complain of oral problems. There are some reports on the relationship between IL-6 in the lungs and smoking. Higher IL-6 and exhaled carbon monoxide (CO) concentrations were found in the exhaled breath condensate of smokers than in that of nonsmokers. In addition, there was a correlation between IL-6 concentrations, number of cigarettes smoked per day, exhaled CO, leukotriene, and lung function [20]. In bronchoalveolar lavage (BAL), statistically greater concentrations of neutrophils, macrophages, IL-1 beta, IL-6, IL-8, and monocyte chemotactic protein-1 (MCP-1) were observed among smokers compared with nonsmokers [21]. Smoking increases peptidylarginine deiminase 2 enzyme expression in the human lungs and increases citrullination in BAL cells [22]. Snelgrove reported that cigarette smoke selectively inhibited leukotriene A(4) hydrolase aminopeptidase activity, which led to the accumulation of the neutrophil chemoattractant proline-glycine-proline and neutrophils, and made inflammation become chronic such as chronic obstructive pulmonary disease (COPD) and cystic fibrosis [23]. Cigarette smoke induces proinflammatory cytokines and chemokines, including IL-1 beta, and IL-6 from synovial fibroblast-like cells (SFCs) [24]. And blood leukocytes, platelets, C-reactive protein (CRP), and fibrinogen were reported to be significantly high in smokers [25]. Mean platelet volume increased significantly with acute exposure to smoking [26]. IL-6 stimulates thrombopoiesis through thrombopoietin [27], and IL-6 activates platelets [28]. Boilard et al. surveyed the capacity of collagen-stimulated human platelet microparticles (MPs) to elicit a range of cytokines and chemokines from fibroblast-like synoviocytes (FLSs) and observed prominent production of the broadly inflammatory cytokine IL-6 and the neutrophil chemoattractant IL-8 without production of TNF alpha [29]. Therefore, the positive feedback of IL-6 through fibroblast-like synoviocytes and platelets is formed in the human body. In this case report, cases 1 and 3 showed elevation of platelet count.

Smoking is an established risk factor of RA and may cause prominent production of cytokines especially IL-6 (as described above). An IL-6 blockade might be suitable for treating these 3 cases. But this is a case report; however, further study of a large series of cases is required to determine the efficacy of an IL-6 blockade for patients with RA who smoke.

References

[1] D. L. Mattey, A. Brownfield, and P. T. Dawes, "Relationship between pack-year history of smoking and response to tumor necrosis factor antagonists in patients with rheumatoid arthritis," *Journal of Rheumatology*, vol. 36, no. 6, pp. 1180–1187, 2009.

[2] A. Abhishek, S. Butt, K. Gadsby, W. Zhang, and C. M. Deighton, "Anti-TNF-α agents are less effective for the treatment of rheumatoid arthritis in current smokers," *Journal of Clinical Rheumatology*, vol. 16, no. 1, pp. 15–18, 2010.

[3] S. Saevarsdottir, S. Wedrén, M. Seddighzadeh et al., " Patients with early rheumatoid arthritis who smoke are less likely to respond to treatment with methotrexate and tumor necrosis factor inhibitors. observations from the epidemiological investigation of rheumatoid arthritis and the Swedish rheumatology register cohorts," *Arthritis and Rheumatism*, vol. 63, no. 1, pp. 26–36, 2011.

[4] M. K. Söderlin, I. F. Petersson, and P. Geborek, "The effect of smoking on response and drug survival in rheumatoid arthritis patients treated with their first anti-TNF drug," *Scandinavian Journal of Rheumatology*, vol. 41, no. 1, pp. 1–9, 2012.

[5] N. G. Papadopoulos, Y. Alamanos, P. V. Voulgari, E. K. Epagelis, N. Tsifetaki, and A. A. Drosos, "Does cigarette smoking influence disease expression, activity and severity in early rheumatoid arthritis patients?" *Clinical and Experimental Rheumatology*, vol. 23, no. 6, pp. 861–866, 2005.

[6] S. Musich, S. D. Faruzzi, C. Lu, T. McDonald, D. Hirschland, and D. W. Edington, "Pattern of medical charges after quitting smoking among those with and without arthritis, allergies, or back pain," *The American Journal of Health Promotion*, vol. 18, no. 2, pp. 133–142, 2003.

[7] E. W. Karlson, I. M. Lee, N. R. Cook, J. E. Manson, J. E. Buring, and C. H. Hennekens, "A retrospective cohort study of cigarette smoking and risk of rheumatoid arthritis in female health professionals," *Arthritis & Rheumatism*, vol. 42, no. 5, pp. 910–917, 1999.

[8] N. Nishimoto, J. Hashimoto, N. Miyasaka et al., "Study of active controlled monotherapy used for rheumatoid arthritis, an IL-6 inhibitor (SAMURAI): evidence of clinical and radiographic benefit from an x ray reader-blinded randomised controlled trial of tocilizumab," *Annals of the Rheumatic Diseases*, vol. 66, no. 9, pp. 1162–1167, 2007.

[9] M. de Bandt and B. Saint-Marcoux, "Tocilizumab for multirefractory adult-onset Still's disease," *Annals of the Rheumatic Diseases*, vol. 68, no. 1, pp. 153–154, 2009.

[10] K. Matsumoto, T. Nagashima, S. Takatori et al., "Glucocorticoid and cyclosporine refractory adult onset Still's disease successfully treated with tocilizumab," *Clinical Rheumatology*, vol. 28, no. 4, pp. 485–487, 2009.

[11] M. Yoshimura, J. Makiyama, T. Koga et al., "Successful treatment with tocilizumab in a patient with refractory adult-onset Still's disease (AOSD)," *Clinical and Experimental Rheumatology*, vol. 28, no. 1, pp. 141–142, 2010.

[12] K. Perdan-Pirkmajer, S. Praprotnik, and M. Tomšič, "A case of refractory adult-onset Still's disease successfully controlled with tocilizumab and a review of the literature," *Clinical Rheumatology*, vol. 29, no. 12, pp. 1465–1467, 2010.

[13] J. Rech, M. Ronneberger, M. Englbrecht et al., "Successful treatment of adult-onset Still's disease refractory to TNF and IL-1 blockade by IL-6 receptor blockade," *Annals of the Rheumatic Diseases*, vol. 70, no. 2, pp. 390–392, 2011.

[14] S. L. Tomar and S. Asma, "Smoking-attributable periodontitis in the United States: findings from NHANES III," *Journal of Periodontology*, vol. 71, no. 5, pp. 743–751, 2000.

[15] B. H. Mullally, "The influence of tobacco smoking on the onset of periodontitis in young persons," *Tobacco Induced Diseases*, vol. 15, no. 2, pp. 53–65, 2004.

[16] Y. Yamamoto, N. Nishida, M. Tanaka et al., "Association between passive and active smoking evaluated by salivary cotinine and periodontitis," *Journal of Clinical Periodontology*, vol. 32, no. 10, pp. 1041–1046, 2005.

[17] R. A. Reinhardt, M. P. Masada, W. B. Kaldahl et al., "Gingival fluid IL-1 and IL-6 levels in refractory periodontitis," *Journal of Clinical Periodontology*, vol. 20, no. 3, pp. 225–231, 1993.

[18] A. I. Dongari-Bagtzoglou and J. L. Ebersole, "Increased presence of interleukin-6 (IL-6) and IL-8 secreting fibroblast subpopulations in adult periodontitis," *Journal of Periodontology*, vol. 69, no. 8, pp. 899–910, 1998.

[19] W. Nesse, J. Westra, J. E. van der Wal et al., "The periodontium of periodontitis patients contains citrullinated proteins which may play a role in ACPA (anti-citrullinated protein antibody) formation," *Journal of Clinical Periodontology*, vol. 39, no. 7, pp. 599–607, 2012.

[20] G. E. Carpagnano, S. A. Kharitonov, M. P. Foschino-Barbaro, O. Resta, E. Gramiccioni, and P. J. Barnes, "Increase inflammatory markers in the exhaled breath condensate of cigarette smokers," *The European Respiratory Journal*, vol. 21, no. 4, pp. 589–593, 2003.

[21] W. G. Kuschner, A. D'Alessandro, H. Wong, and P. D. Blanc, "Dose-dependent cigarette smoking-related inflammatory responses in healthy adults," *European Respiratory Journal*, vol. 9, no. 10, pp. 1989–1994, 1996.

[22] D. Makrygiannakis, M. Hermansson, A.-K. Ulfgren et al., "Smoking increases peptidylarginine deiminase 2 enzyme expression in human lungs and increases citrullination in BAL cells," *Annals of the Rheumatic Diseases*, vol. 67, no. 10, pp. 1488–1492, 2008.

[23] R. J. Snelgrove, P. L. Jackson, M. T. Hardison et al., "A critical role for LTA4H in limiting chronic pulmonary neutrophilic inflammation," *Science*, vol. 330, no. 6000, pp. 90–94, 2010.

[24] M. Shizu, Y. Itoh, R. Sunahara et al., "Cigarette smoke condensate upregulates the gene and protein expression of proinflammatory cytokines in human fibroblast-like synoviocyte line," *Journal of Interferon and Cytokine Research*, vol. 28, no. 8, pp. 509–521, 2007.

[25] H. Yasue, N. Hirai, Y. Mizuno et al., "Low-grade inflammation, thrombogenicity, and atherogenic lipid profile in cigarette smokers," *Circulation Journal*, vol. 70, no. 1, pp. 8–13, 2006.

[26] M. Yarlioglues, I. Ardic, O. Dogdu et al., "The acute effects of passive smoking on mean platelet volume in healthy volunteers," *Angiology*, vol. 63, no. 5, pp. 353–357, 2012.

[27] A. Kaser, G. Brandacher, W. Steurer et al., "Interleukin-6 stimulates thrombopoiesis through thrombopoietin: role in inflammatory thrombocytosis," *Blood*, vol. 98, no. 9, pp. 2720–2725, 2001.

[28] L. Oleksowicz, Z. Mrowiec, D. Zuckerman, R. Isaacs, J. Dutcher, and E. Puszkin, "Platelet activation induced by interleukin-6: evidence for a mechanism involving arachidonic acid metabolism," *Thrombosis and Haemostasis*, vol. 72, no. 2, pp. 302–308, 1994.

[29] E. Boilard, P. A. Nigrovic, K. Larabee et al., "Platelets amplify inflammation in arthritis via collagen-dependent microparticle production," *Science*, vol. 327, no. 5965, pp. 580–583, 2010.

21

Large Pyoderma Gangrenosum-Like Ulcers: A Rare Presentation of Granulomatosis with Polyangiitis

Basheer Tashtoush,[1] Roya Memarpour,[1] Yasmin Johnston,[2] and Jose Ramirez[1]

[1] *Department of Pulmonary and Critical Care Medicine, Cleveland Clinic Florida, 2950 Cleveland Clinic Boulevard, Weston, FL 33331, USA*
[2] *Department of Clinical Pathology, Cleveland Clinic Florida, 2950 Cleveland Clinic Boulevard, Weston, FL 33331, USA*

Correspondence should be addressed to Basheer Tashtoush; tashtob@ccf.org

Academic Editor: Tsai-Ching Hsu

Granulomatosis with polyangiitis (GPA), formerly known as Wegener's granulomatosis (WG), is a rare systemic vasculitis that classically manifests as necrotizing granulomas of the upper and lower respiratory tract, kidneys, and blood vessels; however, it may affect any organ system, including the skin. Cutaneous manifestations occur in up to 45% of patients during the disease course, and are the presenting feature in 9% to 14% of patients. The most common skin lesion specific to GPA is palpable purpura, with the histopathologic correlate of leukocytoclastic vasculitis. However, a wide range of clinical and histologic features may be seen. We herein report a case of a previously healthy 52-year-old Caucasian man who presented with multiple progressively enlarging painful ulcers on his face, upper extremities, back, and abdomen over a two-month period. Skin biopsies revealed pyoderma gangrenosum-like features. Serological tests were positive for PR3/c-ANCA. Six months later, the patient developed recurrent episodes of sinusitis associated with nasal bleeds and eventually nasal septum perforation. Despite aggressive treatment with Cyclophosphamide and steroids over one year, the patient had persistent nonhealing large ulcers and developed multiple lung nodules with cavitary lesions.

1. Introduction

The hallmarks of GPA are systemic necrotizing vasculitis, necrotising granulomatous inflammation, and necrotising glomerulonephritis. The etiology of GPA is thought to be linked to environmental and infectious triggers inciting onset of disease in genetically predisposed individuals. Antineutrophil cytoplasmic antibodies (ANCAs) play an important role in the pathogenesis of this disease, although ANCA positivity is not essential for a clinical diagnosis of GPA. The diagnosis is based on clinical manifestations of systemic vasculitis and histological evidence of necrotizing vasculitis or granulomatous inflammation.

2. Case Presentation

A 52-year-old Caucasian man presented with multiple large nonhealing ulcers on his upper extremities and back that started two months earlier. He stated that he was previously healthy when he bumped into a shelf at the supermarket and superficially scratched his arm. Over the next week, his wife noticed that the scratch became erythematous and increased in size. After completing treatment with a course of antibiotics, the scratched area soon became tender and black in color. A skin biopsy showed areas of acute and chronic inflammation with dermal necrosis and negative for microorganisms on stains and cultures. At the site of the biopsy purulent drainage was noted and an ulcer developed. Over the next two months, the patient developed multiple painful ulcers over the face, back, and abdomen. These ulcers all began as areas of intense erythema and tenderness with subsequent purulent drainage and ulceration (Figures 1(a) and 1(b)).

Repeated microbial stains and cultures showed negative results, and repeated biopsies from several ulcers (Figures 2, 3, and 4) showed pyoderma gangrenosum-like features with

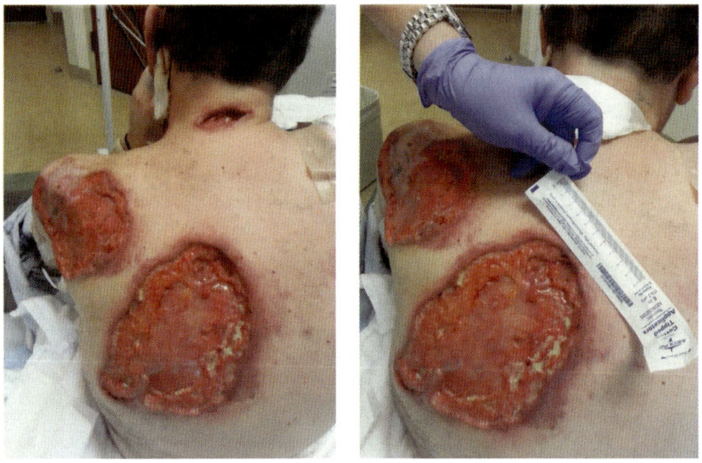

(a) (b)

Figure 1: (a) and (b) Multiple large ulcers with irregular, violaceous, undermined borders and yellow necrotic centers, with the largest measuring 20×10 cm.

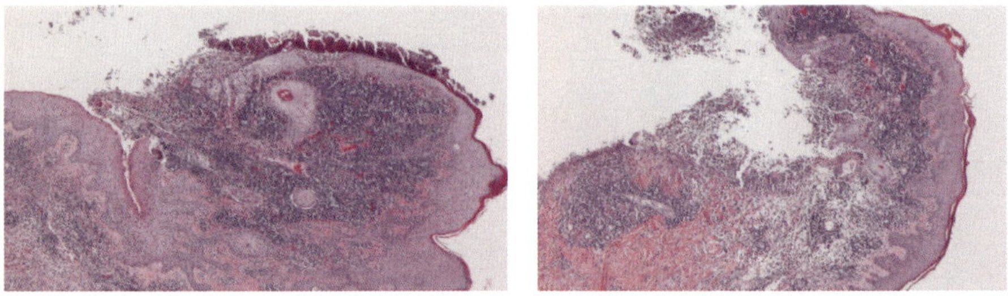

(a) (b)

Figure 2: (a) and (b) (4x) Surface ulcerations with mixed acute and chronic inflammation and overlying fibrinopurulent exudate.

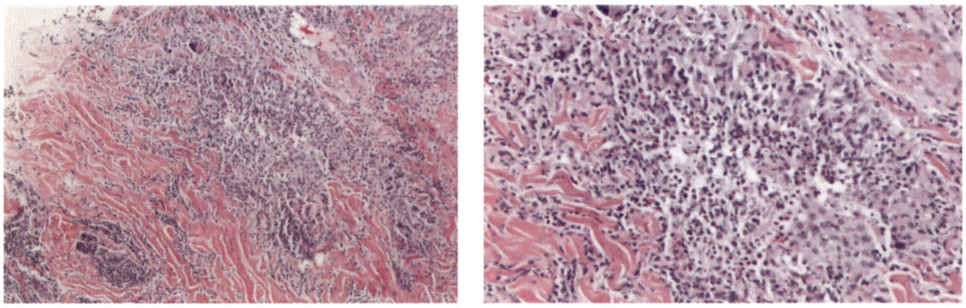

(c) (d)

Figure 3: (c) (10x) and (d) (20x) Microgranulomas with suppurative necrosis. Small foci of tissue necrosis with acute inflammation, surrounded by histiocytes and multinucleated giant cells (arrows).

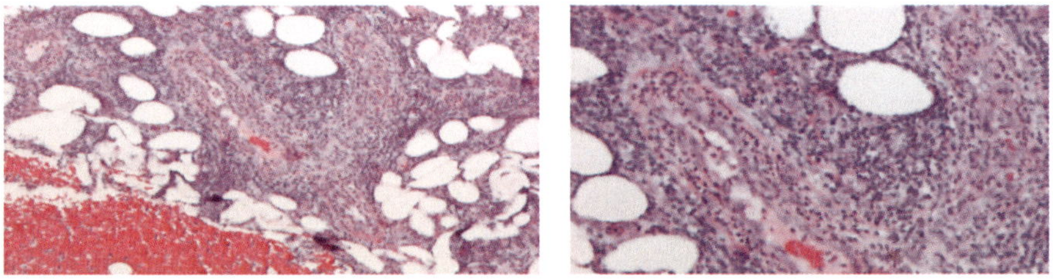

(e) (f)

Figure 4: (e) (10x) and (f) (20x) Vessels in the deep dermis and subcutis are infiltrated by neutrophils and have fibrin in their walls.

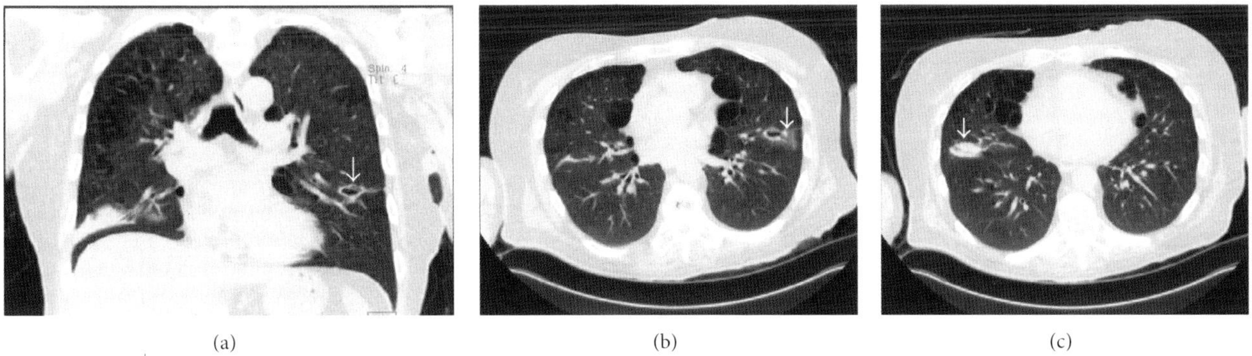

FIGURE 5: Chest CT scan. Coronal view (a) and axial views ((b) and (c)) showing a right lower lobe mass-like dense opacity with a left lower lobe cavitary lesion (arrows) and upper lobe predominant paraseptal emphysema.

foci of prominent granulomatous and neutrophilic necrotizing vasculitis with basophilic collagen degeneration. Serological testing was positive for PR3/c-ANCA. Treatment was initiated with Cyclophosphamide and steroids, but persistent nonhealing ulcers remained and became infected requiring frequent antimicrobial treatment and careful debridement.

Six months after the first ulcer, recurrent episodes of purulent nasal discharge and epistaxis were reported by the patient and a perforated nasal septum was seen on physical exam. Pulmonary evaluation revealed multiple lung opacities with cavitary lesions (Figure 5).

The patient underwent a bronchoscopy procedure with a bronchoalveolar lavage (BAL) from the lung segments corresponding to the cavitary and mass-like lesions, with negative results on gram stain, cultures, and acid fast bacilli staining, as well as absent growth on fungal and mycobacterial cultures. However, the BAL samples showed neutrophil predominant cells, 52% neutrophils, with no evidence of malignant cells on cytological exam, indicating an inflammatory lung disease. The clinical history and BAL results were supportive of GPA lung disease.

The patient had a modest response to treatment with Methotrexate, characterized by reduced inflammation at the ulcer margins, and repeated serological tests 3 months after initiating Methotrexate showed negative PR3/c-ANCA results; however Methotrexate was discontinued for gastrointestinal side effects and treatment with Rituximab was initiated.

A reduction in the size of ulcers and surrounding inflammation was described a few months after initiating Rituximab.

3. Discussion

No reliable test can identify which patients with GPA skin lesions will eventually show systemic signs and symptoms [1, 2].

The presence of compatible histologic features of GPA, cutaneous manifestations, and positive c-ANCA/PR3-ANCA serologic test results should raise clinical suspicion for the subsequent development of systemic disease. Such patients should have frequent follow-up evaluations to be screened for internal organ involvement, and appropriate management should be initiated early in the disease course. Serial tests for ANCAs are recommended because ANCA levels correlate with disease activity [3].

Differential diagnosis for refractory cases of cutaneous GPA must include indolent infectious etiologies, such as mycobacterial infections and cutaneous leishmaniasis, where biopsies also show a granulomatous inflammation [4].

The most common skin lesions are palpable purpura, necrotic ulcerations, papules and nodules with many histological patterns, leukocytoclastic vasculitis, granulomatous vasculitis, and palisading granulomas [5].

In a retrospective analysis by Daoud et al. on 244 cases of GPA, necrotizing ulcerations resembling pyoderma gangrenosum were not uncommon. Leukocytoclastic vasculitis was the most common cutaneous pathologic pattern. Findings of c-ANCA were positive in 81% of patients with cutaneous GPA [6].

Treatment strategies are tailored to the severity of the disease. They are based on published evidence of the efficacy and safety of the immunosuppressive drugs indicated to manage active vasculitis and maintain clinical remission.

Currently, hopes are raised by biological agents. Rituximab is one of the best studies of monoclonal antibodies used as an alternative treatment for patients with refractory disease [7, 8].

4. Conclusion

Pyoderma gangrenosum-like lesions in GPA have been rarely reported. In these cases, multiple devastating pyoderma gangrenosum-like lesions and disease activity were controlled with biologic agents, which may prove to be effective in this subcategory of patients who are refractory to standard immunosuppressive therapy.

References

[1] J. B. Hall, B. M. Wadham, C. J. Wood, V. Ashton, and W. R. Adam, "Vasculitis and glomerulonephritis: a subgroup with an antineutrophil cytoplasmic antibody," *Australian and New Zealand Journal of Medicine*, vol. 14, no. 3, pp. 277–278, 1984.

[2] F. J. Van Der Woude, N. Rasmussen, S. Lobatto et al., "Autoantibodies against neutrophils and monocytes: tool for diagnosis and marker of disease activity in Wegener's granulomatosis," *The Lancet*, vol. 1, no. 8426, pp. 425–429, 1985.

[3] J. D. Finkielman, P. A. Merkel, D. Schroeder et al., "Antiproteinase 3 antineutrophil cytoplasmic antibodies and disease activity in Wegener granulomatosis," *Annals of Internal Medicine*, vol. 147, no. 9, pp. 611–619, 2007.

[4] E. Brahn, D. A. Pegues, Q. Yao, and N. Craft, "Mucocutaneous leishmaniasis masquerading as Wegener granulomatosis," *Journal of Clinical Rheumatology*, vol. 16, no. 3, pp. 125–128, 2010.

[5] A. S. Fauci, B. F. Haynes, P. Katz, and S. M. Wolff, "Wegener's granulomatosis: prospective clinical and therapeutic experience with 85 patients for 21 years," *Annals of Internal Medicine*, vol. 98, no. 1, pp. 76–85, 1983.

[6] M. S. Daoud, L. E. Gibson, R. A. DeRemee, U. Specks, R. A. El-Azhary, and W. P. D. Su, "Cutaneous Wegener's granulomatosis: clinical, histopathologic, and immunopathologic features of thirty patients," *Journal of the American Academy of Dermatology*, vol. 31, no. 4, pp. 605–612, 1994.

[7] P. Seo, U. Specks, and K. A. Keogh, "Efficacy of rituximab in limited Wegener's granulomatosis with refractory granulomatous manifestations," *Journal of Rheumatology*, vol. 35, no. 10, pp. 2017–2023, 2008.

[8] S. Donmez, O. N. Pamuk, M. Gedik, R. Ak, and G. Bulut, "A case of granulomatosis with polyangiitis and pyoderma gangrenosum successfully treated with infliximab and rituximab," *International Journal of Rheumatic Diseases*, 2014.

22

Acute Hemorrhagic Myositis in Inflammatory Myopathy

Howard Van Gelder,[1] Kim M. Wu,[1] Nayiri Gharibian,[2] Dharmi B. Patel,[2] Philip J. Clements,[1] Emil R. Heinze,[1,2] Robert I. Morris,[1] and Andrew L. Wong[1,2]

[1] *UCLA-Olive View Rheumatology Program, Division of Rheumatology, Olive View-UCLA Medical Center, 14445 Olive View Drive, 2B182, Sylmar, CA 91342, USA*
[2] *UCLA-Olive View Internal Medicine Program, Department of Medicine, Olive View-UCLA Medical Center, 14445 Olive View Drive, 2B182, Sylmar, CA 91342, USA*

Correspondence should be addressed to Andrew L. Wong; alunwong@ucla.edu

Academic Editor: Masataka Kuwana

We describe two patients with dermatomyositis that presented with interstitial lung disease, positive V and Shawl sign who developed acute spontaneous abdominal/retroperitoneal bleed. Both patients expired despite aggressive treatment and resuscitation. Hemorrhagic myositis in these two patients with inflammatory myopathy is a very rare complication. The association of anti-Ro52 with this potentially very serious complication remains unclear. This potential relationship should be further evaluated in future studies.

1. Introduction

Dermatomyositis is an autoimmune idiopathic inflammatory myopathy (IIM) with characteristic skin manifestations, classically heliotrope rash, V, shawl, and Holster sign, and Gottron's papules [1]. Up to 30 percent of patients with dermatomyositis (DM) or polymyositis (PM) have a constellation of clinical findings termed the "antisynthetase syndrome" [2–4]. Findings include constitutional symptoms such as fever, interstitial lung disease (ILD), myositis, Raynaud's phenomenon, mechanic's hands, and arthritis [5]. Dermatomyositis can be associated with systemic manifestations including ILD, pneumomediastinum, and cardiomyopathy [6]. We present two cases of inflammatory myopathy (Dermatomyositis) complicated by acute spontaneous hemorrhage of the iliopsoas, psoas, and pectineus muscles. To our knowledge, there are only a handful of cases of myositis complicated by hemorrhage.

2. Case 1

A 50-year-old African-American male with a history of borderline diabetes presented with three weeks of myalgia, a fifteen-pound weight loss, arthralgia, odynophagia, fatigue, dyspnea on exertion, and progressive nonproductive cough in early 2012. These symptoms coincided with a new erythematous rash on the back of his scalp, neck, and inner left ear and over the knuckles of his hands. A short trial of 4 mg of oral methylprednisolone was given at a previous urgent care visit with some improvement in the rash. Review of systems confirmed intermittent subjective fever, hoarseness, and tea color urine for 4 days. Medications included over-the-counter smooth move for constipation, multivitamins, and fish oil.

Initial exam showed normal vital signs. His voice was hoarse. His lung exam revealed mild crackles bilaterally. Muscle strength testing of the neck flexors and proximal upper and lower extremities was 4/5 with bilateral distal upper and lower extremities scoring 5/5. Skin exam showed malar erythema, erythematous patches over the scalp and behind the ears, minimal heliotrope rash, mild erythema over his chest (V sign), and diffuse erythematous hypopigmented macules over his proximal interphalangeal joints (PIPs) and metacarpal phalangeal joints (MCPs) bilaterally. He had "mechanic's hands" and periungal erythema. There was

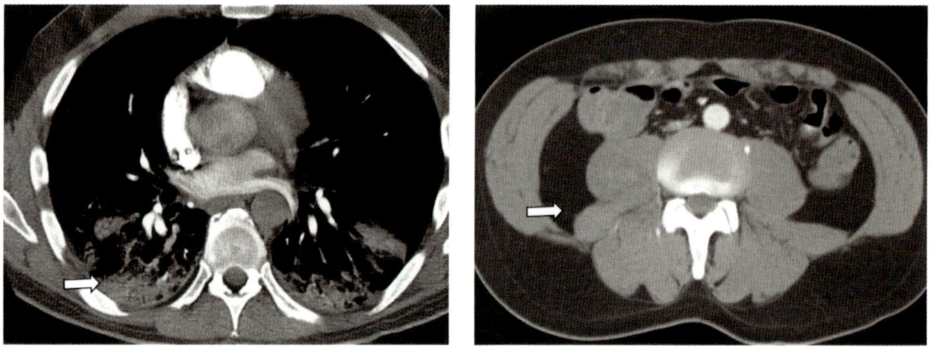

(a) (b)

Figure 1: (a) CT chest on admission. Axial contrast enhanced images through the chest in the pulmonary phase demonstrate a normal main pulmonary artery trunk and normal segmental pulmonary arterial branches extending to the superior segment of the right upper lobe. Lung windows reveal lower lobe consolidation (see arrow). (b) Normal appearance of the retroperitoneum at that time (see arrow).

a small hard papule along the medial aspect of the right 3rd PIP, which was suspected of being calcinosis.

Initial laboratory results revealed elevated creatine phosphokinase (CPK) of 1123 units/L (reference: 26–174 units/L) with mild elevation of transaminases but unremarkable complete blood count (CBC), chemistry panel, and coagulation studies. Chest X-ray showed patchy consolidations of the right upper lung and posterior lung bases suggestive of possible pneumonia. CT chest showed right upper lobe ground-glass opacity and bilateral lower lobe consolidations with mildly enlarged mediastinal lymph nodes (Figure 1). He was started on ceftriaxone and azithromycin for empiric coverage of community acquired pneumonia. He was admitted for treatment and workup of a possible inflammatory myopathy.

During the initial hospitalization, the patient's CPK improved with bed rest and normal saline infusion. CT abdomen and pelvis ordered to evaluate persistent constipation was unremarkable except for a small hepatic cyst. EMG/NCS showed no electrodiagnostic evidence of a polyneuropathy or myopathy. MRI-STIR of the thighs showed no convincing evidence of an inflammatory myopathy other than minimal muscle edema of the iliopsoas muscles. Given no clear focus of inflammatory muscle seen on MRI or EMG, a muscle biopsy was deferred. For continued hoarseness of voice, laryngoscopy was performed and showed postcommissure edema and erythema involving the laryngeal epiglottis and false cords. For evaluation of continuing dyspnea with gradual worsening hypoxia, a bronchoscopy was performed that visualized signs of mild inflammation in the lungs. Bronchoalveolar lavage returned numerous WBCs with normal respiratory flora present. Transbronchial biopsy of the right lower lung was consistent with organizing pneumonia and was negative for fungi and acid fast bacilli (Figure 2). A transthoracic echocardiogram was read as within normal limits and a CT angiogram was negative for pulmonary embolism. Immunofluorescence for antinuclear antibodies (ANA), serum for anti-RNP/Sm, anti-phospholipid antibodies, anti-Mi-2, anti-SRP, anti-Jo-1, anti-neutrophil cytoplasmic antibodies (ANCA), HIV, hepatitis panel, aldolase, and sputum for AFBx3 all returned normal.

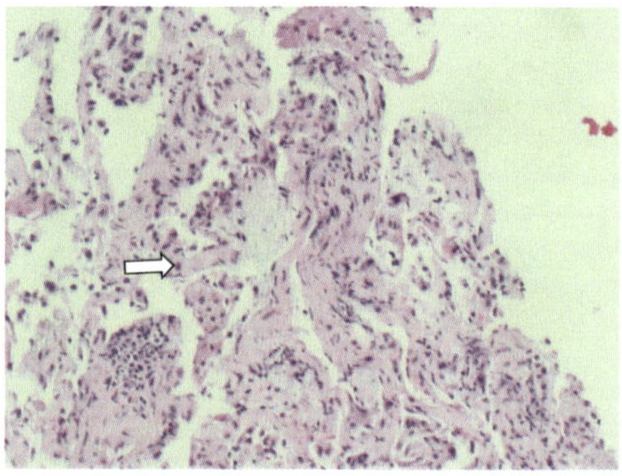

Figure 2: Lung biopsy (mild chronic interstitial pneumonitis with focal fibroblastic foci, consistent with organizing pneumonia; stains for fungi and AFB were negative) (see arrow).

In the interim, the patient developed persistent fever thought likely to be secondary to an underlying inflammatory process. Solumedrol 60 mg IV q 12 hours was started after one week into his hospitalization with near immediate resolution of fevers and improvement of the rash. Given the likely diagnosis of dermatomyositis, two doses of intravenous immunoglobulin (IVIG) were given to treat his persistent dysphagia and unresolving organizing pneumonia. Patient reported improved strength after receiving IVIG and steroid therapy, but he remained hypoxic. Repeat CT scans of chest/abdomen/pelvis were performed and showed no progression of disease on day 15 (Figure 3). On day 17 of hospitalization, the patient began complaining of right hip pain for which an MRI was ordered to rule out avascular necrosis. Later that evening, the patient was found to be uncomfortable in bed and only partially responsive. He became hypotensive, tachycardic, and tachypneic. CBC revealed hemoglobin of 4.1 gm/dL and platelet count of 50,000/μL. The patient was intubated, started on vasopressors, and transferred to the intensive care unit (ICU). He was aggressively resuscitated with IV fluid and blood products. He was also noted to have increasing abdominal girth. Stat CT abdomen/pelvis showed

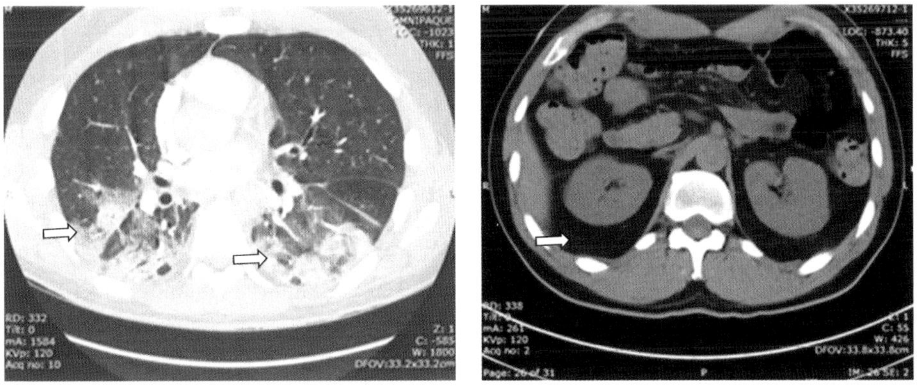

(a) (b)

FIGURE 3: (a) CT chest/abdomen/pelvis. No evidence for pulmonary embolism. Patchy peribronchiolar consolidations are worsened in the right upper lobe, right lower lobe, and left lower lobe (see arrow). (b) No abdominal masses/hemorrhage is seen (see arrow).

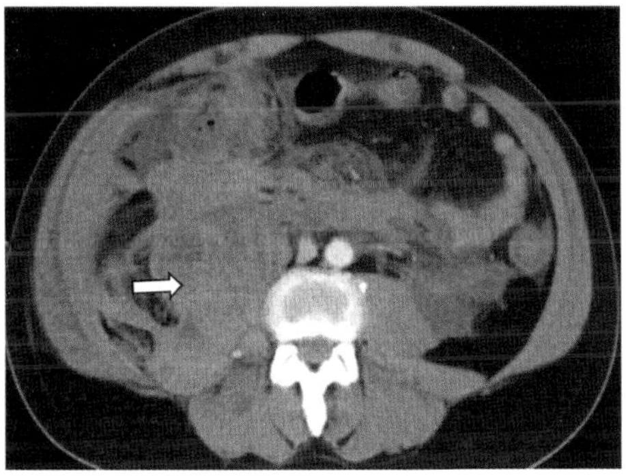

FIGURE 4: Stat CT abdomen/pelvis. Interval development of a large retroperitoneal hemorrhage centered around the right psoas muscle, with extension to the right spinous erector and iliacus musculature (see arrow).

large retroperitoneal bleeding involving the right iliacus and psoas muscles, extending into the retroperitoneum and along the right paracolic gutter (Figure 4). Interventional radiology could not locate a focal source of bleeding and suggested aggressive medical resuscitation. Solumedrol was also increased to 250 mg IV Q6 for possible dermatomyositis associated vasculitis. The patient received a total of 20 units of pack red blood cells, fresh frozen plasma, cryoprecipitate, and 3 units of platelets but ultimately progressed into multiorgan failure. On day 19, the patient was found to be in asystole and expired that day.

The family subsequently agreed to a partial autopsy limited to the chest and abdomen. The autopsy results showed a massive retroperitoneal hematoma, segmental myofiber necrosis in the psoas muscle without lymphocytic infiltrate, and perifascicular atrophy or necrosis (Figure 5). The patient's serum was sent to a reference lab where anti-Ro52 returned positive.

3. Case 2

A 63-year-old Filipino female with a history of diabetes, hypertension, and hyperlipidemia presented to our hospital for new throat pain, fevers, and oral sores for four weeks in early 2013. She had difficulty swallowing to the point where she could no longer eat solid foods and had lost 10–15 lbs. She developed new painful mouth sores involving her lips along with low grade subjective fevers and joint swelling of the fingers during the same time period. She reported a new rash around her eyes and chest that was not itchy or painful. She complained of worsening fatigue over the past week, required assistance to eat and go to the bathroom, and was bedbound on presentation. ROS confirmed a dry cough for four weeks not improved with oral azithromycin prescribed by her PMD. She had been seen in the ED one month ago for the joint pains where a hand XR reportedly showed osteoarthritis of her hands and a chest X-ray noted prominent interstitial lung markings. Medications included amlodipine, metformin, quinapril, ezetimibe, glipizide, aspirin, calcium, and fish oil.

Upon presentation she was afebrile with a blood pressure of 140/80 mmHg, pulse of 107 beats/minute, respiratory rate of 26 breaths/minute, and oxygen saturation of 86% on room air that improved to 95% with 2 L nasal cannula oxygen. She was found to be severely hyponatremic with poor PO intake and have a new bilateral infiltrate on CT angiogram (Figure 6) of the chest, and thus she was admitted for further care. Initial exam was significant for hoarse voice, oropharyngeal ulcerations/erythema, heliotrope rash around the eyes, positive shawl and V sign, and bilateral crackles at the lung bases. Her hand examination showed distal cracking of her skin (mechanic's hands) along with purpuric lesions. Strength testing showed initially 5/5 in all muscle groups but decreased in the lower extremities to 3/5 early in the course of her hospital stay.

Initial labs were significant for CPK level of 2246 IU/I, aldolase of 14.2 IU/L, LDH 498 IU/L, AST 310 IU/L, ALT 77 IU/L, alkaline phosphatase 309 IU/L, T. bilirubin 0.7 mg/dL, and CRP 41.5 mg/mL. All testing for bacterial/fungal pneumonia, urine histoplasmosis antigen, viral hepatitis antibody/antigens, aspergillosis antigen, legionella antigen, influenza A/B antibody, syphilis (RPR) antibody, coccidioidomycosis antibody, and cryptococcus antibody

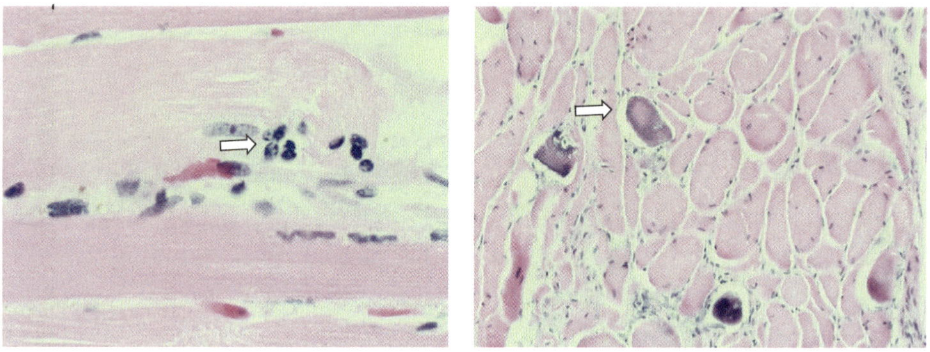

(a) (b)

FIGURE 5: (a) Autopsy of the psoas muscle. Skeletal muscles: nonuniform degree of interior scattered segments of necrotic myofibers in the psoas fascicles without perifascicular myofiber atrophy or necrosis. Extensive morular aggregation of myofiber nuclei in the damaged myofibers (see arrow). Minimal perimysial and endomysial fibrosis, suggesting an acute process. Finding may suggest possible sepsis with intravascular coagulation and capillary disruption. (b) Calcium deposition found in myofiber (see arrow).

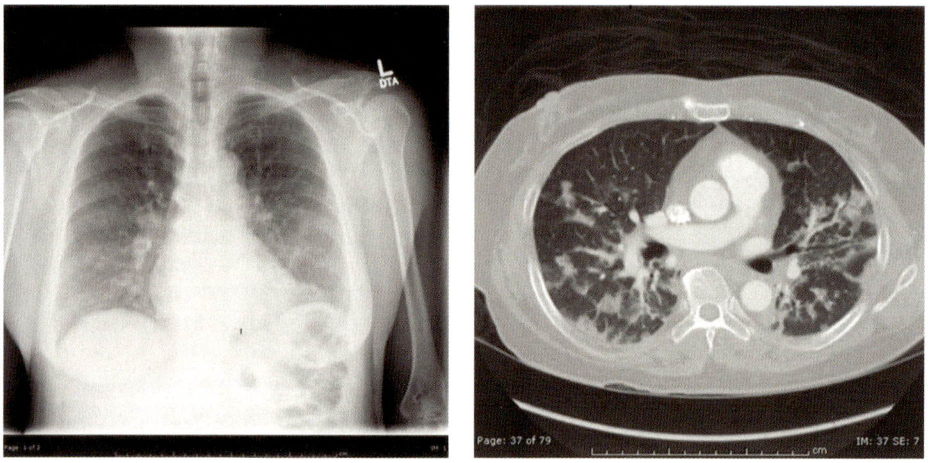

(a) (b)

FIGURE 6: Lung imaging on admission. (a) Chest radiograph showing prominent interstitial lung markings. (b) CT pulmonary angiogram showing multifocal opacities and consolidation.

was negative. ANA, anti-RNP/Sm, anti-dsDNA, anti-Scl70, anti-centromere B, anti-smooth muscle, anti-histone, anti-CCP, ANCA, anti-Mi-2, anti-Jo-1, and anti-SSB antibodies were all negative. Anti-SSA was mildly positive at >1.2 (normal < 1.0 IU). Magnetic resonance imaging (MRI) with short tau inversion recovery (STIR) imaging of the pelvis and shoulders showed diffuse edema in symmetric distribution throughout the shoulder girdles and pelvis bilaterally (Figure 7). Electromyogram with nerve conduction study revealed sharp waves and irritable myopathy consistent with inflammatory myopathy.

A diagnosis of dermatomyositis was made based on the presence of typical rash, mechanic's hands, muscle weakness, elevated muscle enzymes, abnormal EMG/MRI studies, and probable interstitial lung disease. The patient was started on solumedrol 80 mg IV BID and empiric levofloxacin for possible pneumonia. Her CPKs downtrended and her facial and body rashes began to resolve but she remained weak with worsening hypoxia and dysphonia. Given the aggressive nature of her disease, she was given IVIG infusion on consecutive days beginning approximately six days after admission while awaiting a planned muscle biopsy. She had a CT abdomen and pelvis, to search for possible malignancy during the second day of her IVIG infusion, which was read as negative for acute pathology (Figures 8(a)–8(c)). One day after finishing her second dose of IVIG, she became altered with a rapid drop of Hgb from 10.3 to 6.1 gm/dL. A repeat CT scan of the abdomen and pelvis revealed new areas of intramuscular hematomas that were not seen 24 hours ago on the prior CT (Figures 8(d)–8(f)). During her hospitalization, she had only been on prophylactic doses of subcutaneous dalteparin of 5000 units/day with a normal platelet count of 176 on the day of the bleeding event with an INR of 1.21 seconds on admission. Steroid therapy was increased to full 1-gram pulse doses and one dose of IV Cytoxan was given, but eventually the patient slowly decompensated and died of

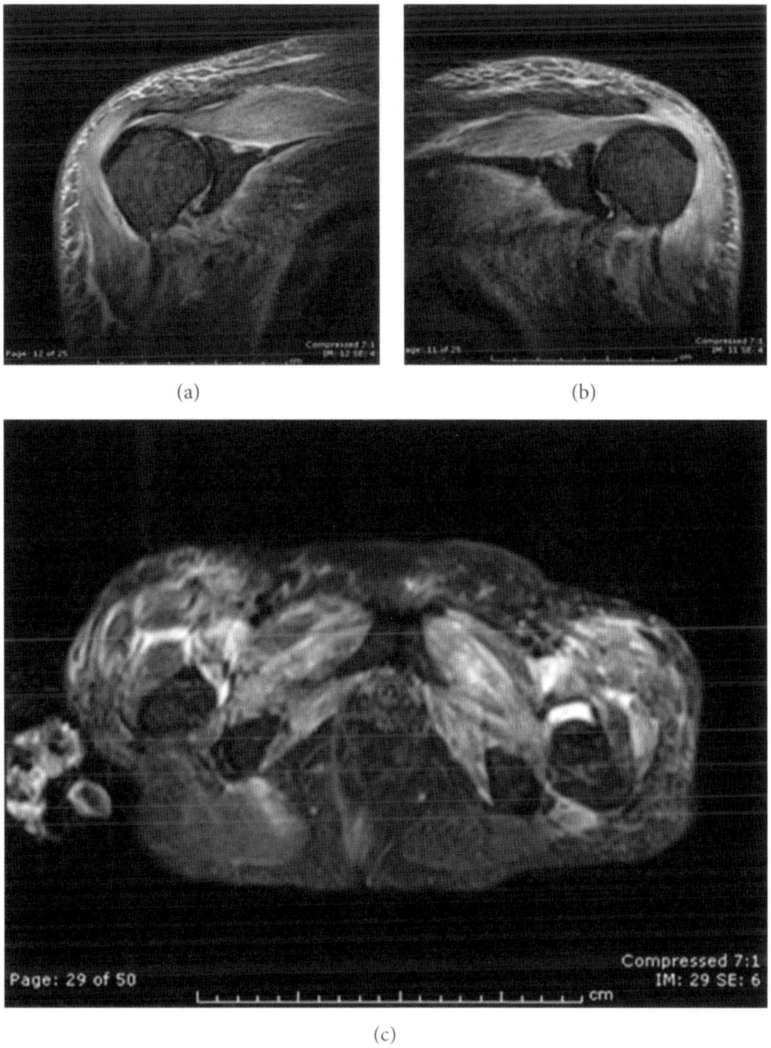

Figure 7: MRI with short tau inversion recovery (STIR) image showing diffuse symmetrical proximal muscle edema. (a) Right shoulder, (b) left shoulder, and (c) pelvis.

multiorgan failure a week later. A sample of her serum early in her hospital course was sent to a reference lab where notably she tested positive for anti Ro/SSA-52 antibodies.

4. Discussion

Here we present two cases of idiopathic inflammatory myopathy (dermatomyositis) complicated by acute severe hemorrhagic myositis. The diagnosis of hemorrhagic myositis is rare and has been reported only several times in the literature but is a serious, often fatal, complication that has been associated with inflammatory myopathies (Table 1). Orrell et al. in a paper in 1998 discussed two cases in Rochester, NY, where patients with DM developed abdominal hematomas [7]. In the first case, a patient with biopsy proven DM for 11 years was started on IVIG monthly for active DM despite steroids and azathioprine. Five years later while on this regimen she developed acute left upper abdominal pain with Hgb drop from 12.9 to 9.1 g/dL and was found to have a large left rectus abdominis muscle hematoma. The patient did well with blood transfusion. The second patient was 11 years old with stable DM diagnosed at the age of 8 who presented with pain in the right hip for 3 days. She was taken to the OR for presumed appendicitis but was found to have retroperitoneal bleeding located from a hematoma posterior to the ascending colon and did well after surgery. A third case report by Fang et al. in Kaohsiung, Taiwan, 2008, described a 65-year-old female patient with polymyositis who developed retroperitoneal bleeding from the superior duodenal-pancreatic artery after a flare of her myopathy [8]. Although the bleeding stabilized with angiography, rebleeding occurred in the superior mesenteric artery that was again stabilized by angiography, but the patient expired from sepsis 10 days later. A fourth case presented by Yamagishi et al. in Niigata, Japan, in 2008 described a 64-year-old female with newly diagnosed DM with ILD who developed bleeding in her right psoas and iliacus muscles after 10 days of treatment with pulse steroids, oral cyclosporine, and IV

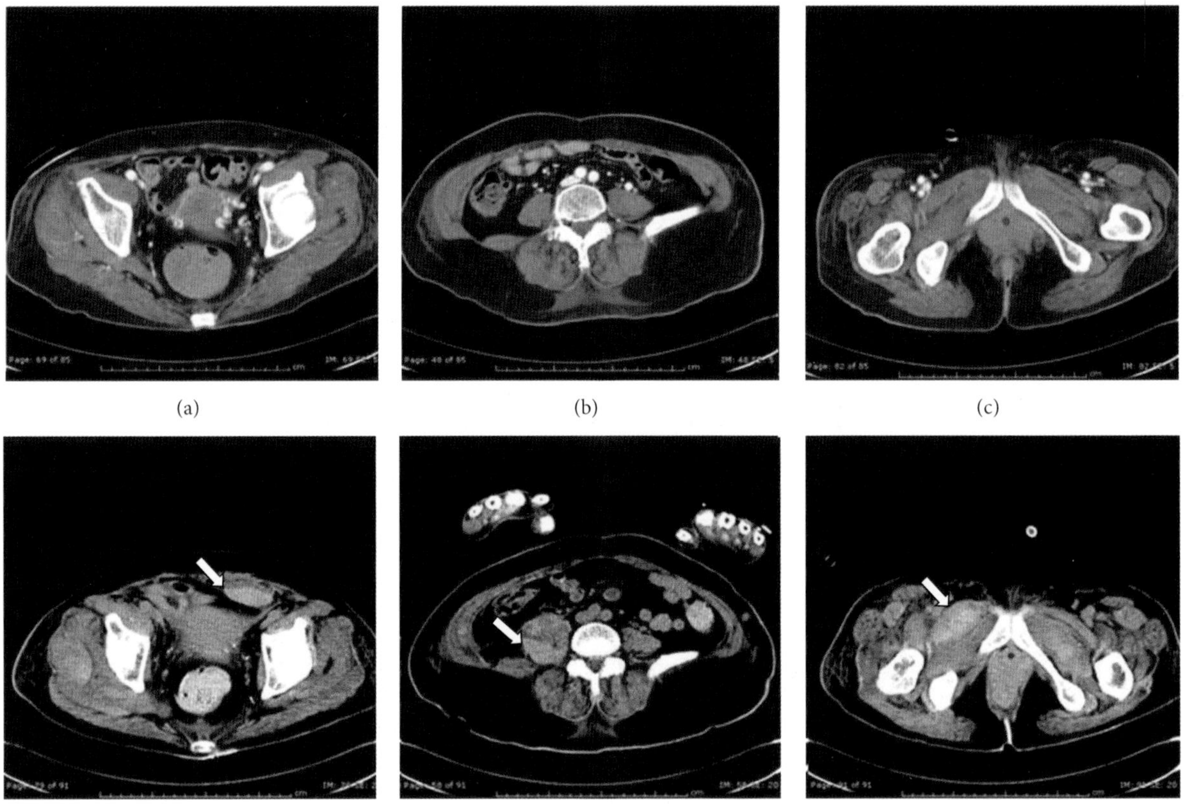

(a) (b) (c)

(d) (e) (f)

Figure 8: CT scan of the abdomen and pelvis before and after bleeding. (a–c) CT scan with contrast shows (a) normal rectus, (b) normal iliopsoas, and (c) normal pectineus muscles. (d–f) CT scan without contrast shows bleeding into (d) rectus sheath (arrow), (e) iliopsoas (arrow), and (f) pectineus muscles (arrow).

cyclophosphamide [9]. Angiography localized the lesions to small aneurysms in the retroperitoneum that were embolized, with rebleeding occurring a week later that was again stopped by angiography, but the patient expired weeks later from TTP and multiorgan failure. Other case reports exist in the literature for hemorrhagic myositis, with a report from Higashi et al. in 2009 on a 77-year-old patient with DM who was on heparin for unstable angina [10].

Both of the cases presented in our study were consistent with dermatomyositis (and probably the antisynthetase syndrome) based on clinical features of rash, mechanic's hands, muscle weakness, ILD, elevated muscle enzymes, abnormal EMG/MRI (Case 2 only), and positive antibodies to anti-RO/SSA-52 from the same reference lab. The sites of bleeding in Case 1 (iliopsoas) and in Case 2 (rectus sheath and iliopsoas) were areas frequently reported in the other case reports. The finding of bleeding frequently in these areas but not in other muscle groups seems to be a possible unique finding in hemorrhagic myositis with inflammatory myopathy.

Both patients were given IVIG infusion for rapidly progressive disease. In Case 1, IVIG preceded the bleeding by several days and in Case 2 it followed directly the next day after IVIG infusion. In the past case reports, only one patient was receiving IVIG and had been doing so monthly for 5 years before the bleeding event. Reports of IVIG causing massive intravascular hemolysis are known but are rare, with the usual hemolysis reported as mild and self-limited [11]. Review of the literature did not show an association with IVIG bleeding into the muscle. More frequently reported IVIG complications include renal failure, anaphylaxis, aseptic meningitis, and thrombosis (up to 13% in one series of patients with autoimmune disorders) [12]. In that same review, it was notable that IVIG thrombotic events favored more arterial involvement (MI, CVA, and peripheral arteries) perhaps hinting at a possible role for enhanced arterial clotting or injury that could relate to hemorrhagic events in our cases.

Finally, both of our cases tested positive for anti-Ro/SSA-52 antibody, which is included among the myositis associated antibodies (MAA) [13]. Among autoantibodies in autoimmune disease, the Ro/SSA (made up of Ro60 and Ro52) antibody is the most common one to extractable nuclear antigens. Antibodies to Ro-52 (a tripartite motif protein/TRIM) can be found independent of antibodies to Ro-60 (a small cytoplasmic ribonucleoprotein/scRNP) in certain autoimmune disorders. Expression of isolated anti-Ro52 alone is mainly seen in certain connective tissue diseases (including myositis), but with unclear clinical significance with an overall prevalence of 0.5% [14]. The anti-Ro52 antibody occurs in about 30%

TABLE 1: Clinical features of selected case reports of hemorrhagic myositis in inflammatory myopathies.

Author	Age (yrs) (at event)	Gender	Clinical history and prebleeding therapies	Antibody profile	Site of bleeding(s)	Treatment	Outcome (as reported)
Orrell et al. [7]	50	Female	DM age 34 Corticosteroid Azathioprine IVIG	None specified	Left rectus abdominis	Blood transfusions Prednisone Azathioprine	Survived, no recurrent bleeding
Orrell et al. [7]	11	Female	DM age 8 Prednisone	ANA 1 : 320 speckled	Retroperitoneum, posterior to right ascending colon	Supportive	Survived without recurrence
Fang et al. [8]	65	Female	PM age 65 Hydrocortisone Prednisone	ANA 1 : 320 speckled	Retroperitoneum, superior duodenal pancreatic artery, SMA	Angiography with embolization	Expired from sepsis without rebleeding
Yamagishi et al. [9]	64	Female	DM/ILD age 64 Solumedrol Prednisone Cyclosporine Dalteparin	ANA positive Elevated serum KL-6	Retroperitoneum, right psoas, right iliacus, left rectus sheath	Angiography with embolization with rebleeding and repeat embolization	Expired from TTP and multiorgan failure
Higashi et al. [10]	77	Female	DM age 77 Solumedrol Prednisone Cyclosporine Heparin	Elevated serum KL-6	Retroperitoneum, left iliopsoas, left iliacus, right sternomastoid	Supportive	Expired from DIC
Van Gelder et al.	50	Male	DM/ILD age 50 Solumedrol IVIG	Anti-Ro52	Retroperitoneum, right iliacus, right psoas	Transfusions Solumedrol	Expired from multiorgan failure
Van Gelder et al.	63	Female	DM/ILD age 63 Solumedrol IVIG	Anti-SSA Anti-Ro52	Retroperitoneum, right pectineus, right iliopsoas	Transfusions Solumedrol Cytoxan	Expired from multiorgan failure

of patients with inflammatory myopathy and up to 72% of those that are also positive for anti-Jo-1, a myositis specific antibody (MSA) associated with ILD. However, since both our cases were negative for selected MSAs including anti-Jo-1, it is unclear whether the positive testing for anti-Ro52 may be associated with inflammatory myopathy and ILD or possibly overlapping with additional, nondetected antibodies more specific for inflammatory myopathy associated with this serious complication.

5. Conclusion

In summary, we present two cases of inflammatory myopathy (dermatomyositis with ILD) complicated by severe hemorrhagic myositis. The pattern of bleeding in our cases, as in the previous literature, seems to favor the retroperitoneum or rectus abdominis muscles. The possibility of hemorrhagic myositis should always be entertained as a possible complication of inflammatory myopathy, especially in the setting of an acute drop in the hemoglobin. It remains to be seen if the anti-Ro52 antibody may play an accessory role in predicting which patients may be at risk for this potentially very serious complication.

References

[1] A. Bohan and J. B. Peter, "Polymyositis and dermatomyositis," *The New England Journal of Medicine*, vol. 292, no. 7, pp. 344–347, 1975.

[2] L. A. Love, R. L. Leff, D. D. Fraser et al., "A new approach to the classification of idiopathic inflammatory myopathy. myositis specific autoantibodies define useful homogeneous patient groups," *Medicine*, vol. 70, no. 6, pp. 360–374, 1991.

[3] T. Mimori, Y. Imura, R. Nakashima, and H. Yoshifuji, "Autoantibodies in idiopathic inflammatory myopathy: an update on clinical and pathophysiological significance," *Current Opinion in Rheumatology*, vol. 19, no. 6, pp. 523–529, 2007.

[4] I. N. Targoff, "Autoantibodies and their significance in myositis," *Current Rheumatology Reports*, vol. 10, no. 4, pp. 333–340, 2008.

[5] E. Katzap, M. L. Barilla-Labarca, and G. Marder, "Antisynthetase syndrome," *Current Rheumatology Reports*, vol. 13, no. 3, pp. 175–181, 2011.

[6] A. J. Rodrigues, M. Jacomelli, P. R. Scordamaglio, and V. R. Figueiredo, "Spontaneous pneumomediastinum associated with laryngeal lesions and tracheal ulcer in dermatomyositis," *Revista Brasileira de Reumatologia*, vol. 52, no. 5, pp. 796–799, 2012.

[7] R. W. Orrell, H. M. Johnston, C. Gibson, R. M. Cass, and R. C. Griggs, "Spontaneous abdominal hematoma in Dermatomyositis," *Muscle & Nerve*, vol. 21, no. 21, pp. 1800–1803, 1998.

[8] T.-J. Fang, S.-C. Hsu, M.-C. Shih et al., "Spontaneous retroperitoneal hemorrhage in a mediastinal tumor in a patient with polymyositis: a case report," *Kaohsiung Journal of Medical Sciences*, vol. 24, no. 8, pp. 436–440, 2008.

[9] M. Yamagishi, S. Tajima, A. Suetake et al., "Dermatomyositis with hemorrhagic myositis," *Rheumatology International*, vol. 29, no. 11, pp. 1363–1366, 2009.

[10] Y. Higashi, K. Mera, T. Kanzaki, and T. Kanekura, "Fatal muscle haemorrhage attributable to heparin administration in a patient with dermatomyositis," *Clinical and Experimental Dermatology*, vol. 34, no. 3, pp. 448–449, 2009.

[11] M. Mohamed, G. Bates, and B. Eastley, "Massive intravascular haemolysis after high dose intravenous immunoglobulin therapy," *British Journal of Haematology*, vol. 160, no. 5, p. 570, 2013.

[12] I. Marie, G. Maurey, F. Hervé, M.-F. Hellot, and H. Levesque, "Intravenous immunoglobulin-associated arterial and venous thrombosis: report of a series and review of the literature," *The British Journal of Dermatology*, vol. 155, no. 4, pp. 714–721, 2006.

[13] C. Defendenti, F. Atzeni, M. F. Spina et al., "Clinical and laboratory aspects of Ro/SSA-52 autoantibodies," *Autoimmunity Reviews*, vol. 10, no. 3, pp. 150–154, 2011.

[14] B. Hervier, M. Rimbert, F. Colonna, M. A. Hamidou, and M. Audrain, "Clinical significance of anti-Ro/SSA-52 kDa antibodies—a retrospective monocentric study," *Rheumatology*, vol. 48, no. 8, pp. 964–967, 2009.

23

Diffuse Large B Cell Lymphoma Mimicking Granulomatosis with Polyangiitis

Mohammad E. Naffaa,[1,2] Alexander P. Rozin,[1,2] Netanel Horowitz,[2,3] Ofer Ben-Itzhak,[2,4] Yolanda Braun-Moscovici,[1,2] and Alexandra Balbir-Gurman[1,2]

[1] *The B. Shine Rheumatology Unit, Rambam Health Care Campus, 31096 Haifa, Israel*

[2] *Rappaport Faculty of Medicine, Technion-Israel Institute of Technology, 31096 Haifa, Israel*

[3] *Hematology Institute, Rambam Health Care Campus, 31096 Haifa, Israel*

[4] *Pathology Institute, Rambam Health Care Campus, 31096 Haifa, Israel*

Correspondence should be addressed to Mohammad E. Naffaa; m_naffaa@rambam.health.gov.il

Academic Editor: Gregory J. Tsay

In a patient with systemic multiorgan disease with overlapping features, the differential diagnosis included infectious diseases, malignancies, and systemic autoimmune or inflammatory diseases. We present an unusual case of a young male with B cell lymphoma who presented with symptoms mimicking systemic vasculitis and review the existing literature.

1. Introduction

Granulomatosis with polyangiitis (GPA) is a small and medium-sized vessels vasculitis which is highly associated with positive anti-neutrophil cytoplasmic antibodies (ANCA), mainly with antibodies against proteinase 3 (PR3) [1]. Among reported clinical manifestations of GPA, necrotizing granulomatous inflammation in the upper respiratory tract, pulmonary nodules (often with cavitations), and necrotizing glomerulonephritis are prominent; their combination is a classic GPA triad [1]. Involvement of other organs and systems, such as the skin, eyes, ears, and peripheral nervous system, is less specific but definitely is not rare. The involvement of gastrointestinal tract (GIT) in GPA is infrequent [2].

2. Case Presentation

A 22-year-old male was admitted because of fever (39.5°C), weakness, excessive sweating, vomiting, and weight loss during the previous month. His medical history was unremarkable, and physical examination did not show any pathological signs. Laboratory data revealed white blood count 2100 (WBC, 4000–10800/μL), hemoglobin 12.5 (Hb, 13–17 g/dL), and platelet count 113000 (PLT, 130000–350000/μL); aspartate aminotransferase 65 (AST, 5–40 U/L), alanine aminotransferase 63 (ALT, 30–65 U/L), alkaline phosphatase 123 (AlkPh, 30–115 U/L), lactate dehydrogenase 997 (LDH, 60–225 U/L), creatinine 0.73 (0.4–1.3 mg/dL), blood urea nitrogen 8 (BUN, 5–20 mg/dL), creatine kinase 20 (CK, 35–300 U/L), albumin 3.9 (3.4–5 g/dL), and ferritin 469 (15–300 ng/mL); erythrocyte sedimentation rate 24 mm/1 hour (ESR, <20 mm/1 hour) and C-reactive protein 18 mg/L (CRP, 0–5 mg/L). Coagulation profile and thyroid function tests were normal. Urine dip-stick was negative for protein or blood. Blood, urine, throat, and stool cultures were all sterile. Serology tests, including human immunodeficiency virus, hepatitis B and C virus, *Cytomegalovirus*, Epstein Barr virus (EBV), *Rickettsia*, *Chlamydia*, *Toxoplasma*, *Brucella*, and Q-fever, were negative. Anti-nuclear (ANA) and anti-dsDNA antibodies were positive; anti-cardiolipin, and B_2-glycoprotein antibodies and cryoglobulins were negative; complements C3 and C4 levels were normal; protein electrophoresis and immunoelectrophoresis were within normal limits. Test for anti-neutrophil cytoplasmic antibodies (ANCA) was positive for myeloperoxidase (MPO) and negative for proteinase 3 (PR3). Computed tomography (CT)

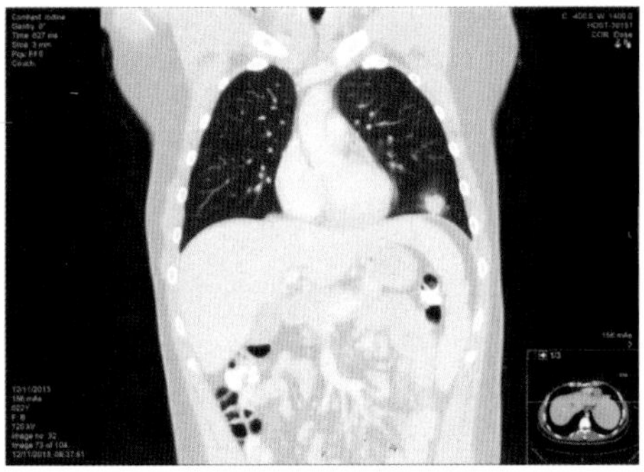

Figure 1: Coronal reconstruction of thoracic CT scan in lung window irregular pulmonary nodule with surrounding ground glass opacity in the left lower lobe of the lung.

demonstrated several bilateral peripheral nodular infiltrates in the lungs (Figure 1) and several nodular lesions in the liver and kidney; the spleen was mildly enlarged. Bone marrow biopsy was negative for granulomas and mycobacterium tuberculosis as well as for malignancy. The patient was discharged with a recommendation for ambulatory treatment with doxycycline for suspected atypical infection.

One month later, due to the ongoing fever, abdominal pain, repeated vomiting, constipation, weight loss, and loss of smelling ability, he was admitted again. Repeated CT scan showed resolution of previous pulmonary nodules with the concomitant appearance of several new ones. The number of hepatic nodules had increased with further enlargement of the spleen and the appearance of mild mesenteric lymphadenopathy. CT-guided fine needle aspiration of the pulmonary lesion failed and an open lung biopsy was performed. At that time, the patient was transferred to our hospital.

On admission the patient looked ill, pale, and weak. Heart and lung evaluation was unremarkable. There was mild tenderness of the upper abdomen without signs of peritoneal irritation or liver enlargement; the spleen was mildly enlarged and palpable. Repeated blood tests showed WBC 4200/μL, HB 12.4 g/dL, PLT 248000/μL, creatinine 0.65 mg/dL, albumin 3.9 g/dL, AST 25 U/L, ALT 43 U/L, GGT 52 U/L, ALKP 123 U/L, LDH 234 U/L, CK 20 U/L, CRP 16.43 mg/L, and ESR 24 mm/1 hour. Repeated ANA and anti-dsDNA were negative; the test for ANCA was pending. Gastroscopy showed only a small sliding hiatal hernia. Otolaryngologist assessment and brain magnetic resonance imaging were normal. Fundus evaluation did not show signs of retinal vasculitis. Transthoracic echocardiography was normal.

During the next several days the patient's condition deteriorated due to progressive weakness, abdominal pain, and repeated vomiting. After receiving the lung biopsy results which were summarized as necrotizing vasculitis and taking into account the existing findings from previous assessments (positive MPO, pulmonary nodules), the working diagnosis of ANCA-associated vasculitis was suggested and pulse therapy with methylprednisolone 1000 mg/day for 3 consecutive days was introduced. After the first infusion the patient continued to complain of abdominal pain, constipation, and vomiting, and he refused to eat. Serial clinical abdominal assessments revealed epigastric tenderness without signs of peritoneal irritation. X-ray did not show free air in the abdominal cavity or signs of bowel obstruction. Abdominal ultrasonography demonstrated multiple hypoechoic hepatic lesions with mild ascites. Suddenly, the patient developed acute and severe epigastric pain, diffuse abdominal wall rigidity and rebound, marked tachycardia, and hypotension.

CT angiography of the abdomen demonstrated large amount of free air in the upper abdomen, peritoneal effusion, and a thickened small and large bowel wall with no signs of mesenteric arteries or veins thrombosis. The patient underwent emergent laparotomy which revealed multiple small necrotic areas in different segments of the small bowel; the involved part of small bowel was resected. The postoperative period was unremarkable. Pathologic examination of the resected small bowel showed high-grade EBV-associated diffuse large B cell lymphoma with signs of lymphomatoid granulomatosis and positive IgH rearrangement (Figure 2). The intestinal wall and the blood vessels showed extensive lymphoid infiltration. Later, repeated ANCA revealed negative results for MPO and PR3. The patient was treated with the CHOP-R protocol (cyclophosphamide, doxorubicin, vincristine, prednisone, and rituximab) with achievement of rapid clinical and hematological remission.

3. Discussion

We describe a unique case of a young male who developed high-grade EBV-associated diffuse large B cell lymphoma mimicking granulomatosis with polyangiitis (GPA). Our patient presented with constitutional symptoms (prolonged fever, severe fatigue, and weight loss), nasal involvement (anosmia), multiple pulmonary, hepatic, and spleen nodules, elevated inflammatory markers, anemia, transiently positive MPO, and findings on open lung biopsy suggestive of necrotizing vasculitis. All together, these findings were "strong" clues for the diagnosis of ANCA-associated vasculitis.

GPA is a small and medium-sized vessels vasculitis which is highly associated with positive ANCA, mainly with antibodies against PR3 [1]. Among reported clinical manifestations of GPA, necrotizing granulomatous inflammation in the upper respiratory tract, pulmonary nodules (often with cavitations), and necrotizing glomerulonephritis are prominent; their combination is a classic GPA triad [1]. Involvement of other organs and systems, such as the skin, eyes, ears, and peripheral nervous system, is less specific but definitely is not rare. The involvement of gastrointestinal tract (GIT) in GPA is infrequent [2]. Akbulut reported a patient with severe GPA who developed bowel perforation and sepsis and eventually died. The author reviewed thirteen similar cases and summarized the main clinical features of GIT involvement in GPA as follows: gingivitis, peptic ulcers, bloody diarrhea, bowel ulcerations, persistent perianal ulcers, pancreatitis, cholecystitis, small bowel perforations, and colitis [2]. Involvement of the GIT in GPA has been usually reported during relapses, in uncontrolled diseases, and late in the disease course (2-3 years later or more). The most common GIT complications in vasculitis in general and in GPA particularly are oral ulcers, intestinal ulcerations, bleeding,

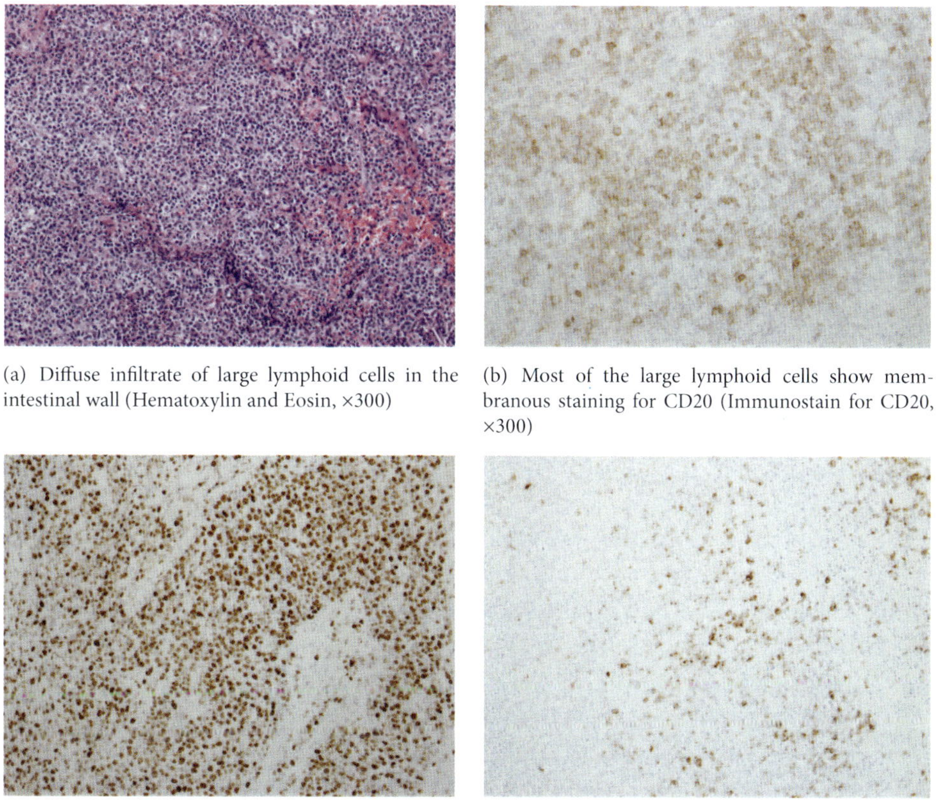

(a) Diffuse infiltrate of large lymphoid cells in the intestinal wall (Hematoxylin and Eosin, ×300)

(b) Most of the large lymphoid cells show membranous staining for CD20 (Immunostain for CD20, ×300)

(c) Ki67 index over 90% of the large lymphoid cells (Immunostain for Ki67, ×200)

(d) Many of the large lymphoid cells show positive cytoplasmic staining for latent membrane protein of EBV (Immunostain for LMP-1, ×200)

FIGURE 2: Histopathologic examination of intestinal biopsy.

and perforations. In this regard, treatments such as corticosteroids and non-steroidal inflammatory drugs have been suggested as triggering agents. The presence of active vasculitis-related changes at the sites of bowel perforations in about 61% of reported cases supports the idea that uncontrolled vasculitis in the intestinal wall was the main reason for perforation and not corticosteroids as was presumed previously [2]. Involvement of the GIT as a presenting symptom of GPA is extremely rare. We could find in the English language literature only 20 cases with GIT involvement as an early (less than one-year disease duration) or even initial GPA presentation (Table 1). Patients were mainly males (15/20) with the mean age of 41.7 years (our patient was much younger) [3–22]. According to case descriptions, 4 (20%) patients had appetite and weight loss, 9 (45%) patients had oral and/or tongue ulcers, 6 (30%) had diarrhea, 9 (45%) had blood in stool, melena, or bloody diarrhea, 2 (10%) had anal ulcers, and 1 had odynophagia (2%); 9 (45%) patients developed "acute abdomen" due to perforation, intra-abdominal bleeding, or obstruction. Our patient had abdominal symptoms for more than two months but never had oral ulcers, diarrhea, or GIT hemorrhage. Only in one reported patient was the GIT involvement an isolated GPA feature but was accompanied by fever [3] while, in the majority of cases, there were signs of multiorgan disease with almost an obligatory involvement of the upper airways (our patients had anosmia but not involvement of sinuses, eyes, or ears) and lungs (our patient had nodules without cavitations) and less often the kidneys (our patient did not have signs of nephritis).

Walton analyzed clinical and pathology features in 56 cases of GPA (Wegener's granulomatosis at that time). He found granulomatous lesions in the spleen (55.6%), kidney (66.7), and liver (16.7%) and fibrinoid necrosis in blood vessels in the spleen (77.8%), kidney (77.8%), liver (18.5%), intestine (24.1%), pancreas, and gallbladder (7.4% each) [23]. One patient had severe refractory anosmia which later was complicated by nasal septum destruction and deafness (our patient also had anosmia but not structural or mucosal damage in the oral or nasal cavity). Described liver and spleen nodules were mainly microscopic findings but not macroscopic lesions on imaging films. Although the classic splenic manifestations of GPA are splenic infarcts, hemorrhage and spleen necrosis may also occur [24–27]. In one GPA case, multiple small bowel ulcers and perforations were accompanied by spleen infarctions [9]. Walton and Leggat described a patient with anosmia, lung involvement, multiorgan failure, and spleen granulomas [15].

Involvement of the liver is extremely rare in the course of GPA. Among liver manifestations, nonspecific nontraumatic hepatic hematoma and incomplete septal cirrhosis were

Table 1: Analysis of cases with gastrointestinal symptoms in the early course of granulomatosis and polyangiitis (one year or less).

Author, year of publication	Gender, age (years)	Presenting symptoms	Disease duration	APR elevation	Concomitant respiratory system/kidney/other involvement	CT/endoscopic findings	Biopsy findings	ANCA
Yoshikawa et al., 2014 [3]	Male, 30	Oral ulcer, bloody stool	1 month	ESR, CRP	Fever	CT: thickening of the transverse colon wall	Superficial inflammatory cell infiltration and edema noted in lamina propria mucosae	PR3
Sinnott et al., 2013 [4]	Male, 29	Bloody diarrhea	2 months	ESR, CRP	Lung/kidney	CT: inflammatory changes in caecum and ascending colon	No bowel biopsy	PR3
Dag et al., 2013 [5]	Male, 29	Bloody stool, rectal bleeding	6 months	CRP, ESR	Lung, kidney, joints, skin	CT: distal ileum perforations Colonoscopy: ulcers in ileum, cecum, colon	Active chronic inflammation and ulcer bases	PR3
Qian et al., 2010 [6]	Female, 79	Bloody diarrhea	Presenting symptom	Not reported	Pulmonary hemorrhage, acute renal failure	Colonoscopy: pancolitis with numerous ulcers of varying sizes	Mucosal ulcerations with foci of acute inflammation and hemorrhage Kidney biopsy: crescentic and necrotizing glomerulonephritis	PR3
Samim et al., 2010 [7]	Male, 35	GI bleeding	1-2 weeks	CRP	Sinusitis/kidney/arthritis/skin rash	CTA: bleeding from one mesenteric artery Endoscopy: mucosal ulcerations	Central ulcerative inflammation and occluded small arteries in intestinal wall	PR3
Marie et al., 2010 [8]	Male, 31	Epigastric pain, rectal bleeding	Before diagnosis of GPA	ESR, CRP	Arthritis, purpura	Colonoscopy: multiple rectal and sigmoidal ulcerations with spontaneous bleeding	Inflammatory cell infiltrates surrounding small vessels	PR3
Deniz et al., 2007 [9]	Male, 44	Acute abdomen	4 weeks	Not reported	Sinusitis, lung cavitation nodules	CT: intra-abdominal free air and fluid, small bowel wall thickening, chronic splenic infarction	Ulcerations, necrotizing transmural granulomatous inflammation, fibrinoid necrosis of small to medium-sized submucosa vessels	ANCA
Kuwahara et al., 2006 [10]	Male, 30	Bloody diarrhea, oral and anal ulcers	Before diagnosis of GPA	CRP	Nasal bleeding, skin and mucosal ulcers, conjunctivitis	Colonoscopy: multiple ulcerations with irregular shapes, macroscopic bleeding, pseudopolyposis in terminal ileum, colon, rectum	Inflammation and epithelioid granuloma with multinuclear giant cells	PR3

Table 1: Continued.

Author, year of publication	Gender, age (years)	Presenting symptoms	Disease duration	APR elevation	Concomitant respiratory system/kidney/other involvement	CT/endoscopic findings	Biopsy findings	ANCA
Socas Macías et al., 2005 [11]	Male, 28	Oral ulcers, diarrhea, recurrent bowel obstruction	Before diagnosis of GPA	Not reported	Nasal and upper airway, skin rash with necrosis, glomerulonephritis	Colonoscopy and GIT X-rays: ulcers and structures due to ulceration in terminal ileum and colon (signs compatible with Crohn's disease)	Endoscopic biopsy: features compatible with Crohn's disease in large bowel and terminal ileum Autopsy: small vessel vasculitis (arterioles and venules), occasional histiocytes around vessels forming loose granulomas with scattered multinuclear giant cells	Negative
Chow et al., 2003 [12]	Male, 45	Melena	4 weeks	Not reported	Sinusitis, glomerulonephritis	Endoscopy: patchy ulceration of small bowel mucosa Nuclear medicine scan: proximal jejunal blood loss	Resected jejunum: small vessel vasculitis of bowel, mucosal ulceration, submucosa inflammation, fibrosis	c-ANCA
Fallows et al., 2000 [13]	Female, 34	Odynophagia	4 weeks	ESR	Otitis, conjunctivitis, skin rash and ischemia, arthritis, mild kidney involvement	Esophagoscopy: multiple punch-out ulcers	Fibrinoid necrosis with ulcerations and inflammatory cells infiltration surrounding small blood vessels	c-ANCA
Shaikh et al., 2006 [14]	Male, 44	Abdominal pain, peritonitis	Several weeks	ESR	Polyarthralgia, skin rash, polyneuropathy	X-ray and abdominal CT: pneumoperitoneum Laparotomy (three times): multiple perforations in ileum, colonic ischemia	Resected ileum: vasculitis with fibrinoid necrosis	c-ANCA
Walton and Leggat, 1956 [15]	Female, 42	Oral and tongue ulcers	10 months	Not reported	Fever, anosmia and nasal ulcers, deafness, lung infiltrates and pleurisy, arthritis, rash, neuritis, kidney involvement	ND	Autopsy (data restricted to GIT): multiple spleen solitary granulomata similar to those in lung, signs of vasculitis in pancreas	ND
Tokuda et al., 1989 [16]	Male, 37	Gingival ulcers, weight loss, abdominal pain, distention, ascites, peritonitis due to ileum perforation	Nasal symptoms 2 years; systemic disease several weeks	CRP	Rhinorrhea, arthralgia, fever, nasal blockade, necrotizing glomerulonephritis	X-ray: abdominal ascites	Biopsy from perforated ileum, granulomatous vasculitis	ND
Srinivasan and Coughlan, 1999 [17]	Female, 55	Crampy abdominal pain, perforation, weight loss	8 weeks	ESR, CRP	Rhinorrhea, arthralgia, fever, nasal bridge swelling	Barium study: normal Laparotomy: areas of perforation	Granulomatous reaction surrounding perforation without inflammation	c-ANCA

Table 1: Continued.

Author, year of publication	Gender, age (years)	Presenting symptoms	Disease duration	APR elevation	Concomitant respiratory system/kidney/other involvement	CT/endoscopic findings	Biopsy findings	ANCA
Geraghty et al., 1986 [18]	Male, 46	Weight loss, palate ulcerations, peritonitis	4–8 weeks	ESR	Fever, lung and kidney involvement, fingers and toes ischemia	Chest X-ray: free air in abdominal cavity Laparotomy: inflammation of entire small bowel with numerous areas of necrotic ulceration, multiple perforations in terminal ileum	Autopsy: large perforations of ascending colon and multiple punched out ulcers of distal small bowel and proximal large bowel; granulomata in lungs, spleen, and prostate	RF
Haworth and Pusey, 1984 [19]	Female, 43	Mouth ulcer, bloody mucous diarrhea, weight loss, anorexia	11 months	Not reported	Sinusitis, otitis, deafness, arthritis, iritis, rash, kidney involvement	Sigmoidoscopy: ulcerated rectal mucosa with spontaneous bleeding Barium meal: narrowed terminal ileum and cecum Barium enema: ulcerated and ragged cecum	Biopsy: neutrophilic infiltration in rectal and sigmoid mucosa	RF
McNabb et al., 1982 [20]	Male, 50	Pharyngeal and mouth ulcers, abdominal pain, vomiting, peritonitis	Nine months symptoms, GIT symptoms a week after diagnosis	ESR	Arthralgia, nasal blockade, epistaxis, pleurisy, hemoptysis, fingers nodules, proteinuria, renal failure	Laparotomy: multiple ileum ulcers	Biopsy: nonspecific ulcerations	RF
Aymard et al., 1990 [21]	Male, 46	Anal ulcerations	Six months before systemic vasculitis	ESR	Weight loss, polyarthralgia, otalgia, hearing loss, lt. peripheral fascial nerve palsy, hemoptysis	Colonoscopy: normal X-rays of small intestine normal Chest X-ray: right pulmonary apical lesion with cavitation CT: mastoiditis and otitis media	Necrotizing vasculitis, ulcerations and microgranuloma	ANCA
Akça et al., 2005 [22]	Male, 56	Tongue plaques, intestinal perforation	Before diagnosis	ESR, CRP	Pulmonary nodules, severe skin vasculitis	Chest and abdomen X-ray: free air under the diaphragm	Mucosal ulceration, mixed inflammatory cells infiltration and transmural infarcts	c-ANCA

Notes. APR = acute phase reactant; CT = computed tomography; ANCA = anti-neutrophil cytoplasmic antibody; ESR = erythrocyte sedimentation rate; CRP = C-reactive protein; PR3 = proteinase 3; GI = gastrointestinal; CTA = computed tomographic angiography; GPA = granulomatosis with polyangiitis; c-ANCA = cytoplasmic anti-neutrophil cytoplasmic antibody; ND = not done.

reported [28, 29]. Holl-Ulrich and Klass described a patient with necrotizing granulomatous changes in the liver, lungs, parotid glands, and skin in a GPA patient with fatal liver failure [30]. Our patient had multiple nodules in the liver, spleen, and kidneys. Liver biopsy in our patient demonstrated interface hepatitis without granulomas.

Before the 1990s, the main tools for assessment of GPA patients were X-rays with contrast and endoscopy. CT imaging became available later and was found to be very useful. It was obvious from analyzed cases that endoscopy had limited value in the diagnosis of vasculitis, as the main findings were mucosal ulcerations which are not specific for GPA (our patient did not have mucosal damage on endoscopy). In cases with active GIT bleeding on endoscopy, the diagnosis of vasculitis was more reasonable. Inability to perform the deep transmural biopsy during endoscopy also limited the diagnostic value of endoscopy; in the majority of reported cases GPA diagnosis was confirmed in resected bowel specimens or, unfortunately, in autopsies. In the 1980s, the main immunologic abnormality was positive rheumatoid factor (three cases); later, ANCA became a standard diagnostic tool and was reported positive in all but one case, c-ANCA or PR3 in particular (our patient had a transient MPO positive test).

The definitive diagnosis of GPA is based on tissue biopsy, mainly from upper respiratory tract or lung tissue. It is very clear from the Walton report that the presence of granulomas with neutrophils accumulation is a prominent and specific sign, while vascular wall fibrinoid necrosis is nonspecific and probably could only reflect the damage to the blood vessel wall by granuloma [23].

The diversity of GPA clinical manifestations that includes systemic signs (sort of "B-signs") and multiple organ and tissue involvement placed GPA in the list of great "imitators", as it shares various clinical features with other systemic diseases such as hematologic malignances and infections, making the definite diagnosis very challenging. Given the fact that our patient had a combination of listed features, positive ANCA, and findings on open lung biopsy suggestive of necrotizing vasculitis, the working diagnosis of GPA was justified, as was treatment with glucocorticoid pulse therapy. Our patient developed intestinal perforations. "Acute abdomen" with intestinal perforations has been described in GPA patients with GIT involvement [9, 16, 17, 22]. In cases with acute abdomen, laparotomy is mandatory. In our patient, biopsies from resected bowel segments showed signs of diffuse large B cell lymphoma cells. Retrospective revision of lung pathology confirmed that the damage to the blood vessels was mainly due to an accumulation of lymphocytes in the involved tissue but not neutrophil accumulation or granulomas.

Different types of lymphoma may mimic different types of vasculitis. Lymphoma may be associated with ANCA positivity for both PR3 and MPO without vasculitis [31]. In a series of 119 patients with non-Hodgkin's lymphoma and 60 patients with Hodgkin's lymphoma, ANCA positivity was found in 8 patients (6 with p-ANCA and 2 with c-ANCA) with Hodgkin's lymphoma. None had vasculitis or rheumatic manifestations [32]. We could not explain the inconsistent results of positive MPO; in our institution the test for ANCA was negative. Despite the rare association between lymphoma and vasculitis, vasculitis in lymphoma patients mainly presents with skin purpuric rash and leukocytoclastic vasculitis on biopsy; our patient did not have any rash.

In searching the literature, we were able to find three cases of diffuse large B cell lymphoma mimicking GPA [33–35]. All these patients, like our patient, were males, aged between 20 and 40 years of age, and had pulmonary involvement; all had negative ANCA. None of these patients, in contrary to our patient, had liver or spleen involvement; one patient had renal involvement. In the case reported by Cohen et al., the patient was diagnosed with GPA and initially "responded" well to steroids and cyclophosphamide; only because of severe relapse under the treatment, revision of the biopsy leads to the proper diagnosis of lymphoma.

Did we have some clues to doubt the diagnosis of vasculitis in a patient who presented with systemic signs, multiorgan clinical presentations, presence of pulmonary nodules, positive MPO, and signs of vascular damage on open lung biopsy? A retrospective analysis of the case could teach us to pay attention to tiny discrepancies in the patient's condition: the anosmia in the absence of upper respiratory tract involvement was probably a "red herring"; the presence of multiple small and not consistent pulmonary nodules without cavitation is not a typical GPA feature; the presence of nodular lesions on CT imaging ("macroscopic") in the spleen, kidneys, and liver without signs of hemorrhage is not typical for GPA; severe dyspepsia (abdominal pain, vomiting, and constipation) without any mucosal damage (ulceration or bleeding) on upper endoscopy could not be explained by vasculitis, especially in the absence of diarrhea or intestinal/rectal bleeding. GPA is a disease with neutrophils activation and accumulation in organs and tissues; our patient did not have leukocytosis. Also, he had only mildly elevated ESR and CRP in contrast to very high levels in patients with GPA. It is unusual not to find c-ANCA (especially PR3) in patients with active GPA and multiorgan involvement as in our patient. Finally, the absence of granulomas in the involved lung tissue with only the pathological finding of vessel wall damage should raise the question regarding a diagnosis of vasculitis or a search for an alternative diagnosis.

We believe that in cases of atypical clinical course of systemic illness suggestive of vasculitis (GPA), the differential diagnosis should include lymphoma. Prompt efforts should be invested to confirm the diagnosis of vasculitis or to ensure that another condition, such as lymphoma, is not the cause of the disease. Our report pointed out the difficulties and obstacles on the way to making the correct diagnosis in patients with B cell lymphoma mimicking systemic GPA-like vasculitis.

Competing Interests

All authors declare no competing interests.

Acknowledgments

The authors thank Dr. Natalia Puchkov of the Department of Medical Imaging, Rambam Health Care Campus, who provided the CT images and their relevant legends.

References

[1] P. M. K. Lutalo and D. P. D'Cruz, "Diagnosis and classification of granulomatosis with polyangiitis (aka Wegener's granulomatosis)," *Journal of Autoimmunity*, vol. 48-49, pp. 94–98, 2014.

[2] S. Akbulut, "Multiple ileal perforations in a patient with Wegener's granulomatosis: a case report and literature review," *Journal of Gastrointestinal Surgery*, vol. 16, no. 4, pp. 857–862, 2012.

[3] A. Yoshikawa, S. Yoshida, T. Takeuchi, Y. Fujiki, S. Makino, and T. Hanafusa, "Gastrointestinal involvement at the onset of granulomatosis with polyangiitis: a case report," *Modern Rheumatology*, 2015.

[4] J. D. Sinnott, P. Matthews, and S. Fletcher, "Colitis: an unusual presentation of wegener's granulomatosis," *BMJ Case Reports*, 2013.

[5] M. S. Dag, Y. Pehlivan, E. Tutar, and B. Kisacik, "Rituximab seems a promising therapeutic option in granulomatosis with polyangiitis with intestinal perforation: a case report and literature review," *BMJ Case Reports*, 2013.

[6] Q. Qian, L. Cornell, V. Chandan, R. Hartman, and S. Caples, "Hemorrhagic colitis as a presenting feature of Wegener granulomatosis," *Journal of Gastrointestinal and Liver Diseases*, vol. 19, no. 4, pp. 445–447, 2010.

[7] M. Samim, A. Pronk, and P. M. Verheijen, "Intestinal perforation as an early complication in Wegener's granulomatosis," *World Journal of Gastrointestinal Surgery*, vol. 2, no. 5, pp. 169–171, 2010.

[8] I. Marie, L. Lahaxe, S. Josse, T. Lequerre, O. Vittecoq, and G. Savoye, "Rectal involvement revealing Wegener's disease," *Scandinavian Journal of Rheumatology*, vol. 39, no. 4, pp. 346–348, 2010.

[9] K. Deniz, H. S. Özşeker, Ş. Balas, E. Akpýnar, and C. Sökmensüer, "Intestinal involvement in Wegener's granulomatosis," *Journal of Gastrointestinal and Liver Diseases*, vol. 16, no. 3, pp. 329–331, 2007.

[10] Y. Kuwahara, Y. Shima, T. Tanaka et al., "Successful treatment with intravenous cyclophosphamide pulse therapy of severe intestinal involvement in Wegener's granulomatosis," *Scandinavian Journal of Rheumatology*, vol. 35, no. 3, pp. 243–245, 2006.

[11] M. Socas Macías, M. L. Sánchez Bernal, G. Suárez Artacho et al., "Severe intestinal involvement in Wegener's granulomatosis with negative c-ANCAs," *Revista Espanola de Enfermedades Digestivas*, vol. 97, no. 9, pp. 670–671, 2005.

[12] F. Y. F. Chow, D. Hooke, and P. G. Kerr, "Severe intestinal involvement in wegener's granulomatosis," *Journal of Gastroenterology and Hepatology*, vol. 18, no. 6, pp. 749–750, 2003.

[13] G. A. Fallows, S. F. Hamilton, D. S. Taylor, and S. B. Reddy, "Esophageal involvement in Wegener's granulomatosis: a case report and review of the literature," *Canadian Journal of Gastroenterology*, vol. 14, no. 5, pp. 449–451, 2000.

[14] F. M. Shaikh, C. B. Sabu, T. H. Peirce, and S. A. Naqvi, "Extensive intestinal ischaemic necrosis in Wegener's granulomatosis," *Gut*, vol. 55, no. 9, pp. 1368–1369, 2006.

[15] E. W. Walton and P. O. Leggat, "Wegener's granulomatosis," *Journal of Clinical Pathology*, vol. 9, no. 1, pp. 31–37, 1956.

[16] M. Tokuda, N. Kurata, H. Daikuhara et al., "Small intestinal perforation in Wegener's granulomatosis," *Journal of Rheumatology*, vol. 16, no. 4, pp. 547–549, 1989.

[17] U. Srinivasan and R. J. Coughlan, "Small intestinal perforation complicating Wegener's granulomatosis," *Rheumatology*, vol. 38, no. 3, pp. 289–290, 1999.

[18] J. Geraghty, I. R. Mackay, and D. C. Smith, "Intestinal perforation in Wegener's granulomatosis," *Gut*, vol. 27, no. 4, pp. 450–451, 1986.

[19] S. J. Haworth and C. D. Pusey, "Severe intestinal involvement in Wegener's granulomatosis," *Gut*, vol. 25, no. 11, pp. 1296–1300, 1984.

[20] W. R. McNabb, M. S. Lennox, and J. A. Wedzicha, "Small intestinal perforation in Wegener's granulomatosis," *Postgraduate Medical Journal*, vol. 58, no. 676, pp. 123–125, 1982.

[21] B. Aymard, M. A. Bigard, H. Thompson, J. L. Schmutz, J. F. Finet, and J. Borrelly, "Perianal ulcer: an unusual presentation of Wegener's granulomatosis. Report of a case," *Diseases of the Colon & Rectum*, vol. 33, no. 5, pp. 427–430, 1990.

[22] T. Akça, T. Çolak, M. Çglikulekçi, K. Öcal, and S. Aydin, "Intestinal perforation in Wegener's granulomatosis: a case report," *Ulusal Travma ve Acil Cerrahi Dergisi*, vol. 11, no. 4, pp. 348–351, 2005.

[23] E. W. Walton, "Giant-cell granuloma of the respiratory tract (Wegener's granulomatosis)," *The British Medical Journal*, vol. 2, article 265, 1958.

[24] J. C. Lee, I. Bringmann, and A. Aly, "Asymptomatic splenic infarct and retroperitoneal sepsis in patient with Wegener's granulomatosis," *International Journal of Surgery Case Reports*, vol. 3, no. 4, pp. 137–138, 2012.

[25] M. Martusewicz-Boros, I. Baranska, E. Wiatr, I. Bestry, and K. Roszkowski-Sliz, "Asymptomatic appearance of splenic infarction in Wegener's granulomatosis," *Polish Journal of Radiology*, vol. 76, no. 2, pp. 43–45, 2011.

[26] A. Ghinoi, N. Pipitone, A. Cavazza, L. Boiardi, and C. Salvarani, "Wegener granulomatosis with spleen infarction: case report and review of the literature," *Seminars in Arthritis and Rheumatism*, vol. 37, no. 5, pp. 328–333, 2008.

[27] D. Papaioannides, S. N. Nikas, M. Fotinou, and N. K. Akritidis, "Asymptomatic splenic infarction in Wegener's granulomatosis," *Annals of the Rheumatic Diseases*, vol. 61, no. 2, pp. 185–186, 2002.

[28] S. Doganay, E. Kocakoc, and M. Balaban, "Nontraumatic hepatic hematoma caused by Wegener's granulomatosis: an unusual cause of abdominal pain," *New Zealand Medical Journal*, vol. 123, no. 1318, pp. 73–78, 2010.

[29] Y. Zen, H. Sunagozaka, K. Tsuneyama et al., "Incomplete septal cirrhosis associated with Wegener's granulomatosis," *Liver*, vol. 22, no. 5, pp. 388–393, 2002.

[30] K. Holl-Ulrich and M. Klass, "Wegener's granulomatosis with granulomatous liver involvement," *Clinical and Experimental Rheumatology*, vol. 28, no. 1, supplement 57, pp. S88–S89, 2010.

[31] K. K. Zuckerman, L. Leventhal, and C. Wynne, "Positive c-ANCA in a patient with lymphoma and without vasculitis," *Journal of Clinical Rheumatology*, vol. 3, no. 5, pp. 279–281, 1997.

[32] T. Cil, A. Altintas, A. Isikdogan, and S. Batun, "Prevalence of antineutrophil cytoplasmic antibody positivity in patients with Hodgkin's and non-Hodgkin lymphoma: a single center experience," *International Journal of Hematology*, vol. 90, no. 1, pp. 52–57, 2009.

[33] Y. Cohen, G. Amir, G. Schibi, N. Amariglio, and A. Polliack, "Rapidly progressive diffuse large B-cell lymphoma with initial clinical presentation mimicking seronegative Wegener's granulomatosis," *European Journal of Haematology*, vol. 73, no. 2, pp. 134–138, 2004.

[34] D. Gawryluk, J. Słodkowska, P. Dobkowski, and E. Wiatr, "Diffuse large B-cell lymphoma mimicking Wegener's granulomatosis," *Pneumologia i Alergologia Polska*, vol. 70, pp. 210–215, 2002.

[35] N. Miyahara, R. Eda, Y. Umemori et al., "Pulmonary lymphoma of large B-cell type mimicking Wegener's granulomatosis," *Internal Medicine*, vol. 40, no. 8, pp. 786–790, 2001.

24

RHUPUS Syndrome in Children

Vahid Ziaee,[1,2,3] Mohammad Hassan Moradinejad,[1,3,4] and Reyhaneh Bayat[4]

[1] *Department of Pediatrics, Tehran University of Medical Sciences, Tehran, Iran*
[2] *Pediatric Rheumatology Research Group, Rheumatology Research Center, Tehran University of Medical Sciences, Tehran, Iran*
[3] *Division of Pediatric Rheumatology, Children's Medical Center, Pediatrics Center of Excellence, Tehran 14194, Iran*
[4] *Growth and Development Research Center, Tehran University of Medical Sciences, Tehran, Iran*

Correspondence should be addressed to Vahid Ziaee; ziaee@tums.ac.ir

Academic Editors: H. Alexanderson, C. Orellana, and G. J. Tsay

Objective. Overlap of juvenile idiopathic arthritis (JIA) and juvenile systemic lupus erythematosus (JSLE) is a rare clinical condition in children. This condition has been described as RHUPUS syndrome. Prevalence of this syndrome and 3 cases are reported in this paper. *Cases Presentation.* During 10 years, 3 patients with SLE had chronic arthritis before or after diagnosis of SLE. Prevalence of this disorder in JSLE was 2.5%. Two patients were females and one of them was a male. According to our review, mean delay between chronic joint involvement and JSLE diagnosis was 50.1 months. In our case report, two females had joint erosion and one of them died due to heart failure, but in the literature review, just 45% cases had joint erosion and 70% cases were polyarticulare form. *Conclusion.* RHUPUS is unusual presentation of lupus in children. It seems that clinical feature and outcome of RHUPUS syndrome are different in children due to difference between RA and JIA. We suggest juvenile RHUPUS for overlap of JIA and JSLE.

1. Introduction

Juvenile idiopathic arthritis (JIA) is the most common type autoimmune rheumatic disease in children. It is a chronic non infectious synovitis that can affect joints in any part of the body. Organs involvement is common in systemic onset type but it decreases after control of inflammation [1].

Systemic lupus erythematosus (SLE) is the most important, multisystem, autoimmune rheumatic disease characterized by both clinical and immunological abnormalities [2].

The peak incidence of childhood SLE occurs around puberty and predominantly involves young women in reproductive age, and in 10%–20% of SLE patients, diagnosis is made for the first time in childhood onset [2]. Arthritis is one of the earliest symptoms in juvenile SLE (JSLE) but it is characteristically short in duration and can be migratory [2]. Although the synovitis of JSLE may be minimally proliferative, it is only occasionally erosive and usually does not result in permanent deformity. JSLE can mimic JIA, especially when it is presented as chronic and erosive arthritis [3].

Overlapping JIA and JSLE is a rare clinical condition in children [4, 5]. RHUPUS syndrome has been defined as an overlap between RA and SLE in adult patients [6]. Although serological overlap between RA and SLE is common in adult patients, clinical overlap between RA and SLE is a rare manifestation of rheumatologic disorders. For the first time, RHUPUS syndrome was described by Schur in 1971 [7], but first clinical observation of this syndrome has been described in 1960 by Toone. He identified this clinical manifestation with this entity [8].

For diagnosis of RHUPUS syndrome, erosive polyarthritis and clinical symptoms of SLE as well as positive dsDNA or anti-Sm autoantibodies are necessary [9].

In this paper, we described the presence of three children with RHUPUS syndrome. Finally we reviewed all cases that have been reported in the literature with clinical picture of JIA as first presentation and eventually turned out to be typical systemic lupus erythemaosus, during follow-up.

2. Case Report

During 10 years, 120 patients with systemic lupus erythematosus who had been referred to our tertiary pediatric medical center were evaluated. Three patients (2 girls and 1 boy) had chronic joint involvement and JSLE (prevalence rate 2.5%).

2.1. Case 1. An 8 year-old girl was referred with pain, swelling, and motion limitation of both knees and left ankle lasting for more than 6 months. She has morning stiffness without fever. She did not have complaints in any other joints. On her first examination, she had bilateral effusions of the knees and swelling of left ankle, but the other joints and systems were normal. There were no skin rashes or mucosal lesions. Initial laboratory results revealed normal complete blood count (CBC), complement levels, and immunoglobulin levels. But RF and ANA were positive. In MRI, chronic inflammation with synovial thickening was seen in both knees, suggesting erosive arthritis. She was diagnosed as oligoarticular JRA and started treatment with prednisolone (7.5 mg/day), Methtrexate (7.5 mg/Week), and hydroxycholoroquine (200/mg/day), and she was regularly followed up at 1.5–2 months intervals. After two years of follow up, at the age of 10 years, she had a flare-up of disease with clinical manifestation (fever, fatigue, and malaise), malar rash, and arthritis in the knees, ankle, oral ulcer, pethecia, and purpura. At that time, laboratory results revealed (pancytopenia), coombs negative anemia (Hb: 9.7 g/dL), thrombocytopenia (30,000/mm3) and leukopenia (WBC count 2900/mm3) (predominant lymphopenia). F-ANA was positive (1/1280, speckled pattern), anti-dsDNA level was positive 1/80, rheumatoid factor level (RF) was 7.88 IU/mL (0–14 IU/mL), and C3 (65.7 mg/dL) and C4 (4.4 mg/dL) levels were low. Antiphospholipid antibodies (aPL) level was negative and urinalysis showed microscopic hematuria (5-10 RBC in hpf) and trace proteinuria (1+). She was diagnosed as JSLE, with more than five criteria, after two years of ongoing chronic arthritis. Treatment was started with new diagnosis of SLE with Prednisolone (1 mg/kg/day), Azathioprine (50 mg/d), and Hydroxycholoroquine (200/mg/day). She was under observation and she had a systemic flare-up of lupus when she was 12 years old which has been controlled with increasing dosage of drugs. When she was 13 years old, she found renal involvement in this course of the illness with clinical manifestations of SLE, hypertension, proteinuria, urine protein 24 hours more than 2300 mg/day, microscopic hematuria, cellular casts, and elevated serum blood nitrogen and creatinine concentration.

She was treated with azathioprine (50 mg/d) with oral prednisolone (50 mg/day) hydroxycholoroquine (400/mg/day). After 4-year followup, she is 17 years old and she is under observation and she was on low dose prednisolone (0.5 gr/kg/day), azathioprine (50 mg/d), and hydroxycholoroquine (400/mg/day).

2.2. Case 2. A 10-year-old girl was referred with morning stiffness and arthralgia in the both knees and ankles. In physical examination, she had sometimes fever, but there was not effusion and swelling in the joints or other systemic manifestation of rheumatologic disorders. In laboratory investigation, she had normal CBC, elevated ESR (40), and positive ANA (1/80). Other tests such as Anti ds-DNA, RF, VDRL, Urinalysis, BUN, and Creatinine were negative. She was under observ for 6 months and she was on naproxen 10 mg/kg during this time. After 6 months, joint effusion in both knees, ankles, and wrists was added to her symptoms. She was diagnosed as JRA polyarticuler form and she was treated with prednisolone (7.5 mg/day), Methtrexate, (7.5 mg/Week), and hydroxycholoroquine (100/mg/day) as well as Naproxane, and she was under observation every 2 months. When she was 12, she was referred to emergency clinic with chief complaint of abdominal pain and acute anemia and splenomegalia. Joint involvement in large joints (knees, elbow, and ankles) and small joints (MCPs and PIPs) was there. In laboratory study, we found an acute hemolytic anemia (Hgb = 5.2, Retic = 6%) with positive direct coombs (2+), positive VDRL (1.32), decreased complements (C3 = 21, C4 = 3, CH50 = 0%), and positive ds-DNA (100). She was diagnosed as an overlap syndrome (RAPUS syndrome) between JRA and JSLE, with more than four criteria, after 24 months ongoing chronic arthritis. Treatment was started with new diagnosis SLE with Prednisolone (2 mg/kg/day) and Hydroxycholoroquine (200/mg/day). After 1 month, anemia was resolved and joint symptoms reduced. During followup, she had multijoints involvement, when we reduced the dosage of prednisolone to less than 0.5 mg/kg/day.

After 2 months, she was referred to clinic with abnormal movement without history of streptococcal infection. In physical examination, cardiac examination was normal and there was not any abnormality in neurologic examaination exept chorea athetosis. Laboratory investigation showed elevation in anti ds-DNA titer, decrement of complements, and normal MRI. The dosage of prednisolone was increased to 2 mg/kg/day and haloperidol and Artan was started. After 2 weeks, abnormal movement was controlled and the dosage of prednisolone was decreased after 4 weeks. She had a relapsing in chorea athetoeid movement after 3 months, and reevaluation did not show any new findings. After 12-month followup, she was under control with prednisolone (0.5 mg/kg/day), Hydoxychlroquine (200 mg/daily), valporate sodium, and haloperidol, but she had on and off joints effusion and in radiographic evaluation, and there is some evidence to erosion in her knees.

After 5 months, she was admitted to hospital with fever (39.5), vomiting and tachypnea, and large joints effusion. Treatment with antibiotics was started based on diagnosis of flare-up of disease because of infection. In second day, the decreased levels of consciousness, low cardiac output, GI bleeding, and anuria were presented. In heart echocardiography, she had ejection fraction: 10%, left ventricle, transverse diameter systole: 10%, dilated cardiomyopathy without pericardial effusion and/or vegetation. Blood culture was negative, and after starting pulse therapy with methylprednisolone, she died due to heart failure.

2.3. Case 3. An 11-year-old boy was referred with pain and swelling of right knee and swelling in the back of the ankle for 2 months, with no abnormal findings in physical exam. In laboratory investigation, he had anemia (HB: 8.8 and thrombocytosis (PLt: 569000), elevated ESR (59) and CRP (3+)

Table 1: Clinical and paraclincal features and outcome of cases with RHUPUS syndrome in this case report and previous reports in children.

Report	Sex	JIA Characteristics					Delay in SLE
		Age at onset (y)	ANA	RF	Subtype	Erosion	diagnosis (mo)[†]
Unsal et al. [10]	Female	8.5	–	–	Oligoarticular	No	24
Bazsó et al. [4]	Female	12	–	–	Polyarticular	No	120
Cavalcante et al. [5]	Female	10	+	+	Polyarticular	No	11
	Female	10	+	+	Polyarticular	Yes	9
	Male	5	+	+	Polyarticular	Yes	15
Takei et al. [11]	Female	15	–	–	Polyarticular	No	96
	Female	3	–	–	Polyarticular	?	120
Martini et al.* [12]	Female	5	?	?	?	?	72
Our study	Female	8	+	+	Oligoarticular	Yes	24
	Female	10	+	+	Polyarticular	Yes	24
	Male	11	–	+	Oligoarticular	No	36
Total cases	82% female	8.1	50% positive	60% positive	70% polyarticular	45% erosion	50.1

*We did not access full text of this report.
[†]Delay between beginning of chronic arthritis and SLE diagnosis.

and positive RF (3+). The patient's brother and sister were known lupus cases, and his brothers were died due to SLE complication; so investigations for finding lupus were done, and in laboratory tests, he had negative FANA and normal ds-DNA. He was treated with methotrexate, prednisolone (2.5 mg daily), and hydroxychloroquine (100 mg/day). After one year, he had a flare-up with no systemic problems and/or abnormal laboratory tests. In third year, he was in full remission and treatment was stopped. After 2 years of followup, he found joint effusion and mallar rash and positive FANA (1/320) and Anti ds-DNA. Regarding positive family history, diagnosis of JSLE was suggested and he was treated with prednisolone (5 mg TDS), hydroxychloroquine (100 mg daily) and azathioprine (1/2 tab daily). There is no evidence of joint erosion in radiologic evaluation. His symptoms were controlled after 2 months and the dosage of treatment was reduced, gradually. After 2 years of followup, he was 18 and he had no problems and was in remission.

3. Discussion

RHUPUS (RA and SLE) is a rare clinical condition in adult. First description of RHUPUS was done by Toone in 1960 [8]. In SLE, joint involvement may range from minor joint pain to severe deforming arthritis as well as Jaccoud's arthropathy, but sometimes joint pain is more severe than joint objective findings [13–15]. The diagnosis of RHUPUS is made when it becomes difficult to support the diagnosis of any of these diseases as an isolated entity. There are three viewpoints on RHUPUS. Some authors such as Fernandez believe that RHUPUS arthropathy is a serious articular involvement of lupus and it is different from a superposition or overlap of RA and SLE [16, 17], while other authors believe that RHUPUS syndrome is combination of SLE and chronic erosive polyarthritis [5, 9, 15], and the last group believes that RHUPUS is overlap of RA or JIA and SLE (regardless to poly or oligoarthritis and erosive or nonerosive) [4, 18]. We agree with last group about RHUPUS syndrome in children. Since, RHUPUS is overlap of RA or RA and SLE, we suggested juvenile RHUPUS for overlap of JIA and JSLE. RHUPUS in children presents with features of JRA but later on develops features of SLE [4]. Although, few cases of RHUPUS syndrome present simultaneously with features of JRA and SLE as overlap syndrome, JRA and SLE as a presenting manifestation may not be complete [5]. In adult the majority polyarticular erosive arthritis is most common manifestation, but in children, features of JIA dominating asymmetrical erosive and/or nonerosive oligoarticular involvement may be common manifestation [10, 11]. All cases with RHUPUS syndrome in this study and previous report in children were compared in Table 1. In this case report, two cases were oligoarticular subtype and one of them had joint erosion. Another case was polyarticular subtype with joint erosion. In the literature review, 70% of cases were polyarticular subtype.

Panush et al. in 1988 in an observational study reviewed approximately 7000 new patients who were evaluated for more than over 11 years [6]. They found 6 patients who had both RA and SLE (the prevalence 0.09%). However, it seems that the prevalence of this presentation of SLE is more common than previously reported. In our study, the prevalence of this syndrome was 2.5%. Similarly, Cavalcante et al. reported the prevalence of chronic polyarthritis in 2.6% of JSLE patients and in all patients, joint involvement was the initial manifestation [5]. It can be due to better management and decreases in mortality of SLE during recent decades.

There are few reports on RHUPUS syndrome in children [10–12]. Martini et al. reported an 11-year-old girl who presented initially as JRA patient at 5 years old, but she developed clinical manifestation of SLE after 6 years [12]. Similarly, Unsal et al. reported an 8.5 year old girl with JIA who developed criteria of SLE after 2 years [10]. In another report, Takei et al. introduced two cases with JRA who developed SLE criteria and after 8 years with ANA and anti ds-DNA positivity and clinical picture of SLE [11]. Our cases fulfilled JSLE criteria after 2-3 years of first manifestation of joint involvement and JIA diagnosis. The mean delay of SLE diagnosis in all reported cases was 50.1 months (Table 1).

Most common features of SLE in our cases were cutaneous involvement in 2 patients and hematologic manifestations in one case, but all of them had ANA and RF positivity before SLE diagnosis.

Similar to our study, in most cases with RHUPUS syndrome, ANA and RF have been positive or they get positivity during followup [11, 19]. Similar with Panush report, our patients have increased frequency of positivity in high titers of ANA. Totally, the rate of positive ANA and RF at the onset of chronic arthritis was 50% and 60%, respectively (Table 1).

It seems that articular erosion is less common in children than adult with RHUPUS syndrome. In our case report, one case had erosive arthritis before completing JSLE, and in our litrature review, just 45% cases had joint erosion (Table 1). Recently, Amezcua-Guerra studied the prevalence of antibodies against anti-CCP antibodies in RHUPUS [18], and they concluded that RHUPUS is an overlap between RA and SLE.

4. Conclusion

Overlap of JIA and JSLE is a rare syndrome in childhood and there is a few case report on this syndrome in children. It seems that clinical feature and outcome of RHUPUS syndrome are different in children due to difference between RA and JIA. Juvenile RHUPUS is suggested for overlap of JIA and JSLE. We recommend all patients with JRA and positive ANA to have followup for long time (at least 4 years) for Juvenile RHUPUS syndrome and to be evaluated for JSLE, if they developed cutaneous or hematological symptoms.

References

[1] R. E. Petty and J. T. Cassidy, "Chronic arthritis in childhood," in *Textbook of Pediatric Rheumatology*, J. T. Cassidy, R. E. Petty, R. M. Laxer, and C. B. Lindsley, Eds., pp. 211–235, Elsevier Saunders, Philadelphia, Pa, USA, 6th edition, 2011.

[2] R. E. Petty and R. M. Laxer, "Systemic lupus erythematosus," in *Textbook of Pediatric Rheumatology*, J. T. Cassidy, R. E. Petty, R. M. Laxer, and C. B. Lindsley, Eds., pp. 342–383, Elsevier Saunders, Philadelphia, Pa, USA, 6th edition, 2011.

[3] M. R. Cohen, G. Steiner, J. S. Smolen, and D. A. Isenberg, "Erosive arthritis in systemic lupus erythematosus: analysis of a distinct clinical and serological subset," *British Journal of Rheumatology*, vol. 37, no. 4, pp. 421–424, 1998.

[4] A. Bazsó, K. Sevcic, I. Orbán, G. Poór, Z. Balogh, and E. Kiss, "Overlapping juvenile idiopathic arthritis and systemic lupus erythematosus: a case report," *Rheumatology International*, vol. 31, no. 5, pp. 695–698, 2011.

[5] E. G. Cavalcante, N. E. Aikawa, R. G. Lozano, A. P. Lotito, A. A. Jesus, and C. A. Silva, "Chronic polyarthritis as the first manifestation of juvenile systemic lupus erythematosus patients," *Lupus*, vol. 20, no. 9, pp. 960–964, 2011.

[6] R. S. Panush, L. Edwards, S. Longley, and E. Webster, "RHUPUS syndrome," *Archives of Internal Medicine*, vol. 148, no. 7, pp. 1633–1636, 1988.

[7] P. H. Schur, "Systemic lupus erythematosus," in *Cecil-Loeb Texbook of Medicine*, P. B. Beeson and W. McDermott, Eds., p. 821, Sanders, Philadelphia, Pa, USA, 1971.

[8] E. C. Toone, R. Irby, and E. L. Pierce, "The L.E. cell in rheumatoid arthritis," *The American Journal of the Medical Sciences*, vol. 240, pp. 599–608, 1960.

[9] M. Satoh, A. K. Ajmani, and M. Akizuki, "What is the definition for coexistent rheumatoid arthritis and systemic lupus erythematosus?" *Lupus*, vol. 3, no. 2, pp. 137–138, 1994.

[10] E. Unsal, A. O. Arli, and H. Akman, "Rhupus arthropathy as the presenting manifestation in Juvenile SLE: a case report," *Pediatric Rheumatology*, vol. 5, p. 7, 2007.

[11] S. Takei, N. Maeno, M. Shigemori et al., "Two cases with SLE and MCTD developed after a long period of chronic arthritis that was initially diagnosed as JRA," *Ryumachi*, vol. 37, no. 5, pp. 702–708, 1997.

[12] A. Martini, A. Ravelli, S. Viola, and R. G. Burgio, "Systemic lupus erythematosus with Jaccoud's arthropathy mimicking junvenile rheumatoid arthritis," *Arthritis and Rheumatism*, vol. 30, no. 9, pp. 1062–1064, 1987.

[13] B. Ostendorf, A. Scherer, C. Specker, U. Mödder, and M. Schneider, "Jaccoud's arthropathy in systemic lupus erythematosus: differentiation of deforming and erosive patterns by magnetic resonance imaging," *Arthritis and Rheumatism*, vol. 48, no. 1, pp. 157–165, 2003.

[14] R. Labowitz and H. R. Schumacher, "Articular manifestations of systemic lupus erythematosus," *Annals of Internal Medicine*, vol. 74, no. 6, pp. 911–921, 1971.

[15] R. M. Van Vugt, R. H. W. M. Derksen, L. Kater, and J. W. J. Bijlsma, "Deforming arthropathy or lupus and rhupus hands in systemic lupus erythematosus," *Annals of the Rheumatic Diseases*, vol. 57, no. 9, pp. 540–544, 1998.

[16] A. Fernández, G. Quintana, F. Rondón et al., "Lupus arthropathy: a case series of patients with rhupus," *Clinical Rheumatology*, vol. 25, no. 2, pp. 164–167, 2006.

[17] A. Fernández, G. Quintana, E. L. Matteson et al., "Lupus arthropathy: historical evolution from deforming arthritis to rhupus," *Clinical Rheumatology*, vol. 23, no. 6, pp. 523–526, 2004.

[18] L. M. Amezcua-Guerra, R. Springall, R. Marquez-Velasco, L. Gómez-García, A. Vargas, and R. Bojalil, "Presence of antibodies against cyclic citrullinated peptides in patients with 'rhupus': a cross-sectional study," *Arthritis Research and Therapy*, vol. 8, no. 5, p. R144, 2006.

[19] B. Sharma, "RHUPUS: report of 3 cases," *Journal of Indian Rheumatology Association*, vol. 11, pp. 51–54, 2003.

25

Efficacy of Cyclosporine in the Induction and Maintenance of Remission in a Systemic Lupus Erythematosus Patient Presenting with Macrophage-Activating Syndrome

Franchesca Cruz-Pérez, Salvador Vilá, Grissel Ríos, and Luis M. Vilá

Division of Rheumatology, Department of Medicine, University of Puerto Rico Medical Sciences Campus, San Juan, PR, USA

Correspondence should be addressed to Salvador Vilá; salvador.vila@upr.edu and Luis M. Vilá; luis.vila2@upr.edu

Academic Editor: Tsai-Ching Hsu

Macrophage-activating syndrome (MAS) is a rare condition characterized by dysfunctional macrophage activation leading to overproduction of cytokines and phagocytosis of erythrocytes, leukocytes, and platelets. MAS is associated with infectious diseases, malignancies, and autoimmune rheumatic disorders. Herein, we present a 22-year-old Hispanic woman with SLE who was hospitalized because of a three-week history of fever, fatigue, polyarthralgia, nausea, and abdominal pain. Initial laboratories showed severe pancytopenia with marked elevation of liver enzymes and ferritin levels. Bone marrow biopsy revealed macrophages with engulfed erythrocytes consistent with MAS. The patient was treated with high-dose corticosteroids, intravenous immunoglobulins, and cyclosporine 3 mg/kg/day. She had a remarkable clinical response to this therapy. She was continued on cyclosporine, and prednisone dose was gradually decreased to 7.5 mg daily without experiencing recurrent disease. She remained in full clinical remission for 12 months. Our case, together with other reports, suggests that combination therapy with corticosteroids, immunoglobulins, and cyclosporine appears to be effective for patients with SLE-associated MAS. Furthermore, cyclosporine seems to be a good drug for maintenance of remission.

1. Introduction

Macrophage-activating syndrome (MAS) is an uncommon and life-threatening complication of infectious diseases, malignancies, and rheumatic diseases that results from uncontrolled production of proinflammatory cytokines leading to overactivation of T lymphocytes and macrophages [1, 2]. MAS has been reported in patients with various rheumatic diseases, such as systemic juvenile idiopathic arthritis (sJIA), adult-onset Still's disease, dermatomyositis, and systemic lupus erythematosus (SLE) [1]. SLE-associated MAS is a rare complication that usually occurs in young adults with high lupus activity [1–3]. Women are more affected than men [2–4]. Patients commonly present with fever, fatigue, arthralgia, pancytopenia, elevated liver enzymes, hypertriglyceridemia, hyperferritinemia, and the presence of serological markers related to SLE activity such as elevated anti-dsDNA antibodies and C3 and C4 hypocomplementemia [1–3]. High-dose corticosteroids, cyclophosphamide, cyclosporine, intravenous (IV) immunoglobulins, and etoposide have been used for SLE-associated MAS [3–7]. However, there are no established treatment guidelines regarding the induction and maintenance of remission for these patients. Herein, we report a Hispanic SLE patient with MAS who was treated with high-dose corticosteroids, immunoglobulins, and cyclosporine. She had a remarkable response to this therapy without adverse events and has remained in clinical remission for one year.

2. Case Presentation

A 22-year-old Puerto Rican woman with SLE was hospitalized to our institution in August 2016 because of a three-week history of fever, chills, polyarthralgia, anorexia, nausea, and marked pancytopenia. Seven years before admission, she was diagnosed with SLE manifested by fatigue, anorexia, anemia, leukopenia, thrombocytopenia, positive antinuclear

Table 1: Results of selected blood tests before and after cyclosporine treatment.

Laboratory test	Two weeks prior to admission	On admission	One day after admission	Five days after cyclosporine therapy	At discharge
WBC (10^9/L)	3.03	1.4	0.57	14.30	17.1
Hemoglobin (g/dL)	7.7	9.6	7.8	10.1	10.1
Platelet (10^9/L)	216	51	85	68	83
AST (U/L)	138	451	—	38	20
ALT (U/L)	73	138	—	58	24
ESR (mm/hr)	56	70	53	—	—
Ferritin (ng/mL)	1,290	5,602	—	3,960	802
Triglycerides (mg/dL)	122	211	—	—	150

WBC: white blood cell; AST: aspartate aminotransferase; ALT: alanine aminotransferase; ESR: erythrocyte sedimentation rate (by Westergren).

antibodies (ANAs), elevated anti-dsDNA antibodies, positive anti-RNP antibodies, and hypocomplementemia (C3 and C4). Initially, she was treated with corticosteroids, hydroxychloroquine, and mycophenolate mofetil having a good clinical response. However, she had poor adherence to these medications and self-discontinued her treatment after one year of therapy.

Two weeks prior to hospitalization at our institution, she was admitted to a community hospital due to high-grade fever (40.1°C), nausea, pancytopenia, and elevated liver enzymes, erythrocyte sedimentation rate (ESR), and ferritin levels. Anti-nuclear antibodies (ANAs) were positive at a titer of 1 : 1280 with a homogeneous pattern. Serum complements levels were normal. Blood cultures were negative, as well as tests for hepatitis B and C, human immunodeficiency virus, varicella-zoster virus IgM, herpes simplex virus IgM, cytomegalovirus IgM, and Epstein–Barr virus IgM. She was treated with methylprednisolone 60 mg IV daily and broad-spectrum antibiotics including vancomycin and cefepime. Also, fluconazole and acyclovir were added. The hospitalization was complicated with ventricular fibrillation which responded to nonsynchronized cardioversion. She had partial clinical improvement to this therapy and was discharged home, but three days later, she developed worsening of fever and malaise associated with abdominal pain, nausea, and diarrhea.

Upon admission to our institution, she appeared acutely ill. Vital signs showed temperature of 39.5°C, heart rate of 110 beats per minute, blood pressure of 120/65 mmHg, and respiratory rate of 18 per minute. Physical examination disclosed right upper quadrant abdominal pain without rebound tenderness or organomegaly. Bowel sounds were normal. She had symmetric polyarthritis involving the hands, wrists, and knees. She had petechial lesions on lower extremities and muscle wasting of upper and lower extremities. She had diffuse hair loss. No nasal or oral ulcers were observed. The rest of the physical exam was unremarkable.

Table 1 shows the laboratories tests during the course of disease. Initially, she presented with leukopenia and anemia that worsened within 24 hours and thrombocytopenia. A peripheral smear revealed poikilocytosis, macrocytosis, anisocytosis, and ovalocytes. No schistocytes were seen. The reticulocyte count was normal at 1.6%. Alanine and aspartate aminotransferase, triglycerides, and ferritin levels were elevated as well as the erythrocyte sedimentation rate. Amylase and lipase levels were negative. Her renal function and urinalysis were within normal limits. Serum C3 complement levels were low at 70 mg/dL. Antinuclear, anti-ribonucleoprotein (97.4 U/mL) and anti-Ro antibodies (>100 U/mL) were elevated. Anti-dsDNA, anti-Smith, anti-La, and anti-citrullinated peptide antibody levels were negative. Rheumatoid factor was negative. Workup for herpes simplex virus IgM, cytomegalovirus IgM/IgG, and Epstein–Barr virus IgM and *Histoplasma* urine antigen, *Aspergillus* antigen, and *Legionella* urine antigen was negative. The tuberculin test and blood, urine, and sputum cultures were negative. Chest radiograph, electrocardiogram, and echocardiogram showed no abnormalities. Abdominal pelvic computer tomography disclosed an enlarged liver measuring 20.4 cm with fatty infiltration. Broad-spectrum antibiotics and antifungal treatment were started without improvement. Bone marrow biopsy revealed macrophages with engulfed erythrocytes consistent with MAS.

The patient was treated with cyclosporine 3 mg/kg/day and methylprednisolone 500 mg IV every day for 3 days, followed by 2 mg/kg/day IV every day. Also, she received IV immunoglobulins 20 g daily for 5 days. One day after initiating treatment, fever subsided. Five days after initiation of treatment, WBC count and hemoglobin levels continued to increase and liver enzymes returned to normal limits.

Upon discharge, WBC count, hemoglobin levels, platelet count, and ferritin levels continued to normalize. She was discharged on prednisone of 60 mg daily and cyclosporine 125 mg orally daily. She was continued on cyclosporine (3 mg/kg/day), and prednisone was gradually tapered down to 7.5 mg daily. After 12 months of follow-up, the patient remained in complete clinical remission of her MAS with normal WBC, hemoglobin, platelet count, liver enzymes, and ferritin levels. Also, she has not presented clinical manifestations of active SLE.

3. Discussion

We describe a Hispanic woman with SLE-associated MAS who was effectively treated with high-dose corticosteroids,

IV immunoglobulins, and cyclosporine. After one year of follow-up, she has remained in complete clinical remission of both her SLE and MAS. Although the mainstay of treatment of SLE-associated MAS consists of high-dose corticosteroid therapy, the optimal dose, combination with other immunosuppressive drugs, or treatment duration has not been clearly established [2–4, 8–10]. Moreover, no treatment guidelines for refractory cases have been proposed.

Our patient fulfilled the 2016 Classification Criteria for Macrophage Activation Syndrome Complicating Systemic Juvenile Idiopathic Arthritis (criteria met: ferritin > 684 ng/mL, platelet count $\leq 181 \times 10^9$/L, AST > 48, and triglycerides > 156 mg/dL) [11]. Although these classification criteria were validated for patients with sJIA, recent studies have shown that this classification is useful to identify MAS in patients with adult-onset Still's disease and SLE [12, 13]. In addition, our patient met the Systemic Lupus International Collaborating Clinics (SLICC) classification criteria for SLE (criteria met: leukocyte count < 4,000/mL, platelet count $< 100 \times 10^9$/L, positive ANA, elevated anti-dsDNA antibodies, and C3 and C4 hypocomplementemia) [14].

Based on previous reports, we used combination of high-dose corticosteroids, IV immunoglobulins, and cyclosporine as the induction therapy for our patient. In a case series of 103 episodes of MAS in 89 patients with SLE, the majority were initially treated with high-dose IV methylprednisolone [6]. Thirty-two episodes that were refractory to the corticosteroids required other immunosuppressive treatments. Cyclophosphamide, etoposide, and cyclosporine were most commonly used as second- and third-line therapy. Three episodes were treated with cyclosporine with favorable outcomes without serious side effects after two years of follow-up. Similarly, Liu et al. reported 32 patients with SLE-associated MAS treated with IV pulse corticosteroid therapy alone or in combination with other immunosuppressive agents including cyclosporine (43.8%), cyclophosphamide (28.1%), or etoposide (21.9%), among others [7]. Cyclosporine was given in combination with cyclophosphamide or etoposide in nearly 25% of patients. IV immunoglobulin therapy was used in 47.9% of patients. This study reported the death of four patients; three were due to severe infections and one died of multiple organ failure as a consequence of MAS. Additionally, Ravelli et al. described a lupus pediatric patient with MAS treated with cyclosporine after failing several immunosuppressive treatments including high-dose intravenous corticosteroids, IV immunoglobulins, and plasma exchange therapy [5]. This patient experienced a rapid and full recovery without reported side effects. Besides SLE, cyclosporine has shown to be effective for other rheumatic diseases associated with MAS such as sJIA [15, 16]. Minoia et al. described 213 patients with sJIA complicated with MAS in which cyclosporine was the most commonly used drug for those refractory to corticosteroids [15]. In another study, Boom et al. reported that cyclosporine, alone or in combination with other immunosuppressive drugs, was effective to induce remission in the majority of patients with sJIA-associated MAS [16]. On the other hand, the use of biologic agents including infliximab, tocilizumab, anakinra, and canakinumab in patients with MAS is still controversial as data confirming their efficacy are limited and needs further investigation [17, 18].

The pathogenesis in SLE-associated MAS is not well understood. However, it has been proposed that autoantibodies mediate phagocytosis of hematopoietic cells. In addition, the deposition of immune complexes on the bone marrow and oversecretion of cytokines by uncontrolled T-cell activation stimulate the uncontrolled phagocytosis [8, 9, 19]. Consistent with these hypotheses, SLE-associated MAS is associated with higher clinical and serological disease activity and with renal involvement [3, 4, 6, 7].

It can be argued that the prompt clinical response observed in our patient was attributable to corticosteroid and immunoglobulin therapy and not to cyclosporine. However, a study conducted in healthy volunteers and transplant recipients showed marked suppression of interleukin 2, interferon-gamma, and granulocyte-macrophage colony-stimulating factor after only two hours of cyclosporine ingestion [20]. Additionally, this calcineurin inhibitor suppresses the production of TNF-α, IL-1, and IL-6 [21, 22]. Therefore, it is expected that cyclosporine would be effective in the treatment of SLE-associated MAS in which T-cells have a central pathogenic role. Nonetheless, cyclosporine use is limited in the SLE general management because of its side effects which include nephrotoxicity, severe hypertension, and hyperlipidemia [23]. These side effects are usually dose-related. Our patient was treated with low-dose cyclosporine (3 mg/kg/day) for 12 months without adverse events. On the other hand, tacrolimus, which is another calcineurin inhibitor, is more widely used for SLE than cyclosporine, particularly for those complicated with lupus nephritis [24, 25]. However, it is unknown if tacrolimus would also be helpful for SLE-associated MAS.

In summary, we report a woman with SLE-associated MAS who responded well to combination therapy with corticosteroids, IV immunoglobulins, and cyclosporine without adverse events. Furthermore, cyclosporine seems to be a good agent for maintenance of remission, as our patient did not experience any exacerbation even after decreasing prednisone to 7.5 mg daily. Our case, together with other reports, reaffirms the importance of early recognition and aggressive treatment for patients with SLE-associated MAS.

References

[1] S. Kumakura and Y. Murakawa, "Clinical characteristics and treatment outcomes of autoimmune-associated hemophagocytic syndrome in adults," *Arthritis & Rheumatology*, vol. 66, no. 8, pp. 2297–2307, 2014.

[2] O. Lambotte, M. Khellaf, H. Harmouche et al., "Characteristics and long-term outcome of 15 episodes of systemic lupus erythematosus associated hemophagocytic syndrome," *Medicine*, vol. 85, no. 3, pp. 169–182, 2006.

[3] N. Jiang, M. T. Li, D. Wu, and X. F. Zeng, "The clinical characteristics of macrophage activation syndrome secondary

to systemic lupus erythematosus," *Zhonghua Nei Ke Za Zhi*, vol. 55, no. 11, pp. 840–844, 2016.

[4] J. M. Kim, S. K. Kwok, J. H. Ju, H. Y. Kim, and S. H. Park, "Reactive hemophagocytic syndrome in adult Korean patients with systemic lupus erythematosus: a case-control study and literature review," *Journal of Rheumatology*, vol. 39, no. 1, pp. 86–93, 2012.

[5] A. Ravelli, S. Viola, F. De Benedetti, S. Magni-Manzoni, C. Tzialla, and A. Martini, "Dramatic efficacy of cyclosporine A in macrophage activation syndrome," *Clinical and Experimental Rheumatology*, vol. 19, no. 1, p. 108, 2001.

[6] P. E. Gavand, I. Serio, L. Arnaud et al., "Clinical spectrum and therapeutic management of systemic lupus erythematosus-associated macrophage activation syndrome: a study of 103 episodes in 89 adult patients," *Autoimmunity Reviews*, vol. 16, no. 7, pp. 743–749, 2017.

[7] A. C. Liu, Y. Yang, M. T. Li et al., "Macrophage activation syndrome in systemic lupus erythematosus: a multicenter, case-control study in China," *Clinical Rheumatology*, 2017.

[8] G. S. Schulert and A. A. Grom, "Pathogenesis of macrophage activation syndrome and potential for cytokine- directed therapies," *Annual Review of Medicine*, vol. 66, no. 1, pp. 145–159, 2015.

[9] K. F. Wong, P. K. Hui, J. K. Chan, Y. W. Chan, and S. Y. Ha, "The acute lupus hemophagocytic syndrome," *Annals of Internal Medicine*, vol. 114, no. 5, pp. 387–390, 1991.

[10] R. Dhote, J. Simon, T. Papo et al., "Reactive hemophagocytic syndrome in adult systemic disease: report of twenty-six cases and literature review," *Arthritis & Rheumatism*, vol. 49, no. 5, pp. 633–639, 2003.

[11] A. Ravelli, F. Minoia, S. Davì et al., "2016 Classification Criteria for Macrophage Activation Syndrome Complicating Systemic Juvenile Idiopathic Arthritis: a European League Against Rheumatism/American College of Rheumatology/Paediatric Rheumatology International Trials Organisation Collaborative Initiative," *Annals of the Rheumatic Diseases*, vol. 75, no. 3, pp. 481–489, 2016.

[12] S. S. Ahn, B. W. Yoo, S. M. Jung, S. W. Lee, Y. B. Park, and J. J. Song, "Application of the 2016 EULAR/ACR/PRINTO classification criteria for macrophage activation syndrome in patients with adult-onset Still disease," *Journal of Rheumatology*, vol. 44, no. 7, pp. 996–1003, 2017.

[13] S. Ahn, B. W. Yoo, S. M. Jung, S. W. Lee, Y. B. Park, and J. J. Song, "In-hospital mortality in febrile lupus patients based on 2016 EULAR/ACR/PRINTO classification criteria for macrophage activation syndrome," *Seminars in Arthritis and Rheumatism*, vol. 47, no. 2, pp. 216–221, 2017.

[14] M. Petri, A. M. Orbai, G. S. Alarcón et al., "Derivation and validation of the Systemic Lupus International Collaborating Clinics classification criteria for systemic lupus erythematosus," *Arthritis & Rheumatism*, vol. 64, no. 8, pp. 2677–2686, 2012.

[15] F. Minoia, S. Davì, A. Horne et al., "Clinical features, treatment, and outcome of macrophage activation syndrome complicating systemic juvenile idiopathic arthritis: a multinational, multicenter study of 362 patients," *Arthritis & Rheumatology*, vol. 66, no. 11, pp. 3160–3169, 2014.

[16] V. Boom, J. Anton, P. Lahdenne et al., "Evidence-based diagnosis and treatment of macrophage activation syndrome in systemic juvenile idiopathic arthritis," *Pediatric Rheumatology*, vol. 13, no. 1, p. 55, 2015.

[17] T. Henzan, K. Nagafuji, H. Tsukamoto et al., "Success with infliximab in treating refractory hemophagocytic lymphohistiocytosis," *American Journal of Hematology*, vol. 81, no. 1, pp. 59–61, 2006.

[18] M. Durand, Y. Troyanov, P. Laflamme, and G. Gregoire, "Macrophage activation syndrome treated with anakinra," *Journal of Rheumatology*, vol. 37, no. 4, pp. 879-880, 2010.

[19] T. Papo, M. H. Andre, Z. Amoura et al., "The spectrum of reactive hemophagocytic syndrome in systemic lupus erythematosus," *Journal of Rheumatology*, vol. 26, no. 4, pp. 927–930, 1999.

[20] T. Giese, M. Zeier, P. Schemmer et al., "Monitoring of NFAT-regulated gene expression in the peripheral blood of allograft recipients: a novel perspective toward individually optimized drug doses of cyclosporine A," *Transplantation*, vol. 77, no. 3, pp. 339–344, 2004.

[21] A. Mak and N. Y. Kow, "The pathology of T cells in systemic lupus erythematosus," *Journal of Immunology Research*, vol. 2014, Article ID 419029, 8 pages, 2014.

[22] G. Moroni, A. Doria, and C. Ponticelli, "Cyclosporine (CsA) in lupus nephritis: assessing the evidence," *Nephrology Dialysis Transplantation*, vol. 24, no. 1, pp. 15–20, 2009.

[23] B. Griffiths, P. Emery, V. Ryan et al., "The BILAG multi-centre open randomized controlled trial comparing ciclosporin vs azathioprine in patients with severe SLE," *Rheumatology*, vol. 49, no. 4, pp. 723–732, 2010.

[24] N. Miyasaka, S. Kawai, and H. Hashimoto, "Efficacy and safety of tacrolimus for lupus nephritis: a placebo-controlled double-blind multicenter study," *Modern Rheumatology*, vol. 19, no. 6, pp. 606–615, 2009.

[25] T. Kraaij, O. W. Bredewold, S. Trompet, T. W. Huizinga et al., "TAC-TIC use of tacrolimus-based regimens in lupus nephritis," *Lupus Science & Medicine*, vol. 3, no. 1, p. e000169, 2016.

26

A Case of Hyperimmunoglobulinemia D Syndrome Successfully Treated with Canakinumab

Elena Tsitsami,[1] Charis Papadopoulou,[1] and Matthaios Speletas[2]

[1] Pediatric Rheumatology Unit, 1st Department of Pediatrics, Children's Hospital "Aghia Sophia", University of Athens, 115 27 Athens, Greece
[2] Department of Immunology & Histocompatibility, School of Medicine, University of Thessaly, 411 10 Biopolis, Larissa, Greece

Correspondence should be addressed to Elena Tsitsami; etsitsami@med.uoa.gr

Academic Editors: G. S. Alarcon, D. R. Alpert, A. Chalmers, and C. Saadeh

Hyperimmunoglobulinemia D syndrome is a rare autosomal recessive autoinflammatory disorder caused by mutations in the mevalonate kinase gene (*MVK*). In a proportion of patients, however, no *MVK* mutations are detected. Although various standard anti-inflammatory drugs have been tried, until now there is no consensus about how HIDS should be treated. We present a case of HIDS in an 8-year-old girl whose clinical picture had started before the end of the first year of life. The patient had consistently elevated IgD levels but no mutations were found after a full-length analysis of the *MVK* gene. The method of *MVK* mutational analysis is presented in details. Treatment with canakinumab in a final single dose of 4 mg/kg every 4 weeks resulted in the disappearance of febrile attacks and a considerable improvement of patients' quality of life during a 12-month follow-up period. The drug has been well tolerated, and no side effects were observed.

1. Introduction

Hyperimmunoglobulinemia D and periodic fever syndrome (HIDS) is a rare autosomal recessive autoinflammatory disorder, characterized by recurrent febrile attacks associated with lymphadenopathy, abdominal pain, diarrhea, arthralgia, and skin rash [1, 2]. HIDS is caused by mutations in the mevalonate kinase gene (*MVK*) resulting in deficient activity of the mevalonate kinase enzyme [3, 4]. Until the discovery of the *MVK* gene as underlying HIDS, the presence of a high level of serum IgD was necessary to establish the diagnosis of HIDS, but since, several cases of HIDS with *MVK* mutations and normal IgD serum levels have been described [3, 5]. On the other hand, Ammouri et al. [6] described 14 patients who had a recurrent fever syndrome with high level of IgD without *MVK* mutations and proposed to use the term of mevalonate kinase deficiency (MKD) for patients who have a biochemical deficiency of mevalonate kinase and *MVK* mutations and the term HIDS for the group of patients who have a recurrent fever syndrome and an elevated IgD concentration. A wide variety of immunomodulatory drugs was tried to treat and prevent attacks in these patients, including colchicine, steroids, and nonsteroidal anti-inflammatory drugs. Anakinra, a IL-1 receptor antagonist, has also been tested in a small number of patients [7–9].

We are reporting a case of HIDS in an 8-year-old girl treated with canakinumab, a newer IL-1 receptor antagonist, with an excellent response.

2. Case Presentation

An 8-year-old girl of central Greek ancestry was admitted to the hospital because of periodic fever spikes, which occurred every 3-4 weeks and lasted 3–5 days. Since the first months of life she had experienced characteristic febrile attacks. She had a surgery history of tonsillectomy and adenoidectomy at the age of 2 and 6, respectively. During fever flare ups, she usually developed chills, malaise, and abdominal pain with diarrhoea and vomiting. Between attacks the patient was

TABLE 1: Primers and PCR conditions used for the detection of *MVK* mutations.

Exon(s)	Primer	Sequence	PCR conditions	PCR product
1	forward reverse	5′-GAGTGGAAGAGCTGGCATTTGAA-3′ 5′-GCCTCAGGGTGTCCTTTTACCTTCT-3′	94°C for 2 min, followed by 32 cycles (94°C for 30 s, 56°C for 30 s, 72°C for 30 s) and a final elongation at 72°C for 5 min. $MgCl_2$: 1.5 mM	381 bp
2	forward reverse	5′-TGGCCTCTGTGCTTATGTTTG-3′ 5′-AAGCTAATTTTATGAGGTCAGGGTA-3′	94°C for 2 min, followed by 30 cycles (94°C for 30 s, 58°C for 30 s, 72°C for 30 s) and a final elongation at 72°C for 5 min. $MgCl_2$: 1.5 mM	386 bp
3	forward reverse	5′-AAAGTCCCTCTCACCCACTTGTGTT-3′ 5′-CCAGCAGCAATGACAGAAACTCTTC-3′	94°C for 2 min, followed by 30 cycles (94°C for 30 s, 55°C for 30 s, 72°C for 45 s) and a final elongation at 72°C for 5 min. $MgCl_2$: 2.5 mM	271 bp
4	forward reverse	5′-GAATTTGAAGACGCACATTATTACA- 3′ 5′-GGCCACTATGACACCTCTCAC-3′	94°C for 2 min, followed by 32 cycles (94°C for 30 s, 55°C for 30 s, 72°C for 70 s) and a final elongation at 72°C for 5 min. $MgCl_2$: 1.5 mM	1010 bp
5 & 6	forward reverse	5′-AGCTGGAGAGGTTCAGAGTGGACTT-3′ 5′-GGGAGAAGGAGAGAGCAGGTCT-3′	94°C for 2 min, followed by 32 cycles (94°C for 30 s, 58°C for 30 s, 72°C for 70 s) and a final elongation at 72°C for 5 min. $MgCl_2$: 2.0 mM	1116 bp
7 & 8	forward reverse	5′-TGCCTCCCTTCTTCCTCCGTATC-3′ 5′-CCTCCCTTGCACTCTCCCAATTACT-3′	94°C for 2 min, followed by 30 cycles (94°C for 30 s, 57°C for 30 s, 72°C for 70 s) and a final elongation at 72°C for 5 min. $MgCl_2$: 1.5 mM, 10% DMSO	932 bp
9	forward reverse	5′-GTCTCCAGCCAACAACTGTCAGATG-3′ 5′-TTCCAGGTCTCTTTTTCCTTTCAA-3′	94°C for 2 min, followed by 30 cycles (94°C for 30 s, 57°C for 30 s, 72°C for 30 s) and a final elongation at 72°C for 5 min. $MgCl_2$: 2.5 mM	352 bp
10	forward reverse	5′-TTGCCTTGAATATGATGAGCTTC-3′ 5′-GCCAGCACAGAGTCGAACTG-3′	94°C for 2 min, followed by 30 cycles (94°C for 30 s, 57°C for 30 s, 72°C for 30 s) and a final elongation at 72°C for 5 min. $MgCl_2$: 2.5 mM	306 bp

free of symptoms. From her family history, recurrent febrile episodes during childhood were reported both to her mother and maternal grandmother.

On admission, her blood pressure and temperature were normal. Physical examination showed normal findings, except from small aphthous ulcers in her mouth. No symptoms suggestive of respiratory, abdominal, or urinary infection were apparent. Chest radiography and abdominal ultrasonography scan revealed no abnormalities. Laboratory investigations revealed marked increase of erythrocyte sedimentation rate and C-reactive protein, a total leukocyte count of 5.710/mm^3, serum amyloid 29.7 mg/L, serum IgD 80 mg/dL (normal range 0.3–11), and creatinine 0.37 mg/dL. Immunological tests, including antinuclear antibodies, rheumatoid factors, complement factors, serum immunoglobulins as well as serology for CMV, parvovirus,

B19, EBV, adenovirus, coxsackie virus, and antistreptolysin O titre resulted negative or within normal limits. Common causes of infections were ruled out. The genetic analysis for familial Mediterranean fever (FMF) and cryopyrin-associated periodic syndromes (CAPS) was negative. A full-length analysis of the *MVK* gene was performed according to the method described below but no mutation was found.

Serum IgD was repeated several times and was always elevated. On this basis, the diagnosis of HIDS was considered and the patient started the therapy with canakinumab, an interleukin-1 receptor antagonist. Initially, a single dose (2 mg/kg) every 4 weeks was administered and resulted in prompt remission of the fever the other symptoms (abdominal pain, diarrhoea, and vomiting). Before, however, the third monthly dose of canakinumab the patient presented a new febrile episode with severe abdominal symptoms and, therefore, duplication of the dose was decided. Thereafter and during a followup of 12 months, the patient continues receiving canakinumab 4 mg/kg per month and remains free of febrile attacks. A considerable improvement of her quality of life was observed but the levels of acute phase reactants, although significantly diminished, remain constantly higher than normal values. The drug has been well tolerated and no side effects were observed.

2.1. Mutational Analysis of MVK Gene. Genomic DNA was extracted from peripheral blood using the QIAamp DNA Blood Mini Kit (Qiagen, UK), according to manufacturer's instructions. Afterwards, an amplification of all 10 (ten) exons, including exon-intron boundaries, of *MVK* gene was performed. The position and the sequences of the utilized primers, designed with the aid of the Oligo-6 software (NBI, Plymouth, MN, USA), as well as the conditions of PCR reactions, are shown in Table 1. For each PCR reaction, a total of 100–200 ng of genomic DNA was amplified in a 30 μL reaction using 62.5 μM of each deoxynucleotide triphosphate, 20 pmoles of each primer and 0.8 U Taq Polymerase (Bioline, UK) in a buffer supplied by the manufacturer. The concentration of $MgCl_2$ used in every PCR reaction is also provided in Table 1. All PCR procedures were carried out in the PCR-engine apparatus PTC-200, MJ-Research (Watertown-Massachusetts, USA), and the PCR products were analyzed in 2% TBE agarose gels, stained with ethidium bromide and visualized under UV light. Afterwards, PCR products were purified by the QIAquick gel extraction kit (Qiagen) and directly sequenced using an ABI Prism 310 Genetic Analyzer (Applied Biosystems, Foster City, CA, USA) and a Big Dye Terminator DNA sequencing kit (Applied Biosystems).

3. Discussion

HIDS is characterized by recurrent, self-limiting attacks of fever occurring since early childhood. Febrile episodes usually last 3–7 days and are usually associated with headache, arthralgias, lymphadenopathy, abdominal pain, diarrhoea, vomiting, and skin lesions. The causative mutations in HIDS are located in the gene encoding *MVK*, an enzyme in the isoprenoid metabolism, the end-products of which include cholesterol, protein isoprenylation, dolichol, and ubiquinone [10].

In our patient, the recurrent and periodic nature of her illness over a period of 7 years was suggestive of a periodic fever syndrome. A number of periodic fever syndromes were excluded based on a combination of laboratory findings, genetic testing, and clinical features. Although no test for *TNFRSF1A* mutation was performed, the patient's clinical features and the lack of family history for an autosomal dominant disorder made TRAPS defect to seem unlikely. Serum IgD values were >11 mg/dL on more than two occasions one month apart. Although this does not completely confirm the diagnosis of HIDS, again the periodicity and patterns of fever and the clinical symptoms in our patient were very suggestive for this syndrome.

The exact pathogenesis of HIDS is unclear. However, several of the isoprenoid end-products have been linked with apoptosis [11]. Evidence exists for a pathologic role of IL-1β activation through caspase-1 [12] and for successful treatment with anakinra in acute crises [7–9]. Treatment of monocytes with simvastatin, an inhibitor of isoprenoid biosynthesis mimicking MKD, resulted in increased activation of caspase-1-mediated IL-1β activation [13]. Canakinumab, another IL-1 receptor antagonist, has been administered to our patient on the basis of its excellent results in patients with other IL-1-mediated syndromes [14]. The pharmacokinetics of this drug is in favour of a good compliance of patients to the long-term treatment although sustained IL-1 suppression may have potentially serious long-term effects, which are currently unknown.

Autoinflammatory syndromes always pose diagnostic and therapeutic challenges to treating clinicians. The clinical description of the diversity of periodic fever syndromes is helpful in the assessment and management of these patients. Our case confirms the previous reports indicating that IL-1 targeting drugs brings substantial benefit to HIDS patients [7, 8]. To the best of our knowledge this is the first report of HIDS treatment with canakinumab indicating that controlled trials are worthy to be undertaken to further assess its clinical benefit and safety in these patients.

References

[1] V. Prietsch, E. Mayatepek, H. Krastel et al., "Mevalonate kinase deficiency: enlarging the clinical and biochemical spectrum," *Pediatrics*, vol. 111, no. 2, pp. 258–261, 2003.

[2] D. Haas and G. F. Hoffmann, "Mevalonate kinase deficiencies: from mevalonic aciduria to hyperimmunoglobulinemia D syndrome," *Orphanet Journal of Rare Diseases*, vol. 1, article 13, 2006.

[3] S. M. Houten, W. Kuis, M. Duran et al., "Mutations in MVK, encoding mevalonate kinase, cause hyperimmunoglobulinaemia D and periodic fever syndrome," *Nature Genetics*, vol. 22, no. 2, pp. 175–177, 1999.

[4] J. P. H. Drenth, L. Cuisset, G. Grateau et al., "Mutations in the gene encoding mevalonate kinase cause hyper-IgD and periodic fever syndrome," *Nature Genetics*, vol. 22, no. 2, pp. 178–181, 1999.

[5] F. T. Saulsbury, "Hyperimmunoglobulinemia D and periodic fever syndrome (HIDS) in a child with normal serum IgD, but

increased serum IgA concentration," *Journal of Pediatrics*, vol. 143, no. 1, pp. 127–129, 2003.

[6] W. Ammouri, L. Cuisset, S. Rouaghe et al., "Diagnostic value of serum immunoglobulinaemia D level in patients with a clinical suspicion of hyper IgD syndrome," *Rheumatology*, vol. 46, no. 10, pp. 1597–1600, 2007.

[7] J. C. H. van der Hilst, E. J. Bodar, K. S. Barron et al., "Long-term follow-up, clinical features, and quality of life in a series of 103 patients with hyperimmunoglobulinemia D syndrome," *Medicine*, vol. 87, no. 6, pp. 301–310, 2008.

[8] M. Cailliez, F. Garaix, C. Rousset-Rouvière et al., "Anakinra is safe and effective in controlling hyperimmunoglobulinaemia D syndrome-associated febrile crisis," *Journal of Inherited Metabolic Disease*, vol. 29, no. 6, p. 763, 2006.

[9] C. Galeotti, U. Meinzer, P. Quartier et al., "Efficacy of interleukin-1-targeting drugs in mevalonate kinase deficiency," *Rheumatology*, vol. 51, no. 10, pp. 1855–1859, 2012.

[10] J. P. H. Drenth and J. W. M. van der Meer, "Medical progress: hereditary periodic fever," *The New England Journal of Medicine*, vol. 345, no. 24, pp. 1748–1757, 2001.

[11] E. J. Bodar, J. C. H. van der Hilst, W. van Heerde, J. W. M. van der Meer, J. P. H. Drenth, and A. Simon, "Defective apoptosis of peripheral-blood lymphocytes in hyper-IgD and periodic fever syndrome," *Blood*, vol. 109, no. 6, pp. 2416–2418, 2007.

[12] L. M. Kuijk, J. M. Beekman, J. Koster, H. R. Waterham, J. Frenkel, and P. J. Coffer, "HMG-CoA reductase inhibition induces IL-12 release through Rac1/PI3K/PKB-dependent caspase-1 activation," *Blood*, vol. 112, no. 9, pp. 3563–3573, 2008.

[13] L. M. Kuijk, S. H. Mandey, I. Schellens et al., "Statin synergizes with LPS to induce IL-1β release by THP-1 cells through activation of caspase-1," *Molecular Immunology*, vol. 45, no. 8, pp. 2158–2165, 2008.

[14] J. B. Kuemmerle-Deschner, E. Hachulla, R. Cartwright et al., "Two-year results from an open-label, multicentre, phase III study evaluating the safety and efficacy of canakinumab in patients with cryopyrin-associated periodic syndrome across different severity phenotypes," *Annals of Rheumatic Diseases*, vol. 70, no. 12, pp. 2095–2102, 2011.

27

Behçet's Disease and Intracardiac Thrombosis: A Report of Three Cases

Nurşen Düzgün,[1] Orhan Küçükşahin,[1] Kayhan Çetin Atasoy,[2] Canan Togay Işıkay,[3] Demet Menekşe Gerede,[4] Ayşe Erden,[2] Seda Kaynak Şahap,[2] Muhammed Arif İbiş,[5] and Aşkın Ateş[1]

[1] *Department of Internal Medicine-Rheumatology, Ankara University, Faculty of Medicine, Akademik Yerleşke, Sıhhıye, 06100 Ankara, Turkey*
[2] *Department of Radiology, Ankara University, Faculty of Medicine, Akademik Yerleşke, Sıhhıye, 06100 Ankara, Turkey*
[3] *Department of Neurology, Ankara University, Faculty of Medicine, Akademik Yerleşke, Sıhhıye, 06100 Ankara, Turkey*
[4] *Department of Cardiology, Ankara University, Faculty of Medicine, Akademik Yerleşke, Sıhhıye, 06100 Ankara, Turkey*
[5] *Department of Internal Medicine, Ankara University, Faculty of Medicine, Akademik Yerleşke, Sıhhıye, 06100 Ankara, Turkey*

Correspondence should be addressed to Nurşen Düzgün; duzgun@medicine.ankara.edu.tr

Academic Editors: G. S. Alarcon and R. Cevik

We present three patients with Behçet's disease associated with intracardiac thrombus and pulmonary vascular involvement. One of these patients had also Budd-Chiari syndrome. All patients were treated with corticosteroid plus monthly intravenous cyclophosphamide as first line treatment and with no recurrences. Immunosuppressive therapy was successful in the treatment of intracardiac thrombus and also in the regression of pulmonary vascular thromboses in these patients. Intracardiac thrombus in Behçet's disease is rarely seen. Behçet's disease should be remembered in the differential diagnosis of the patients with intracardiac mass, especially in patients from the Mediterranean and Middle East populations.

1. Introduction

Behçet's disease (BD) is a multisystemic, chronic, inflammatory disorder of unknown etiology. In 1937, Dr. Behçet first described the disease as a distinct clinical picture with a triple complex of recurrent oral aphthosis, genital ulcer, and iridocyclitis with hypopyon [1]. BD may also involve other locations such as skin, joint, central nervous system, gastrointestinal tract, lung, and cardiovascular system. The diagnosis is primarily based on clinical criteria because there is no specific diagnostic laboratory test. The histopathologic findings are also nonspecific. BD is frequent among the Mediterranean, Middle East, and Far Eastern populations.

Behçet's disease is recognized as a systemic vasculitis involving both arteries and veins of any size. Vascular involvement has occurred in one-third of patients. Most vascular events consist of recurrent superficial or deep vein thrombosis [2–4]. Arterial thrombosis is less frequent [3].

The cardiac findings were found in 1%–6% of BD cases in previous clinical series [5] and in 16.5% of cases in the Japanese autopsy registry [6]. Cardiac manifestations of BD include endocarditis, myocarditis, pericarditis, endomyocardial fibrosis, coronary arteritis with or without myocardial infarction, aneurysms of the coronary arteries, valve dysfunction, conduction system disturbances, and intracardiac thrombosis (ICT) [5, 7–9]. ICT is a rare manifestation of the disease [10–12].

Here we present the characteristic clinical findings in three cases with ICT related to BD and review the approach to treatment of ICT in BD patients.

2. Patient 1

A 22-year-old Turkish male presented to the emergency ward with complaints of fever, hypoesthesia on the left arm, and slurred speech that had lasted for a week. Medical history revealed previous attacks of intermittent fever together with recurrent oral and genital ulcers, abdominal pain, and lack of appetite. The complaints occurred once a month for the past three years and lasted for a few days. On admission, his body temperature was 39.5°C. Physical examination revealed oral and genital ulcers and a bilateral decrease in pulmonary breath sounds. Neurological examination revealed right facial paralysis and dysarthria. There were no motor and sensory deficits.

Laboratory results were as follows: hemoglobin 9.2 gr/dL, white blood cell (WBC) 11 × 10^9/L, platelets 200 × 10^9/L, erythrocyte sedimentation rate (ESR) 120 mm/h, C-reactive protein (CRP) 180 mg/L, and serum albumin 2.5 g/dL. Renal and hepatic functions were normal.

Diffusion-weighted images of the brain demonstrated multiple acute infarcts in the right frontal, parietal, temporal, and occipital regions and right caudate nucleus. Ultrasonographic imaging of the carotid and vertebral arteries, and angiography of the brain were unremarkable. The patient was referred to the stroke unit of the department of neurology. Transthoracic echocardiography revealed a mobile hyperechogenic mass with 12 × 11 mm in size on the apex of the left ventricle (Figure 1(a)). Low molecular weighted heparin and low dose acetylsalicylic acid were started based on the diagnosis of multiple cerebral infarcts due to possible cardioembolism.

The patient was empirically started on wide spectrum antibiotics including ceftriaxone and clarithromycin. Fever persisted under antibiotherapy. Microbiological analyses were negative. The patient was referred to the rheumatology clinic with suspicion of systemic vasculitis. Autoimmune serology (antinuclear antibodies, ANCA, and antiphospholipid antibodies) was all negative.

Cardiac magnetic resonance (MR) showed a thrombus in the left ventricle (Figure 1(b)). Pulmonary CT angiography showed multiple acute emboli and infarctions affecting both lungs and bilateral minimal pleural effusion (Figures 1(c) and 1(d)).

Hereditary thrombotic risk factors including prothrombin gene 20210G-A and factor V Leiden gene mutations were negative. Methylene tetrahydrofolate reductase (MTHFR) mutation was found homozygote positive.

The patient's history of recurrent oral and genital ulcers, the presence of the scrotal ulceration scars, cerebral and pulmonary vascular lesions, and cardiac thrombus supported the diagnosis of BD. There was no evidence of ocular involvement, and the Pathergy test was negative.

The patient was given intravenous high dose methylprednisolone (1 gr/d for three days), followed by oral prednisone (1 mg/kg/d), monthly intravenous cyclophosphamide (500 mg/m^2/for one day), and colchicine (1.5 mg/d). The fever responded well to the corticosteroid and immunosuppressive therapy.

After three months, the intracardiac thrombus was no longer detectable on echocardiography. The neurological examination was unremarkable. Nine months later, the patient was asymptomatic and complete resolution of ICT persisted.

3. Patient 2

A 24-year-old Turkish male with a previous diagnosis of BD for 10 years was admitted to the rheumatology clinic following a 1-month history of fever and dyspnea on exertion.

On physical examination, body temperature was 38°C. Pulmonary sounds were bilaterally decreased. Laboratory results were as follows: hemoglobin 11.1 gr/dL, WBC 10.8 × 10^9/L, platelets 280 × 10^9/L, ESR 103 mm/h, and CRP 148 mg/L. Renal and hepatic functions were normal. Microbiologic studies did not identify any causative organisms.

Echocardiography revealed a mobile mass (13 × 12 mm in size) in the right ventricle attached to the interventricular septum (Figure 2(a)).

Pulmonary CT angiography showed filling defects due to acute embolism in the middle lobe arteries, apical and posterior basal segment arteries of the right lower lobe, as well as small subpleural consolidations in the right middle and lower lobes representing infarcts (Figure 2(b)).

HLA-B51 and Pathergy tests were negative. Hereditary thrombotic risk factors including prothrombin gene 20210G-A, factor V Leiden and MTHFR gene mutations were negative. Ocular examination showed sequel uveitis in the left eye. The patient was given intravenous high dose methylprednisolone (1 gr/d for three days), followed by oral prednisone (1 mg/kg/d), and monthly intravenous cyclophosphamide (500 mg/m^2/for one day) under a diagnosis of BD. Dyspnea and fever regressed with the corticosteroid and immunosuppressive therapy. After nine months, the intracardiac thrombus showed complete resolution on echocardiography.

The patient was continued to be treated with monthly cyclophosphamide, prednisone, and colchicine.

4. Patient 3

A 25-year-old Turkish man who had been followed for one year with a diagnosis of Budd-Chiari syndrome was admitted to the rheumatology clinic with fever up to 40°C and abdominal pain. On admission, his body temperature was 39°C. Physical examination revealed prominent superficial collateral veins in the chest wall and scars of old ulcers in the scrotum and also papulopustular lesions in the extremities and neck.

Laboratory tests on admission revealed WBC of 6.6 × 10^9/L, hemoglobin of 13.1 g/dL, ESR of 36 mm/h, and CRP concentration of 43.5 mg/dL. Urinalysis, kidney, and liver functions were normal. Microbiologic studies were found negative. Autoimmune serologic tests were negative. He was started on tazocin (piperacillin and tazobactam) and clarithromycin as empiric antibiotherapy, but fever persisted under this therapy.

Transthoracic and transesophageal echocardiography showed a mobile mass (4.5 × 3 cm in size) filling half of the right atrium and extending into the right ventricle and

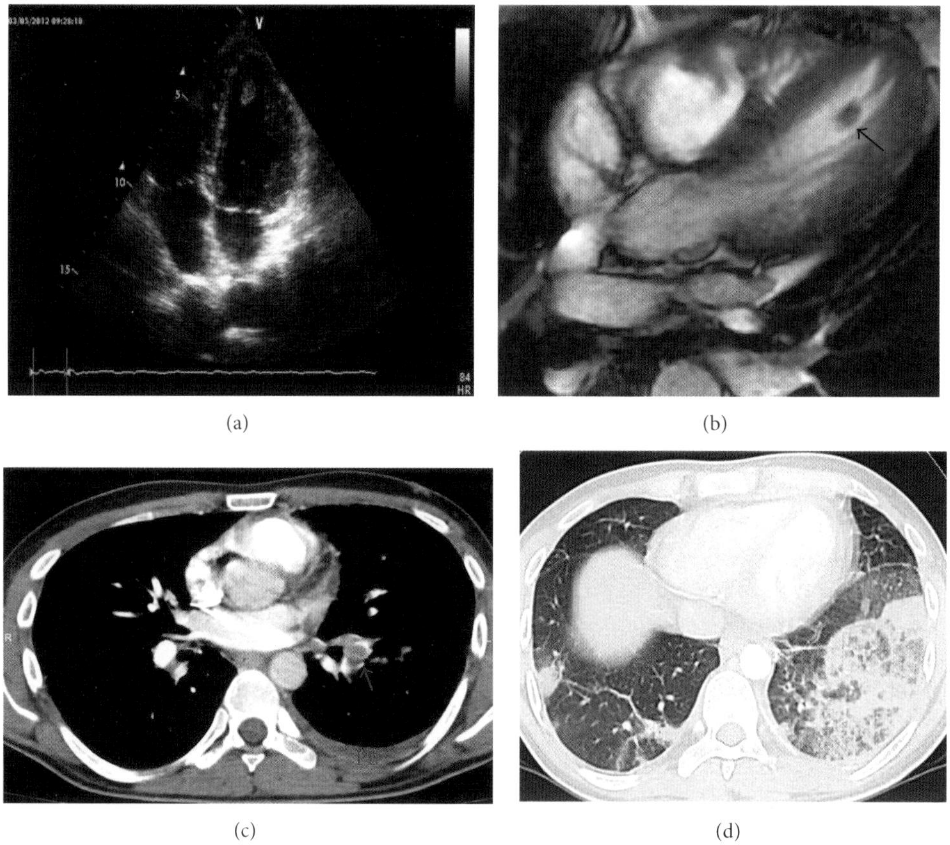

FIGURE 1: (a) Transthoracic echocardiographic apical four-chamber view shows a thrombus in the apex of the left ventricle. (b) Four-chamber-view MR image obtained with fast imaging steady-state free precession sequence shows pedunculated thrombus (arrow) attached to left ventricular apex with a thin stalk (cine images showed mobility of the thrombus throughout the cardiac cycle). (c) Pulmonary CT angiography shows acute embolus as a filling defect in the left lower lobe artery (arrow). Note the associated left pleural effusion (PE). (d) Lung window setting shows bilateral lower lobe infarcts, more prominent in the left lung.

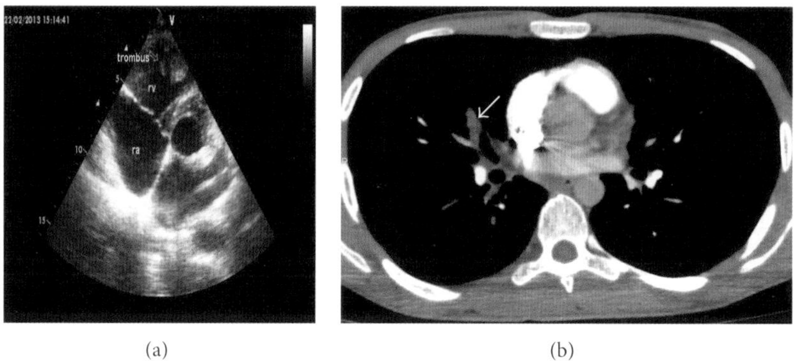

FIGURE 2: (a) Transthoracic echocardiography in the parasternal short-axis view shows a thrombus (arrow) in the right ventricle attached to the interventricular septum. (b) Contrast-enhanced pulmonary CT angiography shows acute embolus filling and mildly enlarging the right middle lobe artery (arrow).

inferior vena cava (Figure 3(a)). Pulmonary arterial pressure by echocardiography was 30 mmHg.

Contrast-enhanced CT angiography confirmed the thrombus in the right atrium that extended into the right ventricle and displayed findings of both chronic and superimposed acute thromboembolism (Figures 3(b) and 3(c)). The right ventricle showed signs of pulmonary hypertension including chamber dilatation, myocardial thickening, and straightening of the interventricular septum.

Medical history revealed complaints of recurrent oral and genital ulcers and papulopustular lesions. HLA-B51 was positive. Pathergy test was negative. The patient was diagnosed

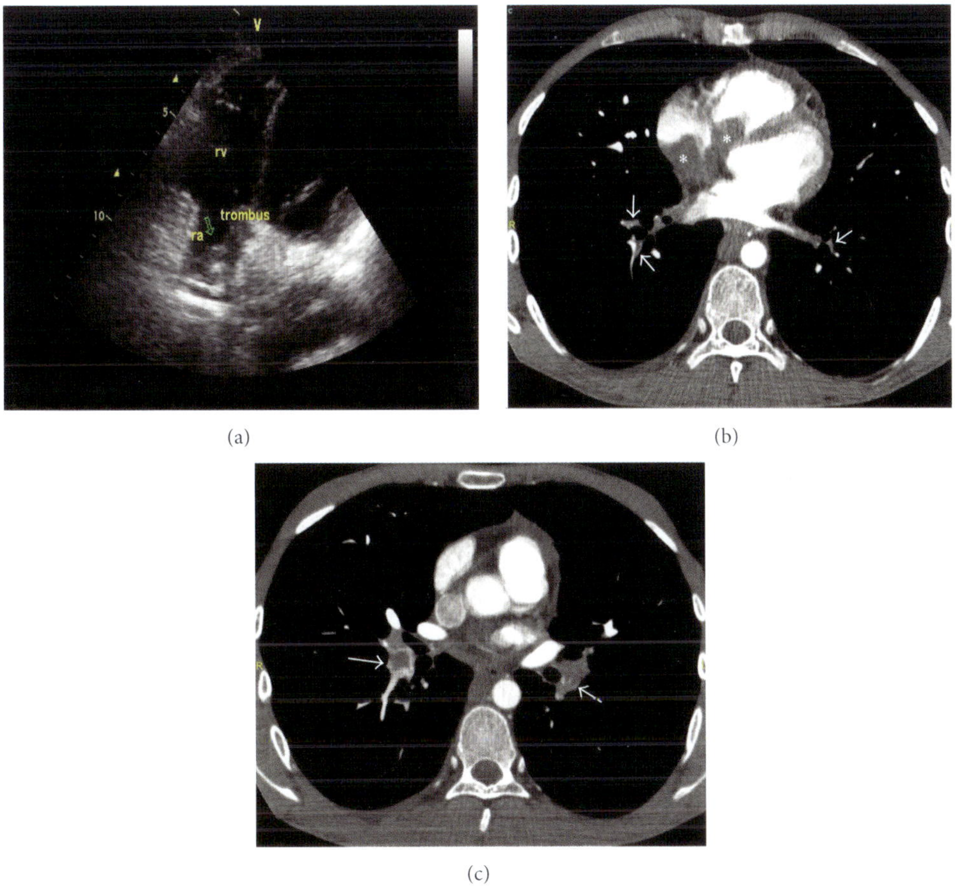

FIGURE 3: (a) Transthoracic echocardiography showed a mobile mass filling the half of the right atrium (4.5 × 3 cm in size) (arrow) extending the right ventricule (1.5 × 1.6 cm in size) and into the vena cava. (b) Contrast-enhanced CT angiographic image shows a large filling defect in the right atrium extending into the right ventricle (asterisks). Segmental arteries in both lower lobes are of small calibre due to chronic thromboembolism (arrows). Pulmonary hypertension resulted in straightening of the interventricular septum. (c) Both lower lobe arteries contain central filling defects (arrows) representing superimposed acute pulmonary embolism.

with BD based on these findings. Hereditary thrombotic risk factors including prothrombin gene 20210G-A, factor V Leiden and MTHFR gene mutations were negative.

The patient was given methylprednisolone (1 mg/kg/d) and monthly cyclophosphamide (500 mg/m^2 for a day). Oral anticoagulant was stopped, and low molecular weighted heparin was started. Clinical findings regressed and laboratory abnormalities returned to normal. Six months later, the ICT was decreased substantially in size. The patient was continued to be treated with monthly cyclophosphamide, prednisone, and colchicine, without recurrence.

5. Discussion

Intracardiac thrombosis is an uncommon complication of BD. Most of the patients are young males and are from the Mediterranean and the Middle East. Though ICT is usually located in the right side of the heart, mainly the right ventricle, thromboses involving both ventricles or limited only to the left ventricle have been also described [10–14]. In two of our patients, ICT was located in the right side of the heart, and one had thrombus in his left ventricle. All our patients had fever and dyspnea, which were the most common presenting symptoms in previously reported cases [5, 10–15]. Sometimes ICT may be the first manifestation of the disease [10, 15].

ICT often coexists with pulmonary involvement such as pulmonary artery aneurysms [16–21] and/or pulmonary artery thrombosis/pulmonary thromboembolism [10–15, 21–24], as was the case in our patients. In a review, pulmonary thromboembolism was reported in 67% of patients with ICT [11].

ICT has been also frequently associated with superficial thrombophlebitis and deep venous thrombosis [15, 23, 24] or thrombosis of vena cava [11], as in patient 3 with Budd-Chiari syndrome, which is an unusual disorder characterised by hepatic venous outflow obstruction either within the liver or in the inferior vena cava. In a study, of 493 patients with BD, 14 patients had Budd-Chiari Syndrome (2.8%) [25]. Association of ICT with Budd-Chiari syndrome seems to be rare. There have been only two cases including our case in the literature [26].

It has been speculated that pulmonary embolism or pulmonary infarction might have originated from deep vein thrombosis or right ventricular thrombi [20, 26–28]. Histopathological studies reveal thrombi and inflammatory infiltrates in vessel walls, which addresses a vasculitic process. Pulmonary vascular inflammation may result in thrombosis, infarction, hemorrhage, or aneurysm. There is no risk of embolic events in BD associated with deep vein thrombosis which is a feature of inflammation and also thrombus strictly adheres to inflamed vessel wall [29–31]. Pulmonary vascular manifestations are a result of in situ pulmonary pathology rather than embolisation from systemic veins [10].

The pathogenetic mechanism of thrombus formation in BD is still unclear. It is attributed to vascular inflammation and endothelial ischemia. High levels of endothelial products such as Von Willebrand factor antigen support endothelial destruction due to vasculitis [32]. Genetic prothrombotic factors such as Factor V Leiden and Prothrombin 20210 G-A gene mutations in BD were found to be markedly increased for the risk of thrombosis [33, 34]. A meta-analysis showed that hyperhomocysteinemia may be associated with thrombosis in BD [35]. Endomyocardial fibrosis may be one of the causes of ICT formation [10].

ICT can be misdiagnosed as an intracardiac tumor such as myxoma or vegetation related to infective endocarditis. Imaging tests such as echocardiography, CT, or MR show the filling defect(s) in the chamber(s). CT and MR also provide information about pulmonary vascular and/or parenchymal lesions. In most cases, ICT is discovered by echocardiography in the workup of fever etiology such as bacterial endocarditis.

Compared with transthoracic echocardiography, cardiac MR imaging is found to be more sensitive for the detection of left ventricular thrombi. The results of the same study also showed that ECG-triggered contrast-enhanced MR imaging is an accurate noninvasive alternative technique for the characterization of intracardiac thrombi, which is important because clots have a higher risk of embolism than that of organized thrombi [36].

There is no consensus for the treatment regimes of ICT associated with BD. There is no randomised controlled study assessing the results of different therapeutic protocols.

ICT in BD has been treated medically and occasionally with surgery and/or thrombolytic therapy. Medical treatment includes colchicine, corticosteroids, immunosuppressive agents, anticoagulants and/or low dose aspirin. It has been concluded that medical treatment should be the first choice of therapy [11, 26].

Immunosuppression is the main therapy for the treatment of vasculitis. Most cases of BD complicating ICT showed complete resolution or decreased in size with systemic corticosteroid and intravenous cyclophosphamide along with anticoagulants [5, 13, 14, 20, 26, 37, 38]. Ahn et al. showed that there were no significant differences in the recurrence rate of thrombosis between immunosuppressive therapy and those combined with anticoagulants therapy [39].

Immunosuppressive therapy without anticoagulation was also associated with complete resolution of the thrombus with no recurrences [40], as in our patients 1 and 2. Anticoagulation therapy can cause life-threatening massive bleeding in the presence of pulmonary aneurysm(s) in patients with ICT. Pulmonary aneurysms and ICT responded well to immunosuppressive therapy without anticoagulation [18], or the anticoagulants may be given after the resolution of hemoptysis with aggressive immunosuppressive treatment [41]. There is no clear evidence to support the benefit of anticoagulation in the treatment of thrombotic lesions in BD. Systemic corticosteroids plus immunosuppressives are highly recommended before anticoagulation in cases of BD [11, 14, 42].

Diagnostic and therapeutic cardiac surgical resection has been performed [11, 19, 28, 42–46]. Surgical treatment may be considered in cases unresponsive to optimal medical treatment, ineffective thrombolysis therapy and impaired hemodynamics or if ICT becomes massive and shows recurrence. Surgery alone does not lead to complete resolution [10, 42, 43]. There is a risk of recurrence after surgery [5]. After surgical removal of ICT, recurrent thrombus successfully resolves with medical treatment including prednisolon and immunosuppressant [22, 44–46]. Some patients underwent surgery before immunosuppressive therapy [10].

Thrombolytic therapy is rarely utilized in BD patients with ICT. Full resolution of thrombosis was reported with intravenous streptokinase plus corticosteroid treatment [12, 23]. A case with multiple ICTs has needed thrombolytic treatment along with anticoagulation, cyclophosphamide, and anti-TNF agent for resolution of ICT [47].

ICT in patients with BD may be resolved with medical treatment including immunosuppressive agents such as cyclophosphamide along with high dose glucocorticoid. Our results show that this combination therapy is the preferred choice of treatment.

References

[1] H. Behçet, "Uber residiverende apthose durchein virus verurschte Geschwure am Mund, am Auge und an den genitalien," *Dermatol Wochenschr*, vol. 105, pp. 1152–1157, 1937.

[2] J. T. Lie, "Vascular involvement in Behcet's disease: arterial and venous and vessels of all sizes," *Journal of Rheumatology*, vol. 19, no. 3, pp. 341–343, 1992.

[3] Y. Koç, I. Güllü, G. Akpek et al., "Vascular involvement in Behçet's disease," *The Journal of Rheumatology*, vol. 19, no. 3, pp. 402–410, 1992.

[4] N. Düzgün, A. Ates, O. T. Aydintug, O. Demir, and U. Olmez, "Characteristics of vascular involvement in Behçet's disease," *Scandinavian Journal of Rheumatology*, vol. 35, no. 1, pp. 65–68, 2006.

[5] G. Geri, B. Wechsler, D. L. Thi Huong et al., "Spectrum of cardiac lesions in Behçet disease: a series of 52 patients and review of the literature," *Medicine*, vol. 91, no. 1, pp. 25–34, 2012.

[6] S. Lakhanpal, K. Tani, J. T. Lie, K. Katoh, Y. Ishigatsubo, and T. Ohokubo, "Pathologic features of Behcet's syndrome: a review of Japanese autopsy registry data," *Human Pathology*, vol. 16, no. 8, pp. 790–795, 1985.

[7] M. Marzban, M. H. Mandegar, A. Karimi et al., "Cardiac and great vessel involvement in Behçet's disease," *Journal of Cardiac Surgery*, vol. 23, no. 6, pp. 765–768, 2008.

[8] F. Atzeni, P. Sarzi-Puttini, A. Doria, L. Boiardi, N. Pipitone, and C. Salvarani, "Behçet's disease and cardiovascular involvement," *Lupus*, vol. 14, no. 9, pp. 723–726, 2005.

[9] A. Hamzaoui, N. Bel Feki, A. Brahem Sfaxi et al., "Chest pain in patients with under undiagnosed of Behçet's disease," *Clinical and Experimental Rheumatology*, vol. 30, supplement 72, pp. S76–S79, 2012.

[10] N. Moğulkoç, M. I. Burgess, and P. W. Bishop, "Intracardiac thrombus in Behçet's disease: a systematic review," *Chest*, vol. 118, no. 2, pp. 479–487, 2000.

[11] T. Kajiya, R. Anan, M. Kameko et al., "Intracardiac thrombus, superior vena cava syndrome, and pulmonary embolism in a patient with Behçet's disease: a case report and literature review," *Heart and Vessels*, vol. 22, no. 4, pp. 278–283, 2007.

[12] P. Hiwarkar, R. Stasi, G. Sutherland, and M. Shannon, "Deep vein and intracardiac thrombosis during the post-partum period in Behçet's disease," *International Journal of Hematology*, vol. 91, no. 4, pp. 679–686, 2010.

[13] E. Seyahi, M. Melikoglu, C. Akman et al., "Pulmonary artery involvement and associated lung disease in Behçet disease: a series of 47 patients," *Medicine*, vol. 91, no. 1, pp. 35–48, 2012.

[14] R. Hammami, L. Abid, F. Frikha et al., "Intracardiac thrombus in young man: don't forget Behçet's disease," *Intern Med*, vol. 51, no. 14, pp. 1865–1867, 2012.

[15] M. Fekih, S. Fennira, L. Ghodhbane, and R. M. Zaouali, "Intracardiac thrombosis: on uncommon complication of Behcet's disease," *Tunisie Medicale*, vol. 82, no. 8, pp. 785–790, 2004.

[16] A. Kaya, C. Ertan, O. U. Gürkan et al., "Behçet's disease with right ventricle thrombus and bilateral pulmonary artery aneurysms: a case report," *Angiology*, vol. 55, no. 5, pp. 573–575, 2004.

[17] K. Marc, G. Iraqui, A. Jniene, J. Benamor, and J. E. Bourkadi, "Intracardiac thrombus and pulmonary artery aneurysm in Behcet's disease," *Revue des Maladies Respiratoires*, vol. 25, no. 1, pp. 69–72, 2008.

[18] J. K. Alkaabi and A. Pathare, "Pattern and outcome of vascular involvement of Omani patients with Behcet's disease," *Rheumatology International*, vol. 31, no. 6, pp. 731–735, 2011.

[19] M. H. Houman, I. Ksontini, I. Ben Ghorbel et al., "Association of right heart thrombosis, endomyocardial fibrosis, and pulmonary artery aneurysm in Behçet's disease," *European Journal of Internal Medicine*, vol. 13, no. 7, pp. 455–457, 2002.

[20] S. Hammami, S. Mahjoub, K. Ben-Hamda et al., "Intracardiac thrombus in Behçet's disease: two case reports," *Thrombosis Journal*, vol. 25, no. 3, pp. 1–9, 2005.

[21] D. Ernam, F. Atalay, A. Alp, and H. C. Hasanoğlu, "A Behçet's disease patient with intracardiac thrombus, pulmonary artery aneurysms complicating recurrent pulmonary thromboembolism," *Tuberkuloz ve Toraks*, vol. 54, no. 2, pp. 168–171, 2006.

[22] L. A. Mendes, L. L. Macgraw, G. S. Aldea, and R. Davidoff, "Right ventricular thrombus: an unusual manifestation of Behçet's disease," *Journal of the American Society of Echocardiography*, vol. 7, no. 4, pp. 438–440, 1994.

[23] M. Piga, F. Puchades, I. Mayo, and D. D'Cruz, "Successful thrombolytic therapy for recurrent right ventricular thrombosis in Behçet's disease," *Clinical and Experimental Rheumatology*, vol. 28, no. 4, supplement 60, pp. S76–S78, 2010.

[24] N. Düzgün, C. Anıl, F. Özer, and T. Acican, "The disapperance of pulmonary artery aneurysms and intracardiac thrombus with immunosuppressive treatment in a patient with Behçet's disease," *Clinical and Experimental Rheumatology*, vol. 20, no. 4, supplement 26, pp. S56–S57, 2002.

[25] Y. Bayraktar, F. Balkancı, M. Bayraktar, and M. Calguneri, "Budd-Chiari syndrome: a common complication of Behçet's disease," *American Journal of Gastroenterology*, vol. 92, no. 5, pp. 858–862, 1997.

[26] F. E. El Louali, A. Tamdy, A. Soufiani et al., "Cardiac thrombosis as a manifestation of Behçet syndrome," *Texas Heart Institute Journal*, vol. 37, no. 5, pp. 568–571, 2010.

[27] M. Yasuo, S. Nagano, Y. Yazaki et al., "Pulmonary embolism due to right ventricular thrombus in a case of Behçet's disease," *Japanese Circulation Society*, vol. 63, no. 11, pp. 909–911, 1999.

[28] O. G. Göktekin, C. Korkmaz, B. Timualp et al., "Wide spread thrombosis associated with recurrent intracardiac thombus in a patient with Behçet's disease," *The International Journal of Cardiovascular Imaging*, vol. 18, no. 6, pp. 431–434, 2002.

[29] G. Hatemi, A. Silman, D. Bang et al., "EULAR recommendations for the management of Behçet disease," *Annals of the Rheumatic Diseases*, vol. 67, no. 12, pp. 1656–1662, 2008.

[30] L. Caspary, "Vasculitides of large vessels," *Vasa*, vol. 40, no. 2, pp. 89–98, 2011.

[31] K. T. Calamia, M. Schirmer, and M. Melikoğlu, "Major vessel involvement in Behçet's disease," *Current Opinion in Rheumatology*, vol. 17, no. 1, pp. 1–8, 2005.

[32] K. Özoran, N. Düzgün, A. Gürler, H. Tutkak, and G. Tokgöz, "Plasma von Willebrand factor, tissue plasminogen activator, plasminogen activator inhibitor, and antithrombin III levels in Behçet's disease," *Scand J Rheumatol*, vol. 24, no. 6, pp. 376–382, 1995.

[33] A. Gul, U. Özbek, C. Özturk, M. Inanç, M. Koniçe, and T. Ozçelik, "Coagulation factor V gene mutation increases the risk of venous thrombosis in Behçet's disease," *British Journal of Rheumatology*, vol. 35, no. 11, pp. 1178–1180, 1996.

[34] P. B. Toydemir, A. H. Elhan, A. Tükün et al., "Effects of factor V gene G1691A, methylenetetrahydrofolate reductase gene C677T, and prothrombin gene G20210A mutations on deep venous thrombogenesis in Behcet's disease," *Journal of Rheumatology*, vol. 27, no. 12, pp. 2849–2854, 2000.

[35] M. la Regina, F. Orlandini, D. Prisco, and F. Dentali, "Homocysteine in vascular Behçet's disease: a metaanalysis," *Arteriosclerosis, Thrombosis, and Vascular Biology*, vol. 30, no. 10, pp. 2067–2074, 2010.

[36] J. Barkhausen, P. Hunold, H. Eggebrecht et al., "Detection and characterization of intracardiac thrombi on MR imaging," *American Journal of Roentgenology*, vol. 179, no. 6, pp. 1539–1544, 2002.

[37] D. Solmaz, I. Sari, E. Ozpelit, and E. Yilmaz, "Intracardiac thrombosis and superior vena cava syndrome in Behçet's disease," *Internal Medicine*, vol. 50, no. 16, pp. 1787–1788, 2011.

[38] S. M. Dogan, A. Birdane, C. Korkmaz, N. Ata, and B. Timuralp, "Right ventricular thrombus with Behçet's syndrome successful treatment with warfarin and immunosuppressive agents," *Texas Heart Institute Journal*, vol. 34, no. 3, pp. 360–362, 2007.

[39] J. K. Ahn, Y. S. Lee, C. H. Jeon, E. M. Koh, and H. S. Cha, "Treatment of venous thrombosis associated with Behçet's disease: immunosuppressive therapy alone versus immunosupressive thearpy plus anticoagulation," *Clinical Rheumatology*, vol. 27, no. 2, pp. 201–205, 2008.

[40] S. M. Samrah, S. S. Saadeh, and K. M. Alawneh, "Resolution of intracardiac and pulmonary thrombi without anticoagulation in a patient with Behçet's disease: a case report," *Clinical and Experimental Rheumatology*. In press.

[41] A. Vivante, Y. Bujanover, J. Jacobson, S. Padeh, and Y. Berkun, "Intracardiac thrombus and pulmonary aneurysms in an adolescent with Behçet disease," *Rheumatology International*, vol. 29, no. 5, pp. 575–577, 2009.

[42] Y. L. Zhu, Q. J. Wo, L. L. Guo et al., "The clinical characteristics and outcome of intracardiac thrombus and aortic valvular involvement in Behçet's disease," *Clinical and Experimental Rheumatology*, vol. 30, no. 3, supplement 72, pp. S40–S45, 2012.

[43] A. Moreno-Rodrigo, J. Muñoz-Sánchez, F. J. B. Bóveda-Romeo, and J. M. Santamaría-Jáuregui, "Intracardiac thrombosis associated with Behçet's disease," *Revista Española de Cardiología*, vol. 63, no. 12, pp. 1513–1515, 2010.

[44] Y. Kaneko, K. Tanaka, A. Yoshizawa et al., "Successful treatment of recurrent intracardiac thrombus in Behçet's disease with immunosuppressive therapy," *Clinical and Experimental Rheumatology*, vol. 23, no. 6, pp. 885–887, 2005.

[45] I. Ben Ghorbel, Z. Ibn Elhadj, M. Khanfir et al., "Intracardiac thrombus in Behçet's disease. A report of three cases," *Journal des Maladies Vasculaires*, vol. 29, no. 3, pp. 159–161, 2004.

[46] K. Kırali, A. Civelek, B. Dağlar et al., "An uncommon complication of Behçet's disease: ıntracardiac thrombosis needing surgical treatment," *The Journal of Thoracic and Cardiovascular Surgery*, vol. 46, no. 2, pp. 102–105, 1998.

[47] L. M. Endo, S. M. Rowe, R. L. Romp, M. A. Buckmaster, and T. P. Atkinson, "Pulmonary aneurysms and intracardiac thrombi due to Behçet's disease in an African-American adolescent with oculocutaneous albinism," *Clinical Rheumatology*, vol. 26, no. 9, pp. 1537–1539, 2007.

Effect of Adalimumab on Refractory Arthritis in Juvenile Idiopathic Inflammatory Myopathy with Anti-MDA5 Autoantibody

Takako Miyamae,[1,2] Takuma Hara,[2] Aki Hanaya,[2] Yumi Tani,[1,2] Takayuki Kishi,[1,2] and Hisashi Yamanaka[1]

[1]*Institute of Rheumatology, Tokyo Women's Medical University, 10-22 Kawada-cho, Shinjuku-ku, Tokyo 162-0054, Japan*
[2]*Department of Pediatrics, Tokyo Women's Medical University, 8-1 Kawada-cho, Shinjuku-ku, Tokyo 162-8666, Japan*

Correspondence should be addressed to Takako Miyamae; tmiyamae@twmu.ac.jp

Academic Editor: Mehmet Soy

A 10-year-old girl manifested persistent fever, skin rash, leg pain, fatigue, and joint pain. Based on muscle weakness, elevated muscle-derived enzymes, magnetic resonance imaging, and skin biopsy results, the diagnosis was juvenile idiopathic inflammatory myopathies (JIIM). Chest CT was normal; the anti-melanoma differentiation-associated protein-5 (anti-MDA5) autoantibody was positive. Initial manifestations subsided after prednisolone (PSL) and methotrexate treatment. After the PSL dosage was decreased, the patient presented with metacarpophalangeal (MCP) joint pain and swelling in both index fingers, synovial fluid, and signals on power Doppler ultrasound. The arthritis was refractory to cyclosporine and tacrolimus. Radiography showed progressive MCP joint space narrowing and joint erosion. Adalimumab was initiated 14 months after disease onset. There was a mildly increased matrix metalloproteinase-3 (MMP3) level, an erythrocyte sedimentation ratio (ESR), and a normal CRP level. Adalimumab resulted in decreased MCP joint pain and swelling. PSL was discontinued 10 months after adalimumab initiation; after 9 more months of adalimumab, there were no significant ultrasonography findings. MMP3 and ESR levels normalized during treatment. Radiography after 2 years of adalimumab showed further progressive MCP joint space narrowing restricting dorsiflexion. This report clarified that anti-MDA5-positive JIIM joint manifestations were due to active synovitis and that adalimumab is required for severe cases. Further experience is needed to determine the pathology, severity, and prognosis of this type of arthritis.

1. Introduction

The juvenile idiopathic inflammatory myopathies (JIIMs) are heterogeneous, systemic, autoimmune diseases with onset in childhood; they are characterized by weakness, chronic inflammation of the skeletal muscles, and typical skin rashes. Recently, new classification criteria for JIIMs have been developed [1], along with an increased understanding of the spectrum of phenotypes associated with JIIMs based on clinicopathologic features and the presence of myositis-specific autoantibodies (MSAs) and myositis-associated autoantibodies (MAAs) [2, 3]. The MAAs seen most frequently in JIIMs are anti-p155/140, anti-MJ, and anti-melanoma differentiation-associated protein-5 (anti-MDA5) autoantibodies [3].

Anti-MDA5 autoantibodies were present in 33% of a Japanese cohort but in only 7% of a UK cohort with JIIMs [4, 5]. Interstitial lung disease was more common in patients from both cohorts with this autoantibody compared with patients without these antibodies. In the UK patients, other common features included oral and cutaneous ulcerations, arthritis, and milder muscle disease, which were similar to findings in the US and European adult cohorts with anti-MDA5 autoantibodies.

With reference to joint manifestations seen among patients with JIIM and anti-MDA5 autoantibodies, the pathology

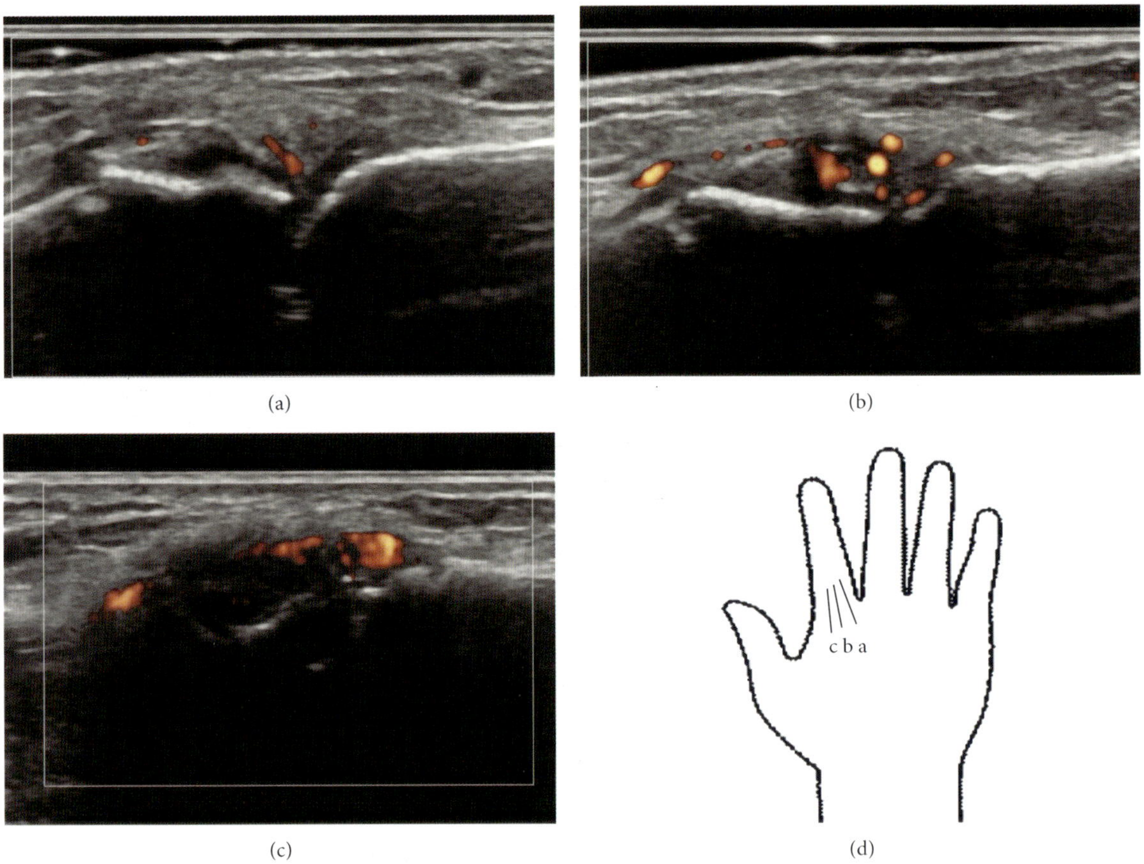

FIGURE 1: Ultrasonography of the metacarpophalangeal joint of the right index finger. No remarkable findings were seen on a midline echo (a), but synovial fluid and power Doppler signals were noted on the radial-shifted view (b) and (c).

and prognosis, including the response to medical treatments for myositis, have not been well described. We report the case of a girl with JIIM presenting with anti-MDA5 autoantibodies who had arthritis refractory to conventional treatments and improvement after adalimumab treatment.

2. Case Presentation

The patient, a 10-year-old Japanese girl, presented with fever and a skin rash after a sunburn due to daily outdoor swimming in July 2013. However, the fever persisted for two months, and she developed multiple symptoms: general fatigue; a skin rash; joint pain in her wrists, elbows, and knees; and pain in the lower extremities. The skin manifestations on the neck, face, upper extremities, and dorsum of the hands were photosensitivity consisting of Gottron's papules and a heliotrope rash, findings consistent with juvenile dermatomyositis. She was diagnosed as having JIIM based on clinical muscle weakness (manual muscle testing-8 score: 68 (range 0–80)), mildly elevated levels of muscle-derived enzymes (creatine kinase, 196 U/L; aldolase, 13.6 IU), the findings on muscle MR imaging, slightly high-signal intensity in the thigh with T2-weighted fat suppression, and skin biopsy. A muscle biopsy was not performed. The patient did not have respiratory symptoms, and a chest CT revealed no abnormality suggesting interstitial lung disease (ILD), though anti-MDA5 autoantibody was positively detected by an immunoprecipitation assay. Hyperferritinemia (773.9 ng/mL) was noted. Daily doses of 75 mg (1.9 mg/kg) of prednisolone (PSL) and weekly doses of 20 mg of oral methotrexate (MTX) were initiated, after which the symptoms improved. Subsequently, the patient visited our institute after 4 months of observation during the corticosteroid taper when 28 mg (0.7 mg/kg) of PSL was given. The Childhood Myositis Assessment Scale (CMAS) was 50 (range of score: 0–52), and a residual skin rash on the dorsum of the hands was seen. No other organ involvement was observed.

Because osteonecrosis of the right talus and both tibia occurred due to the administration of high doses of glucocorticoids, a further taper of PSL was encouraged. MTX was discontinued after 5 months of administration and changed to 200 mg (5 mg/kg)/day of cyclosporine due to the possibility of MTX-induced ILD and the probability of developing anti-MDA5 autoantibody-associated ILD [6]. When the dosage of PSL was decreased to 17.5 mg (0.4 mg/kg)/day, the patient presented with pain and swelling of the metacarpophalangeal (MCP) joints of both index fingers. Ultrasonography of the MCP joints indicated synovial fluid and power Doppler signals (Figure 1). Antinuclear antibody, rheumatoid factor, and anti-citrullinated peptide antibody were not detected. Because the arthritis was refractory to another disease-modifying antirheumatic drug (3 mg/day of tacrolimus) and radiography showed progressive narrowing of the joint space of the MCP joints

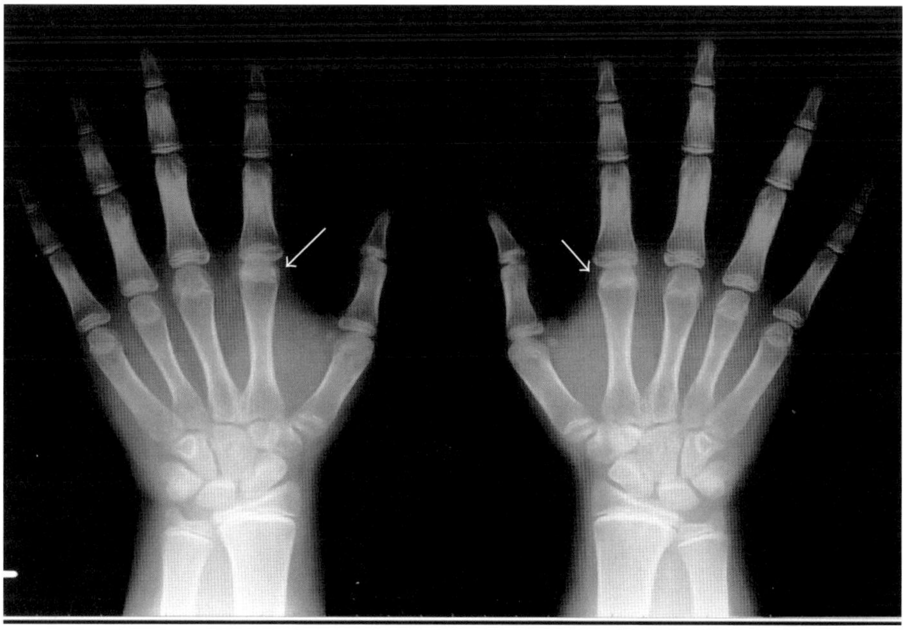

(a)

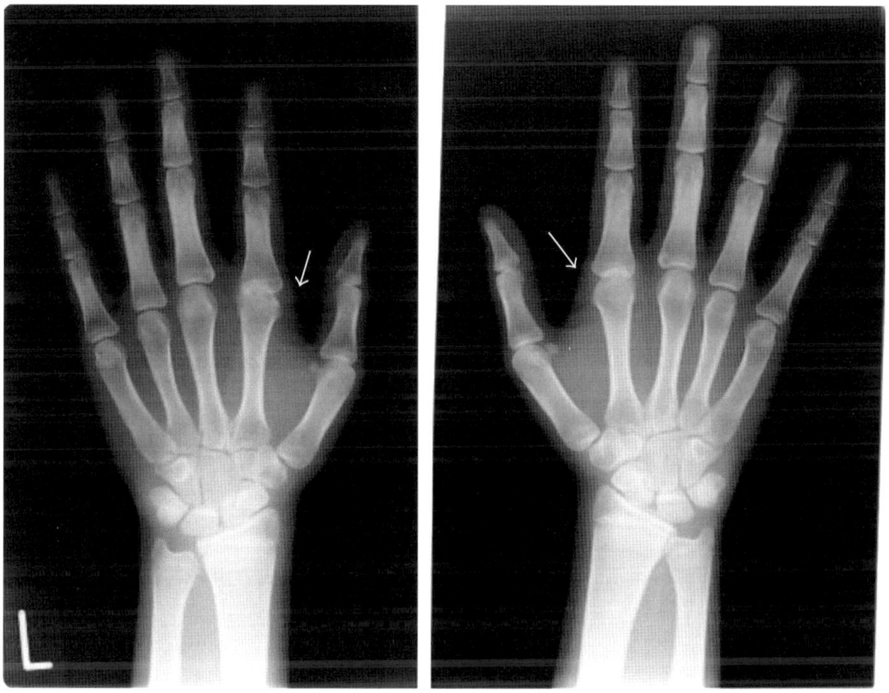

(b)

FIGURE 2: Radiography of both hands. (a) In September 2014, at the initiation of adalimumab when the patient was 12 years and 1 month of age. (b) In September 2016, after 2 years of adalimumab treatment when the patient was 14 years and 1 month of age. Narrowing of the metacarpophalangeal joints of both index fingers was observed when adalimumab was started (a), and more progressive joint space narrowing existed under treatment with adalimumab, whereas insignificant bone erosion was observed (b).

(Figure 2(a)), biweekly administration of 40 mg of adalimumab was initiated in September 2014, 14 months after the initial onset of JIIM when the patient was 12 years old. Laboratory data showed a mildly increased level of matrix metalloproteinase-3 (MMP3) of 105.5 ng/mL, an erythrocyte sedimentation ratio (ESR) of 21 mm/hour, and a normal CRP level (0.08 mg/dL). Adalimumab treatment resulted in the subsidence of pain and swelling of the MCP joints. Oral PSL was discontinued 10 months after initiation of adalimumab, and no significant fluid or power Doppler signals were observed on ultrasonography of the MCP joints performed 19 months after the drug's initiation (Figure 3). The elevated levels of MMP3 and ESR were gradually normalized during the time course of adalimumab administration

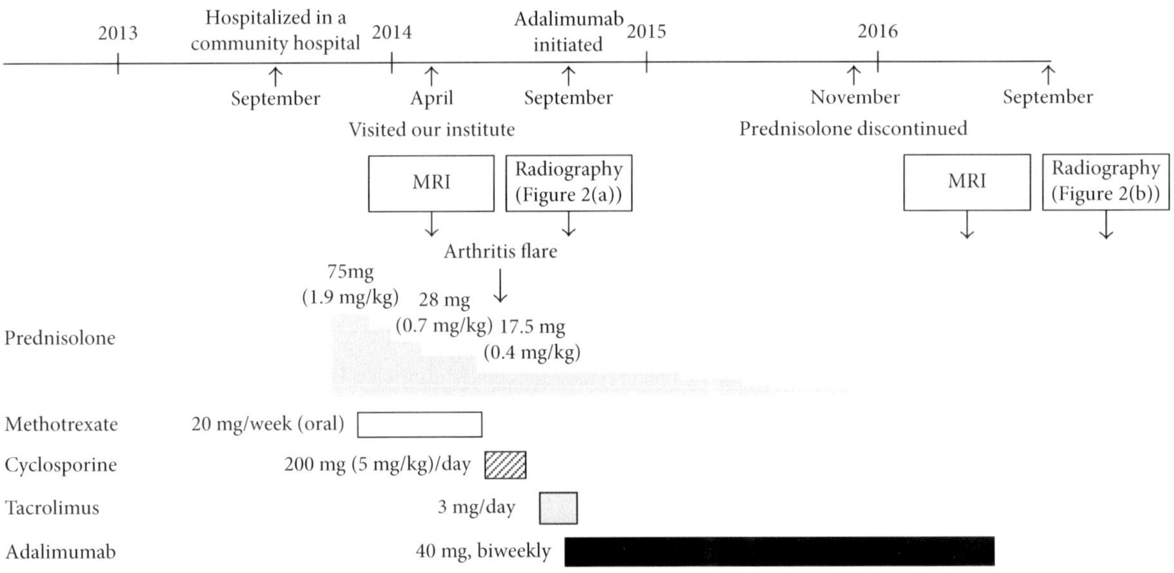

FIGURE 3: Time course of clinical treatments.

without clinical manifestations of active arthritis, such as swelling and pain. However, radiography in September 2016, after 2 years of adalimumab treatment, showed further progressive narrowing of the MCP joints that restricted dorsiflexion, whereas bone erosion was insignificant (Figure 2). Bone erosion was not detected even on an MRI performed almost at the same time as radiography. Myositis and skin manifestations remained stable during adalimumab treatment.

Anti-MDA5 autoantibody levels were measured by qualitative immunoprecipitation assay. It remains unclear whether a correlation exists between anti-MDA5 autoantibody levels and arthritis activity.

3. Discussion

This is the first time that adalimumab was used to treat arthritis associated with JIIM and anti-MDA5 autoantibodies. The initial high doses of corticosteroids prevented the development of ILD and CNS disease but resulted in osteonecrosis. In a series of 54 Japanese patients with JDM, 33% had anti-MDA5 autoantibodies [4], whereas these autoantibodies were present in only 7% of patients in the UK JDM registry [5]. It is also called "an arthro-dermato-pulmonary syndrome" with anti-MDA5 autoantibodies because there was a high rate of interstitial lung disease, arthritis, and distinctive skin lesions, such as ivory-centered papules and/or cutaneous ulcerations, which could develop among the patients [7].

With reference to the joint involvement seen in children with JIIM and anti-MDA5 autoantibodies, few reports have been described so far. In a US cohort study of 160 adult DM patients, anti-MDA5-positive patients were frequently observed with arthritis that was often symmetric, present in the small joints of the hands, and associated with morning stiffness that was clinically similar to rheumatoid arthritis [8]. In the 9 cases with arthritis, a small erosion on the radial site of the 2nd metacarpal head was seen in one patient, but only on MRI of the hands; conventional X-rays did not demonstrate erosive disease in any of the patients.

With regard to joint involvement, the patient in our report met the International League of Associations for Rheumatology (ILAR) classification of juvenile idiopathic arthritis (JIA) [9]. However, the joint manifestation seen in our patient was characteristically limited to the symmetrical small MCP joints of the hands, though the ultrasonography findings were consistent with active synovitis observed in typical JIA. Compared with progressive joint space narrowing on radiography, insignificant bone erosion might be specific to arthritis associated with the disorder. The disease activity of the patient's dermatitis and myositis was relatively mild, and based on our experience, immunosuppressive treatments were mainly required for the refractory arthritis. Considering this patient's joint manifestations, the change in ultrasonography findings, and the time course of the ESR and MMP3 levels, adalimumab apparently contributed to the subsidence of the refractory arthritis and the discontinuation of PSL in this adolescent girl. This case report clarified that the joint manifestations associated with anti-MDA5 autoantibody-positive JIIM were due to active synovitis, although the affected joints were limited to the MCP joints of the index fingers. Although discontinued in this case, MTX is used as a first line immunosuppressant in several treatment algorithms for juvenile dermatomyositis and could be effective against the arthritis independent of PSL [10]. However, this report also indicates the importance of adalimumab treatment in severe cases. Further experience is needed to determine the pathology and prognosis of this type of arthritis.

Abbreviations

JIIM: Juvenile idiopathic inflammatory myopathy
MSA: Myositis-specific autoantibody
MAA: Myositis-associated autoantibodies

MDA-5: Melanoma differentiation-associated protein-5
PSL: Prednisolone
MTX: Methotrexate
MCP: Metacarpophalangeal
MMP-3: Metalloproteinase-3
ESR: Erythrocyte sedimentation ratio
JIA: Juvenile idiopathic arthritis.

Consent

Written informed consent was obtained from the patient and the parents for publication of this case report and any accompanying images.

References

[1] A. Tjarnlund, M. Bottai, L. G. Rider et al., "Progress report on development of classification criteria for adult and juvenile idiopathic inflammatory myopathies," *Pediatric Rheumatology*, vol. 12, no. 1, p. P94, 2014.

[2] L. G. Rider, J. D. Katz, and O. Y. Jones, "Developments in the classification and treatment of the juvenile idiopathic inflammatory myopathies," *Rheumatic Disease Clinics of North America*, vol. 39, no. 4, pp. 877–904, 2013.

[3] L. G. Rider and K. Nistala, "The juvenile idiopathic inflammatory myopathies: pathogenesis, clinical and autoantibody phenotypes, and outcomes," *Journal of Internal Medicine*, vol. 280, no. 1, pp. 24–38, 2016.

[4] N. Kobayashi, S. Takezaki, I. Kobayashi et al., "Clinical and laboratory features of fatal rapidly progressive interstitial lung disease associated with juvenile dermatomyositis," *Rheumatology*, vol. 54, no. 5, pp. 784–791, 2015.

[5] S. L. Tansley, Z. E. Betteridge, H. Gunawardena et al., "Anti-MDA5 autoantibodies in juvenile dermatomyositis identify a distinct clinical phenotype: a prospective cohort study," *Arthritis Research and Therapy*, vol. 16, no. 4, p. R138, 2014.

[6] S. Imokawa, T. V. Colby, K. O. Leslie, and R. A. Helmers, "Methotrexate pneumonitis: review of the literature and histopathological findings in nine patients," *European Respiratory Journal*, vol. 15, no. 2, pp. 373–381, 2000.

[7] R. Goussot, A. Theulin, J. Goetz, J. Sibilia, J. E. Gottenberg, and A. Meyer, "An arthro-dermato-pulmonary syndrome associated with anti-MDA5 antibodies," *Joint Bone Spine*, vol. 81, no. 3, p. 266, 2014.

[8] J. C. Hall, L. Casciola-Rosen, L. A. Samedy et al., "Anti-melanoma differentiation-associated protein 5-associated dermatomyositis: expanding the clinical spectrum," *Arthritis Care and Research*, vol. 65, no. 8, pp. 1307–1315, 2013.

[9] R. E. Petty, T. R. Southwood, P. Manners et al., "International League of Associations for Rheumatology classification of juvenile idiopathic arthritis: second revision, Edmonton, 2001," *Journal of Rheumatology*, vol. 31, no. 2, pp. 390–392, 2004.

[10] K. Barut, P. O. Aydin, A. Adrovic, S. Sahin, and O. Kasapcopur, "Juvenile dermatomyositis: a tertiary center experience," *Clinical Rheumatology*, vol. 36, no. 2, pp. 361–366, 2017.

29

Possible Association of Etanercept, Venous Thrombosis, and Induction of Antiphospholipid Syndrome

Shanti Virupannavar,[1] Anthony Brandau,[2] Carla Guggenheim,[3] and Heather Laird-Fick[1]

[1] *Internal Medicine, Michigan State University, 138 Service Road, A225 Clinical Center, East Lansing, MI 48825, USA*
[2] *Internal Medicine and Hematology/Oncology, McLaren of Greater Lansing, 401 West Greenlawn Avenue, Lansing, MI 48910, USA*
[3] *Internal Medicine and Rheumatology, Michigan State University, 138 Service Road, A225 Clinical Center, East Lansing, MI 48825, USA*

Correspondence should be addressed to Shanti Virupannavar; shantivirup@gmail.com

Academic Editor: Masataka Kuwana

Tumor necrosis factor α (TNF α) inhibitors are commonly used for treatment of aggressive rheumatoid arthritis and other rheumatic diseases. Etanercept is one of the medications approved for treatment of rheumatoid arthritis. Though many studies have documented the safety and efficacy of these medications, evidence for adverse effects is emerging including cancer, infections, and cardiovascular disease. There have been studies showing that these medications induce autoantibody production, including antinuclear antibodies and anti-dsDNA antibodies. Limited data exists, however, regarding induction of antiphospholipid antibodies (APLs) by TNF α inhibitors, including anticardiolipin antibodies (ACLs), lupus anticoagulant (LAC), and anti-β_2-glycoprotein I (anti-β_2 GPI), or an association between antibody development and clinical manifestations. In this case series, we describe five patients who developed venous thromboembolism (VTE) and APLs while receiving etanercept therapy. All five of our patients met the criteria for diagnosis of APS after receiving etanercept. Our case series supports the association between etanercept, APLs, and VTE. We believe that testing for APLs prior to initiation of anti-TNF therapy is reasonable, given this relationship and the risks associated with VTE.

1. Introduction

Tumor necrosis factor α (TNF α) is a cytokine essential to T-cell-mediated inflammatory responses [1–3]. TNF α inhibitors are now widely used for treatment of aggressive rheumatoid arthritis (RA) and other rheumatic diseases. Etanercept is one of the medications approved by the US Food and Drug Administration (FDA) for treatment of RA, psoriatic arthritis, and ankylosing spondylitis. It is a fusion protein produced by recombinant DNA which combines the ligand binding portion of human TNF receptor p75 with the Fc fragment of human IgG1, which binds soluble TNF α, working to block the action on its receptors [4, 5].

While many studies have documented the safety and efficacy of these medications [1, 6, 7], evidence for adverse effects is emerging. These include infections, cancer, lymphoma, demyelinating disorders, and cardiovascular disease [1, 4, 8]. In addition, an association with these medications to autoimmune diseases has been reported [1, 4, 9–12].

TNF α agents induce autoantibody production, including antinuclear antibodies (ANAs) and anti-dsDNA antibodies [2, 4, 5, 11, 13–19]. Eriksson et al. showed that ANA positivity increased from 24% of patients at baseline, to 77% at 30 weeks, and 69% at 54 weeks following initiation of a TNF α inhibitor [20]. Many other studies have confirmed these findings. However, there are limited data regarding the induction of antiphospholipid antibodies (APLs) by TNF α inhibitors, including anticardiolipin antibodies (ACLs), lupus anticoagulant (LAC), and anti-β_2-glycoprotein I (anti-β_2 GPI). Two studies have reported antibody development in RA patients receiving etanercept. Jonsdottir et al. showed that up to 25% of such patients develop IgG or IgM ACL, while Ferraro-Peyret et al. showed that 21% developed APL positivity [17, 21]. The association between antibody development and clinical manifestations remains unclear [21–25].

In this case series, we describe five patients who developed venous thromboembolism (VTE) and APLs while receiving etanercept therapy.

2. Case Presentations

Case 1. A 67-year-old Hispanic man, with a nine-year history of RA, had been treated with multiple combinations of disease-modifying antirheumatic drugs (DMARDs) and corticosteroids. He had been receiving etanercept (25 mg twice weekly) for three years when he presented with dyspnea and right calf swelling. Duplex ultrasound confirmed right femoral deep venous thrombosis (DVT). Computed tomography angiography (CTA) of the chest showed massive filling defects in the right and left pulmonary arteries. He denied any personal or family history of hypercoagulable disorders, immobilization, smoking, trauma, blood clots, or heparin therapy. He had undergone an uncomplicated ankle surgery nine months prior to presentation. He had an elevated activated partial thromboplastin time (aPTT) of 48 seconds prior to initiating anticoagulation therapy. He tested positive for LAC and ANA, with speckled pattern at titer of 1:1280. ACL IgG and IgM were within normal range. LAC, ANA, and aPTT remained persistently elevated one year later. Further thrombophilia workup was negative.

Case 2. A 55-year-old Caucasian female with refractory RA had been on multiple DMARDs, including methotrexate, etanercept, rituximab, leflunomide, adalimumab, azathioprine, and minocycline. One year after restarting etanercept (50 mg every week), she presented to the emergency department with severe palpitations. She was found to have large bilateral VTE secondary to left lower extremity DVT. She had no risk factors for thrombosis. She had a positive ACL IgM, but LAC and the rest of the thrombophilia workup were negative. ACL IgM remained positive 12 weeks later.

Case 3. An 85-year-old Caucasian woman with a remote history of tobacco use had been treated with methotrexate and etanercept for RA for three years when she presented with VTE in the absence of risk factors. She had a positive ACL IgG and LAC at presentation and 12 weeks later. Her aPTT was persistently elevated at 40.9 seconds. The other thrombophilia workup was negative.

Case 4. A 53-year-old Caucasian female with seronegative inflammatory arthritis, poorly controlled by methotrexate, was started on etanercept add-on therapy. She had a negative workup for antiphospholipid syndrome (APS) prior to initiating the new medication. One year later she developed dyspnea and bilateral lower extremity swelling. She was found to have a left lower lobe VTE, along with left tibial DVT. Her only risk factor for thrombosis was a family history of DVT in her mother. At presentation she had a prolonged aPTT of 44 seconds and was positive for LAC. These labs remained persistently positive for more than three months. The other thrombophilia workup was negative.

Case 5. A 61-year-old Caucasian male with psoriatic arthritis had been treated with efalizumab for two years for psoriasis skin involvement. Due to recurrent flares of his arthritis, efalizumab was discontinued. He was started on methotrexate 5 mg per week and prednisone 10 mg daily. After a 25-day washout period, etanercept was started. His arthritis symptoms improved after one week. Eventually methotrexate and prednisone were discontinued. Three years later, he presented with multiple DVTs. He had no risk factors for thrombosis. He had a prolonged aPTT at 51 seconds and a positive LAC and anti-β_2 GPI. All three of these labs remained positive for more than three months.

3. Discussion

Antiphospholipid syndrome is characterized by the occurrence of vascular thrombosis or pregnancy morbidity in the presence of APLs, which include ACL, anti-β_2 GPI, and LAC [26]. According to the revised Sapporo criteria, APS can be diagnosed by one clinical criterion and at least one laboratory criterion. In order to meet the laboratory criteria, the APLs must remain positive on two or more occasions, at least 12 weeks apart [26]. All five of our patients met the criteria for diagnosis of APS after receiving etanercept. Prior to starting anticoagulation for VTE, all of them had tested for aPTT, APL, protein C, protein S, antithrombin III, Factor V Leiden, homocysteine, and prothrombin gene mutation. All had a prolonged aPTT and tested positive for at least one of the APLs prior to initiation of anticoagulation. When present, these tests remained positive for more than three months.

There are several proposed mechanisms by which TNF α inhibitors induce APL. One hypothesis is that the binding of an inhibitor to transmembrane TNF α induces apoptosis, leading to release of nuclear antigens and development of autoantibodies [5, 27]. Only infliximab binds transmembrane TNF α, however, so this hypothesis would not explain the autoantibodies seen with etanercept, which primarily binds soluble TNF α [5]. A second hypothesis is that TNF α inhibitors suppress the T-helper type 1 response, resulting in a T-helper type 2 response; this leads to autoantibody production and lupus-like features [12, 27]. Thirdly, TNF α inhibitors increase the likelihood for bacterial infections, which activate polyclonal B-lymphocytes and result in antibody production [12, 27]. Lastly, Masson suggests that TNF α inhibition results in overproduction of interferon α. This phenomenon, combined with individuals' predisposition to lupus-like syndromes and APS, leads to thromboembolic events [23].

Previous studies have not conclusively shown that TNF α blocker-induced APLs are associated with thrombotic events typical of APS [17, 21, 22, 25]. Two studies have found no association. Davies et al. examined data from the British Society for Rheumatology Biologics Register and found that venous thromboembolism was not increased in patients receiving anti-TNF α treatment [28]. Ferraro-Peyret et al. found no correlation between induction of autoantibodies (ACL or anti-β_2 GPI) and development of APS or lupus-like syndrome over a two-year period [17]. On the other hand, two studies have reported an association. Jonsdottir et al. found that both IgM and IgG ACL antibodies occurred more frequently in patients who received TNF α inhibitors for three months or longer and that positivity was associated with worse clinical outcomes [21]. Finally, Petitpain et al. reported 85 spontaneous cases of TNF α inhibitor-related thromboembolic events from 2000 to 2006 [22]. These events occurred in patients with few or no traditional risk factors for VTE [22]. Unfortunately, the study is limited by variations in how some data, like antibody testing, were assessed and reported. Of the 85 patients, only 23 had documented antibodies, and of those only four had APLs [22].

We believe our findings strengthen the evidence supporting an association of TNF α inhibition with APL antibody induction and VTE. Our series, similar to Petitpain's, identified venous thrombosis in patients with few or no risk factors other than APL. Three of the patients had received etanercept for three years, and a fourth had been on the medication previously. These patients would not have been identified by Ferraro-Peyret, whose analysis was limited to a two-year window of therapy. Strikingly, all five of our cases occurred over a five-year period, in a single private clinic of approximately 500 patients. Unfortunately, four of the five patients did not receive baseline APL testing.

What might be the implications of an association of anti-TNF α therapy with APL antibody induction and VTE? Others have pondered whether patients should be screened for APLs prior to initiating TNF α inhibitor therapy [1, 12, 22, 23, 25], but this is rarely done in the absence of other risk factors for APS [22]. Ramos-Casals et al. recommend performing baseline immunologic studies including ANA, anti dsDNA, APLs, ANCA, and chest X-ray based upon their retrospective study of 233 cases of autoimmune diseases associated with TNF α inhibitor therapy. They also suggest tailoring therapy based upon the severity of autoimmune features. For example, for patients with preexisting autoimmune diseases, Ramos-Casals et al. recommend using anti-TNF α agents with caution.

4. Conclusion

Our case series supports the association between etanercept, APLs, and VTE. We believe that testing for APLs prior to initiation of anti-TNF therapy is reasonable, given the evidence described herein and the morbidity and mortality attendant to VTE. A cohort study that included baseline autoantibody screening could define the benefits and cost of this strategy. As the number of new classes of biologic DMARDS increases, it is also imperative for us to obtain a better understanding of the mechanism of induction of autoantibodies and autoimmunity with these agents.

Authors' Contribution

Shanti Virupannavar and Anthony Brandau collected patient information and wrote the paper. Heather Laird-Fick and Carla Guggenheim helped to edit the paper and collect additional information.

References

[1] M. Ramos-Casals, P. Brito-Zerón, S. Muñoz et al., "Autoimmune diseases induced by TNF-targeted therapies: analysis of 233 cases," *Medicine*, vol. 86, no. 4, pp. 242–251, 2007.

[2] R. Golmia and M. Scheinberg, "Infliximab use and sequential occurrence of autoantibodies and neoplasia in a patient with spondyloarthritis," *Revista Brasileira de Reumatologia*, vol. 50, no. 6, pp. 723–728, 2010.

[3] H. Yoshida, C. E. Yilmaz, and D. N. Granger, "Role of tumor necrosis factor-α in the extraintestinal thrombosis associated with colonic inflammation," *Inflammatory Bowel Diseases*, vol. 17, no. 11, pp. 2217–2223, 2011.

[4] F. Atzeni, M. Turiel, F. Capsoni, A. Doria, P. Meroni, and P. Sarzi-Puttini, "Autoimmunity and anti-TNF-α agents," *Annals of the New York Academy of Sciences*, vol. 1051, pp. 559–569, 2005.

[5] P. Caramaschi, D. Biasi, M. Colombatti et al., "Anti-TNFα therapy in rheumatoid arthritis and autoimmunity," *Rheumatology International*, vol. 26, no. 3, pp. 209–214, 2006.

[6] M. C. Genovese, J. M. Bathon, R. M. Fleischmann et al., "Longterm safety, efficacy, and radiographic outcome with etanercept treatment in patients with early rheumatoid arthritis," *Journal of Rheumatology*, vol. 32, no. 7, pp. 1232–1242, 2005.

[7] M. Lebwohl, A. Gottlieb, W. Wallis, and R. Zitnik, "Safety and efficacy of over 7 years of etanercept therapy in a global population of patients with rheumatoid arthritis," *Journal of the American Academy of Dermatology*, vol. 52, article 195, 2005.

[8] M. Aringer, F. Houssiau, C. Gordon et al., "Adverse events and efficacy of TNF-alpha blockade with infliximab in patients with systemic lupus erythematosus: long-term follow-up of 13 patients," *Rheumatology*, vol. 48, no. 11, pp. 1451–1454, 2009.

[9] T. Reitblat and O. Reitblat, "Appearance of ANCA-associated vasculitis under tumor necrosis factor-alpha inhibitors treatment," *American Journal of Case Reports*, vol. 14, pp. 80–82, 2013.

[10] V. L. Williams and P. R. Cohen, "TNF alpha antagonist-induced lupus-like syndrome: report and review of the literature with implications for treatment with alternative TNF alpha antagonists," *International Journal of Dermatology*, vol. 50, no. 5, pp. 619–625, 2011.

[11] A. T. Borchers, N. Leibushor, G. S. Cheema, S. M. Naguwa, and M. E. Gershwin, "Immune-mediated adverse effects of biologicals used in the treatment of rheumatic diseases," *Journal of Autoimmunity*, vol. 37, no. 4, pp. 273–288, 2011.

[12] M. de Bandt, J. Sibilia, X. le Loët et al., "Systemic lupus erythematosus induced by anti-tumour necrosis factor alpha therapy: a French national survey," *Arthritis Research & Therapy*, vol. 7, no. 3, pp. R545–R551, 2005.

[13] S. Vermeire, M. Noman, G. van Assche et al., "Autoimmunity associated with anti-tumor necrosis factor α treatment in Crohn's disease: a prospective cohort study," *Gastroenterology*, vol. 125, no. 1, pp. 32–39, 2003.

[14] L. de Rycke, E. Kruithof, N. van Damme et al., "Antinuclear antibodies following infliximab treatment in patients

with rheumatoid arthritis or spondylarthropathy," *Arthritis and Rheumatism*, vol. 48, no. 4, pp. 1015–1023, 2003.

[15] M. Antivalle, M. G. Marazza, G. Randisi, P. Sarzi-Puttini et al., "Long term treatment of rheumatoid arthritis with infliximab: efficacy, side effects and autoantibodies induction," *Arthritis & Rheumatology*, vol. 46, article 534, 2002.

[16] J. A. Mendoça, J. F. Marques-Neto, A. M. Samara, and S. Apenzeller, "Increased levels of rheumatoid factors after TNF inhibitor in rheumatoid arthritis," *Rheumatology International*, vol. 32, pp. 815–818, 2012.

[17] C. Ferraro-Peyret, F. Coury, J. G. Tebib, J. Bienvenu, and N. Fabien, "Infliximab therapy in rheumatoid arthritis and ankylosing spondylitis-induced specific antinuclear and antiphospholipid autoantibodies without autoimmune clinical manifestations: a two-year prospective study," *Arthritis Research & Therapy*, vol. 6, no. 6, pp. R535–R543, 2004.

[18] F. Bobbio-Pallavicini, C. Alpini, R. Caporali, S. Avalle, S. Bugatti, and C. Montecucco, "Autoantibody profile in rheumatoid arthritis during long-term infliximab treatment," *Arthritis Research & Therapy*, vol. 6, no. 3, pp. R264–R272, 2004.

[19] F. Atzeni, R. Talotta, F. Salaffi et al., "Immunogenicity and autoimmunity during anti-TNF therapy," *Autoimmunity Reviews*, vol. 12, pp. 703–708, 2013.

[20] C. Eriksson, S. Engstrand, K.-G. Sundqvist, and S. Rantapää Dahlqvist, "Autoantibody formation in patients with rheumatoid arthritis treated with anti-TNFα," *Annals of the Rheumatic Diseases*, vol. 64, no. 3, pp. 403–407, 2005.

[21] T. Jonsdottir, J. Forslid, A. van Vollenhoven et al., "Treatment with tumour necrosis factor α antagonists in patients with rheumatoid arthritis induces anticardiolipin antibodies," *Annals of the Rheumatic Diseases*, vol. 63, no. 9, pp. 1075–1078, 2004.

[22] N. Petitpain, N. Gambier, D. Wahl, I. Chary-Valckenaere, D. Loeuille, and P. Gillet, "Arterial and venous thromboembolic events during anti-TNF therapy: a study of 85 spontaneous reports in the period 2000-2006," *Bio-Medical Materials and Engineering*, vol. 19, no. 4-5, pp. 355–364, 2009.

[23] P. L. Masson, "Thromboembolic events and anti-tumor necrosis factor therapies," *International Immunopharmacology*, vol. 14, pp. 444–445, 2012.

[24] A. Makol, M. Grover, C. Guggenheim, and H. Hassouna, "Etanercept and venous thromboembolism: a case series," *Journal of Medical Case Reports*, vol. 4, article 12, 2010.

[25] L. A. Korswagen, G. M. Bartelds, C. L. M. Krieckaert et al., "Venous and arterial thromboembolic events in adalimumab-treated patients with antiadalimumab antibodies: a case series and cohort study," *Arthritis and Rheumatism*, vol. 63, no. 4, pp. 877–883, 2011.

[26] S. Miyakis, M. D. Lockshin, T. Atsumi et al., "International consensus statement on an update of the classification criteria for definite antiphospholipid syndrome (APS)," *Journal of Thrombosis and Haemostasis*, vol. 4, no. 2, pp. 295–306, 2006.

[27] F. Dedeoglu, "Drug-induced autoimmunity," *Current Opinion in Rheumatology*, vol. 21, no. 5, pp. 547–551, 2009.

[28] R. Davies, J. B. Galloway, K. D. Watson et al., "Venous thrombotic events are not increased in patients with rheumatoid arthritis treated with anti-TNF therapy: results from the British Society for Rheumatology Biologics Register," *Annals of the Rheumatic Diseases*, vol. 70, no. 10, pp. 1831–1834, 2011.

Methotrexate Induced Pancytopenia

Fernando Gonzalez-Ibarra,[1] Sahar Eivaz-Mohammadi,[1] Shiri Surapaneni,[1] Hazem Alsaadi,[2] Amer K. Syed,[3] Simon Badin,[4] Valentin Marian,[5] and Mazhar Elamir[1]

[1] *Department of Internal Medicine, Mount Sinai School of Medicine, Jersey City Medical Center, 355 Grand Street, Jersey City, NJ 07302, USA*

[2] *Department of Internal Medicine, Jersey City Medical Center, St. George's University School of Medicine, Jersey City, NJ 07302, USA*

[3] *Laureate National Institute of Medicine, Jersey City Medical Center, 355 Grand Street, Jersey City, NJ 07302, USA*

[4] *Department of Hematology, Mount Sinai School of Medicine, Jersey City Medical Center, Jersey City, NJ 07302, USA*

[5] *Department of Rheumatology, Mount Sinai School of Medicine, Jersey City Medical Center, Jersey City, NJ 07302, USA*

Correspondence should be addressed to Fernando Gonzalez-Ibarra; drpavelglez@gmail.com

Academic Editor: Geoffrey Owen Littlejohn

The well-reported methotrexate (MTX) toxicities are based on the duration and cumulative dosing of drug. The typical toxicities can be predicted by the timing of drug administration, where mucositis occurs as an earlier effect, while myelosuppression and the sequelae of pancytopenia occur later after MTX administration. Despite these well-known toxicities, low dose MTX therapy can become problematic, in particular with the elderly, who are at a greater risk for significant myelosuppression. We present a case of a 73-year-old female with pancytopenia causing severe neutropenia, mucocutaneous bleeding, and bruising and requiring intravenous antibiotic therapy and limited transfusion dependence as a result of low dose daily MTX for rheumatoid arthritis.

1. Introduction

MTX is a widely used drug most commonly used in the treatment of various malignancies and autoimmune disorders, including rheumatoid arthritis and elective abortions. It is an inhibitor of cellular proliferation. As such, cells with the highest turnover or reduced half-life are most susceptible to its effect. As a consequence, when a patient's oral epithelial cells are affected, mucositis develops. Via the same mechanism, cytopenia leads to increased bleeding, easily bruising, macrocytic erythrocytes, and an increased risk of infections [1–3].

2. Case Report

A 73-year-old African American female with a past medical history of CAD, CVI, hypertension, and rheumatoid arthritis presents to the emergency room with epistaxis and gingival bleeding which initially began as a mild oral mucositis but progressed to odynophagia. She also experienced increased bruising for the last couple of weeks. These bruises progressed to open bleeding ulcerations with minimal trauma. Despite this, the patient had no prior hematological or oncological pathologies. Her home medications included aspirin (81 mg), carvedilol, enalapril, folic acid, furosemide, clopidogrel, MTX, and simvastatin. Her rheumatologist had recently changed her dosage of MTX from 7.5 mg weekly to 2.5 mg daily approximately two months prior due to worsening of her rheumatoid arthritis symptoms. Apparently the patient did not have a proper outpatient monitor of CBC, creatinine, or liver function tests after MTX dose was increased. Vital signs are pulse (68 bpm), respiratory rate (18/minute), blood pressure (152/85), and temperature (98.7°C). Her physical examination is evident for multiple petechiae scattered in the upper body. On admission, patient is pancytopenic: WBC (2.0; differential: polys = 23%, lymphocytes = 55%, monocytes = 2%, and eosinophils = 20%), Hb (7), MCV (89), and platelets (3000). Her last CBC two months prior was WBC (7.6), Hb (10.2), and platelets (194).

The following findings were also present: BUN = 36, creatinine = 1.5, AST = 27, and ALT = 26. Chest X-ray showed multiple scattered pulmonary infiltrates. Given her near normal CBC 2 months prior, we were suspicious of MTX induced myelosuppression. She was immediately started on leucovorin. A bone marrow evaluation was performed to rule out malignancy and myelodysplasia; however, no bone marrow could be aspirated and the biopsy attempt was not tolerated by the patient.

The patient was transfused with blood products including packed red blood cells, platelets, and fresh frozen plasma. She was empirically started on broad spectrum antibiotics for neutropenic fever and MTX was stopped. She improved significantly and pancytopenia resolved with almost normal hematologic parameters in less than a week of followup.

3. Discussion

MTX is a folate antagonist used in the treatment of various malignancies, autoimmune disorders, and abortion. It is transported into cells by an active cellular uptake and an active efflux transporter. Once in the cell, MTX inhibits dihydrofolate reductase (DHFR), an enzyme responsible for the conversion of dihydrofolate (DHF) to tetrahydrofolate (THF) [4, 5]. Consequently, there is a reduction in thymidylate and purine biosynthesis. DNA synthesis eventually halts and cells can no longer replicate [4]. Polyglutamination of this drug prolongs its intracellular presence [6, 7]. Hence, cells with the capability of effective polyglutamination such as leukemic myeloblasts, synovial macrophages, lymphoblasts, and epithelia are more susceptible to this medication [6, 7]. On the contrary, an increase in polyglutamination results in increased risk of toxicity as a result of direct prolonged intracellular exposure. Myeloid lineage megakaryocytes and epithelial polyglutamination increase the intracellular concentration of MTX and consequently patients may experience ulcers and bleeding as in this case. The same is true for WBC and RBC, which may manifest as infections and macrocytic anemia, also present in this case [8].

In addition to antifolate pathway, MTX also works on the adenosine pathway with important anti-inflammatory effects. Inhibition of transformylase (ATIC) by MTX-PG leads to accumulation of 5-aminoimidazole-4-carboxamide ribonucleotide (AICAR) and ultimately leads to increased levels of adenosine. Adenosine is a potent inhibitor of inflammation and induces vasodilation. Adenosine's anti-inflammatory effects include regulation of endothelial cell inflammatory functions, including cell trafficking. This effect of MTX does not seem to be affected by folate supplementation [9].

Resistance to MTX is variable and can include increased DHFR and efflux, as well as decreased polyglutamination and uptake. MTX may be administered orally in low doses (5–10 mg/m^2) or parenterally in high doses (>25 mg/m^2). The starting dose is usually 5 to 10 mg given as a single weekly dose. More frequent administration is associated with a significantly increased risk of liver toxicity. If the oral dose of MTX exceeds 15 mg, consideration should be given to splitting the dose, with each half given 6 to 12 hours apart, for improved bioavailability. The dosage of MTX can be escalated gradually, usually every 4 to 8 weeks up to 25 mg/week [10, 11]. Most MTX is excreted in the urine within the first 12 hours after administration, except for MTX-PG. MTX and metabolites not only are excreted by the kidney by glomerular filtration and proximal tubular secretion but also undergo distal tubular reabsorption. The estimated median half-life of elimination of MTX-PG is 3.1 weeks (ranging from 0.94 to 4.1 weeks), and MTX-PG is undetectable at 15 weeks. Serum half-life is 10 hrs, but tissue half-life of MTX-polyglutamate is more than 3 weeks. At low doses, MTX can be administered either orally or parenterally (subcutaneous or intramuscular), and absorption is rapid, peaking from 1 to 2 or from 0.1 to 1 hour, respectively. The absorption of low-dose oral and parenteral MTX (<15 mg/wk) is roughly equivalent, but once the oral dose exceeds 15 mg/wk, absorption diminishes by as much as 30% [10, 12–15]. Although not prospectively studied in RA patients receiving long-term MTX treatment, the parenteral route should have diminished potential for hepatotoxicity. This effect has been seen in a retrospective study wherein more elevations in transaminases were noted when oral MTX was administered to the same individuals versus when given parenterally [16].

Adverse effects are of vital importance as they can be quickly progressive and fatal. The main ones include myelosuppression as in this case, pneumonitis, hepatotoxicity, and gastrointestinal toxicity [2]. Early toxicity is oral mucositis while severe toxicity includes bleeding, as with our patient. Rash and neurotoxicity (via the intrathecal route) are also observed. Toxicity can be increased in renal impairment or reduced renal blood flow, as with NSAIDs use [17]. In fact, MTX is contraindicated in any patient with eGFR <30 mL/min [18]. It is advised that routine blood count be performed every four to eight weeks [1]. Concomitant administration of folic acid (1 to 3 mg/day) decreases the frequency of toxicities, including mucositis, nausea, hematologic abnormalities, and liver enzyme elevations, without seeming to interfere with clinical efficacy [8, 19].

This case is extraordinary due to an unfortunate chain of events that led to severe toxicity. Despite initial concerns, when given once a week in doses used for rheumatic diseases and monitored correctly, MTX is very well tolerated. Five important events need to be clearly pointed out as critical when we care for patients with rheumatic diseases on therapy with MTX: (1) patients older than 65 years represent a special subset at particular high risk for toxicity (our patient is 75 years old). There are differences among the pharmacokinetic profiles in this group of patients, including drug distribution as a result of decreases in end-organ blood flow and lean body mass, decreased hepatic drug metabolism, and decreased renal drug excretion. The serum creatinine may be a misleading measure of renal function in older patients owing to an overall reduction in lean muscle mass. Dosing recommendations are as follows: initial doses should be around 5 to 7.5 mg/wk and should not exceed 20 mg/wk. Dosage adjustments for CrCl are as follows: for a CrCl of 61 to 80 mL/min, reduce the dose by 25%; for a CrCl of 51 to 60 mL/min, reduce the dose by 30%; for a CrCl of 10 to 50 mL/min, reduce the dose by 50% to 80%; and for a CrCl less than 10 mL/min, avoid use [20]; our patient had a GFR <40 and her dose should have been reduced by 50%. (2) MTX should not be given more frequent than once a week due to increased toxicity risk (our patient received daily dosing); alternatively parenteral dosing could be used for better bioavailability and less GI and liver toxicity. (3) MTX dose should be gradually increased by no more than 2.5 mg every 1 to 2 weeks; our patient dose was increased from 7.5 mg/week to 17.5 mg/week. (4) Monitoring for toxicity should be done every 2 to 4 weeks for the first 3 months of therapy; our patient had no blood work done for 2 months after the dose was increased before she presented to ER.

Bone marrow toxicity, in most cases, is dose dependent and responds to folic acid administration. Pancytopenia, leukopenia, anemia, and thrombocytopenia can occur but are rare. In a review by Gutierrez-Urena and associates, clinically significant pancytopenia was found in 1% to 2% of RA patients on MTX therapy [2]. The mucocutaneous toxicities of MTX, which have been reported to occur in up to one-third of patients, are dose dependent and respond to folate replacement.

4. Conclusions

It is of utmost importance that primary care physicians are aware of these complications and recommendations, because the majority of these serious complications can be detected on time and even prevented. Patients on MTX therapy should be regularly monitored with liver function tests and CBC to identify myelosuppression and avoid the sequelae of pancytopenia. Renal function must also be monitored as this drug uses mainly the kidneys for excretion.

Disclosure

The authors have not received any money for their participation in the study or support in the form of equipment, drugs, or grants related to this paper.

References

[1] R. W. Simms, C. K. Kwoh, L. G. Anderson et al., "Guidelines for monitoring drug therapy in rheumatoid arthritis: American College of Rheumatology Ad Hoc Committee on Clinical Guidelines," *Arthritis and Rheumatism*, vol. 39, no. 5, pp. 723–731, 1996.

[2] S. Gutierrez-Urena, J. F. Molina, C. O. Garcia et al., "Pancytopenia secondary to MTX therapy in rheumatoid arthritis," *Arthritis and Rheumatism*, vol. 39, pp. 272–276, 1996.

[3] A. C. Cannella and J. R. O'dell, "Traditional DMARDs: methotrexate, leflunomide, sulfasalazine, hydroxychloroquine, and combination therapies," in *Kelley's Textbook of Rheumatology*, chapther 61, Elsevier Saunders, Philadelphia, Pa, USA, 9th edition, 2012.

[4] E. Beutler and W. J. Williams, *Williams Hematology*, McGraw-Hill, New York, NY, USA, 2010.

[5] L. Brunton, B. Chabner, and B. Knollman, *Goodman and Gilman's the Pharmacological Basis of therapeutics*, McGraw-Hill, New York, NY, USA, 12th edition, 2013.

[6] A. N. Colebatch, J. L. Marks, and C. J. Edwards, "Safety of non-steroidal anti-inflammatory drugs, including aspirin and paracetamol (acetaminophen) in people receiving methotrexate for inflammatory arthritis (rheumatoid arthritis, ankylosing spondylitis, psoriatic arthritis, other spondyloarthritis)," *Cochrane Database of Systematic Reviews*, no. 11, Article ID CD008872, 2011.

[7] J. M. Kremer and R. A. Hamilton, "The effects of nonsteroidal antiinflammatory drugs on methotrexate (MTX) pharmacokinetics: Impairment of renal clearance of MTX at weekly maintenance doses but not at 7.5 mg," *Journal of Rheumatology*, vol. 22, no. 11, pp. 2072–2077, 1995.

[8] S. L. Morgan, J. E. Baggott, W. H. Vaughn et al., "Supplementation with folic acid during methotrexate therapy for rheumatoid arthritis. A double-blind, placebo-controlled trial," *Annals of Internal Medicine*, vol. 121, no. 11, pp. 833–841, 1994.

[9] S. Bar-Yehuda, M. H. Silverman, W. D. Kerns, A. Ochaion, S. Cohen, and P. Fishman, "The anti-inflammatory effect of A3 adenosine receptor agonists: a novel targeted therapy for rheumatoid arthritis," *Expert Opinion on Investigational Drugs*, vol. 16, no. 10, pp. 1601–1613, 2007.

[10] R. A. Hamilton and J. M. Kremer, "Why intramuscular methotrexate may be more efficacious than oral dosing in patients with rheumatoid arthritis," *British Journal of Rheumatology*, vol. 36, no. 1, pp. 86–90, 1997.

[11] J. M. Kremer, G. S. Alarcón, R. W. Lightfoot Jr. et al., "Methotrexate for rheumatoid arthritis: suggested guidelines for monitoring liver toxicity," *Arthritis and Rheumatism*, vol. 37, no. 3, pp. 316–328, 1994.

[12] P. A. Andersen, S. G. West, J. R. O'Dell, C. S. Via, R. G. Claypool, and B. L. Kotzin, "Weekly pulse methotrexate in rheumatoid arthritis. Clinical and immunologic effects in a randomized, double-blind study," *Annals of Internal Medicine*, vol. 103, no. 4, pp. 489–496, 1985.

[13] M. E. Weinblatt, H. Kaplan, B. F. Germain et al., "Methotrexate in rheumatoid arthritis: a five-year prospective multicenter study," *Arthritis and Rheumatism*, vol. 37, no. 10, pp. 1492–1498, 1994.

[14] H. J. Williams, R. F. Willkens, C. O. Samuelson Jr. et al., "Comparison of low-dose oral pulse methotrexate and placebo in the treatment of rheumatoid arthritis. A controlled clinical trial," *Arthritis and Rheumatism*, vol. 28, no. 7, pp. 721–730, 1985.

[15] J. Dalrymple, L. Stamp, and J. O'Donnell, "Pharmacokinetics of oral Methotrexate in patients with rheumatoid arthritis," *Arthritis and Rheumatism*, vol. 58, pp. 3299–3308, 2008.

[16] J. Wegrzyn, P. Adeleine, and P. Miossec, "Better efficacy of methotrexate given by intramuscular injection than orally in patients with rheumatoid arthritis," *Annals of the Rheumatic Diseases*, vol. 63, no. 10, pp. 1232–1234, 2004.

[17] J. M. Kremer and J. K. Lee, "The safety and efficacy of the use of methotrexate in long-term therapy for rheumatoid arthritis," *Arthritis and Rheumatism*, vol. 29, no. 7, pp. 822–831, 1986.

[18] K. G. Saag, G. T. Gim, N. M. Patkar et al., "American College of Rheumatology 2008 recommendations for the use of nonbiologic and biologic disease-modifying antirheumatic drugs in rheumatoid arthritis," *Arthritis Care and Research*, vol. 59, no. 6, pp. 762–784, 2008.

[19] A. E. Van Ede, R. F. Laan, M. J. Rood et al., "Effect of folic or folonic acid supplementation on the toxicity and efficacy of MTX in rheumatoid arthritis: a forty eight week, multicenter, randomized, double-blinded, placebo-controlled study," *Arthritis and Rheumatism*, vol. 44, pp. 1515–1524, 2001.

[20] F. Bressolle, C. Bologna, J. M. Kinowski, B. Arcos, J. Sany, and B. Combe, "Total and free methotrexate pharmacokinetics in elderly patients with rheumatoid arthritis. A comparison with young patients," *Journal of Rheumatology*, vol. 24, no. 10, pp. 1903–1909, 1997.

Ramsay Hunt Syndrome in a Patient with Rheumatoid Arthritis after Treatment with Infliximab

Yoshio Nagayama,[1] Naoki Matsushiro,[2] Akihide Nampei,[1] Hideo Hashimoto,[3] and Kenrin Shi[4]

[1] *Department of Orthopaedic Surgery, Osaka Rosai Hospital, 1179-3 Nagasonecho, Kita-ku, Sakai 591-8025, Japan*
[2] *Department of Otolaryngology, Osaka Police Hospital, 10-31 Kitayamacho, Tennoji-ku, Osaka 543-0035, Japan*
[3] *Rinku Hashimoto Rheumatology Orthopaedics, 1 Rinku Orai kita, Izumisano, Osaka 598-0048, Japan*
[4] *Department of Orthopaedic Surgery, Osaka University Graduate School of Medicine, 2-2 Yamadaoka, Suita, Osaka, Japan*

Correspondence should be addressed to Akihide Nampei; ak-nampei@orh.go.jp

Academic Editors: R. Cevik, G. O. Littlejohn, J. Mikdashi, L. Stojanovich, and A. Zoli

A 39-year-old female patient with rheumatoid arthritis developed Ramsay Hunt syndrome after infliximab treatment. This condition is caused by the reactivation of varicella zoster virus infection in the geniculate ganglion of facial nerve in the host's immunosuppression. She was treated immediately with valaciclovir and hydrocortisone, and the complete recovery was achieved at 6 months after the onset. This is the first report of Ramsay Hunt syndrome as an adverse effect of infliximab in rheumatoid arthritis.

1. Introduction

Infliximab (IFX) is the firstly introduced biologic agent for the treatment of rheumatoid arthritis (RA) and its successful efficacy for the patients with methotrexate (MTX) resistant RA has been proven over ten years [1–3]. On the other hand, serious opportunistic infection and reactivation of pathogens, such as tuberculosis, *Pneumocystis jiroveci*, hepatitis B virus (HBV), cytomegalovirus (CMV), Epstein-Barr virus (EBV), and human immunodeficiency virus, have been reported to be associated with IFX treatment [4, 5].

Ramsay Hunt syndrome is characterized by herpetic vesicles in or around the ear, facial nerve paralysis, and vestibulocochlear nerve paralysis manifesting hearing loss and vertigo. It is caused by reactivation of varicella zoster virus (VZV) latently and persistently infected in the geniculate ganglion of facial nerve, often in immunosuppressed conditions of the host. Early intervention is important for complete recovery of the paralysis, but if not, it is more likely to remain permanent damage. Although several reports about VZV reactivation in RA patients have been published, reports on Ramsay Hunt syndrome in RA patients are very few. Here we report a case of Ramsay Hunt syndrome recognized in a patient with RA after treatment with IFX.

2. Case Report

A 39-year-old woman, diagnosed as RA in 1997, had been treated with MTX, bucillamine, and prednisolone, but unfortunately was resistant to these medications. In May 2005, her disease activity of RA elevated as high as Disease Activity Score including a 28-joint count (DAS28[6])-erythrocyte sedimentation rate (ESR) of 5.60. Moreover, the progression of joint destruction and functional status was recognized as stage III and class III by Steinbrocker's classification [7, 8], respectively. Then IFX, a biologic agent inhibiting tumor necrosis factor (TNF)-α, was introduced with a dose of 3 mg/kg. After three times of IFX administration at 0, 2, and 6 weeks, DAS28-ESR improved significantly to 3.96.

Ten days after the third infusion of IFX, she felt sore throat, dysphagia, and left otalgia, with development of vesicles on the left pinna. Then three days after these initial symptoms, she felt motor paralysis on the left side of the

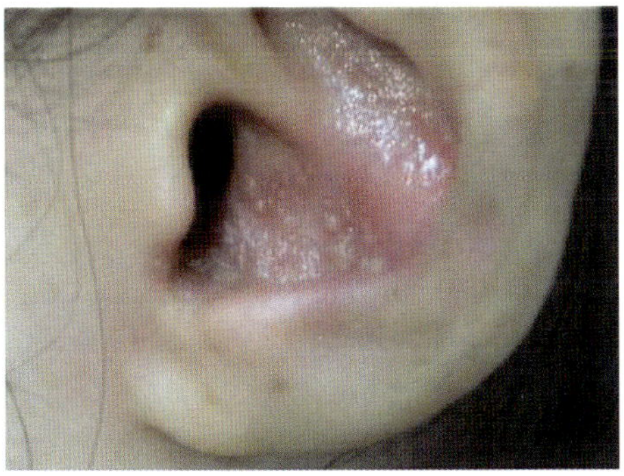

FIGURE 1: Vesicles on the left pinna.

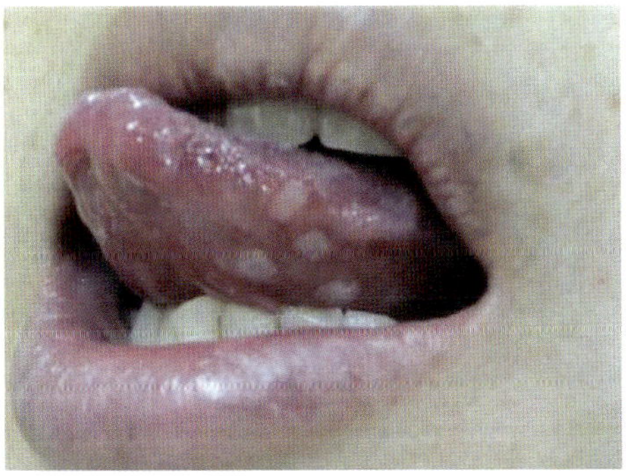

FIGURE 2: Vesicles on the left side of tongue.

face. She visited otolaryngologist in a private clinic who immediately consulted the otolaryngology department in our hospital at the same day; thereafter, she was diagnosed with Ramsay Hunt syndrome. Physical examination presented multiple vesicles on the left pinna, as well as on the left side of soft palate, tongue, and epiglottic vallecula (Figures 1 and 2). Facial nerve score was 4 points with Yanagihara' grading scale ([9]; total, 40 points). Neurootological examination presented sensorineural hearing loss (36.3 dB; normal value, ≤30 dB), nystagmus, and diminished lacrimation (Schirmer test, 7 mm; normal value, >10 mm) on the left side, with the disappearance of the left stapedial reflex and the reduced sense of taste (electrogustometry, 32 dB; normal value, ≤8 dB). Since such symptoms as sternocleidomastoid muscle atrophy, trapezius muscle paralysis, neck stiffness, and Kernig's sign were not recognized, either accessory nerve paralysis or meningitis was not suggested. Serological study by enzyme immunoassay (EIA) for specific antibodies against VZV presented IgM 0.45 (normal value, <0.80 antibody index) and IgG 29.3 (normal value, <2.0 EIA titer). At 12 days after the onset, increased levels of VZV antibodies were recognized: IgM 2.02 and IgG 83.9 (Table 1).

Treatment was started immediately after her visit at our hospital with valaciclovir 3000 mg for 7 days and hydrocortisone sodium succinate for 9 days (500 mg for 3 days, 300 mg for 3 days, and 100 mg for 3 days), while all medications for RA, IFX, MTX, bucillamine, and prednisolone were discontinued. At 6 days after the onset, left recurrent laryngeal nerve paralysis and left glossopharyngeal nerve paralysis, the symptom of which is characterized as "curtain sign", appeared. At 7 days after the onset, electroneurography (ENoG) and nerve excitability test (NET) were performed for prognostic diagnosis [10], and ENoG was 24.5% (excellent, ENoG ≥ 40%; good, 20% ≤ ENoG < 40%; fair, 10% ≤ ENoG < 20%; poor, ENoG < 10%), while NET was 4.2 mA (good, NET ≤ 3.5 mA; fair, 3.5 mA < NET ≤ 20 mA; poor, NET > 20 mA), both indicating unfavorable prognosis of paralysis. Then another course of hydrocortisone sodium succinate with the same dose for 9 days was conducted (Figure 3). After these treatments were introduced, facial nerve paralysis, as graded by Yanagihara's scale, improved successfully to 36 points at 3 months after the onset, and finally to full marks at 6 months (Figure 4). Other cranial nerve symptoms recovered at 2 months after the onset. However, facial synkinesis appeared at 3 months after the onset and remained even at 6 months, though it improved gradually to low grade. As for serological study, levels of VZV antibodies demonstrated a tendency to decrease after the treatment was introduced, and IgM level declined to normal value, 0.55, at 2 months after the onset whereas IgG level still remained high, 47.6 (Table 1).

TABLE 1: Serological study of varicella zoster virus (VZV).

	Day 3	Day 12	Day 25	Day 62
IgM (antibody index)	0.45	2.02	1.35	0.55
IgG (EIA titer)	29.3	83.9	68.6	47.6

Values of specific antibodies against VZV, IgM, and IgG are shown in a time-course manner. Antibodies were studied by enzyme immunoassay (EIA). Normal value; IgM: <0.80 antibody index; IgG: <2.0 EIA titer.

With regard to treatment of RA, prednisolone 10 mg/day and bucillamine 300 mg/day were readministered at 26 days after the onset of Ramsay Hunt syndrome. Then MTX 4 mg/week was readministered at 5 months after the onset and was increased to 8 mg/week at 6 months. Disease activity of RA elevated as high as DAS28-ESR of 4.98 at 3 months after the onset but finally improved to DAS28-ESR of 2.68 after readministration of medications, especially of MTX. Recurrence of Ramsay Hunt syndrome was not recognized, and the patient transferred to another hospital for her own reasons at 9 months after the onset (Figure 4).

3. Discussion

It is over ten years that biological agents such as IFX have been utilized for RA, and there have been many clinical evidences as well as experiences of their efficacy for MTX resistant RA [1–3], leading to the current general concept that they are indispensable medications for RA treatment [11–14]. However, the development of bacterial, viral, and fungal infections is one of the well-known and sometimes severe adverse events of these medications with potent immunosuppressive effect [4, 5, 15, 16], and reactivation of old or resolved infections such as tuberculosis, HBV, CMV, and EBV has been reported [6, 17–21].

Among 5040 RA patients with episodes of herpes zoster in the German biotherapy registry, TNF inhibitors were

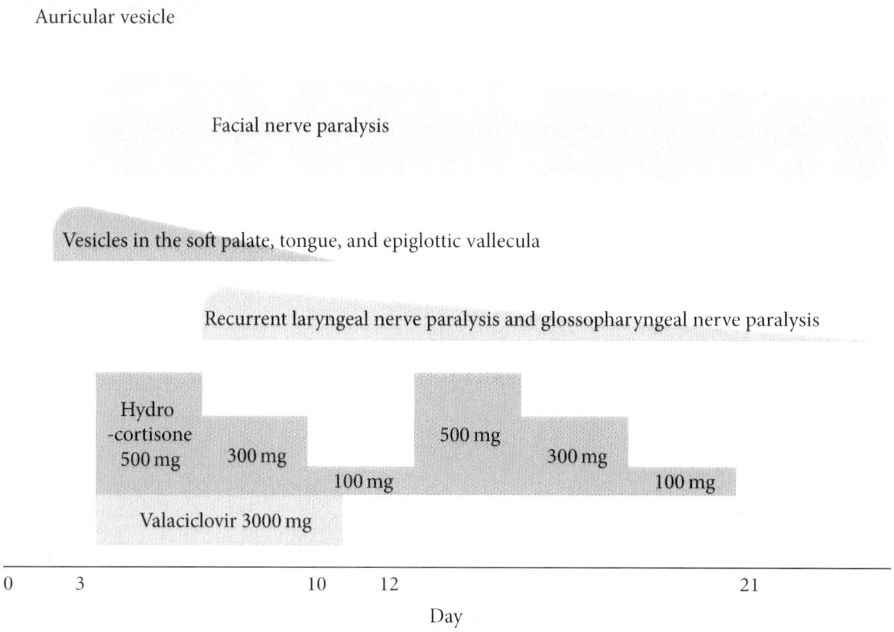

Figure 3: Initial clinical course of Ramsay Hunt syndrome. At 3 days after the onset, the treatment was started with valaciclovir 3000 mg for 7 days and hydrocortisone sodium succinate for 9 days (500 mg for 3 days, 300 mg for 3 days, and 100 mg for 3 days), followed by another course of hydrocortisone sodium succinate with the same dose for 9 days. Vesicles, recurrent laryngeal nerve paralysis, and glossopharyngeal nerve paralysis were relieved soon after the treatment but facial nerve paralysis continued.

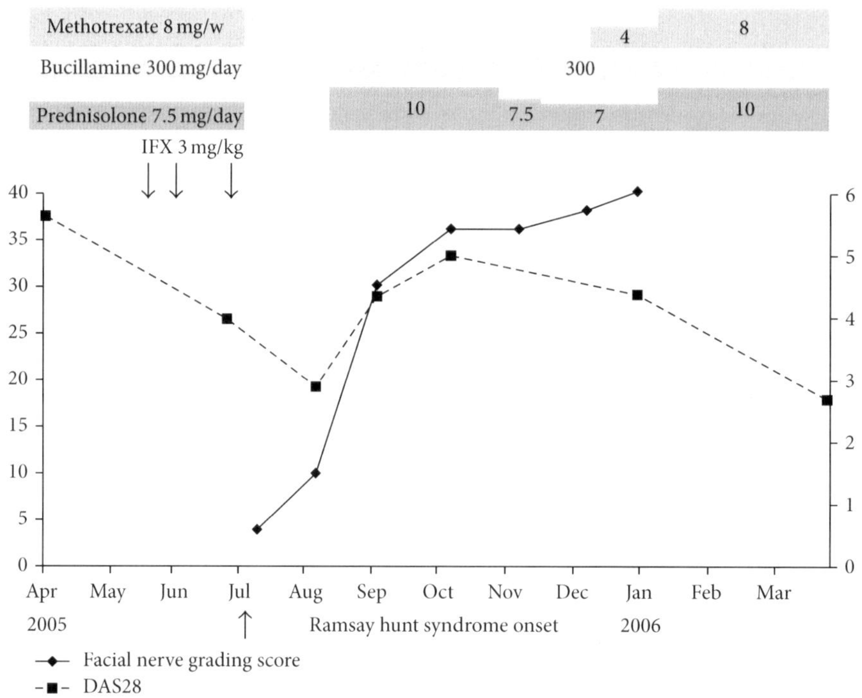

Figure 4: Clinical course of facial nerve paralysis and RA. Facial nerve paralysis as graded by Yanagihara's scale recovered completely at 6 months after onset, except for a slight synkinesis. DAS28-ESR elevated after discontinuation of RA treatment but relieved after readministration of medications including MTX. RA: rheumatoid arthritis; DAS28: Disease Activity Score including a 28-joint count; ESR: erythrocyte sedimentation rate; MTX: methotrexate.

reported to be administered in 3266 patients, among which IFX was reported in 591, as compared to 1774 patients without TNF inhibitors, concluding that TNF inhibitors were significantly associated with herpes zoster (hazards ratio: 2.24) [22]. Also, in a large-scale controlled study of IFX in patients with ulcerative colitis, the incidence of herpes zoster episode increased significantly in the IFX group (1.3%), as compared to the placebo group (0.4%) during 54 weeks [23].

Ramsay Hunt syndrome is a rare condition which is caused by reactivation of latent or persistent infection of VZV in the geniculate ganglion of facial nerve, occurring mostly in the host's immunosuppression [24, 25]. Its major symptoms are herpetic vesicles in or around the ear, facial nerve paralysis, and vestibulocochlear nerve paralysis presenting hearing loss and vertigo, and the annual incidence was reported previously as 5/100,000 person-year [26], much less than that of herpes zoster reported as over 300/100,000 person-year [27, 28]. Moreover, there is only one case report of Ramsay Hunt syndrome occurring in a patient with RA under etanercept treatment [29], and there have so far been no reports on Ramsay Hunt syndrome in RA patients after IFX treatment.

As the grade of facial nerve paralysis in Ramsay Hunt syndrome is severe, the prognosis is worse, and early treatment is thought necessary for complete recovery [30]. Among 28 patients in whom the treatment was started within 3 days from the onset of facial nerve paralysis, complete recovery was observed in 21 patients (75%), while it was observed in 14 (48%) among 29 patients in whom the treatment was started at 4 to 7 days after the onset. Furthermore, among 23 patients in whom the treatment was started later than 7 days, the complete recovery was only in 7 (30%) and permanent as well as none or less severe paralysis remained in other patients [31].

In the case presented in this paper, it is assumed that inhibition of TNF-α by IFX promoted the reactivation of latently infected VZV in the geniculate ganglion of facial nerve and caused Ramsay Hunt syndrome. Fortunately, an otolaryngology specialist appropriately diagnosed and the treatment was started as early as at 3 days after the onset, after which the complete recovery of the paralysis was achieved. In conclusion, this is the first report of Ramsay Hunt syndrome as an adverse effect following IFX treatment. Rheumatologists should be aware of this condition, especially for the patients with immunosuppressive treatments. Also, when this condition is suspected, immediate treatment should be introduced after the proper diagnosis by an otolaryngology specialist.

Authors' Contribution

Yoshio Nagayama and Naoki Matsushiro contributed equally to this paper.

References

[1] P. E. Lipsky, D. M. F. M. van der Heijde, E. W. St. Clair et al., "Infliximab and methotrexate in the treatment of rheumatoid arthritis," *The New England Journal of Medicine*, vol. 343, no. 22, pp. 1594–1602, 2000.

[2] R. Maini, E. W. St Clair, F. Breedveld et al., "Infliximab (chimeric anti-tumour necrosis factor α monoclonal antibody) versus placebo in rheumatoid arthritis patients receiving concomitant methotrexate: a randomised phase III trial," *The Lancet*, vol. 354, no. 9194, pp. 1932–1939, 1999.

[3] P. C. Taylor, "Anti-tumor necrosis factor therapies," *Current Opinion in Rheumatology*, vol. 13, pp. 164–169, 2001.

[4] J. J. Gómez-Reino, L. Carmona, V. Rodríguez Valverde, E. M. Mola, and M. D. Montero, "Treatment of rheumatoid arthritis with tumor necrosis factor inhibitors may predispose to significant increase in tuberculosis risk: a multicenter active-surveillance report," *Arthritis and Rheumatism*, vol. 48, no. 8, pp. 2122–2127, 2003.

[5] T. Takeuchi, Y. Tatsuki, Y. Nogami et al., "Postmarketing surveillance of the safety profile of infliximab in 5000 Japanese patients with rheumatoid arthritis," *Annals of the Rheumatic Diseases*, vol. 67, no. 2, pp. 189–194, 2008.

[6] M. L. L. Prevoo, M. A. van 'T Hof, H. H. Kuper, M. A. van Leeuwen, L. B. A. van de Putte, and P. L. C. M. van Riel, "Modified disease activity scores that include twenty-eight-joint counts: development and validation in a prospective longitudinal study of patients with rheumatoid arthritis," *Arthritis and Rheumatism*, vol. 38, no. 1, pp. 44–48, 1995.

[7] O. Steinbrocker, C. H. Traeger, and R. C. Batterman, "Therapeutic criteria in rheumatoid arthritis," *Journal of the American Medical Association*, vol. 140, no. 8, pp. 659–662, 1949.

[8] M. C. Hochberg, R. W. Chang, I. Dwosh, S. Lindsey, T. Pincus, and F. Wolfe, "The American College of Rheumatology 1991 revised criteria for the classification of global functional status in rheumatoid arthritis," *Arthritis and Rheumatism*, vol. 35, no. 5, pp. 498–502, 1992.

[9] Y. Satoh, J. Kanzaki, and S. Yoshihara, "A comparison and conversion table of "the House-Brackmann facial nerve grading system" and "the Yanagihara grading system"," *Auris Nasus Larynx*, vol. 27, no. 3, pp. 207–212, 2000.

[10] E. Esslen, "Electromyography and electroneurography," in *Proceedings of the 3rd International Symposium on Facial Nerve Surgery, Facial Nerve Surgery*, U. Fisch, Ed., pp. 93–100, Anstelveen, Zurich, Switzerland, August 1976.

[11] R. Koike, T. Takeuchi, K. Eguchi, and N. Miyasaka, "Update on the Japanese guidelines for the use of infliximab and etanercept in rheumatoid arthritis," *Modern Rheumatology*, vol. 17, no. 6, pp. 451–458, 2007.

[12] R. Koike, M. Harigai, T. Atsumi et al., "Japan College of Rheumatology 2009 guidelines for the use of tocilizumab, a humanized anti interleukin-6 receptor monoclonal antibody, in rheumatoid arthritis," *Modern Rheumatology*, vol. 19, no. 4, pp. 351–357, 2009.

[13] J. S. Smolen, R. Landewé, F. C. Breedveld et al., "EULAR recommendations for the management of rheumatoid arthritis with synthetic and biological disease-modifying antirheumatic drugs," *Annals of the Rheumatic Diseases*, vol. 69, pp. 964–975, 2010.

[14] J. A. Singh, D. E. Furst, A. Bharat et al., "2012 update of the 2008 American college of rheumatology recommendations for the use of disease-modifying antirheumatic drugs and biologic agents in the treatment of rheumatoid arthritis," *Arthritis Care and Research*, vol. 64, no. 5, pp. 635–639, 2012.

[15] H. Okubo, M. Iwamoto, T. Yoshio et al., "Rapidly aggravated *Mycobacterium avium* infection in a patient with rheumatoid arthritis treated with infliximab," *Modern Rheumatology*, vol. 15, no. 1, pp. 62–64, 2005.

[16] S. Mori, F. Imamura, C. Kiyofuji et al., "Pneumocystis jiroveci pneumonia in a patient with rheumatoid arthritis as a complication of treatment with infliximab, anti-tumor necrosis factor α neutralizing antibody," *Modern Rheumatology*, vol. 16, no. 1, pp. 58–62, 2006.

[17] Y. Hirano, T. Kojima, Y. Kanayama, H. Ishikawa, and N. Ishiguro, "A case of lung tuberculosis in a patient with rheumatoid arthritis treated with infliximab after antituberculosis chemoprophylaxis with isoniazid," *Modern Rheumatology*, vol. 19, no. 3, pp. 323–328, 2009.

[18] H. Tsuboi, A. Tsujii, A. Nampei et al., "A patient with rheumatoid arthritis treated with tocilizumab together with lamivudine prophylaxis after remission of infliximab-reactivated hepatitis B," *Modern Rheumatology*, vol. 21, no. 6, pp. 701–705, 2011.

[19] A. Tamori, T. Koike, H. Goto et al., "Prospective study of reactivation of hepatitis B virus in patients with rheumatoid arthritis who received immunosuppressive therapy: evaluation of both HBsAg-positive and HBsAg-negative cohorts," *Journal of Gastroenterology*, vol. 46, no. 4, pp. 556–564, 2011.

[20] G. Haerter, B. J. Manfras, Y. de Jong-Hesse et al., "Cytomegalovirus retinitis in a patient treated with anti-tumor necrosis factor alpha antibody therapy for rheumatoid arthritis," *Clinical Infectious Diseases*, vol. 39, no. 9, pp. e88–e94, 2004.

[21] M. Colaci, M. Sebastiani, G. Sandri, M. Meacci, and C. Ferri, "Epstein-barr virus reactivation after infliximab in rheumatoid arthritis: a case report," *Case Reports in Infectious Diseases*, vol. 2011, Article ID 530568, 3 pages, 2011.

[22] A. Strangfeld, J. Listing, P. Herzer et al., "Risk of herpes zoster in patients with rheumatoid arthritis treated with anti-TNF-α agents," *Journal of the American Medical Association*, vol. 301, no. 7, pp. 737–744, 2009.

[23] P. Rutgeerts, W. J. Sandborn, B. G. Feagan et al., "Infliximab for induction and maintenance therapy for ulcerative colitis," *The New England Journal of Medicine*, vol. 353, no. 23, pp. 2462–2476, 2005.

[24] A. Aviel and G. Marshak, "Ramsay Hunt syndrome: a cranial polyneuropathy," *American Journal of Otolaryngology*, vol. 3, no. 1, pp. 61–66, 1982.

[25] D. S. Asnis, L. Micic, and D. Giaccio, "Ramsay hunt syndrome presenting as a cranial polyneuropathy," *Cutis*, vol. 57, no. 6, pp. 421–424, 1996.

[26] K. K. Adour, "Otological complications of herpes zoster," *Annals of Neurology*, vol. 35, pp. S62–S64, 1994.

[27] R. E. HOPE-SIMPSON, "The nature of herpes zoster," *Proceedings of the Royal Society of Medicine*, vol. 58, pp. 9–20, 1965.

[28] R. P. Insinga, R. F. Itzler, J. M. Pellissier, P. Saddier, and A. A. Nikas, "The incidence of herpes zoster in a United States administrative database," *Journal of General Internal Medicine*, vol. 20, no. 8, pp. 748–753, 2005.

[29] D. Kaski, N. Davies, and B. M. Seemungal, "Varicella-zoster virus meningo-rhombencephalitis presenting as Ramsey Hunt," *Neurology*, vol. 4, pp. 2291–2292, 2012.

[30] C. J. Sweeney and D. H. Gilden, "Ramsay Hunt syndrome," *Journal of Neurology Neurosurgery and Psychiatry*, vol. 71, no. 2, pp. 149–154, 2001.

[31] S. Murakami, N. Hato, J. Horiuchi, N. Honda, K. Gyo, and N. Yanagihara, "Treatment of Ramsay Hunt syndrome with acyclovir-prednisone: significance of early diagnosis and treatment," *Annals of Neurology*, vol. 41, no. 3, pp. 353–357, 1997.

32

Streptococcus agalactiae Septic Arthritis of the Shoulder and the Sacroiliac Joints

Yahia Z. Imam,[1] Housam Aldeen Sarakbi,[2,3] Nagui Abdelwahab,[4] and Issa Mattar[1,3]

[1] *General Medicine Division, Department of Medicine, Hamad Medical Corporation, P.O. Box 3050, Doha, Qatar*
[2] *Rheumatology Division, Department of Medicine, Hamad Medical Corporation, P.O. Box 3050, Doha, Qatar*
[3] *Weill Cornell Medical School, Hamad Medical Corporation, P.O. Box 3050, Doha, Qatar*
[4] *Department of Radiology, Faculty of Medicine, Cairo University, Giza, Egypt*

Correspondence should be addressed to Housam Aldeen Sarakbi, sarakbi@yahoo.com

Academic Editors: R. Cevik and T. C. Hsu

Invasive group beta-streptococcal arthritis is being increasingly diagnosed as suggested by recent data. We report a case of a middle-aged lady from Sri Lanka who developed septic arthritis of the right shoulder and the left sacroiliac joint as well as an iliopsoas collection caused by *Streptococcus agalactiae* shortly after labor at Hamad General Hospital in Doha, Qatar. We conclude that *Streptococcus agalactiae* septic arthritis is rare. It can present with invasive disease in adults. It usually targets older females and immuno compromised patients especially those with risk factors for bacteraemia. Therefore a high index of suspicion is needed. Shoulder and sacroiliac joint affection is not uncommon for unknown reasons. Utilizing imaging modalities such as ultrasonography and magnetic resonance imaging is helpful.

1. Introduction

Septic arthritis is a rheumatologic emergency requiring prompt diagnosis and treatment. Streptococci are a well-recognized cause of septic arthritis causing up to 20% of all septic arthritides, ranking second to *Staphylococcus aureus* which accounts for 50–60% of cases, while gram-negative rods account for 5–10% [1, 2].

GBS (also known as *Streptococcus agalactiae*) are prominent veterinary pathogens, because they can cause bovine mastitis in dairy cows. The species name "*agalactiae*" meaning "no milk" alludes to this.

Search of the available literature reveals the rare occurrence of Group B streptococci septic arthritis among immuno competent hosts after uncomplicated vaginal delivery.

2. Case Report

A previously healthy 45-year-old Sri Lankan housewife, who is gravida 5 and para 5 + 0, was admitted for a normal vaginal delivery at Hamad Medical Corporation. She is known to have *Streptococcus agalactiae* colonization of the vagina as was evident by a high vaginal swab done one month prior to the delivery. The patient developed a persistent right shoulder pain and a low-grade fever 12 hours after delivery of her fifth child via an uneventful noninstrumental vaginal delivery. There was no premature rupture of the membrane, nor were there any laceration in the vagina. She did not receive any peripartum antibiotics. She denied any prior trauma or complaints in the right shoulder or any other joint. She denied having any vaginal discharge. She also had a lower back pain to the extent that she could not walk.

She had an unremarkable past medical and surgical history (no steroid use, autoimmune diseases, diabetes, chemotherapy, or history of HIV infection).

On examination, she was febrile with a temperature of 38.9 Celsius, but otherwise hemodynamically stable. The patient had active arthritis of the right shoulder manifesting with joint swelling, joint tenderness, and marked limitation of movement in all planes.

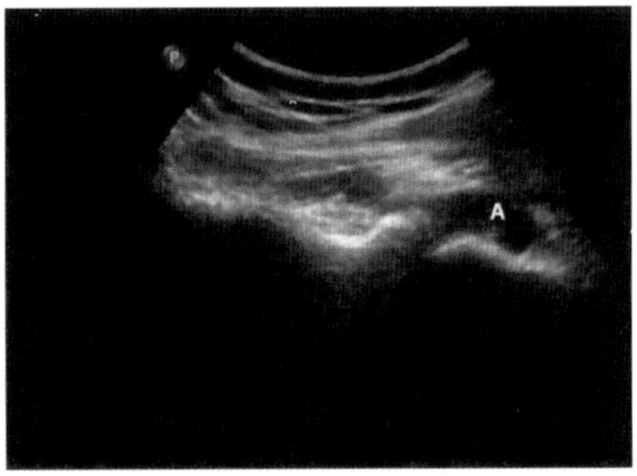

FIGURE 1: Ultrasound of the right shoulder joint using an axial posterior approach to the glenohumeral articulation showing a markedly distended posterior aspect of joint capsule by fluid (A).

The patient had also pain over the left sacroiliac joint and a positive Patrick Fabre's test denoting a sacroiliitis.

Blood cultures were drawn and the patient was admitted to the medical ward.

A complete blood count showed elevated white blood cells (WBCs) of 21,000 with neutrophilia, a hemoglobin of 8.9 gm/dL with normochromic normocytic indices, and a normal platelet count. Serum C reactive protein was severely elevated at 314 (normal < 5). Chemistry and liver function test were within normal values.

Arthrocentesis of the right shoulder attempted blindly on day 1 of the illness produced only 2-3 milliliters of turbid fluid which was only sufficient for a gram staining and culture.

It stained positive for gram-positive cocci in pairs and chains. The patient was started on empirical treatment with ceftriaxone 2 grams intravenously daily.

Ultrasonography of the right shoulder on day 2 of the presentation revealed a distended capsule of the shoulder (Figure 1).

Needle aspiration, attempted on day 4 under ultrasonography guidance, came out as a dry tap because of thick pus.

Culture report from the synovial fluid demonstrated *Streptococcus agalactiae* sensitive to penicillin and ceftriaxone. 2 sets of blood cultures and a high vaginal swap also grew *Streptococcus agalactiae* with similar sensitivity. An echocardiogram was requested and was normal.

The patient was kept on the same antibiotic for ease of administration. She underwent surgical incision and drainage of the right shoulder on day 5. The drainage fluid was turbid but failed to grow any organism. A drain was left in situ, then subsequently removed when no more accumulation was documented via a repeat ultrasound on day 11.

Magnetic resonance imaging (MRI) of the pelvis and the sacroiliac joints (Figure 2) performed on day 10 showed left sacroiliitis with a multiloculated abscess in the anterior superior aspect of the left sacroiliac joint located within the left iliopsoas muscle and extending distally to the level of the left hip joint.

The iliopsoas muscle abscess was drained under radiological guidance on day 12, but the pus also failed to grow the organism; this was attributed to adequate antibiotic coverage.

The patient remained febrile in spite of adequate drainage and 3 weeks of ceftriaxone.

Subsequently the patient was shifted to a once-daily injection of ertapenem. Her fever subsided after 3 days, and she regained some degree of movement in the right shoulder joint.

She received another 5 weeks of ertapenem and continued to have regular physiotherapy sessions.

After one month of physiotherapy and before the course of antibiotics had finished, there was still limitation of movement of the right shoulder joint raising the possibility of a frozen shoulder, a known complication of septic arthritis; at that time an MRI shoulder showed severe inflammatory process involving the shoulder joint (Figure 3).

The patient had a total course of antibiotic (ceftriaxone + ertapenem) of 8 weeks. She continued with regular physiotherapy for a total of 6 months.

Followup after 8 months reveled pain-free joints with no limitation of movement.

3. Discussion

Group B streptococci (GBS) are a common type of the streptococcus bacterium.

Approximately a third of men and women are carriers of GBS in their intestines and a quarter of women carry it in their vaginas. GBS carried in this way can be difficult to detect and does not cause any symptoms [3].

Heavy colonization with this type of bacteria in pregnant women results in adverse outcomes. This includes preterm labor, preterm, and premature rupture of membranes as well as low-birth-weight infants and neonatal disease [4–6].

The current approach to the prevention of Group B streptococcal infection in pregnancy requires intrapartum antimicrobial prophylaxis in term women with microbiological evidence of recent vaginal or rectal Group B streptococcal infection. This is in accordance with the advice from the Center for Disease Control and Prevention (CDC) in 1996 [7].

GBS (also known as *Streptococcus agalactiae*) is now established as a well-known cause of septic arthritis accounting for 5–10% of all septic arthritides [8].

Nolla et al. [9] reported 11 cases over 10 years (1992–2001) where they demonstrated that the organism targeted an older population with those above 60 years of age accounting for 49–91% of cases. They also demonstrated a female preponderance which they attributed to the high rates of vaginal carriage.

Binard et al. [10] reviewed 48 consecutive cases of septic arthritis from May 2000 to May 2004.

Five (10.4%) had arthritis due to Group B streptococci with a mean age of 51.6 ± 18.3 years and a mean hospital stay duration of 13.2 ± 9.23 days.

One of the reported cases was of a 27-year-old lady who developed sacroiliitis postpartum. Specimens from the blood

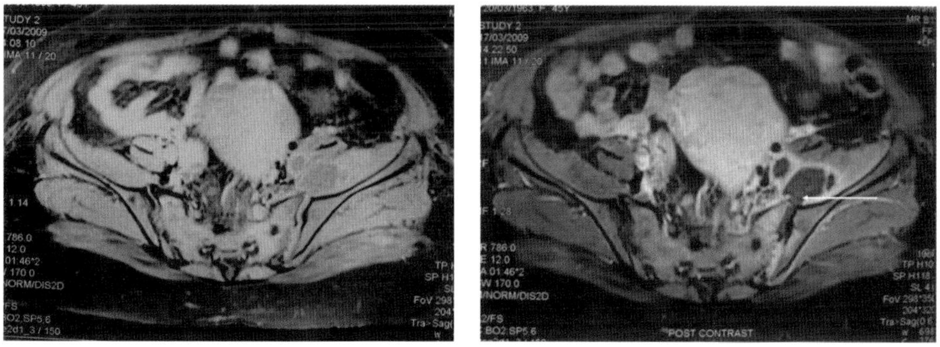

(a) (b)

Figure 2: MRI of the pelvis and sacroiliac joints. Coronal T1-weighted (a) as well as (b) fat-saturated (FS) post IV contrast images of the pelvis and sacroiliac joints; showing a 5 cm in diameter multiloculated collection showing dense marginal enhancement deep to left iliopsoas muscle communicating with underlying left sacroiliac joint cavity (see arrow) with evidence of left sacroiliitis in the form of irregular articular surface with subarticular thickening as well as enhancement.

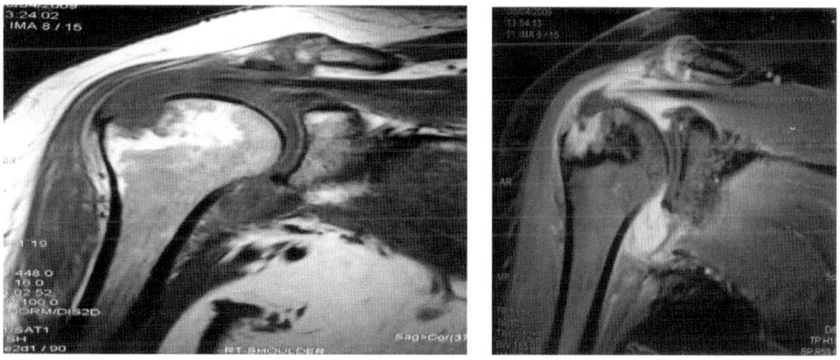

(a) (b)

Figure 3: MRI of the right shoulder joint. Coronal T1-weighted (a) and (b) (FS) after IV contrast images of the right shoulder showing dense enhancement of a markedly thickened shoulder joint synovium as well as the subacromial and the subdeltoid bursae with joint effusion is noted. A focal 1 cm area of erosion and underlying trabecular bone enhancement in the greater tuberosity of the humerus and a full thickness tear of supraspinatus tendon with enhancing edges are evident. There is also associated degeneration of the acromioclavicular joint with hypertrophy of its capsule.

and the vagina showed the same Group B streptococcal strain as in the case of our patient.

Four out of the five cases had either affection of the shoulder, the sacroiliac joints, or both.

In 1984 Small et al. [11] reported 7 cases of septic arthritis caused by *Streptococcus agalactiae*. The shoulder joint was affected in two of them.

A similar case was reported by García et al. [12] where *Streptococcus agalactiae* shoulder arthritis was diagnosed in a 63-year-old female with hepatitis C virus infection.

Similarly Casallo Blanco et al. [13] reported a 47-year-old immunocompetant gentleman with right shoulder arthritis and vertebral osteomyelitis secondary to *Streptococcus agalactiae*.

On the other hand, sacroiliitis was not uncommon as well.

In a review of 13 cases of sacroiliitis caused by *Streptococcus agalactiae* in adults [9, 14–24], there was predominance in the female sex (5 : 1) and the age group from 30 to 40 years. The predisposing factors were in relation to gestation in 4 cases and to cancer of the cervix in another. Other factors implied were a dental handling, a urethral stenosis, and a chronic hepatitis C infection. In 5 cases no factors were identified.

The diagnosis was obtained by means of blood cultures in 12 of the 13 cases and in the remainder by cultivation of the sample obtained by arthrocentesis.

Psoas abscess in a postpartum lady caused by GBS was also reported in the literature [25].

Additionally, this paper emphasizes the contribution of imaging towards the diagnosis. Ultrasonography is a sensitive method for the detection of joint effusions (the hallmark of septic arthritis on ultrasound) in a patient with signs of joint infection before significant lytic lesion in the cartilage or the bone appears as was the case here, It is also helpful for guiding needle aspiration [26].

In the pre-MRI era, imaging of suspected septic arthritis was considered nonspecific. The diagnosis remains a clinical one with the help of arthrocentesis. However, this can be challenging in deep-seated joints such as the shoulder and sacroiliac joints.

MRI can be abnormal as early as 24 hours after the infection, thus becoming a helpful aid to the clinician.

Synovial enhancement, joint effusion (as seen in our patient), and perisynovial edema are typical finding consistent with the clinical diagnosis of a septic joint [27, 28].

4. Conclusion

Streptococcus agalactiae septic arthritis is a rare complication postpartum. It can present with invasive disease in adults. It usually targets older females and immuno compromised patients especially those with risk factors for bacteraemia.

A high index of suspicion is needed. Shoulder and sacroiliac joint involvement is not uncommon for unknown reasons and should raise the suspicion of invasive GBS disease. Microbiological investigation including synovial fluid and blood cultures is indicated and is often rewarding. Ultrasonography and MRI of the joints are helpful diagnostic tools.

Consent

Written informed consent was obtained from the patient for publication of this paper and accompanying images. A copy of the written consent is available for review by the Editor-in-Chief of this journal.

References

[1] L. Le Dantec, F. Maury, R. M. Flipo et al., "Les arthrites septiques périphériques à germes banals étude d'une série de 179 observations," *Revue Du Rhumatisme*, vol. 63, pp. 109–116, 1996 (French).

[2] J. J. Dubost, M. Soubrier, C. De Champs, J. M. Ristori, and B. Sauvezie, "Streptococcal septic arthritis in adults. A study of 55 cases with a literature review," *Joint Bone Spine*, vol. 71, no. 4, pp. 303–311, 2004.

[3] A. Schuchat and J. D. Wenger, "Epidemiology of group B streptococcal disease: Risk factors, prevention strategies, and vaccine development," *Epidemiologic Reviews*, vol. 16, no. 2, pp. 374–402, 1994.

[4] J. A. Regan, M. A. Klebanoff, R. P. Nugent et al., "Colonization with group B streptococci in pregnancy and adverse outcome," *American Journal of Obstetrics and Gynecology*, vol. 174, no. 4, pp. 1354–1360, 1996.

[5] D. R. Feikin, P. Thorsen, S. Zywicki, M. Arpi, J. G. Westergaard, and A. Schuchat, "Association between colonization with group B streptococci during pregnancy and preterm delivery among Danish women," *American Journal of Obstetrics and Gynecology*, vol. 184, no. 3, pp. 427–433, 2001.

[6] M. A. Krohn, S. L. Hillier, and C. J. Baker, "Maternal peripartum complications associated with vaginal group B streptococci colonization," *Journal of Infectious Diseases*, vol. 179, no. 6, pp. 1410–1415, 1999.

[7] Centers for Disease Control and Prevention, "Prevention of perinatal group B streptococcal disease: a public health perspective," *Morbidity and Mortality Weekly Report*, vol. 45, no. RR-7, pp. 1–24, 1996.

[8] A. Schattner and K. L. Vosti, "Bacterial arthritis due to beta-hemolytic Streptococci of serogroups A, B, C, F, and G: analysis of 23 cases and a review of the literature," *Medicine*, vol. 77, no. 2, pp. 122–139, 1998.

[9] J. M. Nolla, C. Gómez-Vaquero, X. Corbella et al., "Group B Streptococcus (Streptococcus agalactiae) pyogenic arthritis in nonpregnant adults," *Medicine*, vol. 82, no. 2, pp. 119–128, 2003.

[10] A. Binard, V. Devauchelle, K. Goulesque, S. Jousse, and A. Saraux, "Group B streptococcal arthritis," *Joint Bone Spine*, vol. 73, no. 4, pp. 465–468, 2006.

[11] C. B. Small, L. N. Slater, and F. D. Lowy, "Group B streptococcal arthritis in adults," *American Journal of Medicine*, vol. 76, no. 3, pp. 367–375, 1984.

[12] S. García, A. Combalía, and J. M. Segur, "Septic arthritis of the shoulder due to Streptococcus agalactiae," *Acta Orthopaedica Belgica*, vol. 62, no. 1, pp. 66–68, 1996.

[13] S. Casallo Blanco, A. I. Muñoz Ruiz, F. Marcos Sánchez, A. Aragón Díez, and A. I. Franco Moreno, "Polyarthritis and vertebral osteomyelitis due to Streptococcus agalactiae," *Revista Clinica Espanola*, vol. 205, no. 12, p. 630, 2005.

[14] A. M. Ramsay, "Puerperal infection associated with haemolytic streptococci other than Lancefield's group A," *Journal of Obstetrics and Gynaecology of the British Commonwealth*, vol. 48, pp. 569–585, 1941.

[15] B. Elgefors, "Another 2 cases of group B streptococcal sacroiliitis," *Scandinavian Journal of Infectious Diseases*, vol. 34, no. 5, p. 399, 2002.

[16] M. Jedwab, S. Ovadia, and M. Dan, "Pyogenic sacroiliitis in pregnancy," *International Journal of Gynecology and Obstetrics*, vol. 65, no. 3, pp. 303–304, 1999.

[17] U. Järvholm, B. R. Bergman, and B. Elgefors, "Bacterial infection of the sacroiliac joint," *Lakartidningen*, vol. 81, no. 22, pp. 2278–2279, 1984.

[18] G. Gordon and S. A. Kabins, "Pyogenic sacroiliitis," *American Journal of Medicine*, vol. 69, no. 1, pp. 50–56, 1980.

[19] G. Matfin, P. Mahfood, P. M. Wallach, and H. M. Adelman, "Arthralgias following dilation and curettage," *Hospital Practice*, vol. 33, no. 5, pp. 31–34, 1998.

[20] C. Perret, B. Hoen, A. Gerard, P. Canton, and J. B. Dureux, "Group B streptococcal sacroiliitis in a patient," *Presse Medicale*, vol. 20, no. 22, pp. 1048–1049, 1991.

[21] H. Corominas, P. Domingo, J. M. Llobet, F. Caballero, C. Díaz, and G. Vázquez, "Group B streptococcal sacroiliitis: case report and review," *Scandinavian Journal of Infectious Diseases*, vol. 33, no. 9, pp. 708–710, 2001.

[22] P. Y. C. Lee, V. Jasani, and R. Bendall, "Group B haemolytic streptococcal sacro-iliitis," *Journal of Infection*, vol. 30, no. 3, p. 263, 1995.

[23] R. A. Yood and K. Kronlund, "An uncommon cause of acute leg and buttock pain," *Hospital Practice*, vol. 29, no. 7, pp. 109–110, 1994.

[24] B. Zimmermann, D. J. Mikolich, and E. V. Lally, "Septic sacroiliitis," *Seminars in Arthritis and Rheumatism*, vol. 26, no. 3, pp. 592–604, 1996.

[25] N. K. Pandya, K. Z. Accardi, and C. Israelite, "Septic arthritis of the hip following group B Streptococcal psoas abscess in a postpartum patient resulting in total hip arthroplasty," *The Internet Journal of Orthopedic Surgery*, vol. 6, no. 2, 2007.

[26] C. L. F. Chau and J. F. Griffith, "Musculoskeletal infections: ultrasound appearances," *Clinical Radiology*, vol. 60, no. 2, pp. 149–159, 2005.

[27] J. Tehranzadeh, F. Wang, and M. Mesgarzadeh, "Magnetic resonance imaging of osteomyletis," *Critical Reviews in Diagnostic Imaging*, vol. 33, no. 6, pp. 495–534, 1992.

[28] M. Karchevsky, M. E. Schweitzer, W. B. Morrison, and J. A. Parellada, "MRI findings of septic arthritis and associated osteomyelitis in adults," *American Journal of Roentgenology*, vol. 182, no. 1, pp. 119–122, 2004.

33

A Rare Case of Digital Ischemia and Gangrene in ANCA-Associated Vasculitis

Richard A. Lau,[1] Ramandeep Bains,[1] Duminda Suraweera,[2] Jane Ma,[2] Emil R. Heinze,[1,2] Andrew L. Wong,[1,2] and Philip J. Clements[1]

[1] *UCLA-Olive View Rheumatology Program, Division of Rheumatology, Olive View-UCLA Medical Center, 14445 Olive View Drive, 2B182, Sylmar, CA 91342, USA*

[2] *UCLA-Olive View Internal Medicine Program, Department of Medicine, Olive View-UCLA Medical Center, 14445 Olive View Drive, 2B182, Sylmar, CA 91342, USA*

Correspondence should be addressed to Emil R. Heinze; emilheinze@gmail.com

Academic Editor: Shigeko Inokuma

This paper describes one patient with Antineutrophil Cytoplasmic Antibody- (ANCA-) associated vasculitis who initially presented with multiple ischemic fingers and toes. On further evaluation, the patient was also found to have pulmonary-renal involvement and episcleritis. The diagnosis was supported with a positive cANCA (anti-proteinase 3) and a bronchoscopy consistent with diffuse alveolar hemorrhage. Although the patient refused a tissue biopsy, clinical presentation including nasal ulceration, sinus congestion, and epistaxis and anti-proteinase 3 antibody were more consistent with Granulomatosis with Polyangiitis (GPA) rather than Microscopic Polyangiitis (MPA) or Eosinophilic Granulomatosis with Polyangiitis (EGPA) based on the recently presented ACR/EULAR Provisional 2017 Classification Criteria for GPA (Luqmani et al., 2016). The patient responded well to therapy including high dose steroids and cyclophosphamide, with improvement of all organs involved and had no further digital ischemia or gangrene on follow-up. We include a review of the English literature summarizing presentation, management, and outcome of 16 similar cases.

1. Introduction

Antineutrophil Cytoplasmic Antibody- (ANCA-) associated vasculitis is a group of autoimmune small to medium vessel necrotizing vasculitides [1–6]. Granulomatosis with Polyangiitis (GPA), previously known as Wegener's, is a type of ANCA vasculitis that is usually associated with cANCA. The range of clinical manifestations of GPA can involve almost any organ system, but the classic organ systems involved include the upper respiratory tract, lower respiratory tract, and kidneys [1–6]. One of the rarer manifestations is digital ischemia and gangrene. We report a rare case of GPA presenting with digital ischemia and gangrene, with a review of the literature.

2. Case

A 62-year-old male with a past medical history of hypertension and vitiligo presented to the hospital with 2 months of worsening left 1st toe, left 3rd finger, and right 2nd, 3rd, and 4th finger pain, swelling, and discoloration. The patient was a mechanic and endorsed an inciting traumatic event from dropping a heavy tool to his left 3rd finger and left 1st toe but denied any preceding trauma to the digits on his right hand. Soon after the initiation of the pain and swelling, there was also associated discoloration, with blue/black color changes with gradual scab formation.

On further review of systems, the patient reported several weeks of diffuse joint pains, intermittent eye pain and red eyes, hemoptysis, epistaxis, nasal congestion, and weight loss (unable to quantify but has decreased several belt notches). The patient otherwise denied any Raynaud's phenomenon, skin tightening, oral ulcerations, genital ulceration, chest pain, shortness of breath, abdominal pain, hematuria, ear pain, sinus pain, fevers, chills, night sweats, or smoking history.

The patient's initial vitals were significant for hypertension only. On physical exam, the patient was in no acute

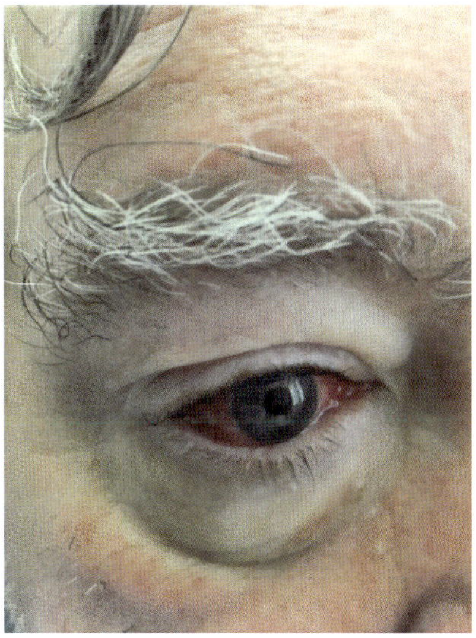

Figure 1

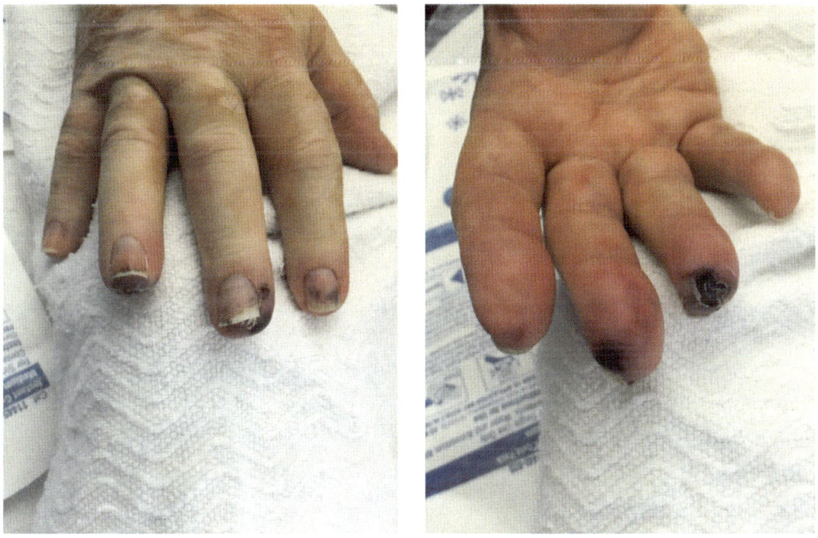

(a) (b)

Figure 2

distress. The head and neck exam was notable for bilateral conjunctivitis (see Figure 1) and right nasal ulceration. The cardiopulmonary exam was notable for poor airflow on lung auscultation. The skin exam was notable for vitiligo. The musculoskeletal exam was significant for diffuse joint tenderness but no joint swelling/warmth. The extremity exam revealed 3+ pitting edema of his lower extremities, right 2nd/3rd/4th finger duskiness and necrosis (see Figures 2(a) and 2(b)), left 3rd finger duskiness and necrosis (see Figures 3(a) and 3(b)), and left 1st toe with duskiness and necrosis (see Figures 4(a) and 4(b)).

The admitting labs were notable for elevated creatinine (1.74 mg/dL [ref 0.6–1.3]), elevated alkaline phosphatase (180 units/L [ref 38–126]), elevated CRP (140 mg/L [ref 0.0–7.0]), elevated ESR (67 mm/hr [ref < 20]), leukocytosis (12.5 thousand cells/uL [ref 3.8–10.9]), and anemia (12.5 gm/dL [ref 13.6–17.3]). Urinalysis revealed the presence of large blood, red blood cells (113 cells/HPF [ref 0–3]), white blood cells (13 cells/HPF [ref 0–5]), protein (100 mg/dL [ref negative]), and cellular casts (4/LPF). Random urine protein/creatinine ratio was 0.959 gm/gm. Initial chest X-ray on admission showed patchy right upper lobe airspace disease.

Given both pulmonary and renal system involvement, there was concern for pulmonary-renal syndromes, including ANCA-associated vasculitides, antiglomerular basement membrane disease, systemic lupus erythematous,

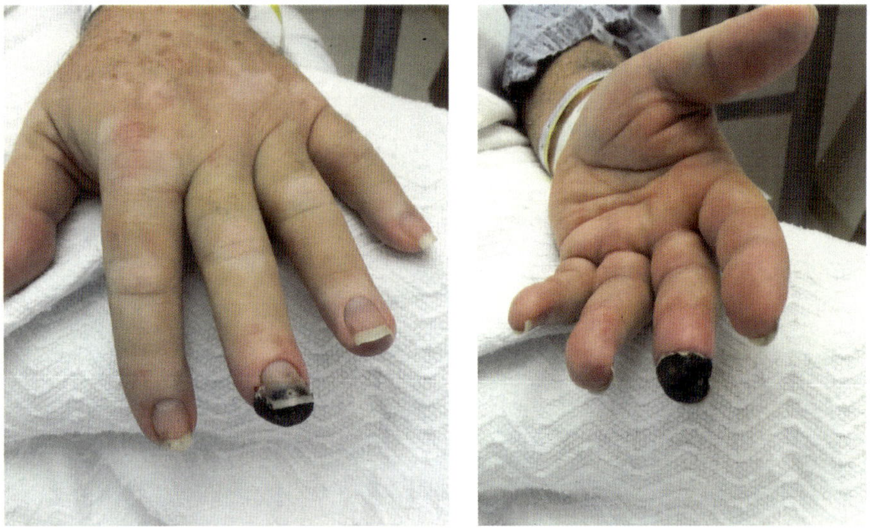

(a) (b)

FIGURE 3

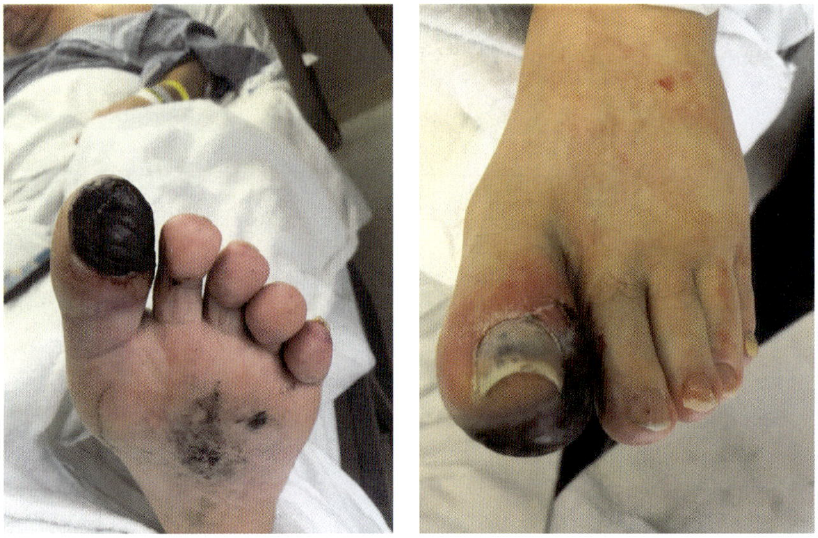

(a) (b)

FIGURE 4

and cryoglobulinemia. Other vasculitides of consideration included polyarteritis nodosum and thromboangiitis obliterans. We also considered that prothrombotic disorders such as antiphospholipid syndrome and embolic phenomenon can occur with cholesterol emboli or atrial myxoma. Infectious etiologies were considered as well, including endocarditis with embolic phenomenon. A paraneoplastic syndrome from a malignancy was entertained as well.

Further investigation was pursued to workup the aforementioned etiologies, including more laboratory evaluation with serologies pertinent for positive c-ANCA (proteinase-3 Ab 3.1 AI [ref < 1.0]), positive rheumatoid factor (80 IU/mL [ref < 14]), negative ANA, negative antiglomerular basement membrane antibody, negative anti-SSA/SSB, negative cryoglobulin screen, negative lupus anticoagulant, negative anti-Beta2 glycoprotein, and negative anticardiolipin. The infectious laboratory workup included multiple blood cultures with no growth. Transthoracic echocardiography did not show any thrombus, valvular disease, or atrial myxoma. Additional imaging was pursued that included computer tomography of the chest, which demonstrated extensive consolidation with air bronchograms predominately involving the right upper lobe and some contiguous involvement of the right middle and lower lobes. Bronchoscopy with serial

TABLE 1: Literature review of digital ischemia and gangrene associated with GPA in adults.

Age/sex	Onset after initial GPA symptoms	cANCA	Biopsy status	Other organ systems involved	Management	Outcome	Reference
30/M	3-4 months	Positive	Skin: nonspecific chronic inflammation Renal: segmental necrotizing GN	Sinusitis, epistaxis, arthralgias, painless oral ulcers, active urine sediment, mild renal insufficiency (creat. 2.3 mg/dL), and left upper lung lobe fibrotic infiltrates	Cyclophosphamide and steroids	Gangrene formation with autoamputation	Handa and Wali [7]
80/M	1-2 years	Positive	Skin: leukocytoclastic vasculitis	Multiple lung opacities with incomplete cavitation, renal insufficiency (creat. 1.5 mg/dL), microscopic hematuria, sensorineural hearing loss, and nasal ulcers	Cyclophosphamide and steroids	Gangrene formation, improvement of reversible tissue ischemia	La Civita et al. [8]
68/M	2 years	Not available	Sural nerve: vasculitis with secondary demyelination Lung: nodular necrotizing granulomatous inflammation with vasculitis	Purulent sinusitis, renal insufficiency (creat. 1.7 mg/dL), right peroneal neuropathy, otitis media, right 7th nerve palsy, pulmonary nodules, left pleural effusion, and pyoderma gangrenosum	Cyclophosphamide and steroids	Gangrene formation with surgical debridement and amputation	Phillips and Twiest [9]
26/F	1-2 years	Positive	Renal: focal crescentic GN Nasopharyngeal: small artery vasculitis	Secretory otitis, conjunctivitis, tonsillitis, arthritis, hematuria, mild renal insufficiency, mucosal ulcerations, and palpable purpura	Not specified	Gangrene formation	Karjalainen and Hakala [10]
48/M	3 months	Positive	Renal: pauci immune GN	Acute kidney injury (creat. 4.6 mg/dL), nasal crusting, hemoptysis, right sided pleuritic chest pain, and active urine sediment	Cyclophosphamide, steroids, heparin, aspirin, calcium channel blockers, nitroglycerin ointment, and plasmapheresis	Gangrene formation with autoamputation	Lim et al. [11]
24/F	On presentation	Positive	Femoral artery: normal	Pulmonary infiltrates, splenic infarcts, hemoptysis, and nodular masses in bilateral lungs with diffuse interstitial lung disease	Cyclophosphamide, steroids, heparin, and thrombectomy	Gangrene formation with surgical amputation	Bessias et al. [12]
55/M	3-4 months	Negative	Nasopharyngeal: epithelial ulceration with vasculitis	Epistaxis, polyarthralgia, bilateral lung nodular densities with cavitations, and small pleural effusion	Cyclophosphamide, steroids, warfarin, thrombectomy, and bypass	Improvement of reversible tissue ischemia	Maia et al. [13]
58/M	Unclear	Not available	Renal: 30% crescents	ENT, sinusitis, bronchiectasis, lung infiltrates, renal insufficiency (creat. 4.7 mg/dL), eye, and joint pain	Immunosuppression (not specified)	Gangrene formation	Pinching et al. [14]
40/M	Unclear	Not available	Renal: granuloma and vasculitis with 30% crescents Respiratory tract: vasculitis	ENT, lung infiltrates, renal failure requiring hemodialysis (creat. 18.43 mg/dL), joint pain, eye, vasculitic skin rash, and mononeuritis multiplex	Immunosuppression (not specified)	Gangrene formation	Pinching et al. [14]

Table 1: Continued.

Age/sex	Onset after initial GPA symptoms	cANCA	Biopsy status	Other organ systems involved	Management	Outcome	Reference
39/F	On presentation	Positive	Lung: patchy nodular fibrotic changes with hemosiderin laden macrophages and diffuse alveolar hemorrhage Left 4th gangrene digit: vasculitic changes with no thrombotic phenomenon	Hemoptysis, decline in respiratory function, and bilateral pulmonary infiltrates	Cyclophosphamide, steroids, and plasmapheresis	Gangrene formation with surgical amputation, improvement of reversible tissue ischemia	Leung et al. [15]
45/M	2 years	Positive	Renal: necrotizing GN	Polyneuropathy, renal injury, arthralgia, mild bloody nasal discharge, and skin vasculitis	Cyclophosphamide, steroids, heparin, aspirin, and iloprost	Improvement of reversible tissue ischemia	Schmidt et al. [16]
41/M	2 years	Positive	Sinus: granulomatous vasculitis	Bloody nasal discharge, inner ear granuloma, polyneuropathy, pulmonary infiltrates, and destructive sinusitis	Cyclophosphamide, steroids, heparin, aspirin, and iloprost	Improvement of reversible tissue ischemia	Schmidt et al. [16]
49/M	On presentation	Positive	Sural nerve: axonal loss	Mononeuritis multiplex with left foot drop, and cavitary nodule in the lung	Cyclophosphamide, steroids	Acroosteolysis, improvement of reversible ischemia	Modi et al. [17]
61/F	4 months	Positive	Renal: focal segmental necrotizing GN	Joint pain, Raynaud's, and acute kidney injury	Cyclophosphamide, steroids	Gangrene formation with autoamputation	Bartsch et al. [18]
46/F	2 months	Positive	Skin: leukocytoclastic vasculitis	Polyarthralgias, epistaxis, sinusitis, mouth ulcers, episcleritis, mononeuritis multiplex, multiple nodules in right lung, and active urine sediment	Cyclophosphamide, steroids, and iloprost	Gangrene formation	Kejriwal et al. [19]
26/M	On presentation	Positive	Skin: superficial dermal blood vessel necrosis	Oligoarthritis, polydipsia, polyuria, lung nodules, and mucosal thickening of maxillary sinus	Cyclophosphamide, steroids, and azathioprine	Gangrene formation with autoamputation	Agarwal and Khan [20]
62/M	On presentation	Positive		Nasal ulceration and congestion, epistaxis, episcleritis, hemoptysis, diffuse alveolar hemorrhage, pulmonary infiltrates, joint pain, renal insufficiency (creat. 1.7), and active urine sediment	Cyclophosphamide, steroids	Improvement of reversible ischemia, gangrene formation with autoamputation	Current case

M: male; F: female; ENT: ear, nose, and throat; GN: glomerulonephritis; IV: intravenous.

bronchial washings by pulmonary consultants was consistent with alveolar hemorrhage. The ocular examination by ophthalmology consultants was consistent with episcleritis.

The patient was diagnosed with ANCA-associated vasculitis. The defining pathological difference between Granulomatosis with Polyangiitis (GPA) and Microscopic Polyangiitis (MPA) is the presence of granulomatous changes on biopsy based on our current classification criteria [1–3]. To support the diagnosis, we were planning on a skin biopsy but the patient refused. A renal biopsy was scheduled but the patient did not show for the procedure. Often even if biopsies are performed, there is a risk of missing definitive granuloma tissue due to sampling error, which makes differentiating the type of ANCA-associated vasculitis difficult. Based on the recently presented ACR/EULAR Provisional 2017 Classification Criteria for GPA, the patient scores 4 points on clinical criteria given his bloody nasal discharge, sinonasal congestion, and red or painful eyes and scores 5 points on serologic criteria with a positive cANCA-PR3 antibody. A combined score of greater than or equal to 5 is needed for classification of GPA [21]. The patient was classified as most likely having GPA and treated with IV methylprednisolone followed by oral prednisone, which was slowly tapered over the next several months. He was also started on monthly IV cyclophosphamide for a total of 6 months. The patient responded well to therapy with improvement of all of his organ dysfunction, including improvement of the reversible tissue ischemia, cessation of digital gangrenous extension, and eventual autoamputation of the irreversible gangrenous parts of his digits.

3. Discussion

Based on our review of the English literature, to the best of our knowledge, only 16 cases have been previously reported describing adult patients with GPA who presented with digital ischemia and gangrene [7–20] (see Table 1). Given the paucity of cases reported, we suspect the prevalence with digital ischemia and gangrene in the GPA population to be <1%. All of the cases in this review, including our case, satisfy the ACR/EULAR Provisional 2017 Classification Criteria for GPA with the exception of the 58-year-old male, patient number 17, in the case series by Pinching et al. where not enough specific case details were reported to confirm the diagnosis. The mean age of patients was 46.9 years and included a range of 24–80 years. Including our patient, 12 of 17 were males (71%) compared to 5 of 17 females (29%). Most patients presented with multiorgan involvement including 14 of 17 with pulmonary involvement (82%), 11 of 17 with kidney disease (65%), and 13 of 17 with sinonasal disease (76%). cANCA was confirmed positive in 13 patients and negative in one patient, and the data was not available in 3 of the cases. Only 3 patients demonstrated granulomas on biopsy. Confounding risk factors were inconsistently reported but include a past medical history of HTN in three cases [9, 16, 19], DM in three cases [13, 15, 16], tobacco use in two cases [13, 18], and dyslipidemia in one case [13]. The clinical phenotype usually involves multiple disparate digits. 10 of 17 cases described isolated involvement of the upper extremities (59%) compared to the 5 of 17 with isolated involvement of the lower extremities (29%). Only two cases (12%), including ours, have described simultaneous involvement of both the upper and lower extremities [20]. The pathophysiology of the digital ischemia and gangrene is thought to be from destruction of medium sized vessels from active vasculitis, which has been demonstrated in case reports where histological examination of affected tissue showed arteritis [9, 15]. However, there is also evidence that in situ thrombosis, as a result of active vasculitis, can lead to ischemia and gangrene, as seen in angiographic examination of affected patients, as well as on histological examination of affected tissue showing arterial thrombi [12, 13]. Initial symptoms in most cases included pain and swelling with eventual gangrene formation if left untreated. Digital ischemia and gangrene can be part of the initial presentation of GPA or develop later in the course of the disease, even while the patient is on active treatment. The diagnosis is usually made based on clinical grounds, but angiographic examination can support vasculitic or thrombotic lesions [7–20]. Pathology can demonstrate either vascular arteritis or thrombi formation [9, 12, 13, 15]. There is no consensus on treatment regarding GPA with digital vasculitis with ischemia and gangrene. However, cyclophosphamide and steroids are the most commonly used treatment in the literature [7–20]. Other therapies that have been used include anticoagulation and vasodilators. Surgical intervention with thrombectomy and bypass have been used as well.

Digital ischemia and gangrene are rare manifestations of GPA. They can have a heterogeneous presentation as demonstrated by the cases in the literature. Diagnosis can be difficult as biopsy of the skin is often nonspecific. Without treatment, ischemia and gangrene can progress and lead to significant disability. Therefore, it is important for clinicians to be aware of this rare manifestation and institute early treatment as indicated.

Competing Interests

The authors declare that there is no conflict of interests regarding the publication of this paper.

References

[1] J. C. Jennette and R. J. Falk, "Small-vessel vasculitis," *New England Journal of Medicine*, vol. 337, no. 21, pp. 1512–1523, 1997.

[2] C. O. S. Savage, L. Harper, and D. Adu, "Primary systemic vasculitis," *Lancet*, vol. 349, no. 9051, pp. 553–558, 1997.

[3] P. M. K. Lutalo and D. P. D'Cruz, "Diagnosis and classification of granulomatosis with polyangiitis (aka Wegener's granulomatosis)," *Journal of Autoimmunity*, vol. 48-49, pp. 94–98, 2014.

[4] P. Lamprecht and W. L. Gross, "Wegener's Granulomatosis," *Herz*, vol. 29, no. 1, pp. 47–56, 2004.

[5] A. D. Mahr, T. Neogi, and P. A. Merkel, "Epidemiology of Wegener's granulomatosis: lessons from descriptive studies and analyses of genetic and environmental risk determinants," *Clinical and Experimental Rheumatology*, vol. 24, no. 2, supplement 41, pp. S82–S91, 2006.

[6] S. West, N. Arulkumaran, P. W. Ind, and C. D. Pusey, "Diffuse alveolar haemorrhage in ANCA-associated vasculitis," *Internal Medicine*, vol. 52, no. 1, pp. 5–13, 2013.

[7] R. Handa and J. P. Wali, "Wegener's granulomatosis with gangrene of toes," *Scandinavian Journal of Rheumatology*, vol. 25, no. 2, pp. 103–104, 1996.

[8] L. La Civita, G. Jeracitano, C. Ferri, R. Pedrinelli, G. Dell'Omo, and G. Catapano, "Wegener's granulomatosis of the elderly: a case report of uncommon severe gangrene of the feet," *Annals of the Rheumatic Diseases*, vol. 54, no. 4, 1995.

[9] R. W. Phillips and M. W. Twiest, "Wegener's granulomatosis and gangrene in the feet," *Annals of Internal Medicine*, vol. 99, no. 4, p. 571, 1983.

[10] A. Karjalainen and M. Hakala, "Still another case of Wegener's granulomatosis with a digital gangrene," *Scandinavian journal of rheumatology*, vol. 25, no. 5, p. 339, 1996.

[11] S. Y. Lim, J. H. Lim, and C. Horn, "Upper-extremity digital ischemia in granulomatosis with polyangiitis," *Journal of Clinical Rheumatology*, vol. 20, no. 3, pp. 155–159, 2014.

[12] N. Bessias, K. G. Moulakakis, C. Lioupis et al., "Wegener's granulomatosis presenting during pregnancy with acute limb ischemia," *Journal of Vascular Surgery*, vol. 42, no. 4, pp. 800–804, 2005.

[13] M. Maia, P. Brandão, P. Monteiro et al., "Upper limb ischemia in a patient with Wegener's granulomatosis," *Interactive Cardiovascular and Thoracic Surgery*, vol. 7, no. 6, pp. 1137–1140, 2008.

[14] A. J. Pinching, C. M. Lockwood, B. A. Pussell et al., "Wegener's granulomatosis: observations on 18 patients with severe renal disease," *Quarterly Journal of Medicine*, vol. 52, no. 208, pp. 435–460, 1983.

[15] A. Leung, C. B. Sung, G. Kothari, C. Mack, and C. Fong, "Utilisation of plasma exchange in the treatment of digital infarcts in Wegener's granulomatosis," *International Journal of Rheumatic Diseases*, vol. 13, no. 4, pp. e59–e61, 2010.

[16] W. A. Schmidt, D. Wernicke, E. Kiefer, and E. Gromnica-Ihle, "Colour duplex sonography of finger arteries in vasculitis and in systemic sclerosis," *Annals of the Rheumatic Diseases*, vol. 65, no. 2, pp. 265–267, 2006.

[17] M. Modi, A. K. Vats, S. Prabhakar, V. Singla, and S. Mishra, "Acro-osteolysis and mononeuritis multiplex as a presenting symptom of systemic angiitis of Wegener's type," *Indian Journal of Medical Sciences*, vol. 61, no. 4, pp. 212–215, 2007.

[18] P. Bartsch, A. Schossee, J. Sitte, P. R. Mertens, and G. H. Neild, "Joint pain, digital necrosis and acute kidney failure in small-vessel autoimmune disease," *Clinical Kidney Journal*, vol. 6, no. 2, pp. 240–242, 2013.

[19] R. Kejriwal, T. M. Lim, and S. Kumar, "Wegener's granulomatosis and acute upper limb digital ischemia," *International Journal of Rheumatic Diseases*, vol. 11, no. 2, pp. 185–187, 2008.

[20] A. Agarwal and N. A. Khan, "Multiple digital gangrene and polyuria," *Mayo Clinic Proceedings*, vol. 87, no. 4, article e25, 2012.

[21] R. Luqmani, P. A. Merkel, and R. Watts, "New classification criteria for ANCA-associated vasculitis: implications for clinical practice," in *Proceedings of the ACR/ARHP Annual Meeting*, J. Robson, Ed., Washington, DC, USA, November 2016.

34

Adult Onset Still's Disease: A Review on Diagnostic Workup and Treatment Options

Rajesh Gopalarathinam,[1] Eric Orlowsky,[2] Ramesh Kesavalu,[3] and Sreeteja Yelaminchili[4]

[1]*Department of Internal Medicine, Allegheny General Hospital, 320 E. North Avenue, Pittsburgh, PA 15212, USA*
[2]*Department of Rheumatology, Allegheny General Hospital, 320 E. North Avenue, Pittsburgh, PA 15212, USA*
[3]*Department of Rheumatology, Lakeside Community Healthcare Medical Group, 1500 S. Central Avenue No. 200, Glendale, CA 91204, USA*
[4]*Department of Internal Medicine, Capital Health Regional Medical Center, 750 Brunswick Avenue, Trenton, NJ 08638, USA*

Correspondence should be addressed to Rajesh Gopalarathinam; dr.rajeshgr86@gmail.com

Academic Editor: Tsai-Ching Hsu

Adult onset Still's disease (AOSD) is a rare systemic inflammatory disease of unknown etiology and pathogenesis that presents in 5 to 10% of patients as fever of unknown origin (FUO) accompanied by systemic manifestations. We report an interesting case of a 33-year-old African-American male who presented with one-month duration of FUO along with skin rash, sore throat, and arthralgia. After extensive workup, potential differential diagnoses were ruled out and the patient was diagnosed with AOSD based on the Yamaguchi criteria. The case history, incidence, pathogenesis, clinical manifestations, differential diagnoses, diagnostic workup, treatment modalities, and prognosis of AOSD are discussed in this case report.

1. Introduction

AOSD is characterized by the classic triad of persistent high spiking fever, arthralgia, and salmon colored skin rash. However, diagnosing AOSD is often difficult due to the presence of several nonspecific symptoms and the absence of characteristic serological biomarkers. AOSD is typically considered as a diagnosis of exclusion and a definitive diagnosis should be made based on the Yamaguchi or Fautrel criteria only after excluding infectious, malignant, and other connective tissue diseases. Timely diagnosis and treatment of the disease with corticosteroids followed by maintenance therapy with disease modifying antirheumatic drugs (DMARDs) or biologic drugs such as tumor necrosis factor- (TNF-) alpha agents or interleukin (IL-1) antagonists can prevent complications and lead to a favorable prognosis.

2. Case Presentation

A 33-year-old African-American male presented to the emergency department with a 4-week history of high-grade fever, sore throat, and dry cough. His fever was accompanied by nonpruritic macular skin rash on his trunk, arthralgia of bilateral ankles and knees, myalgia, and night sweats. He denied the presence of joint stiffness in the mornings, blurry vision, eye pain, oral ulcers, headache, back pain, burning urination, recent travel, sick contacts, decreased appetite, or weight loss. The rest of the review of the systems was negative. He had no significant past medical history, was not taking any medications previously, and had no significant family history. He had no known allergies. On physical exam, patient was febrile with a temperature of 39 degrees Celsius, tachycardic with a heart rate of 110 beats per minute, tachypneic with a respiratory rate of 22 breaths per minute and a blood pressure of 130/80 mmHg. Patient had a maculopapular skin rash on the chest, abdomen, and back. He also had inflamed throat without any exudates or cervical lymphadenopathy. Musculoskeletal exam showed minimal tenderness in bilateral ankles and knees with normal active and passive range of motion. There were no signs of active synovitis in any of his joints. Abdomen exam showed no organomegaly. Cardiovascular, respiratory, and neurological exam were unremarkable. He was admitted to the hospital and his initial workup revealed elevated acute phase reactants (Erythrocyte sedimentation rate (ESR): 47 mm/hr, C-reactive protein (CRP): 80 mg/L, and ferritin > 2000 μg/L), mildly elevated liver function tests (aspartate transaminase: 75, alanine transaminase: 90, and alkaline phosphatase: 100), normocytic anemia with normal white cell count with neutrophilic predominance (80%), and normal platelet count. Rapid strep throat test, HIV, hepatitis panel, blood cultures, throat cultures, and urine analysis were all negative. Antinuclear antibody (ANA), rheumatoid factor (RF), and cyclic citrullinated peptide (Anti-CCP) antibody were negative too. Chest X-ray showed no acute infiltrates. Subsequently, the patient was referred to an infectious disease specialist for his fever of unknown origin (FUO). The patient received a course of antibiotic (levofloxacin) during hospitalization which did not resolve his symptoms. A few days following admission, the patient experienced nausea, vomiting, and left upper quadrant abdominal pain without diarrhea. An abdomen and pelvis CT was done which was normal except for a borderline splenomegaly. An extensive ID workup was ordered which included fungal serologies and gallium scan, all of which turned out to be normal. Hematology was consulted for the patient's FUO and normocytic anemia. Hematological conditions such as leukemias, lymphomas, and hemophagocytic lymphohistiocytosis were ruled out due to the absence of physical and laboratory findings. A 2D echo, which was ordered to rule out endocarditis, came back as a normal study. As several investigations including serum protein electrophoresis and urine protein electrophoresis were nondiagnostic for the patient's FUO and anemia, a bone marrow biopsy with flow cytometry was finally ordered. The bone marrow study showed mildly hypercellular pattern with adequate storage of iron and no evidence of fibrosis or lymphoproliferative disorder. Rheumatology was consulted for his FUO in relation to arthralgia and myalgia. An anti-neutrophil cytoplasmic antibody (ANCA) panel, Lyme disease serology, and HLA-B27 tests were done and the results came back negative. After ruling out sickle cell anemia, tuberculosis, and other infectious causes, a diagnosis of adult onset Still's disease was made based on the Yamaguchi criteria. Subsequently, the patient was started initially on high dose prednisone 60 mg PO daily and then methotrexate 10 mg once weekly was added for steroid sparing effect. Since then, the patient improved and the intensity of his fever, skin rash, and ankle and knee pain came down significantly. The patient was discharged home in a stable condition with outpatient followup instructions. During the next clinic visit in 2 weeks, his fever, rash, and arthralgia subsided completely and his steroid dose was tapered appropriately. He did clinically well on methotrexate 20 mg once weekly.

3. Discussion

AOSD is a rare systemic inflammatory disease of unknown etiology. It was initially described by Bywaters in 1971 as a distinct clinical entity in adults that is quite similar to the one observed in children known as systemic juvenile idiopathic arthritis (sJIA) [1]. It has an estimated prevalence of 1.5 cases per 100,000–1000,000 people. It has been described all over the world and has a bimodal age distribution with 2 peaks, the first peak affecting people within 15–25 years of age and the second peak affecting people within 36–46 years of age [2]. Although it usually affects the younger adult population, it can also affect elderly people [3]. The disease affects predominantly females as compared to males [4].

The exact pathogenesis of AOSD is unknown. Several factors such as genetics, infectious (bacterial and viral) agents, and environmental factors have been thought to play a causative role [5–8]. But there are no strong evidences to suggest their causal relationship with the disease. An important step in the pathogenesis of AOSD is interleukin-18 (IL-18) mediated macrophage and neutrophil activation (evidenced by upregulation of CD 64 in patients with active disease) [9]. The pathogenesis of AOSD involves the interplay of numerous activated cytokines. Serum levels of tumor necrosis factor- (TNF-) alpha, IL-1, IL-6, IL-18, Interferon gamma IFN-γ, IL-8, and Soluble interleukin-2 receptor SIL-2R have been found to be elevated in patients with active AOSD [10]. Among the various cytokines, interleukin 1β (IL-1β) seems to be emerging as a key regulator in the pathogenesis of AOSD. It is involved in proliferation of neutrophils and diapedesis. Several molecular studies have also shown that elevated levels of IL-1β are associated with active and severe disease [11]. It has also been demonstrated in several studies that high levels of IL-18 in AOSD patients are a predictor of liver dysfunction [12].

Clinically, the most classic manifestations of AOSD are fever, rash, sore throat, and arthralgia with fever and arthralgia being the most common among them [13]. The fever is usually a high spiking quotidian fever ($\geq$39°C) that occurs in the evening with return of normal temperature the next day morning. The fever is often accompanied by other symptoms or could present as FUO alone [14]. In our patient, his high-grade fever occurred mostly during the evenings and was accompanied by pharyngitis and maculopapular skin rash. Nonsuppurative pharyngitis is one of the common earlier findings in AOSD and can either precede the development of fever or can occur along with other symptoms. The pharyngitis in AOSD patients is proposed to be from underlying cricothyroid perichondritis [15]. The characteristic rash in Still's disease is a transient, nonpruritic, salmon colored, macular, or maculopapular lesion often observed during febrile episodes (see Figure 1) [16]. The most common locations of the rash include the trunk and proximal extremities. In one-third of patients, the rash maybe mildly pruritic and can develop at sites of cutaneous injury due to pressure or trauma, which is referred to as Koebner's phenomenon [17]. Skin biopsy of the rash shows a mild nonspecific perivascular inflammation. Immunofluorescence of skin biopsy shows perivascular deposition of C3 protein [17]. Another common finding in many AOSD patients is an exaggerated urticarial response to cutaneous stimuli (i.e., the scratch test) which is referred to as dermatographism [18]. Intense arthralgia is ubiquitously seen in all AOSD patients. The most commonly involved joints are the knees, wrists, ankles, and elbows [6]. AOSD often involves the distal interphalangeal joints of the hand, which are commonly

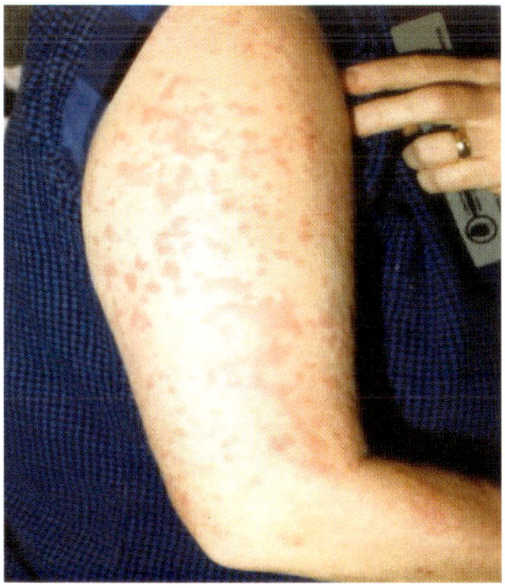

FIGURE 1: Characteristic salmon colored, nonpruritic, and maculopapular rash of Still's disease (source: http://www.stillsdisease.org/).

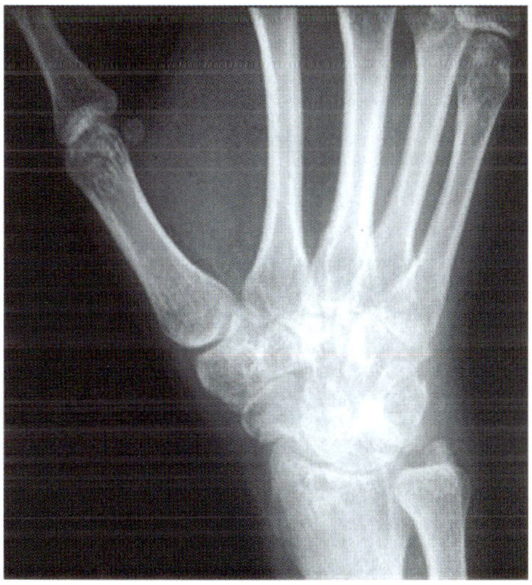

FIGURE 2: Xray of the right wrist showing diffuse narrowing of the radiocarpal and carpometacarpal joints of the wrist which is a characteristic finding in Still's disease. (Source: http://www hopkinsarthritis.org/)

spared in inflammatory joint disease of the young adults (e.g., SLE and rheumatoid arthritis) with the exception of psoriatic arthritis. Narrowing of the carpometacarpal spaces of the hands is also found to be specific for AOSD (See Figure 2) [19]. Joint fluid analysis often shows marked neutrophilic leukocytosis [14]. Our patient had involvement of bilateral ankles and knees with sparing of other joints including hands, wrists, and elbows. Myalgia, which is usually generalized and severe, is a frequently encountered symptom during febrile episodes [6]. In all AOSD patients, throat cultures and viral serologies are negative and, therefore, antibiotic therapy is ineffective [2, 20]. Lymphadenopathy develops in 44–90% of AOSD patients [5, 21] and may raise the suspicion of lymphoma initially [22]. Hepatosplenomegaly can be a common manifestation in the early phase of the disease. Less commonly, pericarditis or pleuritis may occur. Macrophage activation syndrome (MAS) is a life threatening complication seen in AOSD as well as systemic onset juvenile idiopathic arthritis (sJIA). Its pathogenesis is not clearly understood but involves cytokine induced hyperproliferation of activated CD8+ T-lymphocytes and macrophages in the reticuloendothelial system [23]. It should be suspected in ASOD patients who present with fever, hepatosplenomegaly, lymphadenopathy, pancytopenia, transaminitis, coagulopathy, and CNS/pulmonary/renal involvement. Bone marrow aspiration and biopsy which show hemophagocytosis help in establishing the diagnosis of MAS [23]. Another clinical condition that closely mimics macrophage activation syndrome is the reactive hemophagocytic system (RHS) [24].

The laboratory tests in AOSD show features suggestive of an inflammatory process. The most common laboratory abnormalities include

(i) elevated erythrocyte sedimentation rate (ESR),

(ii) leukocytosis (in most cases within 15,000–30,000, mainly neutrophils),

(iii) thrombocytopenia > 400,000,

(iv) elevated ferritin levels.

Elevated ferritin level is a nonspecific but common finding and a helpful feature for diagnosing AOSD [25]. The ferritin levels are often higher (>2000 mg/mL) than the levels found in other autoimmune or inflammatory disease and are likely secondary to cytokine secretion induced by the reticuloendothelial system [25]. Among the several isoforms of ferritin that have been described, one that deserves mention is the glycosylated ferritin which is typically decreased in AOSD patients. Studies have shown that a combination of glycosylated ferritin fraction < 20% and ferritin level above the upper limit of the normal range improved the sensitivity and specificity to 70.5% and 83%, respectively, as compared with using elevated ferritin levels alone [25, 26]. Our patient had a glycosylated ferritin 18%. Although hyperferritinemia is often helpful in diagnosing AOSD, normal levels of serum ferritin should not rule out the diagnosis of AOSD [27]. Glycosylated ferritin should not be used to monitor the disease activity or response to treatment, because it remains low for many months even after the disease goes into remission. Other less common laboratory findings in AOSD include serum albumin < 3.5 gms/dL, anemia of chronic disease, and elevated hepatic transaminase levels [5]. Rheumatoid factor and antinuclear antibody tests are usually negative [5, 6]. Synovial and serosal fluids are inflammatory type with neutrophilic predominance [14]. The radiographic results are generally normal in the early phase of the disease and maybe helpful in the late and chronic phase with worsening erosions and joint space narrowing (carpometacarpal joints are more commonly involved than the tarsometatarsal joints) [19, 28].

Diagnosing AOSD is often difficult due to the presence of several nonspecific symptoms and the absence of characteristic serological biomarkers. The Yamaguchi criteria are the most widely cited criteria and are shown to be the most sensitive ones (93%) [29]. The major and the minor criteria of the Yamaguchi criteria are shown below.

Major criteria are as follows:

(i) Fever of at least 39°C for at least a week.

(ii) Arthralgia or arthritis for at least 2 weeks.

(iii) Nonpruritic salmon colored rash on trunk/extremities.

(iv) Granulocytic leukocytosis (10,000/microL or greater).

Minor criteria are as follows:

(i) Sore throat.

(ii) Lymphadenopathy.

(iii) Hepatomegaly or splenomegaly.

(iv) Abnormal liver function tests.

(v) Negative tests for RF and ANA.

Diagnosis requires at least 5 features, with at least 2 of these being major diagnostic criteria. Our patient had all 4 of the major criteria and all of the minor criteria except lymphadenopathy.

In 2002, Fautrel et al. proposed a new criterion which contained 2 new markers: serum ferritin and glycosylated ferritin. The sensitivity and specificity of Fautrel criteria were 80.6% and 98.5%, respectively [30]. The Fautrel diagnostic criteria for AOSD are shown below.

Major criteria are as follows:

(i) Spiking fever $\geq$ 39°C.

(ii) Arthralgia.

(iii) Transient erythema.

(iv) Pharyngitis.

(v) Neutrophilic polymorphonuclear count $\geq$ 80%.

(vi) Glycosylated ferritin fraction $\leq$ 20%.

Minor criteria are as follows:

(i) Typical Still's rash.

(ii) Leukocytosis (10,000/mm^3).

Diagnosis of AOSD by Fautrel criteria requires 4 or more major criteria or 3 major and 2 minor criteria. Our patient had all 5 major criteria and 2 minor criteria.

AOSD is primarily a diagnosis of exclusion which should be considered only after excluding several other differential diagnoses [2, 5, 14, 31]. Among many differentials, the major diseases that should be excluded are as follows:

(1) Infections: viral infections (Rubella, Epstein-Barr virus, Cytomegalovirus, HIV, hepatitis B and C, coxsackie, and Parvovirus), infective endocarditis, Lyme disease, and tuberculosis.

(2) Granulomatous diseases: Sarcoidosis, Crohn's disease, and idiopathic granulomatous hepatitis.

(3) Malignancy: leukemias and lymphomas.

(4) Connective tissue diseases: systemic lupus erythematosus (SLE), mixed connective tissue disease (MCTD), polyarteritis nodosa (PAN), Wegener's granulomatosis, and Takayasu's arteritis.

Blood cultures and serological tests can be useful to rule out infections. Malignant disorders can be differentiated from AOSD by their hematological profile, but sometimes bone marrow and/or lymph node biopsy may be needed [32]. The familial Mediterranean fever (FMF) and TNF receptor associated periodic syndrome (TRAPS) are two syndromes that fall under the category of periodic fever syndromes that closely resemble the clinical picture of AOSD [33]. Patients with FMF often present with acute, self-limiting episodes of fever that last only for 1–3 days. Unlike AOSD, the fever in FMF does not have the typical quotidian pattern and is accompanied by serositis or acute synovitis of the hip, knee, or ankle. The fever can be accompanied by erysipelas like skin rash. FMF usually starts in childhood. The familial distribution of the disease together with the distinct clinical characteristics and response to Colchicine can help the physician to get the correct diagnosis. Genetic analysis for the MEFV gene is also used to verify the diagnosis in suspected cases. With TRAPS, the fever lasts longer ($\geq$3 to 4 weeks on average) and is associated with ocular manifestations and a characteristic centrifugal erythematous patch. Both FMF and TRAPS often begin during childhood and have a strong familial distribution.

The disease pattern of patients with AOSD can be divided into 3 distinct types [6, 14, 32]:

(1) Monocyclic or self-limiting pattern, which has a single episode of systemic disease of variable duration followed by complete remission.

(2) Polycyclic or intermittent pattern, where 2 or more episodes of systemic disease are separated by symptom-free remission period lasting for a minimum of 2 months.

(3) Chronic articular pattern, which is characterized by the severe articular manifestations causing joint destruction.

In several studies, a poor prognosis is associated in AOSD patients with polyarticular onset, proximal joint arthritis, prior episode in childhood, and requirement of systemic steroids for more than 2 years [6, 34]. In contrast, patients with monocyclic or polycyclic systemic disease, no arthritis at presentation, or an oligoarticular onset and course showed better functional status.

Corticosteroids remain the first-line treatment for AOSD, regardless of the clinical presentation. Usually, prednisolone is preferred among steroids. Steroids control symptoms in about 60% of AOSD patients. Intra-articular steroid injection can be used in the treatment of chronic articular pattern of AOSD [35]. Disease modifying antirheumatic drugs (DMARDs), such as methotrexate (MTX), azathioprine, cyclosporine, and cyclophosphamide, are often used for maintenance therapy of the disease [4, 32]. Sulfasalazine causes severe adverse reactions in AOSD (ranging from gastrointestinal symptoms such as abdominal pain, nausea, and vomiting to severe myelosuppression) and should be avoided [36]. MTX is often used due to its steroid sparing effect and its potential to prevent worsening of arthritis [37]. Cyclosporine can be used for AOSD patients presenting with macrophage activation syndrome (MAS). Since several cytokines such as TNF-alpha, IL-1, and IL-6 are implicated in the pathogenesis of AOSD, biologic agents can be used in refractory AOSD patients [38, 39]. While several studies show the efficacy of anti-TNF agents (infliximab, etanercept, and adalimumab) in refractory AOSD [40–43], IL-1 inhibition is considered the mainstay of treatment for refractory AOSD leading to significant improvement in both clinical and laboratory terms [44, 45]. Three IL-1 antagonists are presently available, that is, a recombinant antagonist of the IL-1 receptor (IL-1Ra, anakinra), a human monoclonal antibody directed against IL-1β (canakinumab), and a soluble IL-1 trap fusion protein (rilonacept). Among the three IL-1 antagonists, anakinra has been used more frequently. Anakinra is particularly efficient in the rapid relief of systemic symptoms. Its effect on articular symptoms is less frequently reported. It is administered subcutaneously once daily, due to its short half-life. In the event of an insufficient response to anakinra, rilonacept and canakinumab can be considered because they have longer half-lives and can be administered every week or every 8 weeks, respectively [46, 47]. Tocilizumab is another monoclonal antibody directed against the IL-6 receptor that has been shown to induce remission in patients with AOSD refractory to standard treatment from several case studies. It is also used in the treatment of systemic onset juvenile idiopathic arthritis (sJIA) and is usually administered as a monthly intravenous infusion or a subcutaneous injection every 1-2 weeks. It has a marked corticosteroid-sparing effect and a good tolerance profile [48, 49]. Plasma exchange and intravenous immunoglobulins are other treatment options in refractory AOSD patients [50, 51].

In conclusion, over the past four decades, AOSD still remains as a diagnostic dilemma for physicians as it presents with a combination of nonspecific symptoms that can be caused by a wide variety of diseases. However, the key point to remember is that, for patients who present with prolonged and unexplained fever combined with musculoskeletal symptoms and macular rash, the differential diagnoses should include AOSD. Timely diagnosis and treatment of the disease can prevent complications and lead to a favorable prognosis with improved quality of life.

References

[1] E. G. Bywaters, "Still's disease in the adult," *Annals of the Rheumatic Diseases*, vol. 30, no. 2, pp. 121–133, 1971.

[2] M. Owlia and G. Mehrpoor, "Adult onset still's disease: a review," *Indian Journal of Medical Sciences*, vol. 63, no. 5, pp. 207–221, 2009.

[3] H. Ichiki, M. Shishido, and S. Nishiyama, "Two cases of adult onset of Still's disease in the elderly," *Nippon Ronen Igakkai Zasshi*, vol. 29, no. 12, pp. 960–964, 1992.

[4] Y. Cagatay, A. Gul, A. Cagatay et al., "Adult-onset still's disease," *International Journal of Clinical Practice*, vol. 63, no. 7, pp. 1050–1055, 2009.

[5] A. Ohta, M. Yamaguchi, H. Kaneoka, T. Nagayoshi, and M. Hiida, "Adult Still's disease: review of 228 cases from the literature," *The Journal of Rheumatology*, vol. 14, no. 6, pp. 1139–1146, 1987.

[6] J. Pouchot, J. S. Sampalis, F. Beaudet et al., "Adult still's disease: manifestations, disease course, and outcome in 62 patients," *Medicine*, vol. 70, no. 2, pp. 118–136, 1991.

[7] F. J. Escudero, Ó. Len, V. Falcó, T. F. de Sevilla, and A. Sellas, "Rubella infection in adult onset Still's disease," *Annals of the Rheumatic Diseases*, vol. 59, no. 6, article 493, 2000.

[8] C. Perez and V. Artola, "Adult Still's disease associated with *Mycoplasma pneumoniae* infection," *Clinical Infectious Diseases*, vol. 32, no. 6, pp. E105–E106, 2001.

[9] A. Komiya, T. Matsui, S. Nogi et al., "Neutrophil CD64 is upregulated in patients with active adult-onset still's disease," *Scandinavian Journal of Rheumatology*, vol. 41, no. 2, pp. 156–158, 2012.

[10] D.-Y. Chen, J.-L. Lan, F.-J. Lin, and T.-Y. Hsieh, "Proinflammatory cytokine profiles in sera and pathological tissues of patients with active untreated adult onset still's disease," *Journal of Rheumatology*, vol. 31, no. 11, pp. 2189–2198, 2004.

[11] C. Giampietro and B. Fautrel, "Anti-interleukin-1 agents in adult onset Still's disease," *International Journal of Inflammation*, vol. 2012, Article ID 317820, 6 pages, 2012.

[12] J. B. Arlet, D. Boutin-Le Thi Huong, J. Pouchot, and J. C. Piette, "Current concepts on the pathogenesis of adult-onset still's disease," *Revue de Medecine Interne*, vol. 26, no. 7, pp. 549–556, 2005.

[13] E. B. Larson, "Adult still's disease-recognition of a clinical syndrome and recent experience," *Western Journal of Medicine*, vol. 142, no. 5, pp. 665–671, 1985.

[14] A. Mert, R. Ozaras, F. Tabak et al., "Fever of unknown origin: a review of 20 patients with adult-onset Still's disease," *Clinical Rheumatology*, vol. 22, no. 2, pp. 89–93, 2003.

[15] D.-Y. Chen, H. H.-C. Lan, T.-Y. Hsieh, H.-H. Chen, and J.-L. Lan, "Crico-thyroid perichondritis leading to sore throat in patients with active adult-onset Still's disease," *Annals of the Rheumatic Diseases*, vol. 66, no. 9, pp. 1264–1266, 2007.

[16] C. Sunderkotter, U. Frieling, D. Nashan, and D. Metye, "Adult onset Still's disease and its characteristic rash," *Hautarzt*, vol. 49, pp. 920–924, 1998.

[17] K. B. Elkon, G. R. V. Hughes, E. G. L. Bywaters et al., "Adult-onset Still's disease: twenty-year follow up and further studies of patients with active disease," *Arthritis and Rheumatism*, vol. 25, no. 6, pp. 647–654, 1982.

[18] G. Mehrpoor, M. B. Owlia, H. Soleimani, and J. Ayatollahi, "Adult-onset Still's disease: a report of 28 cases and review of the literature," *Modern Rheumatology*, vol. 18, no. 5, pp. 480–485, 2008.

[19] A. G. Bjorkengren, M. N. Pathria, D. J. Sartoris et al., "Carpal alterations in adult-onset Still disease, juvenile chronic arthritis, and adult-onset rheumatoid arthritis: comparative study," *Radiology*, vol. 165, no. 2, pp. 545–548, 1987.

[20] J. Kelly, P. Chowienczyk, and T. Gibson, "Sore throat and hyperferritinaemia," *Journal of the Royal Society of Medicine*, vol. 94, no. 8, pp. 400–401, 2001.

[21] J. J. Cush, T. A. Medsger Jr., W. C. Christy, D. C. Herbert, and L. A. Cooperstein, "Adult-onset Still's disease. Clinical course & outcome," *Arthritis & Rheumatism*, vol. 30, no. 2, pp. 186–194, 1987.

[22] M. Kojima, S. Nakamura, S. Miyawaki et al., "Lymph node lesion in adult-onset still's disease resembling peripheral T-cell lymphoma: a report of three cases," *International Journal of Surgical Pathology*, vol. 10, no. 3, pp. 197–202, 2002.

[23] A. G. Tristano, "Macrophage activation syndrome: a frequent but under-diagnosed complication associated with rheumatic diseases," *Medical Science Monitor*, vol. 14, no. 3, pp. RA27–RA36, 2008.

[24] A. A. Grom, "Macrophage activation syndrome and reactive hemophagocytic lymphohistiocytosis: the same entities?" *Current Opinion in Rheumatology*, vol. 15, no. 5, pp. 587–590, 2003.

[25] S. C. A. Meijvis, H. Endeman, A. B. M. Geers, and E. J. ter Borg, "Extremely high serum ferritin levels as diagnosis tool in adult-onset Still's disease," *Netherlands Journal of Medicine*, vol. 65, no. 6, pp. 212–214, 2007.

[26] L. Fardet, P. Coppo, A. Kettaneh, M. Dehoux, J. Cabane, and O. Lambotte, "Low glycosylated ferritin, a good marker for the diagnosis of hemophagocytic syndrome," *Arthritis & Rheumatism*, vol. 58, no. 5, pp. 1521–1527, 2008.

[27] M. Schwarz-Eywill, B. Heilig, H. Bauer, A. Breitbart, and A. Pezzutto, "Evaluation of serum ferritin as a marker for adult Still's disease activity," *Annals of the Rheumatic Diseases*, vol. 51, no. 5, pp. 683–685, 1992.

[28] T. A. Medsger Jr. and W. C. Christy, "Carpal arthritis with ankylosis in late onset Still's disease," *Arthritis & Rheumatism*, vol. 19, no. 2, pp. 232–242, 1976.

[29] M. Yamaguchi, A. Ohta, T. Tsunematsu et al., "Preliminary criteria for classification of adult Still's disease," *Journal of Rheumatology*, vol. 19, no. 3, pp. 424–430, 1992.

[30] B. Fautrel, E. Zing, J.-L. Golmard et al., "Proposal for a new set of classification criteria for adult-onset still disease," *Medicine*, vol. 81, no. 3, pp. 194–200, 2002.

[31] D. Zenagui and J. P. De Coninck, "Atypical presentation of adult Still's disease mimicking acute bacterial endocarditis," *European Heart Journal*, vol. 16, no. 10, pp. 1448–1450, 1995.

[32] P. Efthimiou, P. K. Paik, and L. Bielory, "Diagnosis and management of adult onset Still's disease," *Annals of the Rheumatic Diseases*, vol. 65, no. 5, pp. 564–572, 2006.

[33] S. Padeh, "Periodic fever syndromes," *Pediatric Clinics of North America*, vol. 52, no. 2, pp. 577–609, 2005.

[34] J. M. G. W. Wouters and L. B. A. Van de Putte, "Adult-onset Still's disease; clinical and laboratory features, treatment and progress of 45 cases," *Quarterly Journal of Medicine*, vol. 61, no. 235, pp. 1055–1065, 1986.

[35] B. Fautrel, "Adult onset still's disease," *Best Practice & Research Clinical Rheumatology*, vol. 22, pp. 773–792, 2008.

[36] J. H. Jung, J. B. Jun, D. H. Yoo et al., "High toxicity of sulfasalazine in adult-onset Still's disease," *Clinical and Experimental Rheumatology*, vol. 18, no. 2, pp. 245–248, 2000.

[37] O. Okamoto, M. Oishi, and S. Fujiwara, "Steroid-resistant adult-onset Still's disease which showed a quick response to methotrexate," *Journal of Dermatology*, vol. 35, no. 2, pp. 106–110, 2008.

[38] G. Espinosa and R. Cervera, "Role of biologic therapy in systemic autoimmune diseases," *Medicina Clinica*, vol. 128, no. 12, pp. 456–457, 2007.

[39] P. Efthimiou, A. Kontzias, C. M. Ward, and N. S. Ogden, "Adult-onset Still's disease: can recent advances in our understanding of its pathogenesis lead to targeted therapy?" *Nature Clinical Practice Rheumatology*, vol. 3, no. 6, pp. 328–335, 2007.

[40] A. Kokkinos, A. Iliopoulos, P. Greka, A. Efthymiou, N. Katsilambros, and P. P. Sfikakis, "Successful treatment of refractory adult-onset still's disease with infliximab. A prospective, non-comparative series of four patients," *Clinical Rheumatology*, vol. 23, no. 1, pp. 45–49, 2004.

[41] M. E. Husni, A. L. Maier, P. J. Mease et al., "Etanercept in the treatment of adult patients with Still's disease," *Arthritis and Rheumatism*, vol. 46, no. 5, pp. 1171–1176, 2002.

[42] M. Benucci, G. F. Li, A. Del Rosso, and M. Manfrecli, "Adalimumab (anti-TNF-α) therapy to improve the clinical course of adult onset still's disease: the first case report," *Clinical and Experimental Rheumatology*, vol. 23, no. 5, article 733, 2005.

[43] C. Dechant, P. Schauenberg, C. E. Antoni, H. C. Kraetsch, J. R. Kalden, and B. Manger, "Longterm outcome of TNF blockade in adult-onset Still's disease," *Deutsche Medizinische Wochenschrift*, vol. 129, no. 23, pp. 1308–1312, 2004.

[44] F. M. Vasques Godinho, M. J. Parreira Santos, and J. Canas da Silva, "Refractory adult onset Still's disease successfully treated with Anakinra," *Annals of the Rheumatic Diseases*, vol. 64, no. 4, pp. 647–648, 2005.

[45] I. Kötter, A. Wacker, S. Koch et al., "Anakinra in patients with treatment-resistant adult-onset still's disease: four case reports with serial cytokine measurements and a review of the literature," *Seminars in Arthritis and Rheumatism*, vol. 37, no. 3, pp. 189–197, 2007.

[46] Y. Jamilloux, M. Gerfaud-Valentin, T. Henry, and P. Sève, "Treatment of adult-onset still's disease: a review," *Therapeutics and Clinical Risk Management*, vol. 11, pp. 33–43, 2014.

[47] A. Kontzias and P. Efthimiou, "The use of canakinumab, a novel IL-1β long-acting inhibitor, in refractory adult-onset Still's disease," *Seminars in Arthritis and Rheumatism*, vol. 42, no. 2, pp. 201–205, 2012.

[48] P. Cipriani, P. Ruscitti, F. Carubbi et al., "Tocilizumab for the treatment of adult-onset Still's disease: results from a case series," *Clinical Rheumatology*, vol. 33, no. 1, pp. 49–55, 2014.

[49] F. Ortiz-Sanjuán, R. Blanco, V. Calvo-Rio et al., "Efficacy of tocilizumab in conventional treatment-refractory adult-onset Still's disease: multicenter retrospective open-label study of thirty-four patients," *Arthritis and Rheumatology*, vol. 66, no. 6, pp. 1659–1665, 2014.

[50] T. Ito, Y. Ozaki, K. Shimamoto et al., "Successful treatment with plasma exchange in adult-onset Still's disease with hyper-IL-18-naemia and hyperallergic state," *Modern Rheumatology*, vol. 18, no. 4, pp. 407–410, 2008.

[51] T. Mahmud and G. R. V. Hughes, "Intravenous immunoglobulin in the treatment of refractory adult Still's disease," *Journal of Rheumatology*, vol. 26, no. 9, pp. 2067–2068, 1999.

Atypical Cutaneous Manifestations in Adult Onset Still's Disease

Champa Nataraja[1] and Hedley Griffiths[1,2]

[1]*Barwon Health, Bellerine Street, Geelong, VIC 3220, Australia*
[2]*Barwon Rheumatology Service, 156 Bellerine Street, Geelong, VIC 3220, Australia*

Correspondence should be addressed to Champa Nataraja; champadr@yahoo.co.in

Academic Editor: Tsai-Ching Hsu

Adult Onset Still's Disease (AOSD), an adult variant of systemic onset juvenile idiopathic arthritis, is a rare systemic inflammatory disorder of unknown aetiology. The rarity of this disease is associated with low index of suspicion and delayed diagnosis in patients suffering from it and in the presence of atypical features the diagnosis can be further challenging. This is a case report on a 24-year-old woman, who was a diagnostic dilemma for 2 years due to the nonspecific symptoms of recurrent fever, generalized maculopapular persistent pruritic and tender rash, and polyarthralgia. She was initially diagnosed as leukocytoclastic vasculitis on a skin biopsy and was managed by a dermatologist with various medications including NSAIDs, hydroxychloroquine, dapsone, colchicine, cyclosporine, and high doses of oral steroids with minimal response. Subsequently, she has had multiple admissions with similar symptoms with raised inflammatory markers and negative septic workup. On one occasion, her iron study revealed hyperferritinaemia which led to the suspicion of AOSD. Once the rheumatic fever and infectious, malignant, autoimmune, and lymphoproliferative disorders were excluded, she was diagnosed as probable AOSD and managed successfully with IL-1 (interleukin-1) receptor antagonist, Anakinra, with remarkable and lasting response both clinically and biochemically.

1. Introduction

AOSD is a systemic, inflammatory disorder characterized by spiking fevers, arthritis/arthralgia, and an evanescent salmon-pink maculopapular rash, frequently accompanied by sore throat, myalgia, lymphadenopathies, splenomegaly, and neutrophilic leucocytosis. The aetiology of this disease is unknown with equal distribution between the sexes. There is a bimodal age distribution, with one peak between the ages of 15 and 25 and the second peak between the ages of 35 and 45. The clinical course can be divided into monophasic, intermittent, and chronic pattern. Systemic manifestations predominate in the two former forms while articular involvement predominates in patients with chronic form. AOSD has been associated with markedly elevated serum ferritin level (>3000 ng/mL) in as much as 70% of patients. As there is no diagnostic test, it is a diagnosis of exclusion. The most popular Yamaguchi et al.'s criteria [1] have been proposed for diagnosis which involves four major and five minor criteria. The diagnosis requires the presence of five features with at least two being major criteria. Treatment usually involves NSAIDs, corticosteroids, steroid sparing agents including methotrexate, biological agents including IL-1 receptor antagonist, Anakinra, Canakinumab, IL-6 antagonist, Tocilizumab, and TNF-alpha inhibitors. It is a life-long treatment and prognosis is variable, depending on treatment response.

2. Case Report

A 24-year-old woman initially presented 2 years ago with the widespread pruritic, burning maculopapular rash predominantly involving limbs (Figures 1, 2, and 3), torso, chest, and back associated with high grade fever and polyarthralgia. The rash was tender to palpate. It was diagnosed as leukocytoclastic vasculitis on a skin biopsy and was managed by dermatologist with various medications including antihistamines, NSAIDs, high dose of oral steroids and topical steroids, dapsone, hydroxychloroquine, colchicine, and cyclosporine with minimal response. Her symptoms were intermittent with symptom-free period between the episodes. She was

Table 1

Laboratory tests	Patient's value	Normal value
Full blood count		
WCC ($\times 10^9$)	16.6	4.0–11.0
Neutrophils ($\times 10^9$)	12.6	2.0–8.0
Band cells	2.7	0.0–0.5
Hemoglobin (g/L)	104	115–170
Platelets ($\times 10^9$)	239	150–500
MCV (fl)	64	80–98
MCHC (pg)	20.4	26–34
Liver function tests		
ALP (u/L)	125	8–252
GGT (u/L)	88	<30
ALT (u/L)	12	<45
Albumin (g/L)	26	34–50
Iron studies		
Serum Iron (micromol/L)	5	7–30
Ferritin (microgm/L)	6198	8–252
Acute phase reactants		
CRP (mg/L)	350	<2.9
ESR (mm/hr)	51	0–12
LDH (u/L)	794	80–230

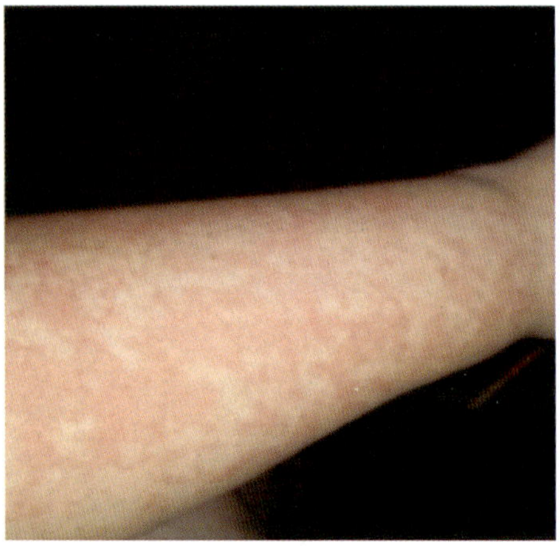

Figure 1: Maculopapular rash involving left forearm.

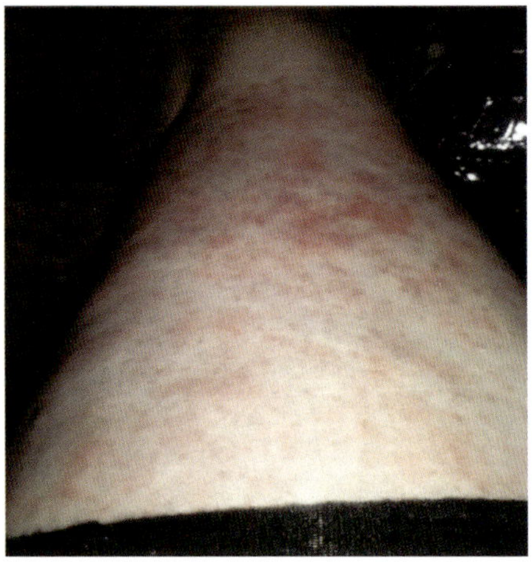

Figure 2: Maculopapular rash involving right leg.

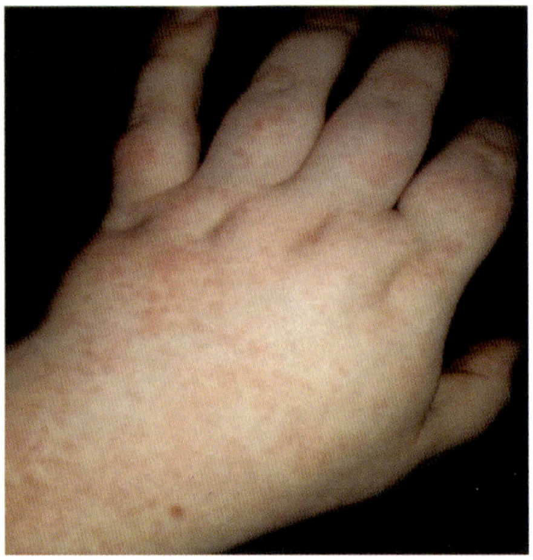

Figure 3: Maculopapular rash involving left hand.

seen once by the rheumatologists in those 2 years, and unfortunately during that consultation, she was symptom-free. She chose to follow up with the dermatologists from then on. She has had several admissions to hospital with similar symptoms and the repeat skin biopsy only revealed features of drug reaction without any evidence of vasculitis. Her last admission was 12 months ago with severe symptoms of widespread persistent, pruritic, and painful rash with high temperatures >39, raised inflammatory markers, and widespread arthralgia; however, there was no evidence of synovitis clinically.

Her laboratory findings were as shown in Table 1.

Her serological test results were as follows: antinuclear antibody (ANA) titre, negative; anti-ds-DNA, 9 units (normal value < 30); ANCA, negative; complements (C3, C4), normal; extractable nuclear antigen (ENA), negative; lupus inhibitor, not detected; immunoglobulin levels were normal with normal cryoglobulin levels.

She had negative hepatitis and HIV serological tests. Thyroid function test was found to be normal. Her extensive septic workup including chest X-ray and urine and multiple blood culture sensitivities were negative; cardiac echocardiogram was normal. PET scan revealed extensive lymphadenopathy involving lymph nodes above and below the diaphragms associated with splenomegaly and hepatomegaly. She subsequently underwent cervical excisional lymph node biopsy which revealed mixed nonspecific paracortical and follicular hyperplasia and excluded lymphoma. There was no family history to suggest a genetic origin to her symptoms. Based on the clinical, laboratory, and pathological examinations, the infectious, malignant, lymphoproliferative, and autoimmune disorders were excluded and probable diagnosis of AOSD was made as per Yamaguchi et al.'s criteria [1]. In our patient, she has had presence of three major criteria (fever > 39, arthralgia lasting 2 weeks or more, and leucocytosis) with an atypical rash and four minor criteria (sore throat, lymphadenopathy, splenomegaly, hepatomegaly, and negative tests for ANA and rheumatoid factor).

Our patient was treated with IL-1 antagonist, Anakinra 100 mg s/c daily (due to the poor response to high dose steroids and other DMARDs in the past). Notable clinical and laboratory regression was observed during her check a month later [2]. Her arthralgia and rash regressed. Laboratory results were serum ferritin 66 micrograms/L, ESR 3 mm/hr, CRP 7.5 mg/L, and haemoglobin 137 g/L. Outpatient follow-up of the patient continues.

3. Discussion

AOSD is rare systemic inflammatory disorder of unknown aetiology. In 1971, the term Adult Still's Disease was used to describe a series of adult patients who had features similar to the children with systemic juvenile idiopathic arthritis and did not fulfil criteria for classic rheumatoid arthritis. The diagnosis is often clinical and often diagnosis of exclusion. The classic skin rash in AOSD is an evanescent, salmon-coloured, macular, or maculopapular cutaneous eruption that is usually nonpruritic and tends to occur with fever and disappear during afebrile episode. The classical features on skin biopsy demonstrate perivascular inflammation of the superficial dermis with invasion of lymphocytes and histiocytes and immunohistochemistry sometimes positive for complement and immunoglobulin [3].

Leukocytoclastic vasculitis is a variant of cutaneous vasculitis. The characteristic features include maculopapular eruption, often painful or burning sensation with pruritus. Some authors state that leukocytoclastic vasculitis is vasculitis limited to skin, and some state that systemic involvement can be mild to moderate [4]. Many medications like penicillins, cephalosporins, sulphonamides, phenytoin, and allopurinol and infections like viral and bacterial infections can cause cutaneous vasculitis. In our case, there were no new medications commenced prior to the appearance of symptoms and all the serological tests for viral and bacterial infections were negative including autoimmune screen. The typical histological features in leukocytoclastic vasculitis include disruption of small vessels by inflammatory cells, deposition of fibrin within the lumen, and/or vessel wall coupled with nuclear debris that allows for the confident recognition of small vessel, mostly neutrophilic vasculitis [5]. The first biopsy in our patient showed features consistent with leukocytoclastic vasculitis as described and the second skin biopsy showed mild spongiotic reaction pattern with dermal inflammation including eosinophils, features suggestive of a drug reaction.

In our case, the rash was persistent, pruritic and tender, and recalcitrant to most medications, which is not a classical feature of AOSD. Even though the initial skin biopsy showed vasculitic picture, subsequent biopsies revealed urticarial reaction/drug reaction without any evidence of vasculitis. The nature of the rash and positive skin biopsy for vasculitis initially delayed the diagnosis of AOSD in our case. Coexistence of leukocytoclastic vasculitis and AOSD is very rare [6, 7]; however, persistent pruritic rash with AOSD is not uncommon [8, 9].

Recent advances revealed a pivotal role of proinflammatory cytokines such as tumour necrosis factor-alpha, IL-1, IL-6, and IL-18 in disease pathogenesis, giving rise to the development of novel targeted therapies aiming at optimal disease control [10].

4. Conclusion

In the initial stages of the disease, the diagnosis of AOSD is challenging due to the absence of specific or diagnostic clinical, serological, and pathological findings. The skin lesions of AOSD are important for the correct diagnosis. Persistent pruritic, erythematous maculopapules and plaques may be an atypical initial presentation of AOSD; therefore, it is important to consider various cutaneous manifestations of AOSD for an early and correct diagnosis [7].

Abbreviations

AOSD:	Adult Onset Still's Disease
NSAIDs:	Nonsteroidal anti-inflammatory drugs
IL-1:	Interleukin-1
IL-6:	Interleukin-6
DMARDs:	Disease modifying antirheumatoid drugs.

Consent

An informed consent was obtained.

References

[1] M. Yamaguchi, A. Ohta, T. Tsunematsu et al., "Preliminary criteria for classification of adult Still's disease," *Journal of Rheumatology*, vol. 19, no. 3, pp. 424–430, 1992.

[2] A. A. Fitzgerald, S. A. LeClercq, A. Yan, J. E. Homik, and C. A. Dinarello, "Rapid responses to anakinra in patients with refractory adult-onset Still's disease," *Arthritis and Rheumatism*, vol. 52, no. 6, pp. 1794–1803, 2005.

[3] P. Efthimiou, P. K. Paik, and L. Bielory, "Diagnosis and management of adult onset Still's disease," *Annals of the Rheumatic Diseases*, vol. 65, no. 5, pp. 564–572, 2006.

[4] S. Kobak, H. Yilmaz, A. Karaarslan, and M. Yalcin, "Leukocytoclastic vasculitis in a patient with ankylosing spondylitis," *Case Reports in Rheumatology*, vol. 2014, Article ID 653837, 3 pages, 2014.

[5] J. A. Carlson, "The histological assessment of cutaneous vasculitis," *Histopathology*, vol. 56, no. 1, pp. 3–23, 2010.

[6] A. V. Elezoglou, E. Giamarelos-Bourboulis, N. Katsilambros, and P. P. Sfikakis, "Cutaneous vasculitis associated with mixed cryoglobulinemia in adult Still's disease," *Clinical and Experimental Rheumatology*, vol. 21, no. 3, pp. 405–406, 2003.

[7] P. Bambery, R. J. Thomas, H. S. Malhotra, U. Kaur, S. R. Bhusnurmath, and S. D. Deodhar, "Adult onset Still's disease: clinical experience with 18 patients over 15 years in northern India," *Annals of the Rheumatic Diseases*, vol. 51, no. 4, pp. 529–532, 1992.

[8] J. Y.-Y. Lee, C.-K. Hsu, M.-F. Liu, and S.-C. Chao, "Evanescent and persistent pruritic eruptions of adult-onset still disease:

a clinical and pathologic study of 36 patients," *Seminars in Arthritis and Rheumatism*, vol. 42, no. 3, pp. 317–326, 2012.

[9] N. Kikuchi, M. Satoh, M. Ohtsuka, and T. Yamamoto, "Persistent pruritic papules and plaques associated with adult-onset Still's disease: report of six cases," *Journal of Dermatology*, vol. 41, no. 5, pp. 407–410, 2014.

[10] S. Kadavath and P. Efthimiou, "Adult-onset Still's disease—pathogenesis, clinical manifestations, and new treatment options," *Annals of Medicine*, vol. 47, no. 1, pp. 6–14, 2015.

36

Axial Spondyloarthritis and Autosomal Dominant Polycystic Kidney Disease in Two Siblings: A Rare Cooccurrence

Ozan Volkan Yurdakul,[1] **Abdulkerim Furkan Tamer**,[2] **Okan Küçükakkaş**,[1] **and Aylin Rezvani**[1]

[1]*Department of Physical Medicine and Rehabilitation, Bezmialem Foundation University, Istanbul, Turkey*
[2]*Department of Nephrology, Gaziosmanpasa Taksim Training and Research Hospital, Istanbul, Turkey*

Correspondence should be addressed to Ozan Volkan Yurdakul; yurdakul_ozan@yahoo.com

Academic Editor: Constantine Saadeh

Autosomal dominant polycystic kidney disease (ADPKD) is the most frequently occurring hereditary kidney disease, and axial spondyloarthritis (SpA) is one of the most frequently occurring rheumatic diseases. Treatment-related decisions for axial SpA may pose a challenge in case of renal involvement. The authors describe two siblings with cooccurrence of these two diseases. The association of these two diseases is not well known. Practitioners should monitor renal function in SpA patients and take treatment-related decisions regarding renal involvement. Antitumor necrosis factor-alpha (anti-TNF-α) agents may be used in case nonsteroidal anti-inflammatory drugs (NSAIDs) cannot be utilized.

1. Introduction

Autosomal dominant polycystic kidney disease (ADPKD), the most common hereditary kidney disease, is characterized by impaired urinary-concentrating ability, hypertension, polyuria, nocturia, nephrolithiasis, hematuria, infections, and progressive loss of kidney function with a prevalence of 2.41–3.89/10000 [1, 2].

ADPKD manifestation is caused either by polycystin-1 (PC-1), encoded by *PKD1* located on chromosome 16p13 in 80%–85% of patients, or by polycystin-2 (PC-2), encoded by *PKD2* located on chromosome 4q21 in 10%–15% of patients [3, 4]. Defects in any of these genes cause abnormal primary ciliary function resulting in cyst formation and growth [5].

Spondyloarthritis is a group of chronic inflammatory diseases primarily affecting the axial skeleton with 0.5%–1.9% prevalence, making it one of the most common rheumatic diseases [6]. Ankylosing spondylitis, the prototype of axial spondyloarthritis, is a polygenic multifactorial disease, and human leukocyte antigen- (HLA-) B27 plays a causal role in its pathogenesis [7]. Axial spondyloarthritis (SpA) treatment includes physical exercise, nonsteroidal anti-inflammatory drugs (NSAIDs), sulphasalazine for peripheral arthritis, and antitumor necrosis factor-alpha (anti-TNF-α) in case NSAIDs are ineffective [8]. Renal involvement is a rare but important complication that is mostly discounted in young patients. Renal complications are estimated to occur in 8%–13.3% of patients with ankylosing spondylitis (AS) [9, 10]. Microscopic hematuria, proteinuria, increased serum creatinine, and nephrotic syndrome are major manifestations, and secondary amyloid A amyloidosis (62%) and immunoglobulin A (IgA) nephropathy (30%) are the two most frequently reported causes of renal involvement [11, 12]. Tubulointerstitial nephritis caused by NSAID use is another cause [8]; renal involvement varies from asymptomatic deterioration of renal function to end-stage renal failure [8].

Although there are numerous articles regarding the general causes of renal involvement in axial SpA in the literature, to our knowledge, association of ADPKD and axial SpA has never been reported. Here, we report two siblings with concurrent ADPKD and axial SpA.

2. Case Report

2.1. Case 1. A 37-year-old male was admitted to the outpatient clinic with back pain lasting for 10 years. He was diagnosed with axial SpA at another center 1 year before and treated with indomethacin 50 mg daily and sulphasalazine 2000 mg daily. He had 20 minutes of morning stiffness and augmented back pain while resting which was indicative of inflammatory back pain. He did not have history of inflammatory bowel diseases, and his examination did not indicate enthesitis or arthritis. His complete blood count was 6,700 cells/μL white blood cells (WBCs) (N: 4,100–11,000), 4,240 cells/μL neutrophils (N: 2,000–8,000), 13.02 g/dL hemoglobin (Hgb) (N: 11–18), 41.3% hematocrit (HCT) (N: 35–55), and 146,000 platelets (PLTs) (N: 150,000–400,000). C-reactive protein (CRP) was 6.71 mg/dL ($N \leq 3.48$), erythrocyte sedimentation rate (ESR) 8 mm/h (N: 0–20), parathyroid hormone (PTH) 36.80 pg/ml (N: 12–88), serum creatinine (sCR) 0.81 mg/dL (N: 0.67–1.17), serum urea 46 mg/dL (N: 17–43), aspartate transaminase (AST) 16.9 U/L (N: 0–50), and alanine transaminase (ALT) 19 U/L (N: 0–50). Total urinalysis findings showed that urine density was 1.011 (N: 1.015–1.020) and other parameters were normal. The Rose Bengal test, hepatitis B surface antigen (HBs-Ag), anti-hepatitis C virus (HCV), and anti-Human Immunodeficiency Virus (HIV) were negative, and the patient was not HLA-B27 positive. A T1-weighted fat-suppressed gadolinium-enhanced MRI of the sacroiliac joints indicated joint space narrowing, bone erosions, subchondral sclerosis, and cortical irregularities in joint margins, indicating chronic damage and contrast agent uptake, both intra-articular and in the subchondral bone marrow, which is favorable for acute sacroiliitis (Figure 1). Lumbar MRI showed fatty degeneration on the anterior vertebral margins indicative of old Romanus lesions as well as multiple cysts and enlarged kidneys (Figures 2 and 3). These findings confirmed axial SpA diagnosis according to the Assessment of SpondyloArthritis international Society (ASAS) axial spondyloarthropathy classification criteria published in 2009 [13]. The clinical features, laboratory findings, and imaging results of the patient are shown in Table 1.

Following consultation with a nephrologist, the patient was diagnosed with ADPKD considering the existing family history of polycystic kidney disease, being asymptomatic until the 4th decade of life and occurring as multiple cysts and enlarged kidneys on MRI. The diagnosis of the ADPKD is based upon family history, clinical features, and imaging [4]. The patient was advised to use NSAIDs with caution as well as with frequent monitoring. Bath Ankylosing Spondylitis Disease Activity Index (BASDAI) was 6.5 and Bath Ankylosing Spondylitis Functional Index (BASFI) was 1.9. His indomethacin dose increased to 75 mg/day, and he was scheduled for a visit after 1 month, when his WBC was 6,300 cells/μL, serum urea 40 mg/dL, uric acid 5.72 mg/dL (N: 3.5–7.2), sCR 0.77 mg/dL, CRP 4.01 mg/dL, and ESR 6 mm/h; total urinalysis showed that density was 1.013 and other parameters were normal; BASDAI was 4.7 and BASFI was 1.5. Hence, his serum CRP levels decreased and activity score improved; considering the patient's renal risk, we maintained daily indomethacin dose and scheduled him for follow-up. Five months later, BASDAI was 6.7 and BASFI was 2 with 1 hour of morning stiffness. Test results indicated that WBC was 6,300 cells/μL, serum urea 29 mg/dL, uric acid 5.62 mg/dL, sCR 0.78 mg/dL, AST 17.4 U/L, ALT 14 U/L,

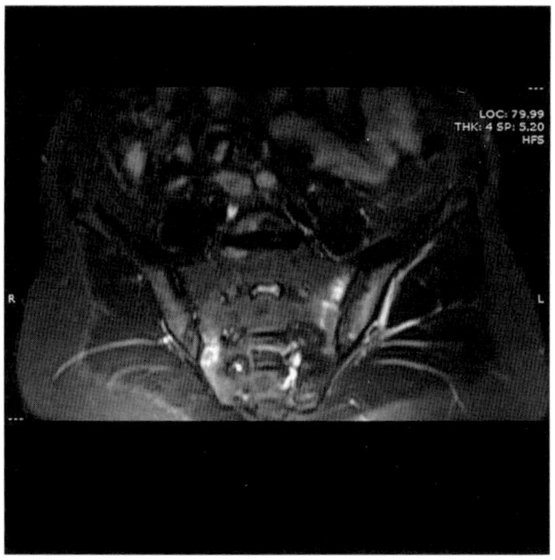

Figure 1: Coronal gadolinium-enhanced fat-suppressed T1-weighted MRI scan of the sacroiliac joints showing chronic degeneration and acute sacroiliitis.

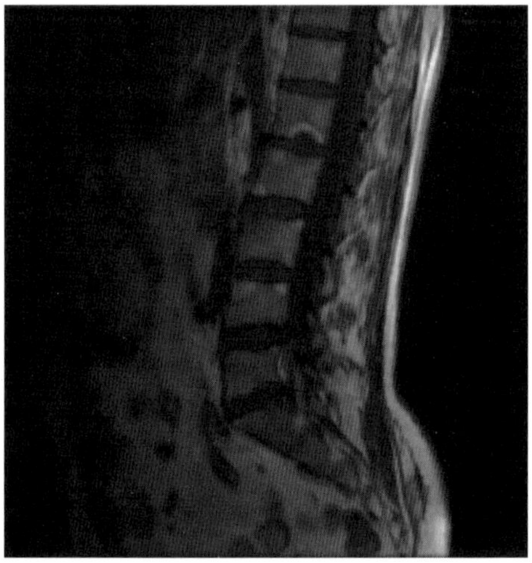

Figure 2: T1-weighted sagittal MRI scan of the lumbar spine indicating old Romanus lesions.

CRP 10.9 mg/dL, and ESR 30 mm/h. Spot urine sample demonstrated a protein-to-creatinine ratio of 0.180. The patient was administered 50 mg/week etanercept due to disease activity deterioration and serum inflammatory markers. Three weeks after the initial etanercept administration, BASDAI was 4.3, BASFI was 1.5, and morning stiffness duration was 30 minutes. Test results showed that WBC was 5,600/μL, serum urea 30 mg/dL, uric acid 6.37 mg/dL, sCR 0.82 mg/dL, serum sodium 138 mmol/L (N: 135–145), serum potassium 3.81 mmol/L (N: 3.5–5.1), AST 14.4 U/L, ALT 11 U/L, CRP 3.11 mg/dL, and ESR 7 mm/h. Total urinalysis findings demonstrated trace proteinuria on strip analysis. Spot urine sample demonstrated a protein-to-creatinine ratio of 0.133. The patient did not experience any side effects of etanercept regarding renal function besides a slight serum uric acid level increase.

One year after initial etanercept administration, the patient had BASDAI of 3.7 and BASFI of 1.4 with 20 minutes of morning stiffness. His final results were WBC 5,700 cells/μL,

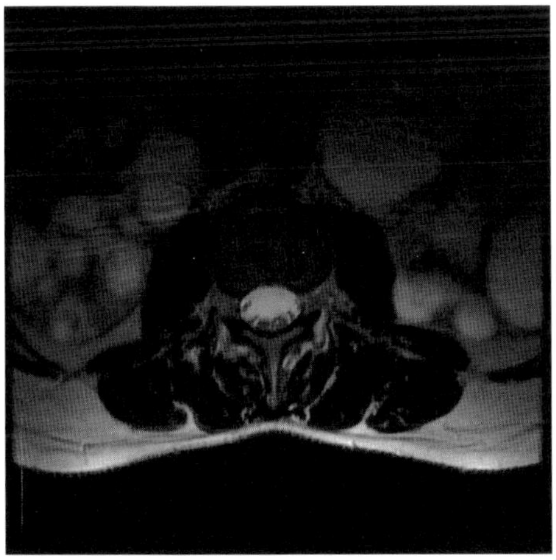

Figure 3: T2-weighted axial MRI scan indicating enlarged kidneys and multiple cysts.

Hgb 14.1 g/dL, PLT 210,000/μL, serum urea 41 mg/dL, sCR 0.88 mg/dL, ALT 8 U/L, CRP 3.14 mg/dL, and ESR 9 mm/h. His final total urinalysis was normal, and uric acid levels slightly increased at follow-up with a final level of 6.8 mg/dL.

2.2. Case 2. A 30-year-old female (the first patient's sister) was admitted to the outpatient clinic with inflammatory back pain complaints for 4 years, morning stiffness lasting 2 hours, a history of transient heel pain, and no history of arthritis. In addition, her examination did not indicate any actual enthesitis despite family history. Complete blood count demonstrated 6,700 cells/μL WBC (N: 4,100–11,000), 4,510 cells/μL neutrophils (N: 2,000–8,000), 12.7 g/dL Hgb (N: 11–18), 38.5% HCT (N: 35–55), and 208,000/μL PLT (N: 150,000–400,000). She had levels of CRP 5.56 mg/dL (N $\leq$ 3.48), ESR 28 mm/h (N: 0–20), sCR 0.54 mg/dL (N: 0.67–1.17), AST 19 U/L (N: 0–50), and ALT 11 U/L (N: 0–50). Total urinalysis findings showed 1.020 density (N: 1.015–1.020), 6.0 pH (N: 5.0–7.0), 10 erythrocytes, and 42 leukocytes. The Rose Bengal test, HBs-Ag, anti-HCV, anti-HIV, and HLA-B27 were negative. A plain anteroposterior radiograph of the patient's pelvis showed grade 3 sacroiliitis on the right side and grade 2 sacroiliitis on the left side (Figure 4). A T2 fat-suppressed sacroiliac joint MRI demonstrated widespread edematous T2 signal augmentation on the sacral sides of the bilateral sacroiliac joints, indicating acute sacroiliitis and bilateral sclerosis (Figure 5). Lumbar MRI revealed Modic type 2 degeneration on the anterior aspects of L1, L2, and L3 vertebrae, indicating old Romanus lesions, multiple cysts, and enlarged kidneys (Figures 6 and 7). She was diagnosed with axial SpA according to ASAS 2009 axial spondyloarthritis classification criteria [13]. The clinical features, laboratory findings, and imaging results of the patient are shown in Table 1. She had a BASDAI of 5.8 and a BASFI of 5.3. After consulting with a nephrologist, she was also diagnosed with ADPKD and started on acemetacin 90 mg daily under strict monitoring. Three weeks after initial treatment, her results were WBC 7,100 cells/μL, neutrophils 4,780 cells/μL, CRP 14.6 mg/dL, ESR 30 mm/h, sCR 0.58 mg/dL, AST 11.4 U/L, and ALT 10 U/L; with the exception of 15 erythrocytes, total urinalysis was within normal limits. Morning stiffness duration improved to 30 minutes, with a BASDAI of 5 and a BASFI of 4.7. Her medication was changed to dexketoprofen trometamol 50 mg/day. One month later, WBC was 8,300 cells/μL, neutrophils 5,330 cells/μL, CRP 3.51 mg/L, ESR 24 mm/h, serum uric acid 5.06 mg/dL, sCR 0.58 mg/dL, AST 10 U/L, and ALT 12 U/L. BASDAI was 5.1, BASFI was 4.2, and morning stiffness duration was 20 minutes. She was followed up for 1 year and did not have any acute episodes, but experienced apparent bacteriuria with symptoms and required antibiotics twice. Her final results were WBC 8,700 cells/μL, neutrophils 6,150 cells/μL, Hgb 12 g/dL, HCT 37.8%, PLT 196,000/μL, CRP 1.26 mg/dL, ESR 15 mm/h, sCR 0.72 mg/dL, serum uric acid 6.6 mg/dL, AST 10 U/L, and ALT 12 U/L, with a spot urine protein-to-creatinine ratio of 0.09. Final total urinalysis showed 5 erythrocytes, 6 leukocytes, and 17 squamous epithelium. BASDAI was 4.3 and BASFI was 4, and the patient had morning stiffness for 1 hour, making her a candidate for an anti-TNF agent.

3. Discussion

Renal involvement among AS patients was reported as high as 13.3% [10–12]. Therefore, patients with AS should be regularly monitored for renal complications. Ironically, NSAIDs are recommended as first-choice drugs for axial SpA, and NSAID-caused tubulointerstitial nephritis is another important cause of renal complications [8, 14]. Also, a recent study demonstrated that frequent NSAID use may cause 2- to 3-fold elevation of kidney injury molecule 1 (KIM1), cystatin C (Cys-C), and neutrophil gelatinase-associated lipocalin (NGAL) in urine and serum due to acute kidney injury; serum levels of these molecules return to normal 12 weeks later following drug cessation [11]. However, end-stage renal disease as a result of long-term NSAIDs is rare without preexisting kidney dysfunction [11, 15]. For patients with impaired renal function, prostaglandin production mediated by cyclooxygenase 1 (COX-1) and COX-2, which are inhibited by NSAIDs, has a major compensatory effect in sustaining renal hemodynamic function [16].

Screening the extra-articular manifestations in axial SpA patients may influence treatment decisions [17]. Physicians may vacillate between types of NSAID used to alleviate disease activity and preserve kidney function. Patients with ADPKD generally progress to end-stage renal disease by 60 years of age, 70% of these patients require renal transplantation by 70 years of age [18]. Delaying the progressive kidney function loss or end-stage renal disease significantly improves quality of life in these patients [4]. In such cases, anti-TNF-α treatment is indicated for conserving renal function. It is not reported to be contraindicated in renal impairment cases, and TNF-α induces glomerular inflammation and permeability [19]. Lee et al. [9] reported significant reduction in proteinuria due to amyloidosis from 3,702 mg/day to 200 mg/day in an AS patient treated with etanercept for 12 months. They reported an AS patient with accompanying IgA nephropathy in whom CRP and BASDAI levels were

Table 1: Clinical features, initial test results, and imaging results of patients.

	Case 1	Case 2
Age	37	30
Gender	Male	Female
Symptoms		
	Inflammatory back pain and 20 minutes of morning stiffness	Inflammatory back pain, 2 hours of morning stiffness, and transient heel pain history
Laboratory findings		
White blood cells (WBCs) (N: 4,100–11,000 cells/μL)	6,700	6,700
Neutrophils (N: 2,000–8,000 cells/μL)	4,240	4,510
Hemoglobin (Hgb) (N: 11–18 g/dL)	13.02	12.7
Hematocrit (HCT) (N: 35–55%)	41.3	38.5
Platelets (PLTs) (N: 150,000–400,000 cells/μL)	146,000	208,000
C-reactive protein (CRP) (N $\leq$ 3.48 mg/dL)	6.71	5.56
Erythrocyte sedimentation rate (ESR) (N: 0–20 mm/h)	8	28
Serum creatinine (sCR) (N: 0.67–1.17 mg/dL)	0.81	0.54
Aspartate transaminase (AST) (N: 0–50 U/L)	16.9	19
Alanine transaminase (ALT) (N: 0–50 U/L)	19	11
Total urinalysis findings	1.011 density (N: 1.015–1.020), and other parameters were normal	1.020 density (N: 1.015–1.020), 10 erythrocytes, and 42 leukocytes
The Rose Bengal test	Negative	Negative
Hepatitis B surface antigen (HBs-Ag)	Negative	Negative
Anti-hepatitis C virus (HCV)	Negative	Negative
Anti-human immunodeficiency virus (HIV)	Negative	Negative
Human leukocyte antigen- (HLA-) B27	Negative	Negative
Imaging		
	T1-weighted, fat-suppressed, gadolinium-enhanced MRI scan showed acute sacroiliitis	Pelvis anteroposterior radiograph showed right grade 3 sacroiliitis and left grade 2 sacroiliitis
	MRI scan indicated old Romanus lesions and polycystic kidneys	MRI scan indicated old Romanus lesions and polycystic kidneys

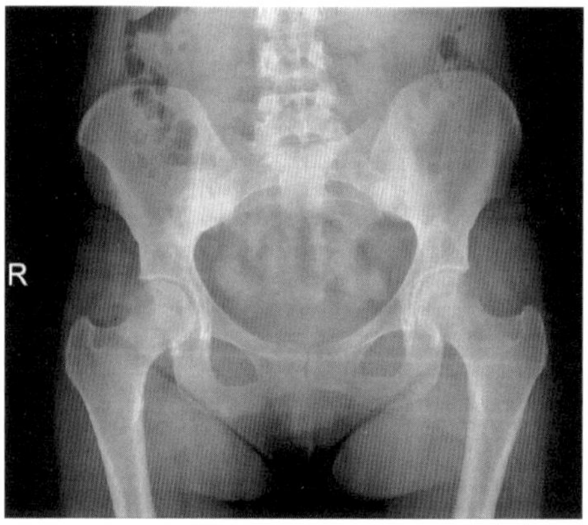

Figure 4: Plain radiograph of the sacroiliac joints demonstrating right grade 3 and left grade 2 sacroiliitis.

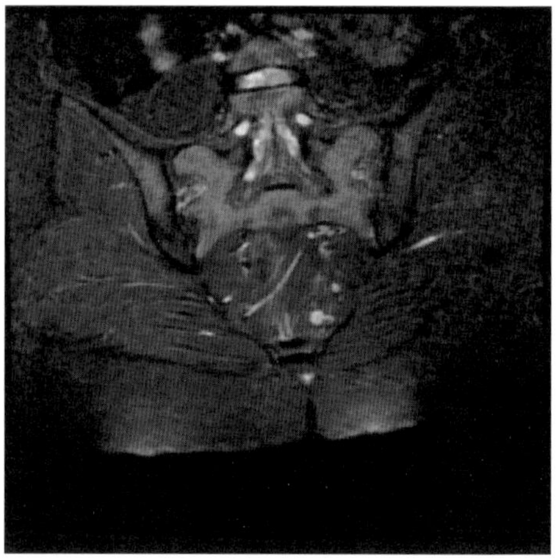

Figure 5: Coronal fat-suppressed T2-weighted MRI scan of the sacroiliac joints in favor of acute sacroiliitis and bilateral sclerosis.

normalized using infliximab although proteinuria was unalleviated. In the same study, another AS patient with IgA nephropathy, who was treated with adalimumab, showed proteinuria alleviation. They concluded that initial serum creatinine levels may be important in predicting anti-TNF-α treatment response [9].

Jacquet et al. [20] reported an AS patient with normal renal function who developed microscopic hematuria and proteinuria after 2-year initial anti-TNF-α treatment and was treated with infliximab. The authors determined that hematuria remained at 3 years and proteinuria increased to 1.75 g/day. Renal biopsy demonstrated IgA nephropathy. Anti-TNF-α treatment induces a shift from T-helper type-1 pattern (e.g., interleukin 1 (IL-1), TNF, and interferon gamma

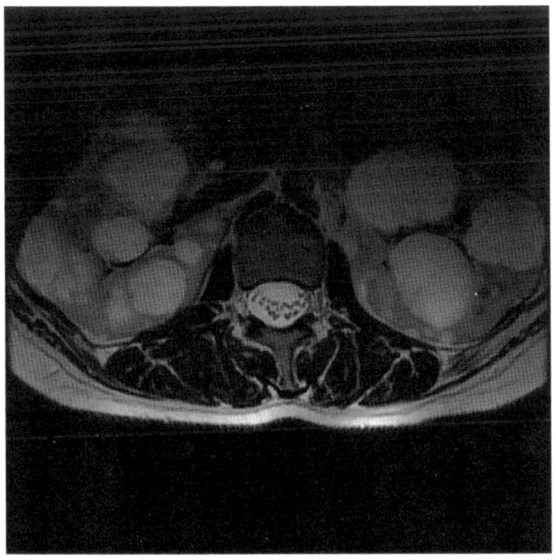

FIGURE 6: T2-weighted axial MRI scan showing polycystic kidneys.

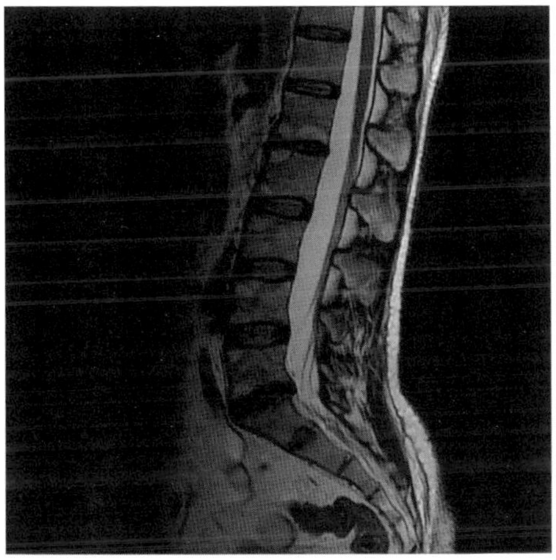

FIGURE 7: T2 sagittal MRI scan of the lumbar spine revealing Modic type 2 degeneration.

(IFγ)) to T-helper type-2 pattern (e.g., IL-4, IL-5, IL-6, IL-10, and IL-13), hence promoting antibody-mediated immunity; this may lead to IgA-mediated renal involvement [20].

Lee et al. [21] monitored a patient with secondary amyloidosis due to AS. Following etanercept treatment for 17 months, amyloid deposits showed slightly regressed histopathology even though proteinuria recovered. Anti-TNF treatment probably alleviates proteinuria by reducing serum amyloid A levels but is insufficient for resolving amyloid deposits [21, 22].

To our knowledge, this is the first case reporting an association between axial SpA and ADPKD. This cooccurrence may be coincidental, or an undiscovered alternate gene or pathway may be responsible for this association considering the HLA-B27 negativity of both patients. Alterations in PC1 and PC2 function result in changes in intracellular calcium and cyclic adenosine monophosphate (cAMP) levels and subsequent mechanistic target of rapamycin (mTOR) pathway alterations [5]. mTOR-controlled metabolic pathways are likely to shape the repertoire of both adaptive and innate inflammatory cells in AS, making the mTOR pathway a possible cause of increased inflammation and AS [23].

In conclusion, although dependency of axial SpA and ADPKD is not well known, this study shows a possible link between these two diseases. Practitioners should consider renal involvement in axial SpA patients and make treatment decisions according to renal complications.

Consent

Informed consent was obtained from all individual participants included in the manuscript.

References

[1] P. A. Gabow, "Autosomal dominant polycystic kidney disease," *New England Journal of Medicine*, vol. 329, no. 5, pp. 332–342, 1993.

[2] C. J. Willey, J. D. Blais, A. K Hall, H. B. Krasa, A. J. Makin, and F. S. Czerwiec, "Prevalence of autosomal dominant polycystic kidney disease in the European Union," *Nephrology Dialysis Transplantation*, vol. 32, no. 8, pp. 1356–1363, 2017.

[3] W. E. Sweeney and E. D. Avner, "Molecular and cellular pathophysiology of autosomal recessive polycystic kidney disease (ARPKD)," *Cell and Tissue Research*, vol. 326, no. 3, pp. 671–685, 2006.

[4] M. B. Lanktree and A. B. Chapman, "New treatment paradigms for ADPKD: moving towards precision medicine," *Nature Reviews Nephrology*, vol. 13, no. 12, pp. 750–768, 2017.

[5] P. C. Harris and V. E. Torres, "Genetic mechanisms and signaling pathways in autosomal dominant polycystic kidney disease," *Journal of Clinical Investigation*, vol. 124, no. 6, pp. 2315–2324, 2014.

[6] M. Rudwaleit, D. van der Heijde, M. A. Khan, J. Braun, and J. Sieper, "How to diagnose axial spondyloarthritis early," *Annals of the Rheumatic Diseases*, vol. 63, no. 5, pp. 535–543, 2004.

[7] E. Dakwar, J. Reddy, F. L. Vale, and J. S. Uribe, "A review of the pathogenesis of ankylosing spondylitis," *Neurosurgical Focus*, vol. 24, no. 1, p. E2, 2008.

[8] C. Mercieca, I. E. van der Horst-Bruinsma, and A. A. Borg, "Pulmonary, renal and neurological comorbidities in patients with ankylosing spondylitis; implications for clinical practice," *Current Rheumatology Reports*, vol. 16, no. 8, p. 434, 2014.

[9] S. H. Lee, E. J. Lee, S. W. Chung et al., "Renal involvement in ankylosing spondylitis: prevalence, pathology, response to TNF-a blocker," *Rheumatology International*, vol. 33, no. 7, pp. 1689–1692, 2013.

[10] C. Ben Taarit, H. Ajlani, F. Ben Moussa, T. Ben Abdallah, H. Ben Maiz, and A. Khedher, "Renal involvement in ankylosing spondylitis: concerning 210 cases," *La Revue de Medecine Interne*, vol. 26, no. 12, pp. 966–969, 2005.

[11] A. Shukla, M. K. Rai, N. Prasad, and V. Agarwal, "Short-term non-steroid anti-inflammatory drug use in spondyloarthritis patients induces subclinical acute kidney injury: biomarkers study," *Nephron*, vol. 135, no. 4, pp. 277–286, 2017.

[12] E. S. Strobel and E. Fritschka, "Renal diseases in ankylosing spondylitis: review of the literature illustrated by case reports," *Clinical Rheumatology*, vol. 17, no. 6, pp. 524–530, 1998.

[13] J. Sieper, M. Rudwaleit, X. Baraliakos et al., "The Assessment of SpondyloArthritis international Society (ASAS) handbook: a guide to assess spondyloarthritis," *Annals of the Rheumatic Diseases*, vol. 68, no. 2, pp. ii1–i44, 2009.

[14] D. van der Heijde, S. Ramiro, R. Landewe et al., "2016 update of the ASAS-EULAR management recommendations for axial spondyloarthritis," *Annals of the Rheumatic Diseases*, vol. 76, no. 6, pp. 978–991, 2017.

[15] A. Whelton, "Nephrotoxicity of nonsteroidal anti-inflammatory drugs: physiologic foundations and clinical implications," *American Journal of Medicine*, vol. 106, no. 5, pp. 13s–24s, 1999.

[16] M. D. Murray and D. C. Brater, "Renal toxicity of the non-steroidal anti-inflammatory drugs," *Annual Review of Pharmacology and Toxicology*, vol. 33, pp. 435–465, 1993.

[17] A. El Maghraoui, "Extra-articular manifestations of ankylosing spondylitis: prevalence, characteristics and therapeutic implications," *European Journal of Internal Medicine*, vol. 22, no. 6, pp. 554–560, 2011.

[18] E. M. Spithoven, A. Kramer, E. Meijer et al., "Renal replacement therapy for autosomal dominant polycystic kidney disease (ADPKD) in Europe: prevalence and survival–an analysis of data from the ERA-EDTA registry," *Nephrology Dialysis Transplantation*, vol. 29, no. 4, pp. iv15–iv25, 2014.

[19] E. T. McCarthy, R. Sharma, M. Sharma et al., "TNF-alpha increases albumin permeability of isolated rat glomeruli through the generation of superoxide," *Journal of the American Society of Nephrology*, vol. 9, no. 3, pp. 433–438, 1998.

[20] A. Jacquet, H. Francois, C. Frangie et al., "IgA nephropathy associated with ankylosing spondylitis is not controlled by infliximab therapy," *Nephrology Dialysis Transplantation*, vol. 24, no. 11, pp. 3540–3542, 2009.

[21] Y. H. Lee, E. Y. Kim, D. W. Jeong et al., "Complete remission of nephrotic syndrome without resolution of amyloid deposit after anti-tumor necrosis factor alpha therapy in a patient with ankylosing spondylitis," *Journal of Clinical Rheumatology*, vol. 22, no. 2, pp. 86–88, 2016.

[22] G. R. Smith, K. E. Tymms, and M. Falk, "Etanercept treatment of renal amyloidosis complicating rheumatoid arthritis," *Internal Medicine Journal*, vol. 34, no. 9-10, pp. 570–572, 2004.

[23] A. Perl, "Activation of mTOR (mechanistic target of rapamycin) in rheumatic diseases," *Nature Reviews Rheumatology*, vol. 12, no. 3, pp. 169–182, 2016.

37

Eosinophilic Esophagitis in Two Patients with Systemic Sclerosis

Tracy M. Frech,[1] Kathleen Boynton,[2] Erinn Downs-Kelly,[3] Bryan Jones,[4] John D. Kriesel,[5] and Kathryn Peterson[2]

[1]*Division of Rheumatology, Department of Internal Medicine, University of Utah School of Medicine, 4B200 30 N. 1900 E., Salt Lake City, UT 84132, USA*
[2]*Division of Gastroenterology, Department of Internal Medicine, University of Utah, 50 N Medical Drive, Salt Lake City, UT 84132, USA*
[3]*Department of Anatomic Pathology, University of Utah, 50 N Medical Drive, Salt Lake City, UT 84132, USA*
[4]*Department of Ophthalmology, University of Utah, 50 N Medical Drive, Salt Lake City, UT 84132, USA*
[5]*Division of Infectious Diseases, Department of Internal Medicine, University of Utah, 50 N Medical Drive, Salt Lake City, UT 84132, USA*

Correspondence should be addressed to Tracy M. Frech; tracy.frech@hsc.utah.edu

Academic Editor: James V. Dunne

The gastrointestinal tract (GIT) is the most common extracutaneous organ system damaged in systemic sclerosis (SSc) and is the presenting feature in 10% of patients. The esophagus as the portion of the GIT is the most commonly affected and there is an association of gastroesophageal reflux (GER) with SSc interstitial lung disease (ILD). Thus, an aggressive treatment for GER is recommended in all SSc patients with ILD; however, it is recognized that a long-term benefit to this treatment is needed to understand its impact. In this case report we discuss the presence of eosinophilic esophagitis (EoE) in two SSc patients and discuss the role for early EGD in SSc patients with moderate-severe GER symptoms for tissue study. Assessment of esophageal biopsy specimens for the presence of eosinophils and possibly ANA can help elucidate disease pathogenesis and direct therapy, as the presence of EoE in SSc has important management considerations, particularly with regards to dietary modification strategies.

1. Introduction

The mechanisms of systemic sclerosis (SSc, scleroderma) which cause vascular changes, immunological abnormalities, and excessive accumulation of collagen in the submucosa are not well understood. The gastrointestinal tract (GIT) is the most common extracutaneous organ system damaged in SSc and is the presenting feature in 10% of patients [1]. Over the course of the disease, GIT complaints occur in almost all of SSc patients [2, 3] and are associated with significant morbidity and mortality [3–5]. The esophagus is most commonly affected by SSc; however the histopathologic changes of smooth muscle atrophy and intestinal wall fibrosis are found throughout the GIT [6].

2. Gastroesophageal Reflux in Systemic Sclerosis

The most common GIT symptom in SSc is gastroesophageal reflux (GER), which is defined as the regurgitation of gastric contents into the esophagus, mainly due to loss of lower esophageal sphincter pressure. A characteristic radiographic feature of SSc is a patulous (i.e., wide open or distended) esophagus [7]. Few objective measures to assess mucosal involvement and motility in GIT have been validated in SSc and most are invasive [5]. Since, GER can be suspected in the presence of a wide open gastroesophageal junction, often this SSc feature is treated with recommendations for dietary changes and avoiding foods that promote reflux and reflux-inducing positions. In addition, acid-reducing treatment, such as proton pump inhibitors (PPI) and/or histamine (H_2) receptor antagonists prior to referral to gastroenterology for endoscopy, is recommended. Due to an association of GER with SSc interstitial lung disease (ILD), an aggressive treatment for GER is recommended in all SSc patients with ILD; however, it is recognized that a long-term benefit to this treatment is needed to understand its impact [8, 9].

Acid suppression for GER, however, is not without risk. The use of acid suppression has been associated with an increased risk of upper and lower respiratory tract infections and small intestine bacterial overgrowth [10]. Nonetheless, SSc is associated with an increased risk of Barrett's esophagus (BE) and esophageal adenocarcinoma (EAC) thought to be related to chronic reflux [11]. However, data suggests that intestinal metaplasia of the squamocolumnar junction in SSc might not be related to GER and may result from other factors in the pathogenesis of SSc [12]. As such, understanding the pathogenesis of esophageal changes is of clinical significance in SSc.

3. The Role of Esophagogastroduodenoscopy in Systemic Sclerosis

Esophagogastroduodenoscopy (EGD) is suggested to be of value both early and late in a SSc patient's course, even if the patient does not report typical symptoms [13]. Endoscopic ultrasound (EUS) in SSc demonstrates that the submucosa and muscularis are enlarged, strengthening the hypothesis that increased matrix deposition is an important aspect in the pathogenesis of GI involvement in SSc [14]. However, the role for esophageal biopsy in SSc has not been established. Commonly mucosal esophageal biopsy results are reported as "long-term changes consistent with SSc"; thus the invasiveness of a procedure must be carefully balanced with the information provided [15]. EGD is often indicated for pneumatic balloon dilatation in SSc [16]. Previous esophageal biopsy studies have helped elucidate aspects of disease pathogenesis, suggesting that SSc is not part of the IgG4-related disease spectrum which is in part characterized by fibrosis [17].

Eosinophilic esophagitis (EoE) has not been previously reported in systemic sclerosis but shares similar disease features. EoE is an allergic inflammatory disease that like SSc leads to esophageal fibrosis and stricture. As detailed by the American College of Gastroenterology guidelines, the diagnosis of EoE is a clinicopathologic correlate with the criteria including symptoms of esophageal dysfunction; eosinophilic inflammation localized to the esophagus, with at least 15 eosinophils per high power field in esophageal mucosal biopsies; and exclusion of other recognized causes of esophageal eosinophilia, including proton pump inhibitor-responsive esophageal eosinophilia [18]. Thus, there may be additional diagnostic roles for EGD in SSc to better assess presence of allergic response, in addition to pneumatic dilatation or Barrett's monitoring.

4. Case Presentation

4.1. Patient 1. A 36-year-old female presented to our SSc clinic with diffuse cutaneous SSc and Raynaud's for 5 years with the onset of rapidly evolving skin thickening over 3 months and a modified Rodnan skin score (mRSS) of 13. Her oral aperture was normal. She had facial telangiectasia. No synovitis or tendon friction rubs were noted. She did not have digital ulcerations or pits but did have abnormal nailfold capillaroscopy. Her antinuclear antibody (ANA) was 1 : 160, but SSc-specific antibodies were negative. At presentation, her University of California Los Angeles Scleroderma Clinical Trials Consortium Gastrointestinal Questionnaire (GIT 2.0) was significant for severe scores for reflux and bloating. She reported a recent EGD at an outside hospital 3-month prior, which revealed eosinophilic esophagitis. Normal upper third of esophagus, middle third of esophagus, and lower third of esophagus were described endoscopically. Biopsies from the stomach and duodenum had no features of *Helicobacter pylori* gastritis or celiac disease, respectively. She was treated with pneumatic dilatation, but she had not received any other treatment, including steroid, prior to presentation to SSc clinic. After her visit to SSc clinic, the patient was referred to an allergist, and she was diagnosed with allergies to peanuts, milk, chocolate, and wheat by radioallergosorbent test. She eliminated these foods from her diet and returned to SSc two months later. Her mRSS had increased to 15; otherwise her physical exam was unchanged. She reported fatigue and Raynaud's as significantly improved (despite no change in seasonal temperatures). Her GIT 2.0 improved from previously severe to now mild scores for reflux and bloating. Remarkably she had repeat endoscopy, which showed resolution of erythema with a report, which read as "normal upper third of esophagus, middle third of esophagus, and lower third of esophagus and stomach". Manometry studies were not done.

4.2. Patient 2. 51-year-old female presented with diffuse cutaneous systemic sclerosis with 2 years of Raynaud's and 6 months of progressive skin thickening and severe GER. Before coming to the University of Utah SSc clinic, she had EGD which noted an esophagitis with a peak density of 20 intraepithelial eosinophils/high powered field (hpf) (Figure 1(a)). Her *Helicobacter pylori* and celiac studies were negative. She was placed on a twice a day PPI. She did not receive steroid therapy. She presented to the SSc clinic 2 months later with a mRSS of 8. She was noted to have normal oral aperture and nailfold capillaroscopy. Her ANA and SSc antibody profile were normal. Her GIT 2.0 was notable for severe reflux, bloating, and diarrhea scores. She was empirically placed on a low Fermentable Oligo-Di-Monosaccharides and Polyols (FODMap) diet and probiotic in addition to the twice a day PPI she was already taking. Due to cough and dyspnea, pulmonary function tests (PFT) and an echocardiogram were obtained. The PFT noted an isolated decrease in diffusion capacity with normal spirometry. The echocardiogram was normal. As such, high resolution computed tomography of the chest was obtained to assess for the presence of early interstitial lung disease, which noted intralobular septal thickening limited to the lung bases with bronchiectasis and a mildly dilated air filled esophagus. She returned to SSc clinic one month later with a mrSS 15 and dysphagia. Her SCTC GIT 2.0 remained moderate-severe

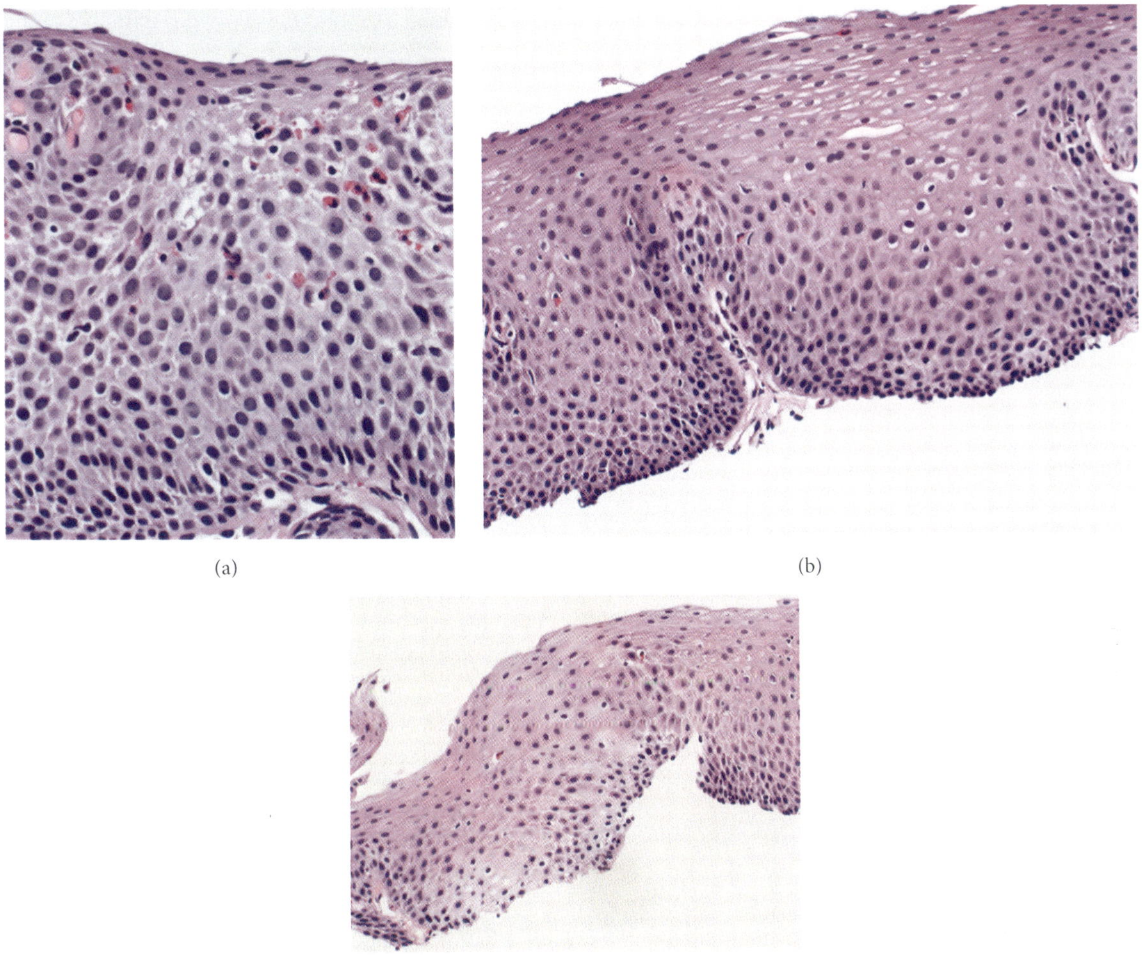

(a) (b) (c)

Figure 1: (a) Patient 2 at time of initial EGD wherein the esophageal squamous epithelium contains a peak density of 20 eosinophils per high power field. (b and c) Esophageal biopsies taken after treatment with a proton pump inhibitor and dietary modification with (b) representing the distal esophagus with a peak density of 5 intraepithelial eosinophils per hpf and (c) representing the proximal esophagus with a peak density of 3 intraepithelial eosinophils per hpf.

for reflux. Flexible laryngoscopy was normal. Manometry was not done. Her repeat EGD reported persistent chronic esophagitis while the corresponding histopathology showed a peak density of 3 intraepithelial eosinophils/hpf within the proximal esophagus and a peak density of 5 intraepithelial eosinophils/hpf within the distal esophagus (Figures 1(b) and 1(c)). Normal upper third of esophagus, middle third of esophagus, and lower third of esophagus were reported. An immunofluorescence for ANA sent on this esophagus biopsy specimen was positive (Figure 2).

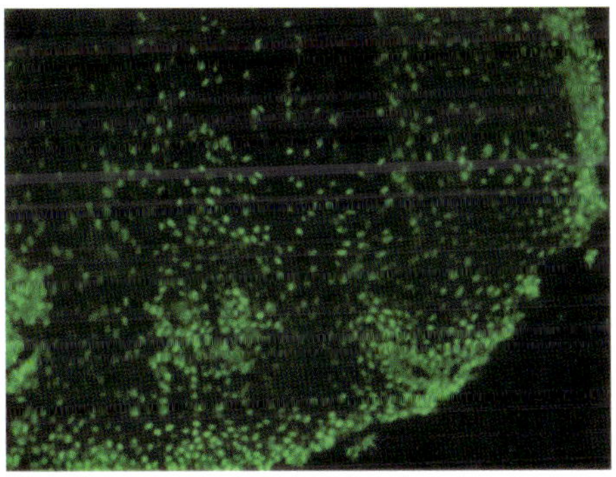

Figure 2: Esophageal tissue stained for ANA.

5. Discussion

These 2 case reports describe the presence of EoE and proton pump inhibitor-responsive esophageal eosinophilia in two diffuse SSc patients. The occurrence of these two conditions highlights the importance of early EGD in SSc patients with esophageal complaints, since tissue is required for diagnosis. The latter case also highlights the potential utility of tissue ANA. In the first patient, elimination diet improved Raynaud's and GIT symptoms and EGD findings dramatically improved. EoE is thought to be primarily a food antigen driven phenomenon and such dietary modification may alleviate symptoms of both EoE and associated diseases. In the second patient, the low FODMAP diet did not significantly improve symptoms, but eosinophils on esophageal biopsy specimen decreased. EoE can be treated with dietary strategies or topical corticosteroids, such as fluticasone and budesonide [19], but steroids are generally avoided because of steroid association with scleroderma renal crisis. Similar to SSc, endoscopic dilation has also become an important tool for treatment of fibrostenotic complications of EoE.

In EoE esophageal epithelial cells are thought to make a mesenchymal cell transition and are the effector cells in EoE-associated fibrogenesis [20]. This is a similar mechanism to that of SSc skin pathogenesis. Since SSc is a rare disease, we were interested whether these two case reports are representative of the SSc population as a whole. We searched the Utah Population Database (UPDB), which is a rich resource for research involving genetic, epidemiological, demographic, public health, and health services delivery studies and has previously been used successfully in studying SSc pedigrees [21, 22]. The majority of families residing in Utah are represented in the database, with a special emphasis on genealogy records of the European founders of Utah and their Utah descendants. Studies using UPDB rely on the linkage between UPDB pedigree structure data, its extensive stores of information about disease incidence and prevalence, and a wide range of additional demographic, geographic, and vital information on more than 7.7 million individuals. For our analysis 2263 well characterized patients with SSc and 4423 patients with EoE were identified, with 11 patients found having diagnostic codes for both SSc and EoE (Table 1(a)). When these patients were age and gender matched for controls (Table 1(b)), the EoE cases were found to have 6 times the risk of SSc (Table 1(c)). While the overlap of EoE and SSc was found to be significant in second-degree relatives (grandparents and cousins), it was not found in first-degree relatives (parents and siblings), making the heritability association of these conditions of question. Nonetheless, this study supports a potential shared pathogenesis between EoE and SSc.

Table 1: Utah population database assessment of eosinophilic esophagitis and systemic sclerosis overlap (a) compared to age and gender matched controls (b) and sorted by heritability (c).

(a)

	Patients with systemic sclerosis	Patients with EoE	Patients with EoE and systemic sclerosis (using EoE diagnosis date)
Age at diagnosis range (median)	1–98 (54)	3–92 (35)	15–83 (66)
Diagnosis year range	1979–2013	2008–2013	2009–2013
Total number of patients	2263	4423	11

(b)

Relationship	Cases		Controls	
	Affected	Unaffected	Affected	Unaffected
Proband	11	4343	10	23937
First degree	18	20204	73	96573
Second degree	44	37934	139	176460

(c)

Relationship	Logistic regression		
	Odds ratio	Confidence interval	*P* value
Proband	6.12	2.59–14.46	$3.57e-05$
First degree	1.19	0.71–2	0.508
Second degree	1.47	1.04–2.06	0.0274

6. Conclusion

This study supports early EGD in SSc patients with moderate-severe GER symptoms for tissue study. Assessment of esophageal biopsy specimens for the presence of eosinophils and possibly ANA can help elucidate disease pathogenesis and direct therapy, as the presence of EoE in SSc has important management considerations, particularly with regards to dietary modification strategies.

Acknowledgments

The University of Utah Center for Clinical and Translational Science and the Program in Personalized Health Collaborative Pilot Proposal supported the protected time for collaborative meetings of these investigators.

References

[1] X.-P. Tian and X. Zhang, "Gastrointestinal complications of systemic sclerosis," *World Journal of Gastroenterology*, vol. 19, no. 41, pp. 7062–7068, 2013.

[2] G. Gyger and M. Baron, "Gastrointestinal manifestations of scleroderma: recent progress in evaluation, pathogenesis, and management," *Current Rheumatology Reports*, vol. 14, no. 1, pp. 22–29, 2012.

[3] T. Schmeiser, P. Saar, D. Jin et al., "Profile of gastrointestinal involvement in patients with systemic sclerosis," *Rheumatology International*, vol. 32, no. 8, pp. 2471–2478, 2012.

[4] V. D. Steen and T. A. Medsger Jr., "Severe organ involvement in systemic sclerosis with diffuse scleroderma," *Arthritis and Rheumatism*, vol. 43, no. 11, pp. 2437–2444, 2000.

[5] D. Khanna, V. Nagaraja, H. Gladue, W. Chey, M. Pimentel, and T. Frech, "Measuring response in the gastrointestinal tract in systemic sclerosis," *Current Opinion in Rheumatology*, vol. 25, no. 6, pp. 700–706, 2013.

[6] R. Domsic, K. Fasanella, and K. Bielefeldt, "Gastrointestinal manifestations of systemic sclerosis," *Digestive Diseases and Sciences*, vol. 53, no. 5, pp. 1163–1174, 2008.

[7] S.-H. Huang, C.-C. Lai, and S.-H. Lin, "Characteristic radiologic features of systemic sclerosis," *Internal Medicine*, vol. 52, no. 18, p. 2167, 2013.

[8] R. B. Christmann, A. U. Wells, V. L. Capelozzi, and R. M. Silver, "Gastroesophageal reflux incites interstitial lung disease in systemic sclerosis: clinical, radiologic, histopathologic, and treatment evidence," *Seminars in Arthritis and Rheumatism*, vol. 40, no. 3, pp. 241–249, 2010.

[9] E. Savarino, M. Bazzica, P. Zentilin et al., "Gastroesophageal reflux and pulmonary fibrosis in Scleroderma: a study using pH-impedance monitoring," *American Journal of Respiratory and Critical Care Medicine*, vol. 179, no. 5, pp. 408–413, 2009.

[10] R. Rosen, J. Amirault, H. Liu et al., "Changes in gastric and lung microflora with acid suppression: acid suppression and bacterial growth," *JAMA Pediatrics*, vol. 168, no. 10, pp. 932–937, 2014.

[11] J. Wipff, R. Coriat, M. Masciocchi et al., "Outcomes of Barrett's oesophagus related to systemic sclerosis: a 3-year EULAR Scleroderma Trials and Research prospective follow-up study," *Rheumatology*, vol. 50, no. 8, pp. 1440–1444, 2011.

[12] R. Vardar, E. Vardar, and S. Bor, "Is the prevalence of intestinal metaplasia at the squamocolumnar junction different in patients with progressive sytemic sclerosis?" *The Turkish Journal of Gastroenterology*, vol. 21, no. 3, pp. 251–256, 2010.

[13] R. Thonhofer, C. Siegel, M. Trummer, and W. Graninger, "Early endoscopy in systemic sclerosis without gastrointestinal symptoms," *Rheumatology International*, vol. 32, no. 1, pp. 165–168, 2012.

[14] I. Zuber-Jerger, A. Müller, F. Kullmann et al., "Gastrointestinal manifestation of systemic sclerosis—thickening of the upper gastrointestinal wall detected by endoscopic ultrasound is a valid sign," *Rheumatology*, vol. 49, no. 2, Article ID kep381, pp. 368–372, 2010.

[15] M. K. Mason, "Looking for trouble—patient preference, misdiagnosis and overtesting: a teachable moment," *JAMA Internal Medicine*, vol. 174, no. 10, pp. 1548–1549, 2014.

[16] R. H. R. Park, J. H. McKillop, J. J. F. Belch, A. Faichney, and J. F. MacKenzie, "Achalasia-like syndrome in systemic sclerosis," *The British Journal of Surgery*, vol. 77, no. 1, pp. 46–49, 1990.

[17] D. M. Reddi, D. M. Cardona, J. L. Burchette, and P. K. Puri, "Scleroderma and IgG4-related disease," *The American Journal of Dermatopathology*, vol. 35, no. 4, pp. 458–462, 2013.

[18] E. S. Dellon, N. Gonsalves, I. Hirano, G. T. Furuta, C. A. Liacouras, and D. A. Katzka, "ACG clinical guideline: evidenced based approach to the diagnosis and management of esophageal eosinophilia and eosinophilic esophagitis (EoE)," *The American Journal of Gastroenterology*, vol. 108, no. 5, pp. 679–693, 2013.

[19] E. S. Dellon and C. A. Liacouras, "Advances in clinical management of eosinophilic esophagitis," *Gastroenterology*, vol. 147, no. 6, pp. 1238–1254, 2014.

[20] A. B. Muir, K. Dods, Y. Noah et al., "Esophageal epithelial cells acquire functional characteristics of activated myofibroblasts after undergoing an epithelial to mesenchymal transition," *Experimental Cell Research*, vol. 330, no. 1, pp. 102–110, 2015.

[21] T. M. Frech, R. Pimentel, G. Mineau, A. Sawitzke, G. Penmetsa, and J. Wong, "Parental influence on systemic sclerosis," *Arthritis Care and Research*, vol. 67, no. 2, pp. 310–312, 2015.

[22] T. Frech, D. Khanna, B. Markewitz, G. Mineau, R. Pimentel, and A. Sawitzke, "Heritability of vasculopathy, autoimmune disease, and fibrosis in systemic sclerosis: a population-based study," *Arthritis and Rheumatism*, vol. 62, no. 7, pp. 2109–2116, 2010.

38

SAPHO Syndrome Masquerading as Metastatic Breast Cancer

Devin Malik,[1] **Richa Handa**,[2] **Andrew Petraszko**,[3] **and Sheela Tejwani**[1]

[1]*Department of Hematology Oncology, Henry Ford Hospital, 2799 W. Grand Blvd., Detroit, MI 48202, USA*
[2]*Department of Internal Medicine, Henry Ford Allegiance Health, 205 N. East Ave., Jackson, MI 49201, USA*
[3]*Department of Radiology, Henry Ford Hospital, 2799 W. Grand Blvd., Detroit, MI 48202, USA*

Correspondence should be addressed to Devin Malik; malikdevin@gmail.com

Academic Editor: Mario Salazar-Paramo

SAPHO syndrome is a rare clinical entity composed of synovitis, acne, pustulosis, hyperostosis, and osteitis (SAPHO). We describe a case of SAPHO syndrome masquerading as metastatic breast cancer in a patient with localized breast cancer who presented with cord compression. There was no pathologic evidence of metastatic cancer; however, a bone scan indicated osseous involvement. After multidisciplinary review of images and with additional findings of pustulosis and acne, a clinical diagnosis of SAPHO was made.

1. Introduction

SAPHO syndrome is a constellation of multiple symptoms and signs including synovitis, acne, pustulosis, hyperostosis, and osteitis. It was first described in 1961 by Windam et al. [1], and the acronym was first coined in 1987 by Chamot et al. [2]. It has different names including nonbacterial osteitis, sternoclavicular hyperostosis, pustulotic arthro-osteitis, spondyloarthritis hyperostotica pustulopsoriatica, and chronic recurrent multifocal osteomyelitis [3, 4]. The annual prevalence of SAPHO syndrome is estimated at 1/10,000 in Caucasians [5]. It is a rare clinical entity, and a high index of suspicion is required to diagnose this disease. We present a case in which a patient with invasive breast cancer had a collection of findings including joint pain, acne, and rash involving palms and soles with imaging showing osseous lesions at multiple sites and diagnosed with SAPHO syndrome.

2. Case

A 59-year-old African American lady with a history of newly diagnosed invasive ductal carcinoma of the breast, stage 1A (pT1b, N0, M0), estrogen receptor and progesterone receptor positive, and Her-2 negative status post lumpectomy and radiotherapy presented to the hospital with complaints of multiple falls and weakness in both arms and legs and incontinence of urine. Complete blood count revealed a neutrophilic leukocytosis of 16.6K/μL (3.8–10.6K/μL), hemoglobin of 13 g/dL (12.0–15.0 g/dL), and platelet of 357K/μL (150–140K/μL). Complete metabolic profile was normal. The patient underwent magnetic resonance imaging which showed osseous lesions involving the cervical spine, thoracic spine, and lumbar spine. Sclerotic lesions were also observed within the left clavicle, sternum, and left T12 proximal rib. The patient underwent X-rays of axial and appendicular skeleton revealing sclerotic appearance of anterior L4 and L5. There was also abnormal appearance of the distal left clavicle, medial right, and left clavicles as well as the sternum. There was no evidence of periostitis. Because of cord compression, the patient underwent vertebral laminectomies which came back negative for metastatic disease and negative for bacteria. The patient also had a bone scan that showed increased radiotracer uptake within the medial left clavicle and manubrium centered upon the left sternoclavicular joint and bilateral 1st costomanubrial joints (Figure 1). There was also increased radiotracer uptake with the cervical spine. The patient also gave a history of rash involving palms and soles (Figures 2 and 3) and facial acne and was seen by a dermatologist in the past and diagnosed with palmoplantar pustular dermatosis. Cultures of these pustules were negative. In light of negative biopsies from

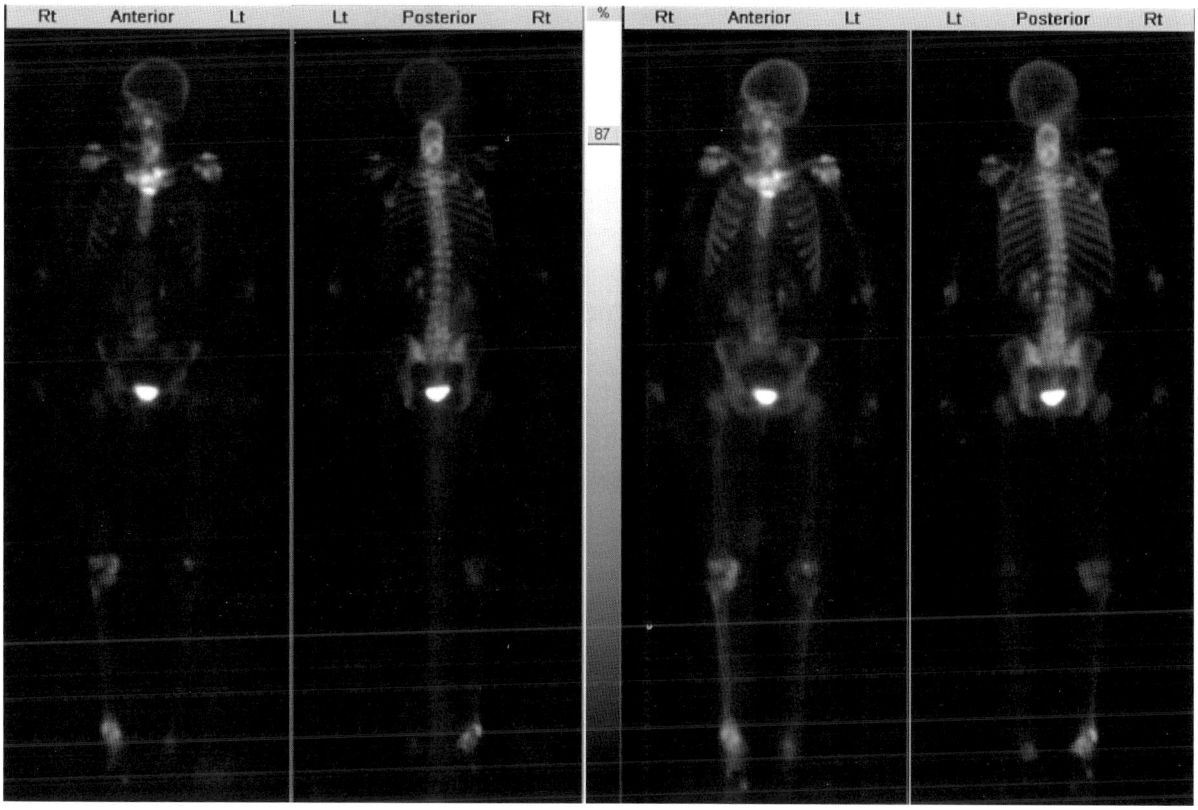

FIGURE 1: Anterior and posterior planar images of a ^{99m}Tc MDP bone scan show increased radiotracer uptake within the medial left clavicle and manubrium centered upon the left sternoclavicular joint and bilateral 1st costomanubrial joints. There is also increased radiotracer uptake with the cervical spine.

surgical specimens and given low-stage breast cancer, an alternative diagnosis for her bone lesions was sought. A comprehensive joint exam was done to evaluate for any bony abnormalities. There was full range of motion of spine, shoulders, elbows, wrists, fingers, hips, knees, and ankles. There was no active swelling, tenderness, soft tissue nodules, or synovitis at any joint. There was tenderness to palpation over the sternum and sternoclavicular joints. There was no malar rash or mouth ulcers, or alopecia.

Plasma cell dyscrasia was ruled out by serum and urine protein electrophoresis and a normal bone marrow biopsy and skeletal radiographic survey. Given her joint pain, bone scan findings, palmoplantar pustulosis, and acne, a diagnosis of SAPHO syndrome was made. The patient was then seen by a rheumatologist and was started on 40 mg of daily prednisone and later transitioned to adalimumab 40 mg every 14 days. She was started on adjuvant Arimidex for her breast cancer and continues to follow with both oncology and rheumatology.

3. Discussion

SAPHO syndrome can present at any age but is most commonly found in children and young adults, and it has a self-limiting, relapsing, and remitting course [6, 7]. Diagnostic criteria for SAPHO syndrome include a combination of acne, palmoplantar pustulosis, hyperostosis with or without dermatosis, and recurrent multifocal chronic osteomyelitis involving the axial or peripheral skeleton, with or without dermatosis [5]. Synovitis of the affected joint is also a common presentation of SAPHO syndrome. Patients can also present with mono or polyarthritis [8]. Various skeletal sites are found to be affected in SAPHO syndrome, including anterior chest wall (65% to 90% of cases), spine (30% of cases with thoracic spine being the most frequently affected part of spine), appendicular skeleton including long bones (5% to 10% of cases), and mandibular area (1% to 10% of cases) [6, 7, 9]. Dermatological manifestations include palmoplantar pustulosis and severe acne [8]. Osteoarticular and dermatological manifestations do not necessarily occur at the same time as the latency period of more than ten years has also been documented [10]. Lab findings generally include moderate leukocytosis, mild anemia, elevated acute phase reactants, elevated immunoglobulin A, and normal or elevated complement levels [11].

Pathogenesis of SAPHO syndrome remains unknown. Multiple mechanisms, including genetic, immunological, and bacterial causes, are found to play an important role in the development of the disease. Regarding infectious etiology, *Propionibacterium* acnes have been isolated in biopsy specimens of both the bone and synovium [7, 8], but despite this, antibiotic trials are not found to be effective [7]. Three hypotheses have been proposed by Hellmann and Schwartz regarding autoimmune response playing an important role in pathogenesis of SAPHO syndrome, which could be triggered by a bacterial or viral pathogen [12, 13]. According

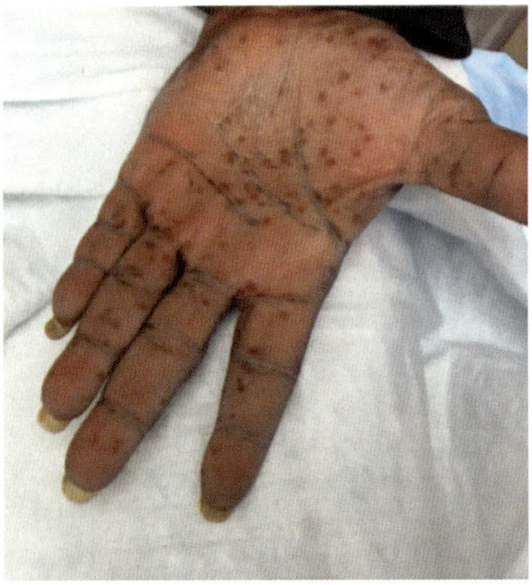

FIGURE 2: Photograph of the left palm demonstrating healed pustules. Similar findings were on the right palm.

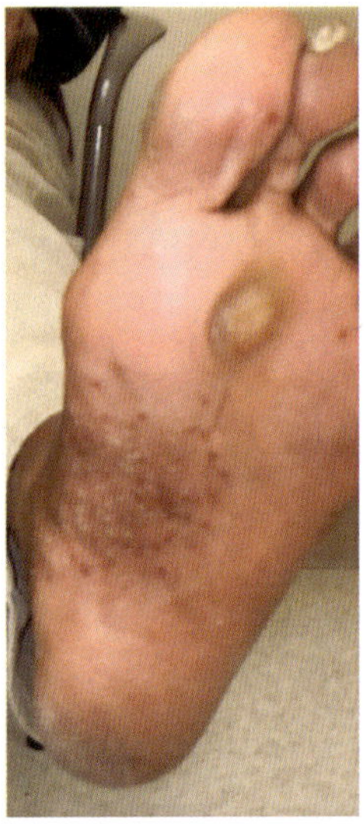

FIGURE 3: Photograph of the left sole lesions demonstrating pustulosis. Similar findings were on the right sole.

to molecular mimicry hypothesis, whenever there is a resemblance between the fragment of microorganism in the skin with the bone or joint, the immune system mistakenly attacks the normal bone or joint causing inflammation of affected joints [14]. According to the second hypothesis, whenever a fragment of microorganism couples with an immunoglobulin, an immune complex is formed which deposits in the bone or joint and can activate a complement cascade, thus causing inflammation [15]. Finally, according to the third hypothesis, which is an immune barrier breakdown hypothesis, whenever a skin infection breaks down a barrier between immune cells and dermatologic tissues, normal antigens in the skin are exposed to the immune system, which may trigger an inflammatory reaction [16]. In some studies, association with seronegative spondyloarthropathies has also been found [7]. HLA B27 has also been found in 30% of SAPHO patients [8]. The main consideration as to why a spondyloarthropathy was not likely in our patient was the absence of several key elements including an antecedent infection, sacroilitis, or ossification of intervertebral ligaments on imaging, no history of inflammatory bowel disease, psoriatic rash or ocular symptoms.

The relationship between cancer and rheumatologic conditions is bidirectional, in that some conditions predispose one to cancer and some cancers may present with rheumatologic features. There is a known association between rheumatoid arthritis, lupus, Sjögren's syndrome, systemic sclerosis, and hematologic malignancies such as lymphoma and leukemia [17]. Furthermore, the presence of dermatomyositis/polymyositis may be a clue for an occult neoplasm [18]. Conversely, paraneoplastic rheumatic syndromes can develop as a result of an underlying malignancy. Hypertrophic osteoarthropathy (HOA) is one such process and has a well-known association with lung cancer. HOA is caused by abnormal growth of bone and skin in the distal extremities and classically presents as digital clubbing, symmetric polyarthritis, and periostitis of long bones [19]. The etiology is unclear, but believed to be caused by tumor-derived growth factors such as platelet-derived growth factor (PDGF) and vascular endothelial growth factor (VEGF) [20]. Typically, signs and symptoms resolve after treatment of the underlying disease. The absence of clubbing, tenderness of long bones, and lack of periosteal reaction on radiographs made HOA in our patient highly unlikely. Carcinomatous polyarthritis (CP) is associated with various solid tumors and can present similar to seronegative rheumatoid arthritis with symmetric involvement of hands, wrists with morning stiffness, or as an asymmetric migratory polyarthritis [21]. The classic presentation, however, is advanced aging, acute onset of symptoms, involvement of lower extremities, and lack of destructive changes on radiographs [22]. Other types of paraneoplastic rheumatic conditions include remitting seronegative symmetrical synovitis with pitting edema which is thought to be related to increased levels of VEGF [23], palmar fibromatosis, and polyarthritis which causes flexion deformities of the hands in patients with certain solid tumors [24]. Our patient's history and symptomatology was not consistent with any of the paraneoplastic rheumatoid conditions.

For diagnosis of SAPHO syndrome, whole-body scintigraphy is useful because in addition to increased tracer uptake in the affected bone, it also reveals clinically silent lesions. The bull's head sign is the pathognomonic of SAPHO syndrome which is characterized by manubrium sterni which represents the upper skull and the inflamed sternoclavicular joint with the adjacent clavicle representing the horns [25]. Though this sign is pathognomonic for SAPHO syndrome, it is not sensitive [26]. Plain radiographs, CT scans, and MRI are also found to be helpful in diagnosing SAPHO syndrome. Histological characteristics of bone lesions involve acute inflammation with predominantly a neutrophilic infiltrate [8]. The differential diagnoses of SAPHO syndrome include osteosarcoma, infectious osteomyelitis, bony metastasis, Ewing's sarcoma, Paget's disease, sternoclavicular osteoarthritis, infectious spondylodiscitis, and many others [8].

Regarding treatment of SAPHO syndrome, nonsteroidal anti-inflammatory drugs (NSAIDs) are the first line of agents [6]. But a lot of patients do not get any relief from NSAIDs alone. *Propionibacterium* acne, which is found to play an important role in pathogenesis of SAPHO syndrome, can be treated with antibiotics that have been found to decrease the disease activity in one of the studies [27]. Corticosteroids, colchicine, and disease-modifying anti-rheumatic drugs (DMARDs), including methotrexate and sulfasalazine, are also found to be effective in some of the case studies [8]. In patients who are refractory to the abovementioned treatment, biological agents such as tumor necrosis factor inhibitors including infliximab, etanercept, or adalimumab have also been used with varying results [6]. Bisphosphonates which inhibit bone resorption and also have probable anti-inflammatory properties have also been used in patients who are refractory to the NSAIDs, corticosteroids, colchicine, and DMARDs [6]. Finally, surgical procedures including partial or complete resection, saucerization, and decortication of the affected bone have also been shown to be useful in some of the cases [6].

4. Conclusion

The course of the disease is highly variable, owing to the fact that not all signs may be present at the same time. Recent studies show that 13% of patients had monophasic disease, and 35% of the patients had relapsing and remitting course [28]. Predictors of chronic disease include female gender, involvement of anterior chest wall, dermatologic lesions, peripheral arthritis, and elevated levels of acute phase reactants [6]. SAPHO syndrome is a distinct clinical entity with characteristic dermatologic and osteoarticular abnormalities and should be considered in the differential diagnosis of sclerotic and hyperostotic bone lesions in low-stage cancers to prevent the use of chemotherapy and radiotherapy in patients with malignancy [8]. Management of a patient with SAPHO syndrome is multidisciplinary in nature [1, 29], and a high index of suspicion is required to diagnose and treat this condition.

References

[1] R. E. Windom, J. P. Sandford, and M. Ziff, "Acne conglobata and arthritis," *Arthritis & Rheumatism*, vol. 4, no. 6, pp. 632–635, 1961.

[2] A. Chamot, C. L. Benhamou, M. F. Kahn et al., "Le syndrome acne pustulose hyperostose osteite (SA-PHO)," *Revue du Rhumatisme*, vol. 54, pp. 187–196, 1987.

[3] K. Hyodoh and H. Sugimoto, "Pustulotic arthro-osteitis: defining the radiologic spectrum of the disease," *Seminars in Musculoskeletal Radiology*, vol. 5, no. 2, pp. 89–93, 2001.

[4] A. F. Jansson, V. Grote, and ESPED Study Group, "Non-bacterial osteitis in children: data of a German Incidence Surveillance Study," *Acta Paediatrica*, vol. 100, no. 8, pp. 1150–1157, 2011.

[5] G. Hayem, "SAPHO syndrome," *La Revue Du Praticien*, vol. 54, pp. 1635-1636, 2004.

[6] M. T. Nhiguyen, A. Borchers, C. Selmi, S. M. Naguwa, G. Cheema, and M. Eric Gershwin, "The SAPHO Syndrome," *Seminars in Arthritis and Rheumatism*, vol. 42, no. 3, pp. 254–265, 2012.

[7] J. W. Earwaker and A. Cotton, "SAPHO: syndrome or concept? imaging findings," *Skeletal Radiology*, vol. 32, no. 6, pp. 311–327, 2003.

[8] I. Rukavina, "SAPHO syndrome: a review," *Journal of Children's Orthopaedics*, vol. 9, no. 1, pp. 19–27, 2015.

[9] R. Depasquale, N. Kumar, R. K. Lalam et al., "SAPHO: what radiologists should know," *Clinical Radiology*, vol. 67, no. 3, pp. 195–206, 2012.

[10] M. F. Kahn, M. B. Bouvier, E. Palazzo, J. Tebib, and E. Colson, "Sternoclavicular pustulotic osteitis (SAPHO): 20 year interval between skin and bone lesions," *Journal of Rheumatology*, vol. 18, pp. 1104–1108, 1991.

[11] P. Kopterides, D. Pikazis, and C. Koufos, "Successful treatment of SAPHO syndrome with zoledronic acid," *American College of Rheumatology*, vol. 50, no. 9, pp. 2970–2973, 2004.

[12] D. B. Hellmann, "Spondyloarthropathy with hidradenitis suppurativa," *JAMA*, vol. 267, no. 17, pp. 2363–2365, 1992.

[13] B. D. Schwartz, "Infectious agents, immunity, and rheumatic diseases," *Arthritis & Rheumatism*, vol. 33, no. 4, pp. 457–465, 1990.

[14] A. Sinha, M. Lopet, and H. McDevitt, "Autoimmune diseases: the failure of self-tolerance," *Science*, vol. 248, p. 1388, 1990.

[15] I. A. Rosner, D. E. Richter, T. L. Huettner, G. H. Kuffner, J. J. Wisnieski, and C. G. Burg, "Spondyloarthropathy associated with hidradenitis suppurativa and acne conglobata," *Annals of Internal Medicine*, vol. 97, no. 4, pp. 520–522, 1982.

[16] R. D. Boutin and D. Resnick, "The SAPHO syndrome: an evolving concept for unifying several idiopathic disorders of bone and skin," *American Journal of Roentgenology*, vol. 170, no. 3, pp. 585–591, 1998.

[17] J. E. Naschitz and I. Rosner, "Musculoskeletal syndromes associated with malignancy (excluding hypertrophic osteoarthropathy)," *Current Opinion in Rheumatology*, vol. 20, no. 1, p. 100, 2008.

[18] J. E. Naschitz, I. Rosner, M. Rozenbaum, E. Zuckerman, and D. Yeshurun, "Rheumatic syndromes: clues to occult neoplasia," *Seminars in Arthritis and Rheumatism*, vol. 29, no. 1, p. 43, 1999.

[19] M. Martinez-Lavin and C. Pineda, "Hypertrophic osteo arthropathy," in *Rheumatology*, M. C. Hochberg, A. J. Silman, J. S. Smolen et al, Eds., p. 1763, Mosby, London, UK, 2003.

[20] Y. Abe, S. Kurita, Y. Ohkubo et al., "A case of pulmonary adenocarcinoma associated with hypertrophic osteoarthropathy due to vascular endothelial growth factor," *Anticancer Research*, vol. 22, no. 6, p. 3485, 2002.

[21] Y. Fatley and M. Luggen, "Seropositive, symmetric polyarthritis in a patient with poorly differentiated lung carcinoma: carcinomatous polyarthritis, hypertrophic osteoarthropathy, or rheumatoid arthritis?," *Arthritis Care & Research*, vol. 11, no. 2, pp. 146–149, 1998.

[22] A. G. Fam, "Paraneoplastic rheumatic syndromes," *Best Practice & Research Clinical Rheumatology*, vol. 14, no. 3, pp. 515–533, 2000.

[23] H. Li, R. D. Altman, and Q. Yao, "RS3PE: clinical and research development," *Current Rheumatology Reports*, vol. 17, no. 8, p. 49, 2015.

[24] A. B. Alexandroff, B. L. Hazleman, M. Matthewson et al., "Woody hands," *The Lancet*, vol. 361, no. 9366, p. 1344, 2003.

[25] M. Q. Rodríguez, I. C. Tormo, M. C. Redal Peña, and L. Castillo, "The importance of bone scintigraphy in the diagnosis of SAPHO syndrome," *Revista Española de Medicina Nuclear*, vol. 29, pp. 127–130, 2010.

[26] A. M. Davies, A. J. Marino, N. Evans, R. J. Grimer, N. Deshmukh, and D. C. Mangham, "SAPHO syndrome: 20-year follow-up," *Skeletal Radiology*, vol. 28, pp. 159–162, 1999.

[27] G. Assmann, O. Kueck, T. Kirchhoff et al., "Efficacy of antibiotic therapy for SAPHO syndrome is lost after its discontinuation: an interventional study," *Arthritis Research & Therapy*, vol. 11, p. R140, 2009.

[28] M. Colina, M. Govoni, C. Orzincolo, and F. Trotta, "Clinical and radiologic evolution of synovitis, acne, pustulosis, hyperostosis, and osteitis syndrome: a single center study of a cohort of 71 subjects," *Arthritis & Rheumatism*, vol. 61, no. 6, pp. 813–821, 2009.

[29] F. Schilling and E. Marker-Hermann, "Chronic recurrent multifocal osteomyelitis in association with chronic inflammatory bowel disease: enteropathic CRMO," *Zeitschrift für Rheumatologie*, vol. 62, no. 6, pp. 527–538, 2003.

Rheumatoid Arthritis, Kartagener's Syndrome, and Hyperprolactinemia: Who Started It?

Hussein Halabi and Israa Mulla

King Faisal Specialist Hospital & Research Center, P.O. Box 40047, Jeddah 21499, Saudi Arabia

Correspondence should be addressed to Hussein Halabi; halabihussein1@gmail.com

Academic Editor: Shigeko Inokuma

We report a case of an 18-year-old girl who presented to our hospital with history of recurrent respiratory infections, amenorrhea, and symmetric polyarthritis. She was diagnosed with rheumatoid arthritis (RA), Kartagener's syndrome (KS), and hyperprolactinemia. There have been very few case reports in the literature of RA occurring in the setting of KS, theoretically proposed to be due to chronic stimulation of the immune system by recurrent infections. Furthermore, hyperprolactinemia has been hypothesized to mirror RA disease activity and case reports of treatment with dopamine agonists have led to the speculation of whether or not they represent a new line of experimental treatment in the future. Our patient was found to have both KS and hyperprolactinemia together in the setting of RA, and based on our literature search, this is the first reported case of such a combination. This strikes a very intriguing question: are these three conditions interlinked by a yet to be defined association? And treatment of which condition leads to the resolution of the other?

1. Introduction

It has been postulated that recurrent bacterial and viral infections are one of the contributing factors to developing autoimmunity in RA, mainly through stimulation of Toll-like receptors expressed in synovial tissue [1]. This in turn will lead to release of various cytokines and inflammatory mediators with constant triggering of the innate immunity, and when this occurs in a genetically susceptible individual, RA is thought to eventually develop. This has led researchers to question whether KS is somehow linked to developing RA. There are nine case reports in the literature of RA and KS occurring together but what's interesting and different about our case is that our patient also had hyperprolactinemia, which up to our knowledge did not occur in any other reported case [2–10]. Prolactin has also been hypothesized as a possible immune stimulatory modulator in RA but its definite role still remains unclear for studies have yielded inconsistent results [11–13]. We describe our case and summarize the previous case reports and their findings including HLA types to help outline a clear association in the future.

2. Case Report

An 18 year old girl with history of chronic sinusitis and repeated childhood chest infections was referred to our hospital for work up of a nonresolving pneumonia.

The patient was first seen and evaluated in Pulmonology Clinic. She had a chronic productive cough but no fever, weight loss, or hemoptysis. Chest X-ray revealed a residual right middle lobe infiltrate with no pleural effusion. Computed tomography (CT) scan of the chest revealed patchy airspace opacities in the right lower lobe associated with bilateral lower lobe bronchiectatic changes. Interestingly, there were multiple structural abnormalities incidentally found in the form of an abdominal situs ambiguous with the liver seen in the midline, a right-sided stomach, and multiple small splenules in the right upper abdomen (Figure 1). Bronchoscopy with bronchoalveolar lavage was positive for *Haemophilus influenzae*. All other differentials including *Mycobacterium tuberculosis*, fungal infections, and malignancy were ruled out.

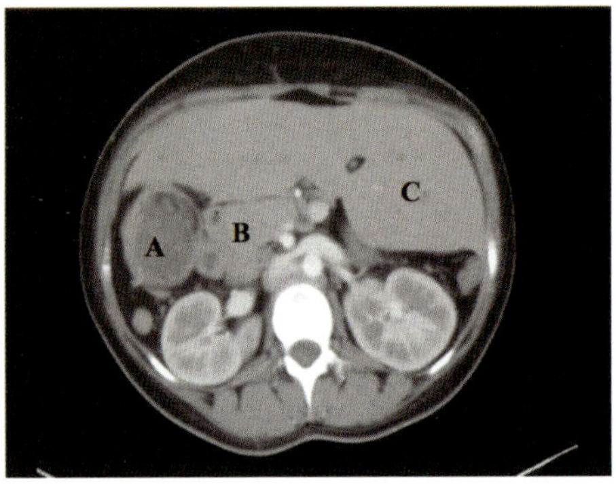

FIGURE 1: CT scan of the chest with contrast demonstrating situs ambiguous: (A) a right-sided stomach, (B) multiple splenules on the right, and (C) the liver in the midline occupying both right and left portions of the abdomen.

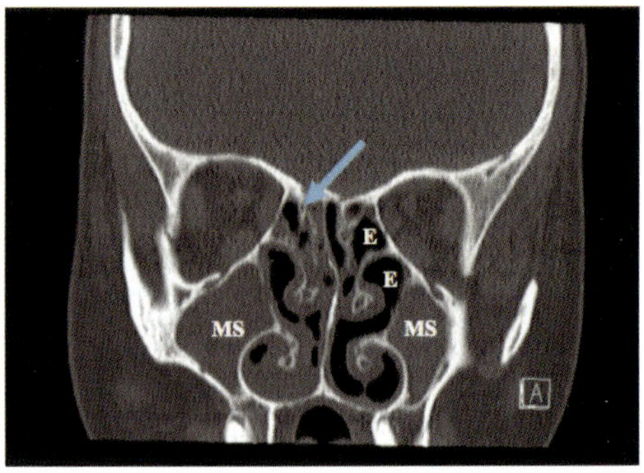

FIGURE 2: CT scan of the paranasal sinuses showing complete opacification of the maxillary sinuses (MS) bilaterally and some of the ethmoid air cells (arrow) including the sphenoid sinuses. There is also obliteration of the osteomeatal complexes bilaterally.

During that same period, the patient gave history of two new complaints: joint pain and swelling and amenorrhea. Regarding her joint complaints, the patient gave history typical of RA with symmetrical joint pain and swelling involving her small and large joints with early morning stiffness of more than an hour. On examination her tender joint count (TJC) was 10 and swollen joint count (SJC) was 7. She had a strongly positive Rheumatoid Factor of 350 and an anti-cyclic citrullinated peptide (Anti-CCP) of 133. Her erythrocyte sedimentation rate (ESR) and C-reactive protein (CRP) were mildly elevated at 21 and 5.27 mg/L, respectively. The rest of her autoimmune panel including ANA and ENA profiles was negative. X-rays of the hands, elbows, shoulders, knees, and feet bilaterally revealed maintained joint spaces and no evidence of erosions. Based on these findings the patient was diagnosed to have RA. Her calculated DAS-28 score was 5.77, her Simple Disease Activity Index (SDAI) 32.5, and her Clinical Disease Activity Index (CDAI) 32, all reflecting high disease activity. She was started on Methotrexate at a dose of 12.5 mg orally once weekly with supplemental folate. She was also kept on Prednisolone 10 mg orally daily with calcium and vitamin D.

As for her amenorrhea symptoms, the patient had irregular periods after menarche but became completely amenorrheic around 8 months prior to presentation. She had been married for one and a half years, had no children, and was not using any method of contraception. She was referred to Obstetrics and Gynecology Team for further evaluation and her work-up revealed the presence of a very high prolactin level of 4425 μg/L (normal range: 3–24 μg/L). another hormonal panel was within normal. She had no symptoms of galactorrhea, was not taking any new drugs, and had no history of renal, thyroid, or liver disease. She had no visual symptoms or headache or vomiting. Pelvic ultrasound showed a retroverted uterus with no abnormalities. She was given an appointment to do pituitary magnetic resonance imaging (MRI) in addition to Endocrinology followup.

Due to the earlier CT findings of situs ambiguous and history of chronic bronchiectasis, the diagnosis of KS was entertained. CT scan of the paranasal sinuses was therefore requested and it confirmed the presence of pansinusitis with complete opacification of the maxillary, sphenoid, and ethmoid sinuses (Figure 2). Based on the presence of this triad, she was diagnosed with KS and was admitted for full work-up and treatment on the 20th of October 2014. Magnetic resonance imaging (MRI) of the pituitary gland was done and it revealed a 2.2 × 2.1 × 1.2 cm intrasellar pituitary macroadenoma (Figure 3). She was seen and evaluated by Endocrinology Team and started on Cabergoline 0.5 mg once weekly and discharged in a stable condition with outpatient followup.

When the patient presented to Rheumatology Clinic the following month, she reported almost 80% improvement of her symptoms with significant reduction in her joint pain and complete resolution of morning stiffness and fatigue. Based on assessment that day, her DAS-28 score was 1.7 and her SDAI and CDAI scores were 4.9 and 3, respectively. Her prolactin level dropped to 293 μg/L. The patient achieved clinical remission and her Methotrexate dose was increased to 15 mg orally once weekly. She was instructed to taper down her steroids until tapering off. During the next visit three months later, she was still in remission with a DAS-28 score of 1.4, SDAI of 2.5, and CDAI of 2. Her Methotrexate dose was maximized to 20 mg once weekly. Repeated MRI of the pituitary gland revealed regression in the size of the macroadenoma to 1.4 × 1.4 cm with a further drop in her prolactin level to 28.9 μg/L. Cabergoline was increased to 1.5 mg orally twice a week on subsequent Endocrinology followup.

3. Case Discussion

RA is a chronic disabling autoimmune disorder, affecting people from all around the world. The annual incidence is around 40 per 100,000 persons but the prevalence varies according to ethnical background, estimated to be around 1% in North Americans [14]. Many theories have been postulated in the pathogenesis of RA but experts generally agree that it is a result of a complex interaction between environmental and genetic factors in an already susceptible individual [15]. Genetic susceptibility to RA has been extensively studied and still remains an area for burning research. Many genes have been identified as conferring a risk, most importantly the HLA Major Histocompatibility Complex (MHC) Genes,

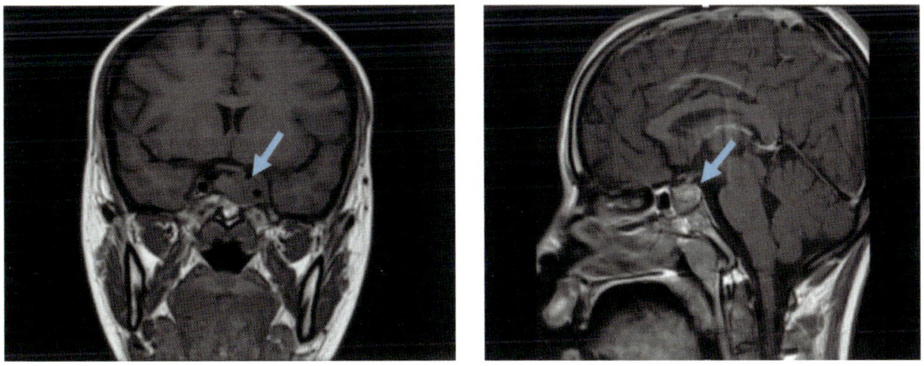

(a) (b)

FIGURE 3: T1 coronal (a) and T1 sagittal (b) sections of the brain on presentation showing a 2.2 × 2.1 × 2.2 cm intrasellar mass in keeping with a pituitary macroadenoma invading the left cavernous sinus and completely encasing the left internal carotid artery.

namely, the HLA-DRB1 gene and the DR4 family of alleles. This in addition to the theory of the shared epitope increases risk of severe erosive disease.

However, genes, although an essential part of the pathogenesis, are not the lone culprits, and other environmental factors play a crucial and influential role in triggering RA. Of these, the most well studied and affirmed is smoking, which can interact with the shared epitope, increasing the risk of developing RA up to 40-fold. Another important and established factor is repeated infection. This will lead to recurrent activation of the immune system ultimately leading to an autoimmune state that gradually ensues. As a matter of fact, in one of the earlier reports of RA and KS occurring concurrently together, Beutler et al. hypothesized this very notion, claiming that it was in fact the repetitive triggering of the immune system by chronic sinusitis and bronchiectasis in patients with KS that eventually led to the unveiling of RA. But if so, does treatment of infection lead to resolution of synovitis and subsequent remission? Of the nine published case reports so far linking RA to KS, and excluding those published in a language other than English, all patients except one presented with erosive disease (Table 1). There has been great emphasis over the past couple of years on early initiation of disease-modifying antirheumatic drugs as soon as a diagnosis of RA is established and delaying RA treatment to test this theory in patients who already have erosions is not always feasible [16]. Our patient had no erosions on X-rays but she had clinically significant synovitis with multiple tender and swollen joints. She was initiated on Methotrexate in addition to steroids and when she presented to the clinic three months after, she was in complete remission with a DAS-28 score of 1.7, SDAI of 4.9, and CDAI of 3. Based on this, it is safe to conclude that treatment with disease-modifying antirheumatic drugs is of utter importance and still remains the cornerstone of therapy.

KS is classically known to present with a triad of chronic sinusitis, bronchiectasis, and situs inversus. Genetically speaking, there has not yet been a clear link between RA and Kartagener's syndrome in terms of a susceptibility gene causatively leading a patient with one condition to develop the other. On reviewing the patients reported in the nine cases aforesaid, and excluding four articles that were not in English, three had undetermined HLA status and two had HLA types not known to be associated with RA (Table 1). Based on these limited results, it is impossible to establish a real connection and data is still insufficient to really prove anything.

What makes our case even more interesting is that our patient had hyperprolactinemia in addition to RA and KS. Based on literature review, this is the first case linking all three. Many studies have been conducted fervently evaluating the role of prolactin and the neuroendocrine system in promoting autoimmunity. Some studies, on the other hand, have claimed a cartilage protective effect. Case reports of experimental treatment with dopamine agonists such as Bromocriptine have also been inconsistent, in some showing improvement in the in vitro immune function and HAQ disability scores, whereas in others exhibiting nonsignificant improvement as compared with placebo [17, 18]. Further studies are definitely warranted to outline the exact role of prolactin in association with autoimmunity but until then its influence still remains elusive.

Our patient was treated with Cabergoline, a dopamine agonist, for her prolactin-secreting macroadenoma and she responded remarkably to treatment with a drop in her prolactin level from 4425 to 293 μg/L when she first achieved clinical remission of RA. But does this drop merely signify response to treatment or does it, in theory, mirror her RA disease activity? Interestingly, when the patient's prolactin dropped further to 28.9 μg/L, her inflammatory markers also dropped (ESR to 5 and CRP to 2.14 mg/L). Moreover, if in fact prolactin does stimulate autoimmunity and RA as proposed by some theories, was the presence of hyperprolactinemia a triggering factor to development of RA or was their concurrence together just a sheer coincidence? Our patient was treated for all of her medical problems so it is difficult to conclude if a specific treatment led to resolution of the other condition(s) or if treatments of everything worked synergistically together.

In summary, we report a case of an 18-year-old girl who presented with RA, KS, and hyperprolactinemia. She was successfully treated with a combination of Methotrexate and Cabergoline. Her macroadenoma regressed in size,

TABLE 1: Summary of reported cases and patient characteristics.

Case report	Race	Age	Sex	Other comorbidities	RF or ACPA	HLA type	Erosions	Other X-ray findings	Treatment received
Kawasaki et al. 2000 [6]	Japan	11	M	None	Negative	—	—	—	MTX, Prednisolone, and NSAIDS (doses not mentioned) and then later MTX changed to Bucillamine
Riente et al. 2001 [7]	Italy	60	F	DM, HTN, heart failure	Positive	A1, B44, B51, DRB1*11 DRB1*16 DRB3, DRB5	No	Symmetric narrowing of MCP + PIP with juxta-articular osteoporosis	Initially Chloroquine 500 mg/day orally + Methylprednisolone 4 mg/d Then Gold IM, low dose steroids + antibiotics
Rébora et al. 2006 [9]	Argentina	38	F	None	Positive	(i) A1, B8, B57 (ii) HLA DR not studied	Yes	Narrowing at the wrists + 3rd MCPs bilaterally with juxta-articular osteopenia	Initially SSZ 1.5 g per day + NSAIDS Later Chloroquine 200 mg and then HCQ 400 mg daily Subsequently shifted to MTX 15 mg/day
Younes et al. 2006 [8]	Tunisia	35	F	None	Positive	—	Yes	Narrowing at the MCPs + 2nd & 3rd PIPs	Indomethacin 100 mg daily, Prednisolone 10 mg orally daily and MTX 10 mg weekly later increased to 15 mg weekly
Takasaki et al. 2014 [10]	Japan	47	F	Periodontitis, smoker	Positive	—	Yes	Joint destruction in the RT thumb MCP + LT thumb MCP and PIP	MTX 12 mg weekly, Tacrolimus 2 mg/daily, Prednisone 4 mg daily Later shifted to Etanercept 50 mg/week + tacrolimus tapered off
Our patient	Saudi Arabia	18	F	—	Positive	—	No	Normal	MTX 12.5 mg PO weekly gradually increased until 20 mg weekly + Prednisolone 15 mg orally daily gradually tapered off

MTX = Methotrexate, HCQ = Hydroxychloroquine, and SSZ = sulfasalazine.

her bronchiectasis was treated, and she achieved clinical remission of her RA. Based on limited evidence from case reports and the fact that these kinds of patients usually need simultaneous treatment for all of their conditions, outlining a clear association still represents a challenge.

References

[1] F. Brentano, D. Kyburz, O. Schorr, R. Gay, and S. Gay, "The role of Toll-like receptor signalling in the pathogenesis of arthritis," *Cellular Immunology*, vol. 233, no. 2, pp. 90–96, 2005.

[2] A. Zangara, "On a case of Kartagener syndrome with associated rheumatoid arthritis," *Reumatismo*, vol. 12, pp. 290–295, 1960.

[3] G. L. Mastaglia and P. Goatcher, "Rare association of rheumatoid arthritis and Kartagener's syndrome: a common denominator?" *Medical Journal of Australia*, vol. 2, no. 7, article 400, 1980.

[4] A. Beutler and S. H. Mackiewicz, "Association of rheumatoid arthritis with Kartagener's syndrome in a patient with HLA-DR1-DR4-B27 haplotype," *Zeitschrift für Rheumatologie*, vol. 51, no. 5, pp. 253–255, 1992.

[5] W. Porawska, K. Swierkocki, A. Marszalek, and S. Mackiewicz, "An unusual case of Kartagener's syndrome associated with rheumatoid arthritis," *Polskie Archiwum Medycyny Wewnętrznej*, vol. 96, no. 6, pp. 577–580, 1996.

[6] Y. Kawasaki, J. Suzuki, T. Sike et al., "Bucillamine-induced nephropathy in a child with juvenile rheumatoid arthritis and Kartagener's syndrome," *Pediatrics International*, vol. 42, no. 3, pp. 316–318, 2000.

[7] L. Riente, P. Fadda, M. Mazzantini, S. Frigelli, B. Fattori, and E. Neri, "Kartagener's syndrome and rheumatoid arthritis: an unusual association," *Clinical Rheumatology*, vol. 20, no. 4, pp. 282–284, 2001.

[8] M. Younes, I. Béjia, S. Zrour-Hassen, M. Touzi, and N. Bergaoui, "Rheumatoid arthritis and Kartagener syndrome: a rare combination," *Joint Bone Spine*, vol. 73, no. 5, pp. 571–572, 2006.

[9] M. E. Rébora, J. A. Cuneo, J. Marcos, and J. C. Marcos, "Kartagener syndrome and rheumatoid arthritis," *Journal of Clinical Rheumatology*, vol. 12, no. 1, pp. 26–29, 2006.

[10] S. Takasaki, S. Yamakage, S. Fukase, and T. Takahashi, "Kartagener's syndrome and rheumatoid arthritis," *Internal Medicine*, vol. 53, no. 3, pp. 269–274, 2014.

[11] N. Adań, J. Guzmán-Morales, M. G. Ledesma-Colunga et al., "Prolactin promotes cartilage survival and attenuates inflammation in inflammatory arthritis," *The Journal of Clinical Investigation*, vol. 123, no. 9, pp. 3902–3913, 2013.

[12] M. Neidhart, R. E. Gay, and S. Gay, "Prolactin and prolactin-like polypeptides in rheumatoid arthritis," *Biomedicine and Pharmacotherapy*, vol. 53, no. 5-6, pp. 218–222, 1999.

[13] S. Ram, D. Blumberg, P. Newton, N. R. Anderson, and R. Gama, "Raised serum prolactin in rheumatoid arthritis: genuine or laboratory artefact?" *Rheumatology*, vol. 43, no. 10, pp. 1272–1274, 2004.

[14] T. D. Spector, "Rheumatoid arthritis," *Rheumatic Disease Clinics of North America*, vol. 16, no. 3, pp. 513–537, 1990.

[15] D. M. Lee and M. E. Weinblatt, "Rheumatoid arthritis," *The Lancet*, vol. 358, no. 9285, pp. 903–911, 2001.

[16] J. S. Smolen, R. Landewé, F. C. Breedveld et al., "EULAR recommendations for the management of rheumatoid arthritis with synthetic and biological disease-modifying antirheumatic drugs: 2013 update," *Annals of the Rheumatic Diseases*, vol. 73, no. 3, pp. 492–509, 2014.

[17] F. E. Figueroa, F. Carrion, M. E. Martinez, S. Rivero, and I. Mamani, "Bromocriptine induces immunological changes related to disease parameters in rheumatoid arthritis," *British Journal of Rheumatology*, vol. 36, no. 9, pp. 1022–1023, 1997.

[18] M. Salesi, S. Sadeghihaddadzavareh, P. Nasri, N. NamdariCharaghani, Z. Farajzadegan, and M. Hajalikhani, "The role of bromocriptine in the treatment of patients with active rheumatoid arthritis," *International Journal of Rheumatic Diseases*, vol. 16, no. 6, pp. 662–666, 2013.

40

Haematological Malignancies in Systemic Sclerosis Patients

M. Colaci, D. Giuggioli, C. Vacchi, and C. Ferri

Rheumatology Unit, Azienda Ospedaliero-Universitaria Policlinico di Modena, University of Modena and Reggio Emilia, Modena, Italy

Correspondence should be addressed to M. Colaci; michelecolaci@virgilio.it

Academic Editor: Jamal Mikdashi

Background. The association of systemic sclerosis (SSc) and haematological cancers was reported in a large number of case reports and cohort studies, describing SSc patients with highly heterogeneous clinical pictures. *Objective.* We reviewed the literature to better describe SSc patients with haematological malignancies. *Methods.* SSc cases complicated by haematological malignancies described in the world literature were collected; other 2 cases referred to our centre were reported. *Results.* One hundred-thirty SSc subjects were collected from 1954 up to date. The mean age of patients at cancer diagnosis was 56.1 ± 16.7 years; 72% of patients were females. In 60% of cases, the diagnosis of haematological malignancy was described within 5 years of SSc diagnosis. In 7.8% of cases, coexistence of Sjögren's syndrome or other autoimmune disorders was cited. Sixty-six cases with lymphoma (in the majority of cases B-cell neoplasms), 28 with leukaemia (chronic lymphocytic form in 9), 14 with multiple myeloma plus one solitary IgM plasmocytoma, and 16 with myeloproliferative disorders were found. No specific SSc subsets seem to be related to haematological malignancies. *Conclusions.* We remarked the importance of clinical work-up in SSc, in order to early diagnose and treat eventual occult haematological malignancies, especially during the first years of the disease.

1. Introduction

The association between malignancies and connective tissue diseases was widely reported in literature [1]; namely, systemic sclerosis (SSc) has showed relatively high incidence of lung, breast (contrasting data), and haematological cancers, as demonstrated by meta-analysis on population-based cohort studies [2, 3]. However, these studies usually reported the frequencies of specific malignancies in the course of SSc, without further characterization of the patients. In this respect, the subset of "haematological tumours" included different types of malignancies that generally were not described in detail. On the other hand, a large number of case reports may be found in literature [4–54], describing SSc patients with highly heterogeneous clinical pictures complicated by the onset of cancer. These reports could potentially contain detailed data that are not included in registry or large cohort studies [55–67].

The haematological neoplasms originate by the myeloid or the lymphoid cell lines, historically named leukaemias or lymphomas, based on the prevalent location in the blood or the lymph nodes, respectively. Afterwards, more than 70 nosological entities were identified, classified according to the 2008 World Health Organization (WHO) classification of neoplasms of the hematopoietic and lymphoid tissues, on the basis of the recognition of distinctive features in terms of morphology, clinical picture, immunophenotype, and genetic and molecular characteristics [68]. Indeed, the systematic categorization of the haematological malignancies evolved during the decades from the Rappaport classification of 1966 to the WHO classification in 2001 [69], lastly updated in 2016 [70], transposing the new knowledge achieved in the field of histology and cytogenetic/immunohistochemical profiling of malignancies.

In these lights, the known association between SSc and haematological malignancies should be better characterized, especially as regards eventual associations between SSc features and specific type of blood neoplasms. Moreover, specific SSc subsets might be associated with peculiar haematological cancers, besides other comorbid predisposing conditions.

Therefore, we aimed to collect all SSc cases complicated by haematological malignancies described in the world literature, searching eventual specific clinical patterns.

2. Patients and Methods

We analysed the whole SSc patients' cohort, recruited in our Rheumatology Centre, including 454 cases referred to our university-based hospital from 1 January 2003 to 31 December 2016, in order to find the patients who presented haematological neoplasms in their clinical history, after SSc diagnosis. For all patients, detailed clinical records were available, which eventually comprehended the documentation regarding the haematological diseases.

Secondly, the electronic databases, including PubMed, Embase, Scopus, Web of Science, SciELO, J-Stage, and Google Scholar, were searched for studies that described the cases with the association between haematological cancers and SSc, including all available previous articles and non-English reports. Search terms were "systemic sclerosis" or "scleroderma" and "h(a)ematological cancer" or "lymphoma" or "leuk(a)emia". Myeloproliferative disorders (search terms: "myelofibrosis", "chronic myelogenous leukaemia", "polycythemia vera", "essential thrombocytemia") were also considered, as well as "MGUS". All available data included in the published studies were analysed, evaluating all the information useful for patients' clinical profiling.

We considered all SSc patients who developed blood cancers; otherwise, the cases describing SSc onset *after* the diagnosis of haematological cancer were excluded. Likewise, the studies that did not exactly indicate the timing of SSc and cancer diagnoses were excluded. On the contrary, the patients with contemporary or very close onset of the two pathologic conditions (blood cancer diagnosis within 1 year from SSc diagnosis) were registered as patients with "probable paraneoplastic" syndrome. Finally, we did not consider studies regarding morphea or localized scleroderma nor sclerodermiform syndromes following antineoplastic treatments.

3. Case Reports

3.1. Case 1. A nonsmoker, 35-year-old male patient referred to our centre in 2008 and received a new diagnosis of SSc. The onset of the disease was few months before, featured by skin thickening of face, hands, forearms, and chest; skin ulcers or calcinosis was absent. He complained of Raynaud's phenomenon, fatigue, and mild sicca syndrome. No anti-topoisomerase I or anti-centromere autoantibodies were found (ANA 1:640 speckled), while anti-Ro/SSA and anti-SSB were present (secondary Sjögren's syndrome). He presented typical oesophageal dyskinesia and interstitial lung disease with reduction of the forced vital capacity to 69% and of the lung diffusion for the carbon monoxide to 33%. Heart function was normal, and no signs of pulmonary hypertension were found, while a slight increase of creatine-kinase was reported. At chest high-resolution CT (HRCT) performed within the first year of follow-up, an enlargement of the thymic shape emerged; the histology confirmed the presence of thymic hyperplasia; thus, the gland was removed, also hoping to counteract SSc progression [71]. After 2 years, the patient presented a deterioration of dyspnea with dry cough, extension of skin thickness to the whole body, increased fatigue, mild fever, and body weight loss. A further chest HRCT revealed a new mediastinal enlargement due to adenopathy (Figure 1); primary mediastinal B cell lymphoma (a type of diffuse large B cell non-Hodgkin lymphoma, NHL) was diagnosed by means of video-assisted thoracoscopic surgery (VATS) lymph node biopsy. The standard CHOP-R (cyclophosphamide, hydroxydaunorubicin, vincristine, prednisone, and rituximab) regimen was chosen; however, after few months, before any clinical improvement, the patient died from sepsis.

3.2. Case 2. A 72-year-old woman referred to our centre in 2012 from another hospital, where she was followed for SSc. The disease's onset dated back to 28 years before. Among SSc features, we emphasize the presence of pulmonary arterial hypertension, treated with sildenafil and, successively, ambrisentan. Calcinosis, telangiectasias, sclerodactyly, and anti-centromere antibodies, but not dysphagia nor interstitial lung disease, were found. As comorbidity, the patient presented severe lower limb arteriopathy obliterans, responsible for digital gangrenous lesions. Moreover, patient's history was marked by the diagnosis of low-grade tubular breast carcinoma in 2006; then, she underwent right quadrantectomy. Six years later, X-ray scan revealed a 2 cm pulmonary opacity in the right lower lobe. After chest CT confirmation, lobectomy was performed; the histological analysis diagnosed an extranodal marginal mature B cell lymphoma (BALToma). Given the absence of metastasis, no radio-/chemotherapy was considered necessary after the lung resection. To date, the patient is doing well, without presenting recidivism.

4. Review of the Literature

Table 1 summarized all cases of SSc patients complicated by haematological malignancies found in literature [4–67]; the studies that do not give any information about SSc features and/or haematological cancer types were excluded. Both case reports and cohort studies were included, even though, usually, only the first ones reported complete description of the clinical histories. To the best of our knowledge, 130 (including our 2 cases) subjects affected by SSc and haematological cancer were collected, from the first case described in 1954 up to date. Majority of patients were from Europe and USA and were Caucasian, while 18% of persons were of Asian ethnicity, coming from the Far Eastern Countries. The mean age of patients was 56.1 ± 16.7 years, without gender difference as regards age, with the higher prevalence of cases in the sixth decade. 72% of the cases were women. The diagnosis of haematological malignancies was frequently close to SSc diagnosis: indeed, in about 30% of cases, scleroderma could be considered as "probable paraneoplastic," while for other 30% of patients the cancer was diagnosed within 5 years of SSc

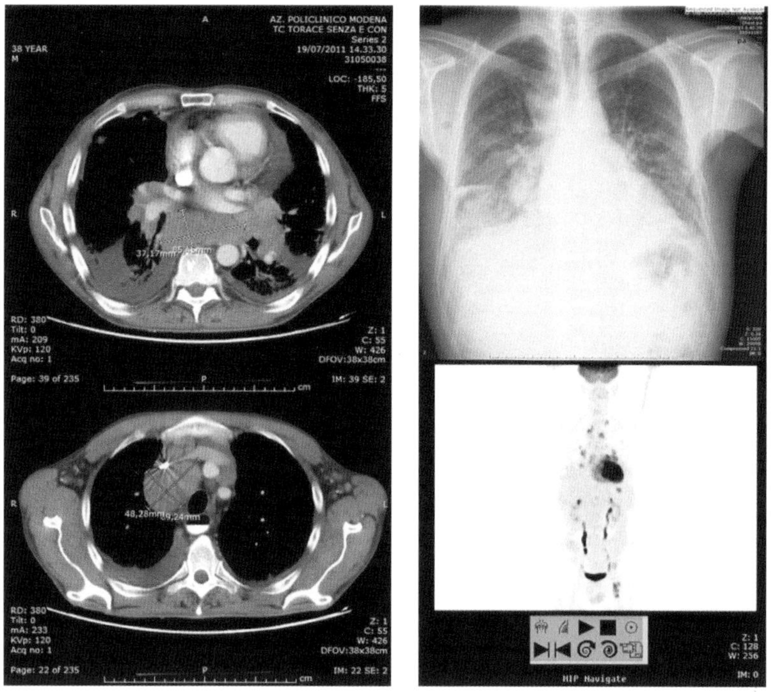

(a) (b)

Figure 1: Radiological chest studies of our patient number 1. (a) Two scans of high-resolution CT, showing the mediastinal adenopathic masses. (b) Standard X-ray and total body PET scan, showing diffuse high-metabolism adenopathies.

diagnosis. Sporadic observations of blood cancer were also reported during the further years, even after several decades.

Among SSc patients with haematological malignancies, the diffuse skin subset was reported in 28% of cases. As regards serology, anticentromere and anti-Scl70 autoantibodies were equally found; of note, a relevant percentage (29%) of specific anti-nuclear autoantibodies (ANA) was observed. Organ SSc involvement was not frequently described; anyway, no peculiar associations may be found, because the malignancies could be observed both in SSc patients with diffuse skin involvement and interstitial lung disease and in the "CREST" patients' subset. In a few cases, overlapping Sjögren's syndrome (a disease with well-known increase of haematological cancer risk) was suspected or clearly reported; moreover, rheumatoid arthritis was recognized in 2 patients, porphyria cutanea tarda in other 2, and pemphigus vulgaris in 1. Finally, only in few patients a detailed clinical history was available, giving the possibility of identifying other eventual cancer risk factors (i.e., smoking).

As regards haematological malignancies, we collected 66 cases with lymphoma (including our 2 cases), 28 with leukaemia, 14 with multiple myeloma (plus one solitary IgM plasmocytoma), and 16 with myeloproliferative disorders; in 3 the exact diagnosis was not expressed. Many types of lymphoma were reported, often not better specified than the mere definition of "non-Hodgkin lymphoma"; in the other cases, the diffuse large B cells lymphoma was the most frequent (8 cases plus 1, our case). With the exception of few patients, all lymphomas described are classifiable as mature B cells neoplasms; in fact, we registered only 3 lymphomas of T cells and 2 from histiocytic cells, while 6 cases of Hodgkin's lymphoma were found.

Considering the 28 cases developing leukaemia, 9 patients showed the chronic lymphocytic form. T cells leukaemia was present in only 2 persons; 8 cases were not better specified. Finally, among myeloproliferative disorders, 4 cases of myelofibrosis and 11 of chronic myelogenous leukaemia were found; just one patient presented polycythemia vera, while no cases of essential thrombocythemia were found.

The clinical courses of the treated patients may be divided into 2 prognostic patterns, substantially equivalent in percentage: (1) rapid improvement up to remission, often associated with SSc features amelioration; (2) rapid deterioration until death from infectious causes. The latter pattern was invariably observed in patients over 50 of age; no other clinical features useful for prognostic purposes were found.

5. Discussion

It is known from the literature that the incidence of haematological malignancies is significantly increased in SSc [1–3]; in this review, we tried to better define this statistical association gathering together all SSc cases complicated by blood cancers previously described. We found that the majority of cases presented the B cells non-Hodgkin lymphoma (especially the diffuse large B cells lymphoma, as well as our case number 1), the multiple myeloma, and the chronic lymphocytic leukaemia; furthermore, also myeloproliferative disorders were frequently described in the course of SSc.

TABLE 1: Haematological diseases in course of systemic sclerosis.

First author/year	Number cases	Study type (country)	Age/sex	Dis. duration	Skin subset	Serology	Visceral inv.	Ass. Sjogren	History notes	Clinical picture	Hematological malignancy	Outcomes
Agard/2000	1	CR (France)	62 F	14	L	ACA	None	No	MGUS	Spleno/lymphoadenop., ascites	Small B cell NHL	Improved with CHOP
Airo'/2011	1	CS (360 Italian pts)	nd	nd	nd	ACA	nd	nd	nd	nd	NHL	nd
Alacacioglu/2005	1	CR (Turkey)	57 M	3	nd	nd	nd	nd	nd	Bilateral upper/lower eyelid hernias	Orbital marginal zone NHL	Improved with chemo/radiotherapy
Angeli/1991	1	CR (France)	42 F	4	L	ACA	nd	No	nd	Splenomegaly	CLL	nd
Arai/2009	1	CR (Japan)	31 F	1	nd	nd	nd	nd	nd	None	Thymic large B-NHL	Remission with CHOP
Arnaud/2006	1	CR (France)	76 F	<1	L	nd	E	nd	*H pylori* +	nd	Gastric MALT lymphoma	nd
Bachleitner-Hofmann/2002	1	CR (Austria)	73 F	14	L	ACA	L, E	nd	MGUS	nd	MM	Marked and sustained improvement with therapy for MM and SSc
Baldini/1994	1	CR (Italy)	59 F	1	nd	ANA	nd	nd	nd	nd	Lymphocytic Ly of intermediate diff.	Improved
Bellis/2014	1	CR (France)	37 M	1	L	ANA	nd	nd	nd	Right axillary lymphoadenopathy	CD30+ anaplastic Ly	Lymphoma and SSc remission with BMT
Ben Ghorbel/2005	1	CR (Tunisy)	70 F	6	L	Scl70	L	No	nd	Generalized lymphoadenopaties	Follicular B NHL	Improved with CHOP
Bielefeld/1996	5	CS (21 French pts)	39 F, 56 F, 69 F, 12 M, 71 M	0, 6, 6, 9, 2	nd	nd	nd	nd	nd	nd	CML, AML, immunocytoma, Burkitt's Ly, Waldenstrom d.	nd
Bistue/1990	1	CR (Argentina)	[illegible]6 F	nd	D	nd	L	No	nd	Dyspnea, splenomegaly, and fever	Myelofibrosis	nd
Cavallero/1994	1	CR (Italy)	79 M	nd	D	ANA	nd	nd	Carpenter	Purpura of legs	Hairy cell leukemia	Died for pneumonia after 3 months
Charlanne/2004	1	CR (France)	72 F	<1	L	ACA	No	Yes	Overlap RA-SS	Neutropenia and lymphocytosis	Large granular lymphocyte leukemia	Sustained (>1 year) improvement with MTX 7.5/week for leukemia and autoimmunity
Chatterjee/2005	5	ES (538 US pts)	2 NHL are F	nd	2 NHL : 1 L, 1 D	nd	nd	nd	nd	nd	NHL (2); MM (2); leukemia (1)	nd
Čolović/2011	1	CR (Serbia)	55 F	20	L	nd	nd	nd	nd	Intense facial pruritus, paraproteinemia	MM	Remission for SSc and MM
Comer/1992	1	CR (UK)	3[illegible] F	1	L	ANA	E, L, H	No	nd	Neck/mediastinum lymphadenopathy	IIb-staged HL	HL remission (MOPP), SSc evolution by 1 year
Constans/1993	1	CR (France)	65 F	0	L	ACA	CREST	No	nd		Hairy cell leukemia	nd
Derk/2003	1	CR (USA)	66 M	2	D	Scl70	E	No	nd	Expanding mass at the tongue base	Large B-NHL	Remission with CHOP
Doyle/1985	5	CS (USA)	10; 22; 31 54; 70 F	4; 9; 9; 40; 57	L	nd	CREST	nd	nd	nd	HL; MM (2); "malignant Ly"; CLL	Variable outcomes

Table 1: Continued.

First author/year	Number cases	Study type (country)	Age/sex	Dis. duration	Skin subset	Serology	Visceral inv.	Ass. Sjogren	History notes	Clinical picture	Hematological malignancy	Outcomes
Duggal/2002	1	CR (India)	42 M	nd	nd	nd	nd	nd	nd	nd	HL	nd
Duncan/1979	7	CS (2,141 USA pts)	50–79 F	2, 0, 1, 3, 0, 61, 1	nd	nd	nd	nd	nd	nd	CLL (3), MM, lymphosarcoma (2), CMML	Died by 1 year (2), alive > 5 years (4)
Dupond/1989	1	CR (France)	73 F	nd	L	ACA	CREST, L	Yes	nd	Splenomegaly	CMML	nd
Ferroir/1991	1	CR (France)	42 M	2	nd	ANA	nd	No	nd	nd	Mixed follicular Ly	Diagnosis at autopsy
Frigui	1	CR (France)	56 F	10	L	Scl70	L, K	No	nd	Skin lesion	Cutaneous B-cell Ly (supraorbital)	Regression after radiotherapy but relapse
Gisser/1979	1	CR (USA)	29 F	4	nd	nd	L, H	nd	Previous chlorambucil treat.	Anemia	CML	Died for bronchopneumonia
Hall/1978	1	CR (USA)	22 F	14	nd	nd	E calcinosis	No	Generalized lipodystrophy	Diffuse lymphoadenopathies	Nodular sclerosing HL	nd
Hasegawa/1999	1	CR (Japan)	43 M	<1	D	ANoA	nd	No	nd	Neck/armpits lymphoadenopathies	Diffuse large T cell NHL	Lymphoma and SSc remission (CHOP 4 cycles)
Haviv/1997	1	CR (Israel)	72 F	1, 5	L	ANA	L, K	No	nd	Fever, wasting, and arthralgias	Diffuse small cell NHL	Death for sepsis
Hill/2003	2	RS (441 Australian pts)	F	nd	nd	nd	nd	nd	nd	nd	Not better specified	nd
Hoshida/2004	7	CS (Japan)	57 (56–65), 2/5 M/F	2.2 (0–12)	nd	nd	nd	2/7	nd	nd	HL (2); diffuse large B cell Ly (5)	All died by 1 year
Kaşifoğlu/2006	1	CR (Turkey)	50 F	7	L	Scl70	L	SSA+	nd	Weakness, weight loss	CML	Improved with HU
Kaşifoğlu/2016	3	CS (340 Turkish pts)	nd	nd	nd	nd	nd	nd	nd	nd	MM, CML, follicular NHL	nd
Katz/1979	1	CR (USA)	57	11	nd	ANA	nd	nd	Pemphigus v.	nd	Diffuse histiocytic Ly	nd
Kyndt/1997	1	CS (123 French pts)	76 F	8	nd	Scl70	L	Yes	nd	nd	CMML	nd
Kojima/2006	2	CS (Japan)	nd	nd	nd	nd	nd	nd	nd	nd	B cell follicular Ly	nd
Kuo/2012	6	RS (2,053 Taiwanese pts)	1 M, 5 F	nd	nd	nd	nd	nd	nd	nd	Ly (3), myeloprolif. dis. (2), CML (2)	nd
Lee/2001	1	CR (Korea)	56 F	15	L	ACA	CREST	No	Porphyria c.t.	Splenomegaly	Myelofibrosis	nd
Marto/2014	1	CR (Portugal)	76 F	0	L	ACA	L	No	Multiple polyps of the colon	Multiple adenop., diarrhea, and rectorrhagia	IIIb-staged mantle cell NHL of the colon	Ly remission with R-CHOP
Miyamoto/2000	1	CR (Japan)	55 F	17	nd	nd	nd	No	nd	Fever, fatigue, pancytopenia, and splenomegaly	Myelofibrosis	Treated with pulse steroids and transfusions
Olesen/2010	18	RS (2,040 Danish pts)	M/F 9/9	2/18 : <1	nd	nd	nd	nd	nd	nd	NHL (10); leukemia (7)	nd

Table 1: Continued.

First author/year	Number cases	Study type (country)	Age/sex	Dis. duration	Skin subset	Serology	Visceral inv.	Ass. Sjogren	History notes	Clinical picture	Hematological malignancy	Outcomes
Owlia/2014	1	CR (Iran)	58 M	15	L	nd	E	No	smoker (30 p-y)	Lumbar pain (extensive bony infiltration)	MM	Death 2 years after VAD/bortezomib
Ozturk/2006	1	CR (Turkey)	54 F	5	L	nd	CREST	No	nd	Sweet syndrome	Myelofibrosis	Improved with steroids and hydroxyurea
Parma/1996	1	CR (Italy)	68	3	nd	nd	nd	nd	nd	Primitive muscle and bone involv.	Large multilobated B-cell NHL	Improved
Prochorec-Sobieszek/2004	1	CR (Poland)	22 F	<1	L	PmScl	nd	No	nd	Parotid swelling	Parotid MALToma	nd
Rodrigues/1989	1	CR (Brazil)	nd	nd	nd	nd	nd	nd	Concom. thyroid adenoca.	nd	Ileal B-cell Ly	Rapid deterioration until death
Rosenthal/1993	3	RS (233 Swedish pts)	nd	<1 (1)	nd	nd	nd	nd	nd	nd	NHL (2), not better specified hematological cancer (1)	nd
Rothfield/1992	1	CS (148 USA pts)	nd	nd	nd	Scl70	nd	nd	nd	nd	Lymphocytic Ly	nd
Roumm/1985	3	CS (262 USA pts)	33 F, 50 F, 71 F	3.5, 5.5, 5.5	nd	nd	nd	nd	nd	nd	CML, AML, and histiocytic Ly	nd
Ryczek/2013	1	CR (Poland)	nd	nd	nd	nd	nd	nd	nd	nd	CML	nd
Schnack/1954	1	CR (Austria)	53 F	8	D	nd	nd	nd	nd	nd	MM	nd
Senel/2006	1	CR (Turkey)	65 F	0	D	Scl70	L, K	No	nd	Weakness, sweating, and weight loss	CML	nd
Shvidel/2002	1	CS (Israel)	71 F	nd	nd	nd	nd	nd	nd	nd	T large granular lymphocytic leukemia	nd
Siau/2011	5	CS (68 UK pts)	nd	0 (case of PC)	L	nd	nd	nd	nd	nd	MM (2), diffuse large B-NHL, thyroid NHL, solitary IgM PC	nd
Sidi/1990	2	CS (Israel)	47 M, 77 M	20; 11	L	nd	CREST	No	nd	Generalized lymphoadenopathy	B-CLL	Alive up to 2 years; death for bronchopneumonia and paralytic ileus
Sugai/1987	1	CR (Japan)	67 F	11	D	ANA	E, L	Yes	nd	Parotid swelling and generalized lymphadenopathy	IIIb-staged NHL	Death after 3 COPP cycles for complicating interstitial pneumonitis
Suzuki/1994	1	CR (Japan)	68 M	3	D	ANA	nd	No	nd	Gait disturbance, anemia, and hemorrhagic stroke	Brain diffuse large B-NHL	Death for pneumonitis during BACOPP chemotherapy
Szekanecz/2008	3	CS (218 Hungarian pts)	53; 67; 69 F	2 1.9; 0.7	D	Scl70;	L-H-E; none; L-H-K-E	nd	nd	nd	(2) b-CLL; (1) chronic small lymphocytic B NHL	Surviving > 5 years

TABLE 1: Continued.

First author/year	Number cases	Study type (country)	Age/sex	Dis. duration	Skin subset	Serology	Visceral inv.	Ass. Sjogren	History notes	Clinical picture	Hematological malignancy	Outcomes
Talbott/1979	2	CS (USA)	64 M; 73 M	<1; 10	L; D	nd	None; L-H	Probable	Pt number 1 coal miner	Backache; generalized weakness	MM	Rapid deterioration and death
Vettori/2010	1	CR (Italy)	45 F		Sine sclerod.					Progressive weight loss	Gastric B-cell Ly	
Watanabe/1994	1	CR (Japan)	44 F	nd	nd	nd	nd	nd	nd	Leukocytosis, thrombocytosis	CML	CML remission and SSc improvement with therapy
William/2011	1	CR (USA)	61 M	30	L	ACA	E, L	No	nd	Thrombocytopenia, cervical adenopathy	Small lymphocytic B-NHL	Remission with FCR
Wooten/1998	1	CR (USA)	nd	3	L		CREST	nd	Porphyria c.t.	nd	CML	nd
Yamamoto/2005	1	CR (Japan)	72 M	5	D	Scl70	L	nd	nd	Multiple lymphoadenopathy	Angioimmunobl. T cell Ly with EBV-assoc. B cell lymphoprol. dis.	Died 6 months after CHOP therapy because of sepsis, initially improved
Present study	2	CR (Italy)	37 M; 72 F	2; 28	D; L	SSA/SSB ACA	E, L; CREST + L	Yes; no	nd; previous breast cancer	Weakness, sweating, and weight loss; asymptomatic	Diffuse large B-NHL; marginal B-NHL	Died few months after during R-CHOP therapy; lung lobe resection and remission
Total	130 pts											

The table included all the case reports and the cohort studies that reported cases of haematological malignancies in the course of SSc [4–67]. Pts = patients; type of study: CR = case report; CS = case series/cohort studies; RS = registry studies; skin subset: D = diffuse, L = limited; serology: ACA = anticentromere, Scl70 = anti-topoisomerase I, ANA = specific antinuclear autoantibodies; organ involvements: K = kidney, L = lung, H = heart, E = esophagus; MGUS = monoclonal gammopathy of undetermined significance; CREST = former acronym for limited SSc form including calcinosis, Raynaud phenomenon, esophageal dysmotility, sclerodactyly, and telangiectasia; CLL = chronic lymphocytic leukemia; CML = chronic myelogenous leukemia; AML = acute myelogenous leukemia; MM = multiple myeloma; PC = plasmacytoma; NHL = non-Hodgkin lymphoma; CMML = chronic myelomonocytic leukemia; Ly = lymphoma; HL = Hodgkin lymphoma; MTX = methotrexate; (R-)CHOP = chemotherapic regimen for NHL; FCR = chemotherapic regimen with fludarabile, cyclophosphamide, and rituximab; BMT = bone marrow transplantation; (BA)COPP = bleomycin, adriamycin, cyclophosphamide, vincristine, procarbazine, and prednisone; MOPP = mustine, vincristine, procarbazine, and prednisone; HU = hydroxyurea; VAD = vincristine, doxorubicin, and dexamethasone.

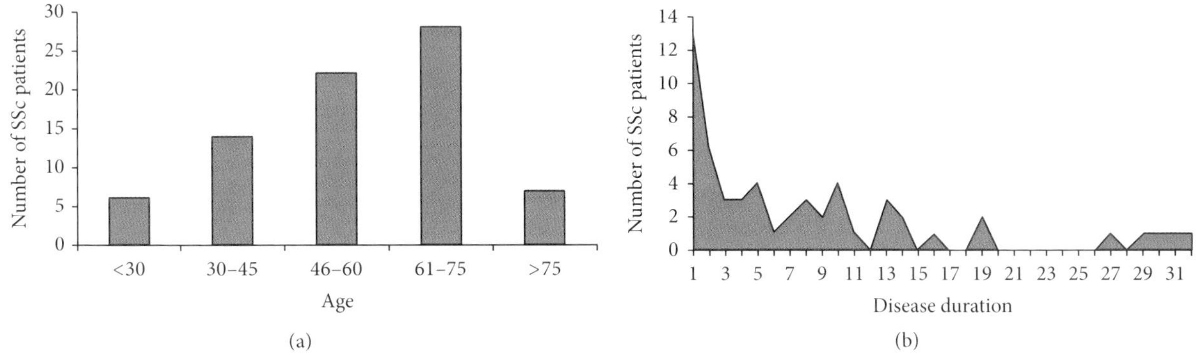

FIGURE 2: Distribution of SSc patients with haematological malignancies on the basis of age at tumour diagnosis (a) and SSc disease duration (b).

Besides the heterogeneity of the cases reported in literature, we found that the diagnosis of haematological neoplasms was a precocious event in SSc patients' clinical histories, particularly within 5 years of SSc diagnosis in the majority of cases (Figure 2). Therefore, given the possibility of successful treatments for a potentially aggressive disease, the clinical-serological surveillance for haematological malignancies in SSc patients should be addressed.

Regarding the demographic characteristics of the SSc patients with blood cancers, we found a higher frequency of males (28%) in comparison to the female/male ratio previously described in large SSc case series [72], probably because of the higher NHL incidence among male subjects [73].

Even though anecdotal in several patients, we underline the coexistence of other autoimmune disorders or pathologic conditions known for their increased risk of cancer. Indeed, the omission of relevant anamnestic information in the descriptions of patients reported in literature is presumable, especially for the registry/large cohort-based studies designed for the statistical analysis of cancers epidemiology. As regards serology, the presence of a specific ANA in SSc patients with haematological cancers was found in 29% of cases, more than generally reported in previous cohort studies [72]. In this respect, Altintas et al. [74] detected ANA in more than 20% of 179 patients affected by lymphomas, even though the majority of them did not show autoimmune diseases. Furthermore, in an elegant study by Guyomard et al. [75], 347 NHL patients and 213 controls were investigated by means of indirect immunofluorescence technique on Hep2 cells. ANA were significantly more frequent in the first group (19% versus 5.6%), before any treatment, particularly in presence of follicular or mantle B cell lymphomas. The latter are characterized by a high rate of cells proliferation and a large number of apoptotic cells, leading to the exposition of large amount of nuclear antigens, eventually targeted by patients' immune system.

The association between autoimmune diseases and haematological neoplasms is an intriguing question; indeed, more than 10% of lymphoid malignancies occur in the setting of an autoimmune disorder [76]. Accumulated evidences indicate that autoreactive B cells are more prone to undergo malignant transformation. In parallel, the chronic activation of the inflammatory response due to autoantigen-driven immune stimulation in specific organ tissues (i.e., the parotid gland in Sjögren's syndrome) is associated with an increased risk of lymphomas [76, 77]. Furthermore, the epidemiological data from large population studies on other autoimmune diseases, such as rheumatoid arthritis or systemic lupus erythematosus, showed a high risk of B cells haematological neoplasms, particularly the diffuse large B cell lymphoma [78, 79]. Consistently, in SSc, we found a clear-cut prevalence of B cells versus the T cells cancers, suggesting that the systemic autoimmune activation plays a pivotal role in the carcinogenetic evolution.

Besides the evidences of pathogenetic and statistical links between SSc and haematological malignancies [1–3], the exact mechanism responsible for cancers is not understood. In other autoimmune disorders specific etiologic factors (i.e., HCV for mixed cryoglobulinemia [80]) lead to persistent stimulation of the immune system and, eventually, to lymphomagenesis. Differently, SSc etiology remains obscure, despite the probable role of a few infectious triggers able to chronically infect immune cells [81]. Overall, a deeper knowledge of the SSc etiopathogenetic processes, probably different for several disease's subsets, could help to better quantify the risk for different types of cancers, including haematological neoplasms.

Since the majority of patients described in the present study developed the tumours in the first years of the disease (Figure 2), including our first case, the possible iatrogenic effect of immunosuppressors may be easily excluded. On the contrary, it was hypothesized that the immune alterations in the early phase of SSc present a different pattern, which tends to change during the disease's follow-up [82].

We previously demonstrated a high prevalence of thymic hyperplasia in SSc patients, particularly during the first years of the disease [71]. Given the fundamental role of the thymus in the maturation of T lymphocytes, it might be assumed that a pathological alteration of the thymic microenvironment could lead to a deficient or incomplete T cell maturation, which might have a role in the immunological alterations of SSc etiopathogenesis. Nonetheless, the autoreactivity of T cells strictly involves also B cells that produce a number of different autoantibodies, which in turn stimulate fibroblasts' toll-like receptors-4 [83] and induce endothelial dysfunction [84]. B cell infiltrates may be detected in SSc patients' skin or in affected areas of the lungs, so giving the rationale for the therapeutic use of rituximab [85]. Therefore, even though T cells are considered the driving force of the autoimmune pathogenesis in SSc, it is not surprisingly the observation of an increased risk for B cells-derived malignancies.

Upon the onset of autoimmune responses, lymphoid tissues undergo histological changes due to the remodelling of the tissue architecture in parallel with the phenotypic transformations of immune cell populations. Recently, Sangaletti et al. [76] hypothesized that an erroneous remodelling of the stromal microenvironment in secondary lymphoid organs could facilitate malignant transformation of lymphocytes, in presence of persistent immune stimulation. Thus, lymphomagenesis would be a result of disrupted myeloid and lymphoid function in lymphoid tissues that harbour autoreactive proliferating T and B cells. In this respect, our paradigmatic case developed a lymphoma that probably rose in the thymus, which was histologically disrupted by the preexistent thymic hyperplasia.

In SSc patients, several studies demonstrated the activation status of the peripheral B lymphocytes with an impaired percentage of apoptotic cells compared to healthy controls [86]. Moreover, Wang et al. [87] found that the levels of histone acetylation and methylation (responsible for increased gene transcription) in B cells from SSc patients correlate with disease activity. Furthermore, serum concentrations of BAFF and APRIL, cytokines regulating B cell activity, survival, and proliferation, are found elevated in SSc in comparison with healthy controls, particularly in patients with active or severe disease [86]. In this light, we might assume that the sclerodermic patients with poorly controlled disease (an occurrence more probable in the early phase of SSc, like in our first case) are more prone to develop haematological malignancies in their clinical histories.

In SSc, the increase of B cells survival and activation sounds apparently in contrast with the finding of augmented Fas (CD95) expression on the surface of memory B cell that facilitate Fas-mediated apoptosis. However, the incessant loss of these lymphocytes is coupled to the increased production of naive B cells and plasma cells in order to maintain B cell homeostasis [88]. Therefore, the amplification of the percentage of less mature B lymphocytes understandably leads to a major risk for lymphoid carcinogenesis.

Finally, as opposite scenario, we briefly mention the possibility that cancer mutations might trigger SSc itself, at least in patients with anti-RNA polymerase III autoantibodies [89]. Neoplasms could harbour missense mutations in the gene coding for the polymerase III polypeptide A, leading to the production of an altered protein. The latter could stimulate an immune response and, possibly, a cross-reaction against the normal protein; this immune response could be relevant in the pathogenesis of a subset of SSc [90].

The present study shows a few limitations. Firstly, even though this review included the higher possible number of studies, several cases of SSc complicated by blood cancers described in literature were lost [91, 92], because of the unavailability of the necessary information for the purposes of our study. This limitation may be exceeded only with further studies designed ad hoc, including large case series.

Secondly, our review included a number of case reports, in which contemporaneous SSc and haematological malignancy are more likely to be reported than cases where the diagnoses are far apart. In particular, SSc patients who suffered from haematological malignancies longer after SSc onset were more unlikely to be published because it was difficult to emphasize the relationship of 'SSc and haematological malignancies.' However, also SSc cohort studies seem to confirm the higher incidence of blood cancers in the first years of SSc. Anyway, the eventual exposure to immunosuppressive therapy in SSc patients with longer disease duration could be considered a further risk factor for cancer development.

In conclusion, SSc may be complicated by several types of cancers, including haematological malignancies. More frequently, B cells-derived lymphomas and leukaemias may be diagnosed in the first years of the disease and represent a significant warning for patients' prognosis. To date, no specific SSc features could predict which subjects present major risk for blood cancer; thus, a careful surveillance of SSc patients should be addressed.

References

[1] N. Zeineddine, L. E. Khoury, and J. Mosak, "Systemic sclerosis and malignancy: a review of current data," *Journal of Clinical Medicine Research*, vol. 8, pp. 625–632, 2016.

[2] A. Onishi, D. Sugiyama, S. Kumagai, and A. Morinobu, "Cancer incidence in systemic sclerosis: meta-analysis of population-based cohort studies," *Arthritis and Rheumatism*, vol. 65, no. 7, pp. 1913–1921, 2013.

[3] M. Bonifazi, I. Tramacere, G. Pomponio et al., "Systemic sclerosis (scleroderma) and cancer risk: systematic review and meta-analysis of observational studies," *Rheumatology*, vol. 52, Article ID kes303, pp. 143–154, 2013.

[4] C. Agard, T. Ponge, B. Mahé, and J. Barrier, "Lymphocytic lymphoma and regenerative liver nodular hyperplasia in systemic scleroderma," *La Revue de Médecine Interne*, vol. 21, pp. 301–303, 2000.

[5] I. Alacacioglu, M. A. Ozcan, N. Kocak et al., "Bilateral primary orbital non-Hodgkin's lymphoma in a patient with scleroderma: a case report," *Leukemia and Lymphoma*, vol. 46, no. 8, pp. 1239–1242, 2005.

[6] C. Angeli, J. P. Lacour, B. Taillan, and J. P. Ortonne, "Chronic lymphoid leukemia in a case of scleroderma," in *Presse Med*, vol. 20, p. 426, 1991.

[7] H. Arai, H. Iso, Y. Arai et al., "Mediastinal large B-cell lymphoma associated with systemic sclerosis," vol. 50, pp. 97–101, Rinsho Ketsueki, 2009.

[8] L. Arnaud, A. Chryssostalis, B. Terris et al., "Systemic sclerosis and gastric MALT lymphoma," *Joint Bone Spine*, vol. 73, no. 1, pp. 105–108, 2006.

[9] T. Bachleitner-Hofmann, K. Machold, R. Knobler, J. Drach, E. Grumbeck, and H. Gisslinger, "Marked and sustained improvement of systemic sclerosis following polychemotherapy for coexistent multiple myeloma," *Clinical and Experimental Rheumatology*, vol. 20, pp. 85–88, 2002.

[10] L. Baldini, A. Guffanti, A. Ferrari et al., "Uncommon clinical presentation of a lymphocytic lymphoma of intermediate differentiation in a patient with systemic sclerosis," *British Journal of Haematology*, vol. 86, no. 3, pp. 657–658, 1994.

[11] R. Bellis, C. Francès, S. Barète, and P. Senet, "Clinical and capillaroscopic regression of CD30 anaplastic lymphoma associated with limited cutaneous systemic sclerosis following autologous bone marrow transplantation," *Annales de Dermatologie et de Venereologie*, vol. 141, pp. 446–451, 2014.

[12] I. Ben Ghorbel, K. Bellil, M. N. Kchir, I. Gharsallah, M. Miled, and M. H. Houman, "Systemic sclerosis and non-Hodgkin lymphoma," *Revue de Medecine Interne*, vol. 26, no. 12, pp. 993–996, 2005.

[13] P. Bielefeld, P. Meyer, D. Caillot et al., "Systemic sclerosis and cancer: 21 new cases and review of literature," *Revue de Medecine Interne*, vol. 17, no. 10, pp. 810–813, 1996.

[14] R. Bistue, M. E. Gallo de Sprazzato, C. D. Scognamillo et al., "Coexistence of myelofibrosis and collagen diseases," *Medicina (B Aires)*, vol. 50, pp. 248–250, 1990.

[15] G. B. Cavallero, M. Bonferroni, A. Gallamini, M. Grasso, and A. Carbone, "Scleroderma and hairy-cell leukemia," *European Journal of Haematology*, vol. 52, no. 3, pp. 189–190, 1994.

[16] H. Charlanne, M. Lambert, E. Hachulla et al., "Large granular lymphocyte leukaemia associated with systemic sclerosis," *Rheumatology*, vol. 43, no. 9, pp. 1197–1198, 2004.

[17] M. Čolović, V. Jurisic, J. Bila, N. Čolović, and V. Palibrk, "FGF-R3 and OPG expression in patient with multiple myeloma following systemic sclerosis: case report and review of the literature," *International Journal of Hematology*, vol. 93, no. 2, pp. 228–231, 2011.

[18] M. Comer and A. R. Harvey, "Remission of scleroderma during chemotherapy for lymphoma," *Annals of the Rheumatic Diseases*, vol. 51, no. 8, pp. 998–1000, 1992.

[19] J. Constans, M. Cadenne, T. Schaeverbeke et al., "Systemic scleroderma and hairy cell leukemia. a new case," *Revue du Rhumatisme (Edition Francaise)*, vol. 60, pp. 371–352, 1993.

[20] C. T. Derk, L. I. Sakkas, M. Rasheed, C. M. Artlett, and S. A. Jimenez, "Autoantibodies in patients with systemic sclerosis and cancer: a case-control study," *Clinical Rheumatology*, vol. 30, pp. 1994–1996, 2003.

[21] J. A. Doyle, S. M. Connolly, and H. C. Hoagland, "Hematologic disease in scleroderma syndromes," in *Acta Dermato-Venereologica*, vol. 65, pp. 521–525, 1985.

[22] L. Duggal, S. Gupta, P. K. Aggarwal, V. P. Sachar, and S. Bhalla, "Hodgkin's disease scleroderma," *J Assoc Physicians India*, vol. 50, pp. 1186–1188, 2002.

[23] J. L. Dupond, P. Humbert, T. Fest, and B. de Wazières, "Scleroderma, Gougerot-Sjögren syndrome and myelomonocytic leukemia," *Rev Rhum Mal Osteoartic*, vol. 56, pp. 425–426, 1989.

[24] J. P. Ferroir, M. H. Nicolle, J. Roland, and A. Guillard, "Generalized scleroderma associated with mixed follicular lymphoma," *Presse Med.*, vol. 20, Article ID 1514, 1991.

[25] M. Frigui, N. Kaddour, M. Mseddi et al., "Lymphome B cutané au cours d'une sclérodermie systémique," *Oncologie*, vol. 12, pp. 21–25, 2010.

[26] S. D. Gisser and K. B. Chung, "Acute myelofibrosis in progressive sclerosis. report of a case developing during long term chlorambucil therapy and discussion of pathogenetic factors," *American Journal of Medicine*, vol. 67, pp. 151–154, 1979.

[27] S. W. Hall, J. J. Gillespie, and T. F. Tenczynski, "Generalized Lipodystrophy, Scleroderma, and Hodgkin's Disease," *Archives of Internal Medicine*, vol. 138, no. 8, pp. 1303–1304, 1978.

[28] M. Hasegawa, S. Sato, H. Sakai, T. Ohashi, and K. Takehara, "Systemic sclerosis revealing T-Cell lymphoma," *Dermatology*, vol. 198, no. 1, pp. 75–78, 1999.

[29] Y. S. Haviv, A. Ben-Yehuda, A. Polliack, and R. Safadi, "Lymphoma and systemic sclerosis—an uncommon association or possible coincidence of two disorders with a fatal outcome," *European Journal of Haematology*, vol. 59, no. 3, pp. 194–196, 1997.

[30] Y. Hoshida, Y. Tomita, D. Zhiming et al., "Lymphoproliferative disorders in autoimmune diseases in Japan: analysis of clinicopathological features and Epstein-Barr virus infection," *International Journal of Cancer*, vol. 108, no. 3, pp. 443–449, 2004.

[31] T. Kaşifoğlu, C. Korkmaz, Ş. Yaşar, and Z. Gülbaş, "Scleroderma and chronic myeloid leukemia: a sheer coincidence, a consequence of long lasting D-penicillamine therapy or a plausible relationship of both diseases?" *Rheumatology International*, vol. 27, no. 2, pp. 175–177, 2006.

[32] A. L. Katz, D. J. Nashel, C. P. Goard, and H. Bauer, "Pemphigus vulgaris and lymphoma in a patient with scleroderma," *Southern Medical Journal*, vol. 72, no. 11, pp. 1463–1466, 1979.

[33] M. Kojima, H. Itoh, K. Shimizu et al., "Malignant lymphoma in patients with systemic rheumatic disease (rheumatoid arthritis, systemic lupus erythematosus, systemic sclerosis, and dermatomyositis): a clinicopathologic study of 24 Japanese cases," *International Journal of Surgical Pathology*, vol. 14, no. 1, pp. 43–48, 2006.

[34] S. C. Lee, S. J. Yun, J.-B. Lee, S.-S. Lee, and Y. H. Won, "A case of porphyria cutanea tarda in association with idiopathic myelofibrosis and CREST syndrome," *British Journal of Dermatology*, vol. 144, no. 1, pp. 182–185, 2001.

[35] G. Marto, R. Aguiar, and A. Barcelos, "Mantle cell lymphoma and acta reumatol port," *Acta Reumatologica Portuguesa*, vol. 39, pp. 82–86, 2014.

[36] Y. Miyamoto, N. Hara, S. Orima, A. Yamakage, and S. Yamazaki, "A case of systemic sclerosis with myelofibrosis," *Nishi Nihon Hifuka*, vol. 62, pp. 454–457, 2000.

[37] Owlia M. B., O. Distler, M. Foratyazdi, and M. Akhtari, "Visual problem and low back pain as initial manifestation of multiple myeloma complicating pre-existing sclerosis," *Journal of the College of Physicians and Surgeons (Pakistan)*, vol. 24, Supplement 1, pp. 29–31, 2014.

[38] M. A. Ozturk, S. Haznedaroglu, Y. Karaaslan, B. Goker, and I. C. Haznedaroglu, "Increased serum thrombopoietin concentration in systemic sclerosis associated with myelofibrosis and thrombocytosis," *Joint Bone Spine*, vol. 73, no. 1, pp. 122–123, 2006.

[39] M. Parma, G. Sita, A. Guffanti, F. Bianchi, M. Colombi, and L. Baldini, "Multilobated B cell lymphoma (Pinkus variant) with isolated muscular localization in a patient with systemic sclerosis: a case report," *Annals of Hematology*, vol. 73, no. 1, pp. 43–45, 1996.

[40] M. Prochorec-Sobieszek, P. Mielnik, T. Wagner, and H. Chwalińska-Sadowska, "Mucosa-associated lymphoid tissue

lymphoma (MALT) of salivary glands and scleroderma: a case report," *Clinical Rheumatology*, vol. 23, no. 4, pp. 348–350, 2004.

[41] C. J. Rodrigues, H. Bisi, N. Yoshinari, P. E. Marchiori, and W. Cossermelli, "Progressive sclerosis, B-cell malignant lymphoma of the ileum and thyroid adenocarcinoma," *Rev Hosp Clin Fac Med Sao Paulo*, vol. 44, pp. 84–86, 1989.

[42] R. Ryczek, J. Góra-Tybor, K. Betkier-Lipińska, and A. Cwetsch, "Reversible pulmonary hypertension as a consequence of dasatinib treatment in a patient with chronic myeloid leukemia and scleroderma," *Polski Merkuriusz Lekarski: Organ Polskiego Towarzystwa Lekarskiego*, vol. 34, pp. 342–344, 2013.

[43] H. Schnack and N. Stefenelli, "A case of diffuse generalized scleroderma and plasmocytoma," *Wien Klin Wochenschr*, vol. 66, pp. 862–864, 1954.

[44] S. Senel, E. Kaya, I. Aydogdu, M. A. Erkurt, and I. Kuku, "Rheumatic diseases and chronic myelogenous leukemia, presentation of four cases and review of the literature," *Rheumatology International*, vol. 26, no. 9, pp. 857–861, 2006.

[45] L. Shvidel, C. Duksin, A. Tzimanis et al., "Cytokine release by activated T-cells in large granular lymphocytic leukemia associated with autoimmune disorders," *The Hematology Journal*, vol. 3, pp. 32–37, 2002.

[46] Y. Sidi, R. Fadilah, J. Pinkhas, and M. Prokocimer, "Systemic sclerosis and chronic lymphocytic leukaemia," *Postgraduate Medical Journal*, vol. 66, no. 782, pp. 1071–1072, 1990.

[47] S. Sugai, J. Tachibana, M. Sawada et al., "Malignant lymphomas in patients with autoimmune diseases: a report of 6 cases and a review of the Japanese literature," *Japanese Journal of Medicine*, vol. 26, no. 3, pp. 339–347, 1987.

[48] A. Suzuki, H. Ohoike, Y. Kitagawa, Y. Matsuoka, and S. Irimajiri, "Progressive systemic sclerosis complicated with primary cerebral malignant lymphoma," *Internal Medicine*, vol. 33, no. 9, pp. 557–559, 1994.

[49] J. H. Talbott and M. Barrocas, "Progressive systemic sclerosis (PSS) and malignancy, pulmonary and non-pulmonary," *Medicine*, vol. 58, pp. 182–207, 1979.

[50] S. Vettori, S. Staibano, M. Mascolo, G. Ilardi, and G. Valentini, "Non-Hodgkin's lymphoma in systemic sclerosis: case and literature review," *Clinical Rheumatology*, vol. 29, no. 1, pp. 1–6, 2010.

[51] S. Watanabe, T. Sugihara, M. Takahashi et al., "Concordant improvement of progressive systemic sclerosis and chronic myelogenous leukemia with interferon-alpha treatment," *Rinsho Ketsueki*, vol. 35, pp. 895–897, 1994.

[52] B. M. William, T. Harbert, A. K. Ganti, and P. J. Bierman, "Small lymphocytic lymphoma in a patient with CREST syndrome," *Hematology/ Oncology and Stem Cell Therapy*, vol. 4, no. 3, pp. 132–135, 2011.

[53] M. D. Wooten, J. W. Scott, A. M. Miller, and E. Boh, "Chronic myelogenous leukemia and porphyria cutanea tarda in a patient with limited systemic sclerosis," *Southern Medical Journal*, vol. 91, no. 5, pp. 493–495, 1998.

[54] H. Yamamoto, H. Miwa, Y. Kato, S. Nakamura, K. Hara, and M. Nitta, "Angioimmunoblastic T cell lymphoma with an unusual proliferation of Epstein-Barr virus-associated large B cells arising in a patient with progressive systemic sclerosis," *Acta Haematologica*, vol. 114, no. 2, pp. 108–112, 2005.

[55] P. Airo', A. Ceribelli, I. Cavazzana, M. Taraborelli, S. Zingarelli, and F. Franceschini, "Malignancies in Italian patients with systemic sclerosis positive for anti-RNA polymerase III antibodies," *The Journal of Rheumatology*, vol. 38, no. 7, pp. 1329–1334, 2011.

[56] S. Chatterjee, G. W. Dombi, R. K. Severson, and M. D. Mayes, "Risk of malignancy in scleroderma: a population-based cohort study," *Arthritis and Rheumatism*, vol. 52, no. 8, pp. 2415–2424, 2005.

[57] S. C. Duncan and R. K. Winkelmann, "Cancer and scleroderma," *Archves of Dermatology*, vol. 115, pp. 950–955, 1979.

[58] C. L. Hill, A. M. Nguyen, D. Roder, and P. Roberts-Thomson, "Risk of cancer in patients with a population based cohort study," *Annals of the Rheumatic Diseases*, vol. 62, pp. 728–731, 2003.

[59] T. Kaşifoğlu, Ş. Yaşar Bilge, F. Yıldız et al., "Risk factors for malignancy in systemic sclerosis patients," *Clinical Rheumatology*, vol. 35, no. 6, pp. 1529–1533, 2016.

[60] X. Kyndt, M. Hebbar, V. Queyrel, E. Hachulla, P. Y. Hatron, and B. Devulder, "Systemic scleroderma and cancer. Search for predictive factors of cancer in 123 patients with scleroderma," *La Revue de Médecine Interne*, vol. 18, no. 7, pp. 528–532, 1997.

[61] C. F. Kuo, S. F. Luo, K. H. Yu et al., "Cancer risk among patients with sclerosis: a nationwide population study in Taiwan," *Scand J Rheumatol*, vol. 41, pp. 44–49, 2012.

[62] A. B. Olesen, C. Sværke, D. K. Farkas, and H. T. Sørensen, "Systemic sclerosis and the risk of cancer: a nationwide population-based cohort study," *British Journal of Dermatology*, vol. 163, pp. 800–806, 2010.

[63] A. K. Rosenthal, J. K. McLaughlin, M. S. Linet, and I. Persson, "Scleroderma and malignancy: An Epidemiological Study," *Annals of the Rheumatic Diseases*, vol. 52, no. 7, pp. 531–533, 1993.

[64] N. Rothfield, S. Kurtzman, D. Vazques-Abad, C. Charron, L. Daniels, and B. Greenberg, "Association of anti-topoisomerase 1 with cancer," *Arthritis and Rheumatism*, vol. 35, Article ID 724, 1992.

[65] A. D. Roumm and T. A. Medsger Jr., "Cancer and systemic sclerosis. an epidemiologic study," *Arthritis & Rheumatology*, vol. 28, pp. 1336–1340, 1985.

[66] K. Siau, C. J. Laversuch, P. Creamer, and K. P. O'Rourke, "Malignancy in from south west England: a population-based cohort study," *Rheumatol Int*, vol. 31, pp. 641–645, 2011.

[67] É. Szekanecz, S. Szamosi, Á. Horváth et al., "Malignancies associated with systemic sclerosis," *Autoimmunity Reviews*, vol. 11, no. 12, pp. 852–855, 2012.

[68] T. I. Mughal, J. M. Goldman, and S. T. Mughal, *Understanding Leukemias, Lymphomas and Myelomas*, CRC Press, 2nd edition, 2009.

[69] E. S. Jaffe, N. L. Harris, Steinm H., and J. W. Vardiman, Eds., *World Health Organisation Classification of Tumours: Tumours of Haematopoietic and Lymphoid Tissue*, IARC Press, Lyon, France, 2001.

[70] S. H. Swerdlow, E. Campo, S. A. Pileri et al., "The 2016 revision of the World Health Organization classification of lymphoid neoplasms," *Blood*, vol. 127, no. 20, pp. 2375–2390, 2016.

[71] M. Colaci, D. Giuggioli, A. Manfredi, C. Vacchi, G. D. Casa, and C. Ferri, "Radiological thymus alterations in systemic sclerosis: our experience and a review of the literature," *Rheumatology*, vol. 53, no. 4, Article ID ket419, pp. 732–736, 2014.

[72] C. Ferri, M. Sebastiani, A. Lo Monaco et al., "Systemic sclerosis evolution of disease pathomorphosis and survival. Our experience on Italian patients' population and review of the literature," *Autoimmunity Reviews*, vol. 13, no. 10, pp. 1026–1034, 2014.

[73] N. Horesh and N. A. Horowitz, "Does gender matter in non-Hodgkin lymphoma? Differences in epidemiology, clinical behavior, and therapy," *Rambam Maimonides Med J*, vol. 5, Article ID e0038, 2014.

[74] A. Altintas, T. Cil, S. Pasa, and et, "Clinical significance of elevated antinuclear antibody test in patients with hodgkin's and non-hodgkin's lymphoma: a single center experience," *Minerva Medica*, vol. 99, pp. 7–14, 2008.

[75] S. Guyomard, G. Salles, M. Coudurier et al., "Prevalence and pattern of antinuclear autoantibodies in 347 patients with non-Hodgkin's lymphoma," *British Journal of Haematology*, vol. 123, no. 1, pp. 90–99, 2003.

[76] S. Sangaletti, C. Tripodo, C. Vitali et al., "Defective stromal remodeling and neutrophil extracellular traps in lymphoid tissues favor the transition from autoimmunity to lymphoma," *Cancer Discovery*, vol. 4, no. 1, pp. 110–129, 2014.

[77] K. E. Smedby, H. Hjalgrim, J. Askling et al., "Autoimmune and chronic inflammatory disorders and risk of non-Hodgkin lymphoma by subtype," *Journal of the National Cancer Institute*, vol. 98, no. 1, pp. 51–60, 2006.

[78] A. G. Singh, S. Singh, and E. L. Matteson, "Rate, risk factors and causes of mortality in patients with sjögren's syndrome: a systematic review and meta-analysis of cohort studies," *Rheumatology*, vol. 55, no. 3, pp. 450–460, 2016.

[79] T. A. Simon, A. Thompson, K. K. Gandhi, M. C. Hochberg, and S. Suissa, "Incidence of malignancy in adult patients with rheumatoid arthritis: a meta-analysis," *Arthritis Research & Therapy*, vol. 17, Article ID 212, 2015.

[80] C. Ferri, M. Sebastiani, D. Giuggioli et al., "Hepatitis C virus syndrome: a constellation of organ- and non-organ specific autoimmune disorders, B-cell non- Hodgkin's lymphoma, and cancer," *World Journal of Hepatology*, vol. 7, no. 3, pp. 327–343, 2015.

[81] C. Ferri, D. Giuggioli, and M. Colaci, "Viral infections and sclerosis.," *Clin Exp Rheumatol*, vol. 32, Supplement 86, no. 6, p. 229, 2014.

[82] M. Cossu, L. van Bon, S. Nierkens et al., "The magnitude of cytokine production by stimulated $CD56^{+}$ cells is associated with sclerosis," *Clinical Immunology*, vol. 173, pp. 76–80, 2016.

[83] C. Chizzolini and F. Boin, "The role of the acquired immune response in systemic sclerosis," *Seminars in Immunopathology*, vol. 37, pp. 519–528, 2015.

[84] N. Del Papa, N. Quirici, C. Scavullo et al., "Antiendothelial cell antibodies induce apoptosis of bone marrow endothelial progenitors in systemic sclerosis," *Journal of Rheumatology*, vol. 37, no. 10, pp. 2053–2063, 2010.

[85] D. Giuggioli, F. Lumetti, M. Colaci, P. Fallahi, A. Antonelli, and C. Ferri, "Rituximab in the treatment of patients with systemic sclerosis. Our experience and review of the literature," *Autoimmunity Reviews*, vol. 14, no. 11, pp. 1072–1078, 2015.

[86] T. Sanges Guerrier, D. Launay et al., "Role of B cells in the pathogenesis of sclerosis," *Rev Med Interne*, 2016.

[87] Y. Wang, Y. Yang, Y. Luo et al., "Aberrant histone modification in peripheral blood B cells from patients with systemic sclerosis," *Clinical Immunology*, vol. 149, no. 1, pp. 46–54, 2013.

[88] A. Yoshizaki, "B lymphocytes in systemic sclerosis: Abnormalities and therapeutic targets," *Journal of Dermatology*, vol. 43, no. 1, pp. 39–45, 2016.

[89] C. G. Joseph, E. Darrah, A. A. Shah et al., "Association of the autoimmune disease scleroderma with an immunologic response to cancer," *Science*, vol. 343, no. 6167, pp. 152–157, 2014.

[90] A. A. Shah and L. Casciola-Rosen, "Cancer and scleroderma: A paraneoplastic disease with implications for malignancy screening," *Current Opinion in Rheumatology*, vol. 27, no. 6, pp. 563–570, 2015.

[91] P. Moinzadeh, C. Fonseca, M. Hellmich et al., "Association of anti-RNA polymerase III autoantibodies and cancer in scleroderma," *Arthritis Research and Therapy*, vol. 16, article R53, 2014.

[92] A. A. Shah, L. K. Hummers, L. Casciola-Rosen, K. Visvanathan, A. Rosen, and F. M. Wigley, "Examination of autoantibody status and clinical features associated with cancer risk and cancer-associated scleroderma," *Arthritis & Rheumatology*, vol. 67, no. 4, pp. 1053–1061, 2015.

41

Sjögren Syndrome Complicated with Cystic Lung Disease and Pulmonary Amyloidosis

Koichiro Takahashi, Hironori Sadamatsu, Shinsuke Ogusu, Kazutoshi Komiya, Tomomi Nakamura, Shinya Kimura, and Naoko Sueoka-Aragane

Division of Hematology, Respiratory Medicine and Oncology, Department of Internal Medicine, Faculty of Medicine, Saga University, 5-1-1 Nabeshima, Saga 849-8501, Japan

Correspondence should be addressed to Koichiro Takahashi; takahak@cc.saga-u.ac.jp

Academic Editor: George S. Habib

A 72-year-old Japanese woman was noted to have multiple cystic lung shadows and infiltrates on chest radiography and computed tomography (CT). She complained of dryness of the mouth and eyes, but she did not have respiratory symptoms, such as cough, sputum production, and dyspnea. Her laboratory findings showed high titers of anti-SSA/Ro and anti-SSB/La antibodies. Surgical lung biopsy was performed and demonstrated pathologic findings of amyloid light-chain deposition and bronchiolitis with lymphocytic infiltration. Taken altogether, she was diagnosed as Sjögren syndrome with bronchiolitis and pulmonary amyloidosis. Since then, she has been carefully followed up without treatment. After 6 years, the cystic lung lesions on CT gradually enlarged and increased in number, but she remained to have no respiratory symptoms and no manifestations of lymphoma. Here, we report a rare case of Sjögren syndrome complicated with cystic lung disease and pulmonary amyloidosis.

1. Introduction

Sjögren syndrome is associated with various respiratory complications; its most common manifestations are interstitial lung disease and tracheobronchial disease [1], but less common manifestations, such as cystic lung lesions and pulmonary amyloidosis, have been reported [2, 3].

Amyloidosis is characterized by extracellular deposition of amyloid in various tissues; the amyloid proteins are fibrillary materials that are mainly classified into about 30 types of proteins [4]. In amyloid light-chain (AL) amyloidosis, the tissue deposits comprise immunoglobulin light chains. Amyloid localized to the respiratory system is classified as tracheobronchial, mediastinal or hilar lymphadenopathy, pleural effusion, and lung parenchymal [5, 6]. When the lung parenchyma is affected, nodules, infiltrates, and interstitial depositions are observed [7]. Interestingly, in the present case, the cystic lung lesions on chest computed tomography (CT) gradually enlarged and increased in number over a 6-year period. The present case is considered to be valuable because it presented evaluation of the progression of the cystic changes in the lung over time. We here report a case of Sjögren syndrome with cystic lung disease and pulmonary amyloidosis.

2. Case Presentation

A 72-year-old Japanese woman visited our hospital because she was noted to have an abnormality on chest radiography upon routine health examination. She recalled having the sensation of dryness of the mouth and eyes for 1 year, but she did not have fever and any respiratory symptoms, such as cough, sputum production, or dyspnea. She had never smoked, and past medical history was significant for uterine fibroid.

Physical examination showed blood pressure of 126/78 mmHg, heart rate of 72 beats per minute, respiratory rate of 16 per minute, body temperature of 36.3°C, and the absence of crackles on auscultation. Chest radiography showed infiltrates on the right lower lung field, and chest CT

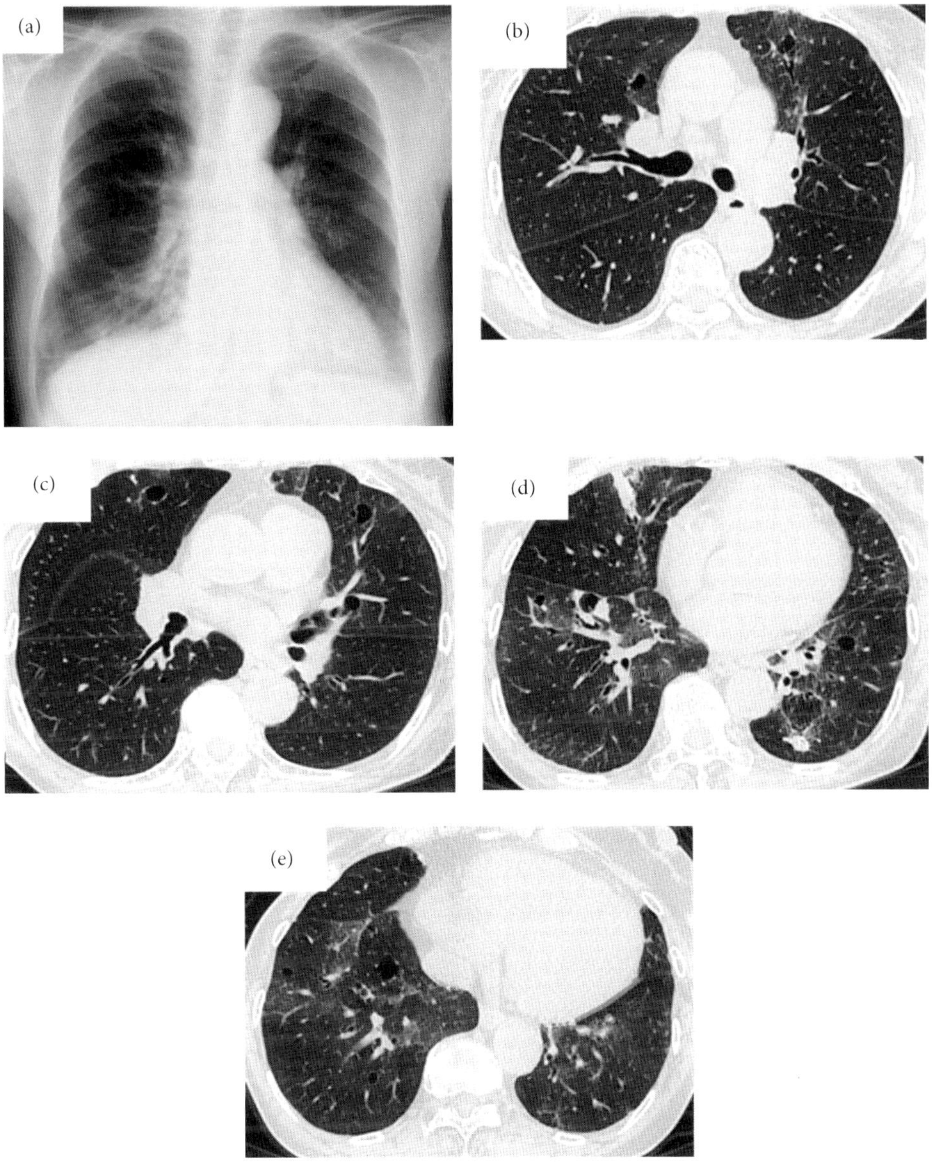

Figure 1: Chest radiograph and CT findings in a 72-year-old woman with Sjögren syndrome and pulmonary amyloidosis. (a) Chest radiograph shows infiltrates in the right lower lung field and ground-glass shadows in the bilateral lower lung fields. Chest CT shows (b, c) multiple cystic lung shadows in the bilateral upper lobes, (d) infiltrates in the right middle lobe and a nodular shadow in the left lower lobe, and (e) ground-glass shadows in the bilateral lower lobes. CT, computed tomography

showed multiple infiltrates and cystic lesions in the bilateral lung (Figure 1). Laboratory findings showed hemoglobin 12.8 g/dL, white blood cell count 5,000/μL, platelet count $24.6 \times 104/\mu$L, C-reactive protein (CRP) 0.04 mg/dL, antinuclear antibody ×160, anti-SSA antibody >500 U/mL, and anti-SSB antibody 101 U/L. The total protein in plasma (8.6 g/dL) comprised 40.7% albumin, 2.7% alpha-1, 7.6% alpha-2, 7.4% beta, and 41.6% gamma-globulin, including immunoglobulin (Ig) G at 2,101 mg/dL, IgG4 at 19.6 mg/dL, and IgA at 999 mg/dL. Serum immunoelectrophoresis showed monoclonal M-protein with IgA-kappa. Coagulation profile, urinalysis, and arterial blood gas were within the normal range. Pulmonary function test revealed small airway obstruction, which showed forced vital capacity (FVC) of 1.73 L (88.7% of predicted), forced expiratory volume in 1 second (FEV1) of 1.20 L (109.0% of predicted), FEV1/FVC of 69.3%, V50 of 1.04 L/sec, V25 of 0.21 L/sec, and V50/V25 of 4.95. She was diagnosed as Sjögren syndrome based on these findings.

Surgical lung biopsy was performed from the left lower lobe, which contained a nodule. The pathologic findings (Figure 2) revealed the presence of amyloid proteins that appeared as homogeneous eosinophilic materials on hematoxylin-eosin and stained on Congo red with apple green birefringence on polarized microscopy (data not shown). Congo red stain performed by standard and polarized light and immunohistochemical staining with AA amyloid and AL-kappa amyloid classified the amyloid protein

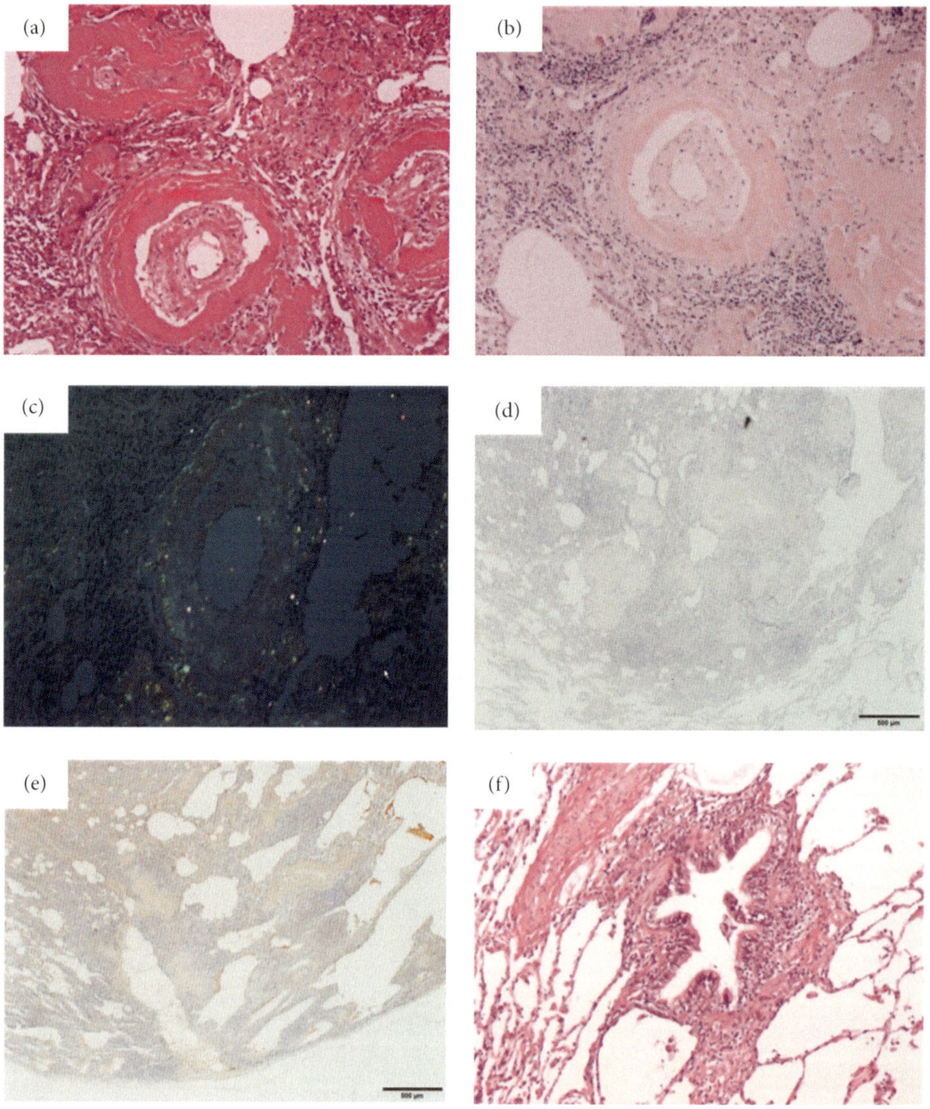

FIGURE 2: Pathologic findings of the surgical lung biopsy in a 72-year-old woman with Sjögren syndrome and pulmonary amyloidosis. (a) There is a homogeneous eosinophilic material in the vascular area (hematoxylin and eosin stain, ×100), which (b) was positive on Congo red stain (×100). (c) Polarizing microscopy shows apple green birefringence (×100). (d) The immunohistochemical staining with AA amyloid (×100) was negative. (e) The immunohistochemical staining with AL-kappa amyloid (×100) was positively stained. (f) There is infiltration of inflammatory cells in the peribronchial areas (hematoxylin and eosin stain, ×100).

as an AL-kappa. Moreover, there was peribronchiolar infiltration of inflammatory cells, mainly lymphocytes. Although we planned salivary gland biopsy, we could not obtain consent from the patient. She was finally diagnosed as Sjögren syndrome with lymphocytic bronchiolitis and pulmonary amyloidosis.

Because of the absence of respiratory symptoms, she was followed by chest CT and pulmonary function test surveillance without treatment. There was no systemic involvement, including the heart, kidney, skin, and gastrointestinal tract during the follow-up period. After 6 years, the cystic lung lesions gradually enlarged and increased in number (Figure 3), but she remained to have no respiratory symptoms, no decrease in FEV1 (1.18 L), and no findings of lymphoproliferative disorder.

3. Discussion

The pulmonary manifestations of Sjögren syndrome include interstitial pneumonia, tracheobronchial disorders, and lymphoproliferative disorders [3]. Interstitial pneumonia and tracheobronchial disorders are common, whereas cystic lung disease and pulmonary amyloidosis are rare manifestations of Sjögren syndrome [1]. Meanwhile, amyloidosis is characterized by extracellular tissue deposition of abnormal amyloid proteins [4]. The World Health Organization classified amyloidosis on the basis of the structure of variable fibrillary proteins and subsequently divided it into primary or secondary disease [8]. The two major forms are AL amyloidosis and reactive amyloidosis or amyloid A (AA) amyloidosis, which is due to chronic inflammation. An AL

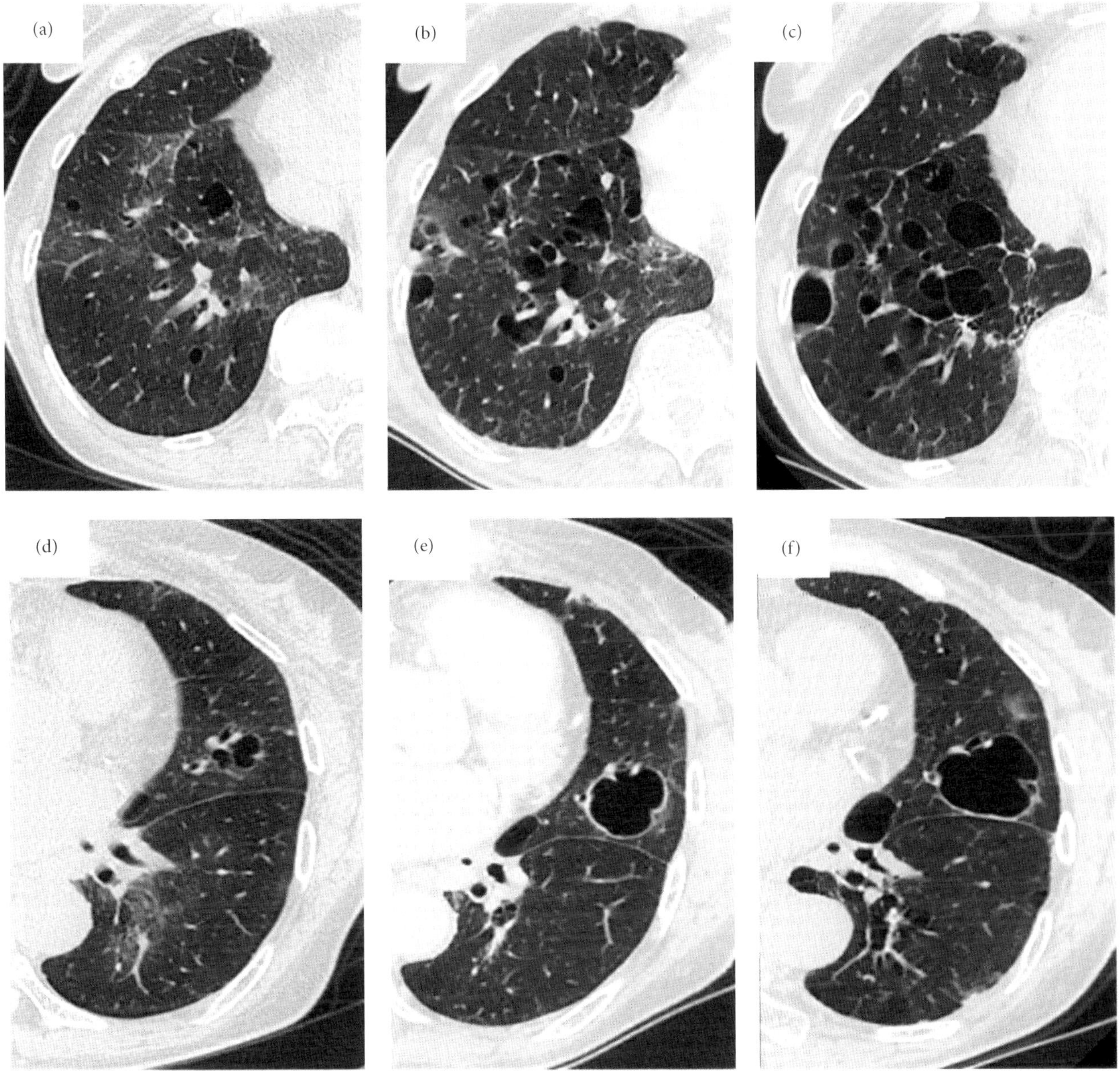

FIGURE 3: Surveillance chest computed tomography in a 72-year-old woman with Sjögren syndrome and pulmonary amyloidosis after 6 years of follow-up. The cystic lung lesions gradually increased in size and number after 6 years. (a–c) The right lower lobe and (d–f) the left upper and lower lobes are shown. (a) and (d) are images taken upon the time of diagnosis, (b) and (e) are images taken after 3 years, and (c) and (f) are images taken after 6 years.

comprises a clonal proliferation of plasma cells, and the fibrillary protein is a fragment of the Ig light chain [9]. On the other hand, AA is an acute-phase protein that is produced in response to systemic inflammation [6, 10]. All types of amyloid protein stain with Congo red and exhibit apple green birefringence on polarized microscopy [4]. Most cases of respiratory tract amyloidosis have been reported to have deposition of the AL-type of amyloid protein [5]. Sjögren syndrome is a chronic inflammatory disease and is also recognized as a lymphoproliferative disorder, similar to monoclonal gammopathy and AL amyloidosis. Lung involvement of amyloidosis in Sjögren syndrome has been reported as AL amyloidosis [11]. Amyloid deposition was considered to be related to the lymphoproliferative process seen in the lung.

Cystic lung disease can be associated with not only Sjögren syndrome with lymphocytic bronchiolitis [2] but also with pulmonary amyloidosis [12]. A previous report stated that among 21 patients with amyloid-associated cystic lung disease, collagen vascular disease (CVD) was present in 12 patients and absent in 9 patients [12]. The group with cystic amyloid and CVD had more women and normal pulmonary function test results than did the cystic amyloid group without CVD. In that report, the patients with amyloidosis without CVD had more obstructive pulmonary function than those with amyloidosis and CVD; this was consistent with the characteristics of the present case. Cystic formation has been suggested to be due to the presence of inflammatory cells or amyloid causing a check valve mechanism, which leads to bronchial obstruction [13]. In one study that analyzed and compared the high-resolution CT (HRCT) and histopathologic findings of amyloidosis in Sjögren syndrome, the cysts appeared to be located in the distal bronchioles that were narrowed by amyloid deposition [11]. In the present case, the cysts were located in the distal bronchioles on sequential HRCT findings (Figure 3). A previous study reported that 12 of 13 patients with cystic lung disease in Sjögren syndrome did not show disease progression after 4 years of follow-up [2]. Interestingly, the present case was observed to have gradual increase in the number and size of the lung cystic lesions for 6 years, which is a rare clinical course. This may indicate the natural progression of interstitial pneumonia to cystic lung disease.

The characteristic pulmonary function test of patients with Sjögren syndrome and cystic lung disease is often an obstructive pattern, which the present case likewise manifested [2]. This obstructive pattern on pulmonary function test is considered to suggest airway narrowing secondary to bronchiolitis. Notably, the FEV1 in the present case did not decline within 6 years of diagnosis.

Sjögren syndrome is associated with increased risk of non-Hodgkin lymphoma [1], the most common subtypes of which are mucosa-associated lymphoid tissue and marginal zone B-cell lymphoma. In fact, the prevalence of pulmonary lymphoma in patients with primary Sjögren syndrome was reported to be 1%-2% [14]. Physicians should also observe for the development of pulmonary lymphoma in these patients.

In conclusion, we reported a rare case of Sjögren syndrome complicated with pulmonary amyloidosis with cystic formation. Physicians should consider amyloidosis in the differential diagnosis of patients with cystic lung shadows and should proactively perform pathologic examination.

References

[1] M. Ramos-Casals, A. G. Tzioufas, and J. Font, "Primary Sjogren's syndrome: new clinical and therapeutic concepts," *Annals of the Rheumatic Diseases*, vol. 64, no. 3, pp. 347–354, 2005.

[2] C. D. Martinez-Balzano, S. Touray, and S. Kopec, "Cystic lung disease among patients with Sjogren syndrome: frequency, natural history, and associated risk factors," *Chest*, vol. 150, no. 3, pp. 631–639, 2016.

[3] T. Flament, A. Bigot, B. Chaigne, H. Henique, E. Diot, and S. Marchand-Adam, "Pulmonary manifestations of Sjogren's syndrome," *European Respiratory Review*, vol. 25, no. 140, pp. 110–123, 2016.

[4] M. B. Pepys, "Amyloidosis," *Annual Review of Medicine*, vol. 57, no. 1, pp. 223–241, 2006.

[5] J. D. Gillmore and P. N. Hawkins, "Amyloidosis and the respiratory tract," *Thorax*, vol. 54, no. 5, pp. 444–451, 1999.

[6] J. L. Berk, A. O'Regan, and M. Skinner, "Pulmonary and tracheobronchial amyloidosis," *Seminars in Respiratory and Critical Care Medicine*, vol. 23, no. 2, pp. 155–165, 2002.

[7] J. D. Gillmore, A. Wechalekar, J. Bird et al., "Guidelines on the diagnosis and investigation of AL amyloidosis," *British Journal of Haematology*, vol. 168, no. 2, pp. 207–218, 2015.

[8] WHO-IUIS Nomenclature Sub-Committee, "Nomenclature of amyloid and amyloidosis," *Bulletin of the World Health Organization*, vol. 71, no. 1, pp. 105–112, 1993.

[9] A. D. Wechalekar, J. D. Gillmore, and P. N. Hawkins, "Systemic amyloidosis," *The Lancet*, vol. 387, no. 10038, pp. 2641–2654, 2016.

[10] M. Baqir, E. M. Kluka, M. C. Aubry et al., "Amyloid-associated cystic lung disease in primary Sjogren's syndrome," *Respiratory Medicine*, vol. 107, no. 4, pp. 616–621, 2013.

[11] Y. J. Jeong, K. S. Lee, M. P. Chung et al., "Amyloidosis and lymphoproliferative disease in Sjogren syndrome: thin-section computed tomography findings and histopathologic comparisons," *Journal of Computer Assisted Tomography*, vol. 28, no. 6, pp. 776–781, 2004.

[12] A. C. Zamora, D. B. White, A. M. Sykes et al., "Amyloid-associated cystic lung disease," *Chest*, vol. 149, no. 5, pp. 1223–1233, 2016.

[13] H. Kobayashi, R. Matsuoka, S. Kitamura, N. Tsunoda, and K. Saito, "Sjogren's syndrome with multiple bullae and pulmonary nodular amyloidosis," *Chest*, vol. 94, no. 2, pp. 438–440, 1988.

[14] L. A. Hansen, U. B. Prakash, and T. V. Colby, "Pulmonary lymphoma in Sjogren's syndrome," *Mayo Clinic proceedings*, vol. 64, no. 8, pp. 920–931, 1989.

Fever, Myositis, and Paralysis: Is This Inflammatory Myopathy or Neuroinvasive Disease?

Aneeta R. Kiran,[1] Richard A. Lau,[1] Kim M. Wu,[1] Andrew L. Wong,[1,2] Philip J. Clements,[1] and Emil R. Heinze[1,2]

[1]*UCLA-Olive View Rheumatology Program, Division of Rheumatology, Olive View-UCLA Medical Center, 14445 Olive View Drive, No. 2B182, Sylmar, CA 91342, USA*
[2]*UCLA-Olive View Internal Medicine Program, Department of Medicine, Olive View-UCLA Medical Center, 14445 Olive View Drive, No. 2B182, Sylmar, CA 91342, USA*

Correspondence should be addressed to Emil R. Heinze; emilheinze@gmail.com

Academic Editor: Mario Salazar-Paramo

West Nile virus (WNV) is a mosquito-borne RNA *Flavivirus* which emerged in North America in 1999. Most patients present with a febrile illness but a few develop WNV neuroinvasive disease. Myopathy is an uncommon manifestation. We describe a case of a 42-year-old male from Los Angeles who presented with 8 days of fever and muscle pain. Initial physical exam was normal except for 4/5 muscle strength testing in his extremity proximal muscles. Laboratory revealed a creatine kinase of 45,000 and a urinalysis with large blood but no red blood cells, suggesting rhabdomyolysis. The patient's condition declined despite aggressive supportive care and hydration, and on hospital day #6 he developed severe altered mental status and progressed to complete right arm paralysis and 2/5 muscle strength in bilateral legs. EMG/NCS showed sensorimotor axonal polyneuropathy and the cerebrospinal fluid was positive for IgM and IgG WNV antibodies. The patient was diagnosed with WNV neuroinvasive disease, poliomyelitis (and encephalitis) type with myopathy/muscle involvement. He was treated supportively and his muscle and neurologic disease gradually improved. At 12-month follow-up his muscle enzymes had normalized and his weakness had improved to 5/5 strength in bilateral legs and 3/5 strength in the right arm.

1. Introduction

West Nile virus (WNV) is an important arthropod-borne human pathogen which is a neurotropic RNA virus of the Flaviviridae family. Most infections are clinically silent or present as a mild febrile illness. However, more severe neuroinvasive disease can occur resulting in meningitis, encephalitis, or acute anterior poliomyelitis [1, 2]. Myopathy is an uncommon presentation and can occur with creatine kinase levels as high as 45,000 U/L suggestive of rhabdomyolysis [3]. We present a case of WNV neuroinvasive disease complicated by sensorineural axonopathy and severe myopathy presenting as progressive paralysis and rhabdomyolysis.

2. Case

A 62-year-old Hispanic male with a past medical history of diabetes, hyperlipidemia, coronary artery disease, and ischemic cardiomyopathy was in his usual state of health until he presented to the emergency room with an eight-day history of fever, rigors, fatigue, whole body muscle pain, and productive cough with yellow sputum. He had decreased appetite and decreased oral intake for seven days. He reported nausea, abdominal discomfort, dark urine, and decreased urinary output for two to three days. On physical exam he was alert and oriented ×4, febrile, and tachycardic and had decreased proximal muscle strength in all his extremities (4/5 in bilateral upper extremities and 3/5 strength in the bilateral lower extremities). The remainder of the physical exam was within normal limits. There was no distal muscle weakness and no sensory deficits. The initial workup included laboratory evaluation which demonstrated WBC of 16.2 thou cells/μL, creatine kinase (CK) of 45,100 U/L, aldolase of 136.8 U/L, elevated aspartate aminotransferase (AST) of 2396 U/L, and alanine transferase (ALT) of 571 U/L, and urinalysis also revealed large blood but no RBCs, all of which was consistent with rhabdomyolysis. The patient was also found to have a troponin leak, with a peak of 2.617 ng/mL, with subsequent transthoracic echocardiogram demonstrating improved ejection fraction of 42% compared to 35% five months priorly and adenosine Myoview stress test showing stable anteroseptal wall defect consistent with previous known myocardial infarction.

The patient was admitted to a monitored bed for management of rhabdomyolysis, likely secondary to statin versus viral induced myopathy, with consideration for autoimmune myopathy as well. Empiric therapy was started for rhabdomyolysis, including statin discontinuation and IV fluid hydration. The patient was also treated with broad spectrum antibiotics until preliminary cultures returned negative, as the patient initially met SIRS criteria at presentation with fevers, tachycardia, and leukocytosis. In regard to the troponin elevation, cardiology consultants treated the patient for a non-ST elevation myocardial infarction secondary to demand ischemia from acute illness with medical optimization of his cardiac medications. The patient responded well to initial medical management, with the creatine kinase trending down after it remained elevated >45,100 U/L during the first four days of admission. The patient's serum creatinine also began trending down after peaking at 4.03 mg/dL, and his troponin trended down to normal after peaking at 2.617 ng/mL. On hospital day #6, however, the patient developed complications of acute mental status change, as well as worsening weakness. On exam, he was noted to be alert and oriented to person only, minimally following commands and with new onset of complete paralysis in the right upper extremity and marked weakness in bilateral lower extremities (2/5 strength). He also had decreased sensation to light touch in bilateral legs and in the right arm. Right biceps and bilateral ankle reflexes were absent. Cranial nerves and fundoscopic exam were normal.

Given the new neurological deficits on top of the existing rhabdomyolysis and nonspecific constitutional symptomology that the patient initially presented with, the differential diagnosis was expanded with the assistance of neurology consultation. Specifically, there was strong concern for possible invasive CNS infections leading to encephalitis, such as HIV, WNV, CMV, EBV, HSV, VZV, HTLV1, Lyme, toxoplasmosis, cysticercosis, mycoplasma, and syphilis, with higher suspicion of viral pathogens, as they are more likely associated with rhabdomyolysis. Possible autoimmune etiologies, mainly idiopathic inflammatory myositis with possible CNS vasculitis involvement, were considered as well. Lastly, toxin mediated myopathy from metal poisoning was considered. Further workup included MRI of the brain and cervical spine which was unremarkable for vasculitis or encephalitis. Electromyogram and nerve conduction study showed a sensorimotor polyneuropathy with predominantly axonal features and moderate irritable myopathy. A lumbar puncture (LP) demonstrated 10 WBC/mm^3 (80% lymphocytes), protein 50 mg/dL, normal glucose, and absence of oligoclonal bands. The lumbar puncture also demonstrated serologies positive for West Nile virus IgG and IgM antibodies but negative for EBV, HSV, VZV, CMV, VDRL, Lyme, toxoplasmosis, cysticercosis, AFB stain, *Cryptococcus*, coccidioidomycosis, bacterial cultures, fungal cultures, and viral cultures. Additional infectious disease workup included negative serologies for HIV screen, HIV RNA PCR, and HTLV I/II. Autoimmune workup demonstrated negative ANA, anti-Jo1, anti-Mi2, and anti-SRP. Other neurological workups performed included mercury levels and heavy metal levels that were undetectable.

The patient was subsequently diagnosed with WNV neuroinvasive disease, specifically West Nile poliomyelitis (WNP) and West Nile encephalitis (WNE) with myopathy/muscle involvement. With supportive care, the patient's CK and renal function trended back to normal over a period of five weeks. At the time of discharge, the patient had normal mental status, 4/5 strength in bilateral lower extremities requiring a cane for ambulation, and persistent right upper extremity weakness with 2/5 strength. At 6-month follow-up, he continued to have normal mental status, 4/5 strength in bilateral lower extremities requiring a cane for ambulation, and persistent right upper extremity weakness with 2/5 strength. At 12-month follow-up, his bilateral lower extremities improved to 5/5 strength and right upper extremity improved to 3/5 strength.

3. Discussion

West Nile virus (WNV) is a mosquito-borne RNA *Flavivirus* and human neuropathogen. During the early discovery of West Nile virus in the mid-1900s, common manifestations described included fevers, chills, malaise, maculopapular rash, headaches, backaches, arthralgia, and myalgia [4]. However, more recently neuromuscular manifestations are being recognized as a prominent feature in patients with WNV infection. The Centers for Disease Control (CDC) now classifies WNV infection into (1) WNV fever and (2) WNV neuroinvasive disease, with further subdivision of the latter group into (a) encephalitis, (b) meningitis, and (c) poliomyelitis. Patients with poliomyelitis commonly have signs of meningitis and encephalitis. Of all the people infected, 25% develop WNV fever [5] and neuroinvasive disease occurs in less than 1% [2]. Advancing age and immunosuppression were the risk factors associated with neuroinvasive disease [6].

More than 50% of patients with confirmed WNV encephalitis can have severe muscle weakness as a cardinal sign [7] which is considered a risk factor for predicting death in patients with WNV encephalitis [7, 8]. However, actual myopathy is an uncommon manifestation, with only several case reports of rhabdomyolysis with creatine kinase levels as high as 45,000 U/L [3, 9, 10]. Muscle biopsies of patients with acute asymmetric paralysis showed scattered necrotic muscle fibers invaded by macrophages [11]. The role of WNV directly invading the muscles remains unclear [4], but there have been case reports where staining with immunohistochemistry for polyclonal antibodies for *Flavivirus* was unremarkable [11]. A muscle biopsy was not pursued for our patient in this case, as our patient began to improve with symptomatic care alone. Additionally, as mentioned, the utility of a muscle biopsy for diagnosing WNV myopathy is still unclear given the rarity of this type of WNV manifestation.

West Nile virus can also cause myocarditis [12, 13] and cardiomyopathy [13, 14], commonly presenting as heart failure symptomology, cardiac arrhythmias, elevated cardiac enzymes, and new global myocardial dysfunction [12–14]. The diagnosis is usually made with the confirmation of WNV and with the exclusion of other etiologies, especially ischemic pathology [12–14]. In our patient, further diagnostics such as cardiac MRI were not pursued, as our patient did not have overt heart failure symptomology or new arrhythmias, and the troponin elevation resolved with symptomatic care. Additionally repeat echocardiogram imaging demonstrated improved ejection fraction compared to 5 months priorly and adenosine myoview showed fixed defect consistent with previous infarction. Our patient was thought to more likely have a non-ST elevation myocardial infarction from demand ischemia from acute illness, which he is at higher risk for given his past medical history of coronary artery disease and ischemic cardiomyopathy.

WNV infections should be considered especially during the summer in patients living in endemic areas presenting with unexplained acute illness or neurological findings. The incubation period ranges from 2 to 14 days. Serum should be tested for WNV IgM antibodies. If there is a neurological manifestation, then the cerebrospinal fluid (CSF) should be tested for WNV IgM antibodies. The CSF analysis will typically reveal increased leukocytes (usually >200 cells/mm^3), increased protein, and normal glucose [4]. Imaging studies in WNV infection are frequently normal but are useful in eliminating other causes of acute meningoencephalitis. When abnormal, the findings are generally nonspecific. T2-weighted magnetic resonance signal abnormalities may be seen in brainstem, deep gray structures, cerebellum, and spinal cord ventral horns [15]. Other infectious entities that can present similarly to WNV should be ruled out as well, including HIV, CMV, EBV, HSV, VZV, HTLV1, Lyme, toxoplasmosis, cysticercosis, mycoplasma, and syphilis, with viral illnesses more likely to lead to rhabdomyolysis. Toxin mediated disease such as heavy metal poisoning should be considered if there is a relevant exposure history. Autoimmune etiologies such as idiopathic inflammatory myositis can be considered as well, but unless there is a concomitant CNS vasculitis, it is unlikely to lead to AMS [16].

The treatment is supportive and full recovery can be seen in uncomplicated cases of WNV fever or meningitis cases. Outcomes of WNV encephalitis are variable and patients can have substantial functional and cognitive difficulties for up to a year [2]. One-third of the patients with WNV poliomyelitis recover strength almost to baseline, one-third have minimal improvement, and one-third have no improvement [17]. Death among the patients with neuroinvasive disease is approximately 10% [6]. No vaccines are available. Mosquito control programs are the mainstay in prevention [2]. Finally, as treatment would be different, rheumatologists should be cognizant of the myopathic complications of WNV neuroinvasive disease as it may simulate an idiopathic inflammatory myopathy early on.

Competing Interests

The authors declare that there is no conflict of interests regarding the publication of this paper.

References

[1] J. J. Sejvar, "Clinical manifestations and outcomes of West Nile virus infection," *Viruses*, vol. 6, no. 2, pp. 606–623, 2014.

[2] L. R. Petersen, A. C. Brault, and R. S. Nasci, "West Nile virus: review of the literature," *The Journal of the American Medical Association*, vol. 310, no. 3, pp. 308–315, 2013.

[3] S. P. Montgomery, C. C. Chow, S. W. Smith, A. A. Marfin, D. R. O'Leary, and G. L. Campbell, "Rhabdomyolysis in patients with West Nile encephalitis and meningitis," *Vector-Borne and Zoonotic Diseases*, vol. 5, no. 3, pp. 252–257, 2005.

[4] A. A. Leis and D. S. Stokic, "Neuromuscular manifestations of West Nile virus infection," *Frontiers in Neurology*, vol. 3, article 37, 2012.

[5] S. Zou, G. A. Foster, R. Y. Dodd, L. R. Petersen, and S. L. Stramer, "West Nile fever characteristics among viremic persons identified through blood donor screening," *Journal of Infectious Diseases*, vol. 202, no. 9, pp. 1354–1361, 2010.

[6] N. P. Lindsey, J. Erin Staples, J. A. Lehman, and M. Fischer, "Surveillance for human West Nile virus disease-United States, 1999–2008," *Morbidity and Mortality Weekly Report*, vol. 59, no. -2, pp. 1–17, 2010.

[7] D. Nash, F. Mostashari, A. Fine et al., "The outbreak of West Nile virus infection in the New York City area in 1999," *The New England Journal of Medicine*, vol. 344, pp. 1807–1814, 1999.

[8] L. R. Petersen and A. A. Marfin, "West Nile virus: a primer for the clinician," *Annals of Internal Medicine*, vol. 137, no. 3, pp. 173–179, 2002.

[9] S. I. Doron, J. F. Dashe, L. S. Adelman, W. F. Brown, B. G. Werner, and S. Hadley, "Histopathologically proven poliomyelitis with quadriplegia and loss of brainstem function due to West Nile virus infection," *Clinical Infectious Diseases*, vol. 37, no. 5, pp. e74–e77, 2003.

[10] M. Gupta, M. Ghaffari, and A. X. Freire, "Rhabdomyolysis in a patient with West Nile encephalitis and flaccid paralysis," *Tennessee Medicine*, vol. 101, no. 4, pp. 45–47, 2008.

[11] J. Li, J. A. Loeb, M. E. Shy et al., "Asymmetric flaccid paralysis: a neuromuscular presentation of West Nile virus infection," *Annals of Neurology*, vol. 53, no. 6, pp. 703–710, 2003.

[12] A. Kushawaha, S. Jadonath, and N. Mobarakai, "West nile virus myocarditis causing a fatal arrhythmia: a case report," *Cases Journal*, vol. 2, no. 5, article 7147, 2009.

[13] L. E. Braun, T. Tsuchida, and H. Spiegel, "Meningoencephalitis in a child complicated by myocarditis, quadriparesis and respiratory failure," *Pediatric Infectious Disease Journal*, vol. 25, no. 9, pp. 853–856, 2006.

[14] R. N. Khouzam, "Significant cardiomyopathy secondary to West Nile virus infection," *Southern Medical Journal*, vol. 102, no. 5, pp. 527–528, 2009.

[15] K. A. Petropoulou, S. M. Gordon, R. A. Prayson, and P. M. Ruggierri, "West Nile virus meningoencephalitis: MR imaging findings," *American Journal of Neuroradiology*, vol. 26, no. 8, pp. 1986–1995, 2005.

[16] I. P. da Costa, E. P. Pradebon, J. V. Campos, F. S. Melo, and F. M. A. A. Tavares, "Polymyositis associated with lymphocytic arteritis of the central nervous system," *Revista Brasileira de Reumatologia*, vol. 50, no. 1, pp. 90–95, 2010.

[17] J. J. Sejvar, A. V. Bode, A. A. Marfin et al., "West nile virus-associated flaccid paralysis outcome," *Emerging Infectious Diseases*, vol. 12, no. 3, pp. 514–516, 2006.

43

Primary Idiopathic Osteoarthropathy: Could It Be Related to Alcoholism?

Yanal Alnimer, Suresh Subedi, Thair Dawood, and Ghassan Bachuwa

Internal Medicine Department, Hurley Medical Center, Flint, MI, USA

Correspondence should be addressed to Yanal Alnimer; yalnime1@hurleymc.com

Academic Editor: Constantine Saadeh

Background. Hypertrophic osteoarthropathy (HOA) is a syndrome characterized by abnormal proliferation of the skin and bony structures at the distal extremities resulting in digital clubbing, periosteal bony reaction, and joint effusion. It can be primary (idiopathic) without any clear identifiable etiology as well as secondary to variety of systemic diseases most notably lung pathology. *Case Presentation.* We describe a rare case of primary idiopathic osteoarthropathy in a male patient who presented with severe pain and tenderness in his legs. His history was significant for long standing alcoholism. Physical examination showed severe fingers and toes clubbing. He reported similar changes in his mother. Clinical and radiological findings were remarkable for distal leg tenderness and diffuse periosteal bony reactions, respectively. Computerized tomography scan failed to show any pathology apart from fatty liver infiltration. In the absence of obesity or diabetes, this was consistent with alcoholic steatosis. He was started on nonsteroidal anti-inflammatory drug which dramatically improved his symptoms. *Conclusion.* Primary hypertrophic osteoarthropathy should be considered in a previously healthy person presenting with bony pain and finger clubbing especially after ruling out the common secondary causes. Moreover, alteration of prostaglandin metabolism secondary to alcoholic consumption might be a contributing factor.

1. Background

Hypertrophic osteoarthropathy (HOA) is a syndrome characterized by abnormal proliferation of the skin and bony structures at the distal extremities manifested by digital clubbing, periosteal bony reaction and joint effusion [1]. It is classified as either primary or secondary; the primary form is considered uncommon and accounts for about 3–5% of all cases. Overproduction of prostaglandin E2 (PGE2) is the proposed mechanism for the primary form. Mutations at hydroxy-prostaglandin dehydrogenase enzyme which is responsible for PGE2 degradation or at SLCO2A1 which is PGE2 transporter result in increase of serum levels of PGE2 that stimulate various intracellular signaling pathways including vascular endothelial growth factor expression (VEGF). The latter stimulates various cellular components of fibrous and bony tissues such as osteoblast, osteoclast, and fibroblast that lead to various bony and dermatological manifestations of hypertrophic osteoarthropathy [2].

Here, we describe a rare case of primary idiopathic osteoarthropathy in a male patient who presented with severe bilateral lower leg pain and tenderness. Clinical and radiological findings were significant for severe digital clubbing and periosteal bony reactions, respectively. Workup was negative for identifying a possible cause. Primary hypertrophic osteoarthropathy should be considered in a previously healthy person who presents with bony pain and finger clubbing.

2. Case Presentation

A 55-year-old male not known to have any previous medical problems presented with worsening bilateral lower leg pain which started couple days prior to his presentation for the first time in his life. He also reported chronic deformities in his fingers, toes, and nails which were present since his teenage, became worse as he grew up, and later stabilized. He denied any pain related to them until this presentation. He also denied any morning stiffness, hand joints pain, recent diarrhea, fever, or chills. He reported drinking alcohol since the age of 12, and he currently drinks 2-3 cans of beer per day. He had no history of smoking or illicit drug use. Family

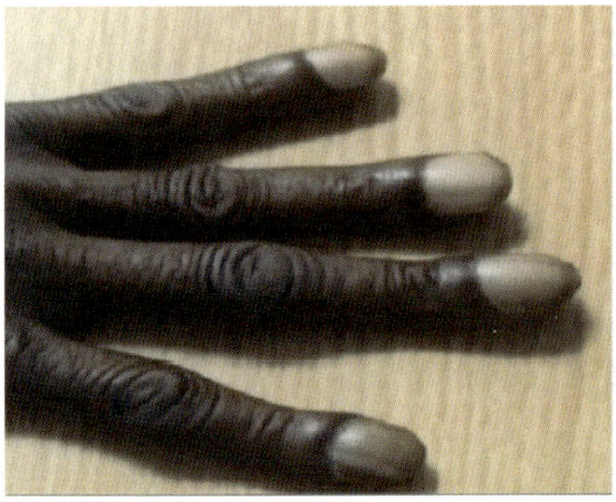

Figure 1: Severe digital clubbing.

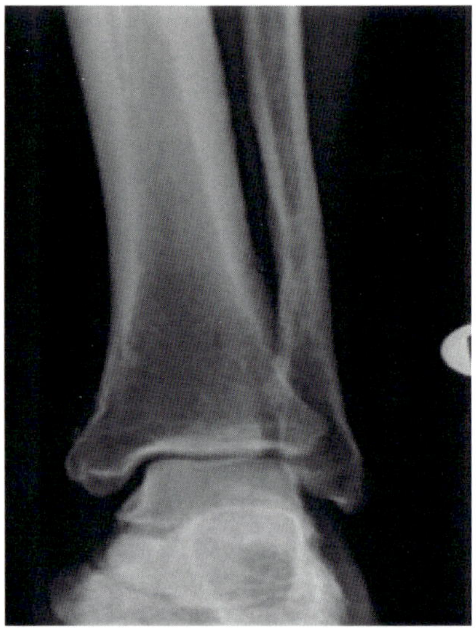

Figure 2: Course periosteal thickening along distal tibia and fibulae.

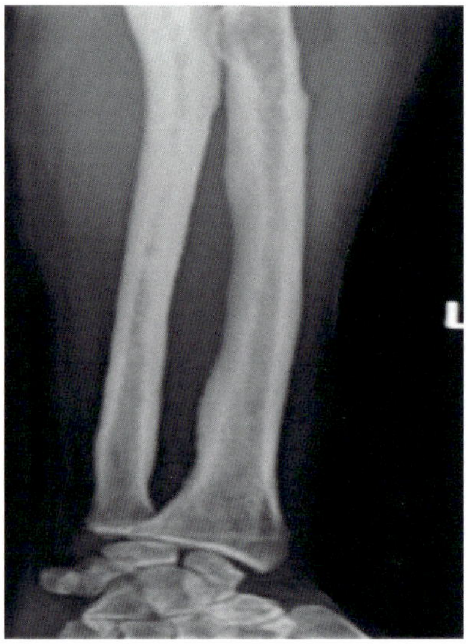

Figure 3: Marked cortical thickening of the radius and ulna.

history was significant for similar hand/nail changes in his mother though he does not remember the age at which it started.

Upon physical examination, the patient looked well-nourished; his vital signs were within normal limits. He was found to have severe bilateral clubbing of the fingernails and toenails along with osteoarthropathic changes in the hand joints (as illustrated in Figure 1). He had severe tenderness at the distal end of his legs, tenderness at the knee joints bilaterally, and mild left knee effusion. He had an antalgic gait secondary to the pain. Heart, lung, and abdominal examinations were unremarkable. There was no lymphadenopathy or hepatosplenomegaly. His skin examination was unremarkable. The patient's blood count and basic metabolic panels were within normal limits. Liver function tests were normal. An x-ray of his legs showed coarse periosteal thickening along the distal ends of the tibia and fibulae (as shown in Figure 2); knee and forearm x-rays (Figure 3) showed periosteal reaction along the long bones with left knee effusion. A chest x-ray and CT scan could not identify any lung pathology or masses. Diffuse fatty infiltration of the liver was noted without evidence of cirrhosis. Due to the presence of severe digital clubbing (Grade 4 as it resembles drumstick appearance) and diffuse long bone periostitis with no apparent secondary cause, the patient was diagnosed to have primary hypertrophic osteoarthropathy, which is also called pachydermoperiostosis. He responded well to NSAIDs and was discharged home in stable condition.

3. Discussion

Both primary and secondary forms have been identified as a cause for HOA. A variety of diseases, including cyanotic heart disease [3], pulmonary metastasis, and notably lung cancer [4], have been recognized as etiologies of the secondary form. Liver cirrhosis has been identified as a culprit in other cases as well [5].

The standard treatment of secondary HOA relies upon removing the underlying cause; however, this is not always curative. Ito et al. found only half of the cases of HOA secondary to lung cancer improved symptomatically and objectively with treatment [6].

The ability of the megakaryocyte to escape degradation in the pulmonary vascular bed due to an underlying lung pathology (lung cancer) or pulmonary arteriovenous shunt (as in the case of liver cirrhosis or cyanotic heart disease) results in platelet clumps at the capillary vascular bed with a subsequent release of a variety of cytokines, including fibroblast growth factor, platelet-derived growth factor, and vascular endothelial growth factors. This results in activation of the platelets and endothelial cells with subsequent proliferation of the skin and osseous structures [7].

Primary hypertrophic osteoarthropathy or pachydermoperiostosis (PDP) (other names include idiopathic hypertrophic osteoarthropathy or Touraine-Solente-Gole syndrome) is a rare disorder that shares some of the manifestations of the secondary form; however, it represents only 3–5% of all cases. Positive family history is found in 25–38%

of the cases, which suggests PDP has familial and idiopathic forms. Castori et al. reviewed 204 patients in 68 published families with PDP and found 37 families had autosomal dominant inheritance while autosomal recessive inheritance was suggested in the rest. Autosomal dominant families showed a variable degree of expression and penetrance. No clear phenotypic differences have been found between the two modes of inheritance [8]; however, Latos-Bielenska et al. proposed that autosomal recessive cases tend to be more severe [9]. Sayli et al. found early onset skin ulcers, acrolysis of distal extremities, and growth retardation present in some of these cases. Nevertheless, the disease usually starts during adolescence and progresses insidiously over a period of 5–10 years before it stabilizes [10].

The familial form of PDP has been mapped to chromosome number 4 (4q33-q34), which encodes the hydroxyprostaglandin dehydrogenase enzyme. Homozygous and combined heterozygous mutation of this enzyme increases the level of PGE2 through impairment of its degradation process; on the other hand, mutation at SLCO2A1 results in impairment of PGE2 cellular uptake. Both of these mutations result in high PGE2 levels which stimulate various intracellular signaling pathways including VEGF which eventually leads to various clinical manifestations of PDP [1, 2].

A wide spectrum of clinical manifestations has been described in the literature. The periosteal bony reaction that occurs at distal tubular bones, particularly the tibia and fibula (less frequently at the radius and ulna), which sometimes leads to adjacent joint effusion is one of the striking features. This periosteal reaction results in symmetrical irregular periosteal hypertrophy and new bone formation between the periosteum and the original cortex, which later fuse together. Distal ends of the tubular bones are most commonly affected, whereas the skull, vertebrae, and articular surfaces tend to be spared in most of the cases [11].

The dermatological manifestations are usually in the form of thickening of facial skin and dorsum of the hands and feet and range from mild to severe skin thickening and puckering. Finger clubbing is present in almost all cases. Pachyderma, hyperhidrosis, and seborrhea are frequently encountered skin changes, while folliculitis is less commonly encountered [12].

Microscopically, these changes result from fibroblast proliferation, thickening, and packing of collagen fibers resulting in acanthotic dermis as well as endothelial cell hyperplasia leading to partial occlusion of the blood vessel lumen. These skin changes are prominent in primary hypertrophic osteoarthropathy while bony changes tend to be more severe in the secondary form [12, 13].

Due to a wide variety of disease manifestations, different diagnostic criteria have been proposed. Touraine et al. recognized three forms of pachydermoperiostosis: a complete form characterized by both pachyderma (thickening of the skin) and periostitis, an incomplete form without pachyderma and a third form having pachyderma with minimal skin changes (Forme Fruste) [14]. However, Borochowitz suggested the diagnosis should be made only if two of the following have been identified: family history, digital clubbing, bony pain/radiographic changes, and hypertrophic changes of the skin [15].

Our patient presented with bilateral lower extremity pain and tenderness which started few days prior to his presentation for the first time in his life. The pain slowly got worse waking him up from sleep and affecting his gait. Radiological images showed diffuse periosteal bony reaction consistent with periostitis. Clinically, in addition to the tenderness, he had severe digital and toe clubbing which had a drumstick appearance (Grade 4) [16] which he said was present since he was a teenager. He did not have any facial features of HOA and he denied excessive sweating. Further questioning revealed his mother had similar finger clubbing changes and she had complained of joint pain too but he was not sure of the age of onset.

The patient was doing clinically well and his physical examination was completely normal apart from distal bony pain, tenderness, left knee effusion, and osteoarthropathic changes in his fingers and toes. His white blood cell count and metabolic panels were within normal limits. A CT scan did not identify any lung pathology or liver cirrhosis; however, it was remarkable for fatty liver infiltration. Of note, Farrús et al. and Mueller and Trevarthen have proposed that excessive alcohol intake with liver steatosis could trigger hypertrophic osteoarthropathy in the absence of significant liver damage or cirrhosis [17, 18]. On the other hand, excessive alcohol consumption alters prostaglandin metabolism and there is consensus data that PGE1 increases in alcoholic patients in the absence of liver cirrhosis [19]. Moreover, PGE1 has been suggested as a cause of hypertrophic osteoarthropathy [20].

The patient reports drinking alcohol since the age of 12; he has been drinking 2-3 cans of beer on a daily basis recently. CT scan showed extensive fatty liver infiltration. In the absence of diabetes and other features of metabolic syndrome, this was consistent with alcoholic steatosis. However, in the previous literature there was no strong association between alcoholic steatosis and osteoarthropathy as it is in liver cirrhosis. On the other hand, the increase production of PGE1 by excessive alcohol drink might be the trigger for our patient presentation.

The patient fits into the incomplete form of primary HOA category according to classification proposed by Touraine et al. He also meets 3 out of 4 of Borochowitz criteria. Nonsteroidal anti-inflammatory drugs are the cornerstone of treatment and intra-articular joint steroid injection, sulfasalazine, methotrexate, and tumor necrosis factor-alpha blockers can be used in resistant cases. The patient's symptoms responded dramatically to ibuprofen and he was discharged home after a couple of days [21].

4. Conclusion

Our case represents the incomplete form of primary hypertrophic osteoarthropathy, which accounts for 3–5% of all cases. It is vital to differentiate it from the secondary form, which requires treatment of the underlying cause. Moreover, the alteration of prostaglandin metabolism due to either excessive alcohol intake or fatty liver disease might trigger bony changes in susceptible patients. Nonsteroidal anti-inflammatory drugs remain the mainstay of treatment and other immunosuppressive agents can be used in resistant cases.

Competing Interests

The authors declare that there is no conflict of interests regarding the publication of this paper.

References

[1] C. Pineda and M. Martínez-Lavín, "Hypertrophic osteoarthropathy. what a rheumatologist should know about this uncommon condition," *Rheumatic Disease Clinics of North America*, vol. 39, no. 2, pp. 383–400, 2013.

[2] S. Lee, S. Y. Park, H. J. Kwon, C. H. Lee, O. H. Kim, and Y. Rhee, "Identification of the mutations in the prostaglandin transporter gene, SLCO2A1 and clinical characterization in Korean patients with pachydermoperiostosis," *Journal of Korean Medical Science*, vol. 31, no. 5, pp. 735–742, 2016.

[3] V. A. Wijesekera and D. J. Radford, "Hypertrophic osteoarthropathy in eisenmenger syndrome," *Congenital Heart Disease*, vol. 8, no. 3, pp. E65–E69, 2013.

[4] N. Sonthalia, K. Mukherjee, A. Saha, and A. Talukdar, "Treatment of hypertrophic osteoarthropathy in the case of pulmonary metastasis secondary-to-nasopharyngeal carcinoma with zoledronic acid: an enlightening experience," *BMJ Case Reports*, vol. 2012, 2012.

[5] I. Nahar, M. Al-Shemmeri, and M. Hussain, "Secondary hypertrophic osteoarthropathy: new insights on pathogenesis and management," *The Gulf Journal of Oncology*, vol. 1, no. 1, pp. 71–76, 2007.

[6] T. Ito, K. Goto, K. Yoh et al., "Hypertrophic pulmonary osteoarthropathy as a paraneoplastic manifestation of lung cancer," *Journal of Thoracic Oncology*, vol. 5, no. 7, pp. 976–980, 2010.

[7] M. Martínez-Lavín, "Digital clubbing and hypertrophic osteoarthropathy: a unifying hypothesis," *The Journal of Rheumatology*, vol. 14, no. 1, pp. 6–8, 1987.

[8] M. Castori, L. Sinibaldi, R. Mingarelli, R. S. Lachman, D. L. Rimoin, and B. Dallapiccola, "Pachydermoperiostosis: an update," *Clinical Genetics*, vol. 68, no. 6, pp. 477–486, 2005.

[9] A. Latos-Bielenska, I. Marik, M. Kuklik, A. Materna-Kiryluk, C. Povysil, and K. Kozlowski, "Pachydermoperiostosis-critical analysis with report of five unusual cases," *European Journal of Pediatrics*, vol. 166, no. 12, pp. 1237–1243, 2007.

[10] U. Sayli, H. Yetkin, O. S. Atik, O. Uluoglu, and S. Bolukbasi, "Pachydermoperiostosis: a case report," *Journal of Foot and Ankle Surgery*, vol. 32, no. 5, pp. 480–483, 1993.

[11] Z. Jajic, I. Jajic, and T. Nemcic, "Primary hypertrophic osteoarthropathy: clinical, radiologic, and scintigraphic characteristics," *Archives of Medical Research*, vol. 32, no. 2, pp. 136–142, 2001.

[12] M. Matucci-Cerinic, T. Lotti, S. Calvieri et al., "The spectrum of dermatological symptoms of pachydermoperiostosis (primary hypertrophic osteoarthropathy): a genetic, cytogenetic and ultrastructural study," *Clinical and Experimental Rheumatology*, vol. 10, supplement 7, pp. 45–48, 1992.

[13] D. M. Thappa, G. Sethuraman, G. R. Kumar, and S. Elangovan, "Primary pachydermoperiostosis: a case report," *Journal of Dermatology*, vol. 27, no. 2, pp. 106–109, 2000.

[14] S. Kumar, S. Sidhu, and B. B. Mahajan, "Touraine-Soulente-Golé syndrome: a rare case report and review of the literature," *Annals of Dermatology*, vol. 25, no. 3, pp. 352–355, 2013.

[15] Z. Borochowitz and D. L. Rimoin, "Pachydermoperiostosis," *Birth Defects Encyclopaedia*, pp. 1349–1350, 1990.

[16] K. A. Myers and D. R. E. Farquhar, "Does this patient have clubbing?" *Journal of the American Medical Association*, vol. 286, no. 3, pp. 341–347, 2001.

[17] M. Farrús, G. Ortiz, R. Pou, J. Ralla, J. Vilaseca, and S. Barluenga, "Hypertrophic osteopathy and acropachy associated with noncirrhotic alcoholic liver disease. Apropos a case," *Atención Primaria*, vol. 6, no. 4, pp. 246–248, 1989.

[18] M. N. Mueller and D. Trevarthen, "Pachydermoperiostosis: arthropathy aggravated by episodic alcohol abuse," *The Journal of Rheumatology*, vol. 8, no. 5, pp. 862–864, 1981.

[19] D. F. Horrobin, "Essential fatty acids, prostaglandins, and alcoholism: an overview," *Alcoholism: Clinical and Experimental Research*, vol. 11, no. 1, pp. 2–9, 1987.

[20] R. Crevenna, M. Quittan, M. Hülsmann et al., "Hypertrophic osteoarthropathy caused by PGE1 in a patient with congestive heart failure during cardiac rehabilitation," *Wiener Klinische Wochenschrift*, vol. 114, no. 3, pp. 115–118, 2002.

[21] G. Giancane, C. P. Diggle, E. G. Legger et al., "Primary hypertrophic osteoarthropathy: an update on patient features and treatment," *The Journal of Rheumatology*, vol. 42, no. 11, pp. 2211–2214, 2015.

44

Hemorrhagic Tamponade as Initial Manifestation of Systemic Lupus with Subsequent Refractory and Progressive Lupus Myocarditis Resulting in Cardiomyopathy and Mitral Regurgitation

Nicole Marijanovich[1,2,3] **and Alexandra Halalau**[1,3,4]

[1]*Internal Medicine Department, Beaumont Hospital, Royal Oak, MI, USA*
[2]*9 North Beaumont Hospital, Royal Oak, MI, USA*
[3]*Oakland University William Beaumont School of Medicine, Rochester, MI, USA*
[4]*General Internal Medicine Division, Beaumont Hospital, Royal Oak, MI, USA*

Correspondence should be addressed to Alexandra Halalau; alexandra.halalau@beaumont.edu

Academic Editor: Jamal Mikdashi

Systemic lupus erythematosus (SLE) is a heterogeneous autoimmune disease with a wide range of clinical and serological manifestations. Cardiac disease among patients with SLE is common and can involve the pericardium, myocardium, valves, conduction system, and coronary arteries. We are reporting a case of SLE in a young woman that is unique is unique in that initial symptoms consisted of pericarditis and hemorrhagic tamponade which remained progressive and resistant to aggressive immunosuppressive treatment and led to severe cardiomyopathy (ejection fraction of 25%) and severe (+4) mitral regurgitation. Her immunosuppressive treatment included hydroxychloroquine, high-dose steroids, intravenous immunoglobulins, azathioprine, and mycophenolate mofetil. Her disease progression was felt to be due to underlying uncontrolled SLE because the complement levels remained persistently low throughout the entire course and PET Myocardial Perfusion and Viability study showed stable persistent active inflammation. Eventually, she was treated with cyclophosphamide which led to improvement in ejection fraction to 55% with only mild mitral regurgitation

1. Introduction

Systemic lupus erythematosus (SLE) is an autoimmune condition that can be associated with significant morbidity and mortality. Pericarditis is the most common cardiac manifestation of SLE; however, pericardial effusions causing pericardial tamponade are rare. There is a 1–2.5% incidence of tamponade in patients with systemic lupus erythematosus [1]. Myocarditis is clinically prevalent in 9% of those who have SLE [2]. Along with congestive heart failure, myocarditis contributes approximately 31% to cardiac deaths in inflammatory myopathies and indicates a poor prognosis [3]. Therefore, prompt recognition, diagnosis, and treatment of pericardial tamponade and myocarditis are imperative.

2. Case Presentation

A 21-year-old female of mixed heritage (Caucasian and African American), with a history of provoked deep venous thrombosis diagnosed six months before, currently treated with warfarin, presented with complaints of acute chest pain. The pain was midsternal, severe, sharp, and worse with inspiration but improved by sitting upright. Vital signs revealed tachycardia (154 beats per minute), tachypnea (30 breaths per minute), and normal blood pressure (136/73 mmHg). The INR was 5.4 on admission. The chest X-ray showed cardiomegaly with a bottle neck sign. The echocardiogram showed a large pericardial effusion, with evidence of right-sided collapse during diastole. Chest, abdomen, and pelvis CT demonstrated a large pericardial effusion, consistent with hemorrhage. There were no pulmonary emboli or signs of pulmonary hemorrhage. The patient was transfused plasma and blood with improvement of the INR to 2.1. Pericardiocentesis was performed with a return of 500 cc of bloody fluid, and a drain was placed. Her vital signs improved and symptoms diminished immediately after the procedure.

She was diagnosed with underlying pericarditis with effusion that converted to a hemorrhage from the anticoagulation. The etiology of her pericarditis was sought. She denied any recent viral illnesses, tuberculosis exposure, malignancy, or fungal infections. She denied any arthritis, oral ulcers, fever, weight loss, night sweats, rash, or family history of autoimmune disease. Pericardial fluid was sent for cytology as well as viral, fungal, aerobic, anaerobic, and AFB cultures that were all negative. No autoimmune testing was performed on the pericardial fluid. Initial laboratory work revealed normal electrolyte panel and renal function and BNP 59 pg/ml (0–100). She had mildly elevated liver function tests with AST 69 U/L (10–37) and ALT 52 U/L (8–37). She was also found to have normocytic anemia. The hemoglobin was 9 g/dl (baseline was 11.1) with a normal white blood cell and platelet count. Inflammatory markers were elevated: erythrocyte sedimentation rate was 35 mm/hr (0–18), C-reactive protein was 10.4 mg/dl (0–0.8), and ferritin was 314 ng/ml (12–207).

Autoimmune evaluation showed an ANA titer of 1 : 1280 with speckled pattern and markedly elevated anti-double-stranded DNA 195 IU/ml (<100). SSA Ab and SSB Ab were also elevated at 187 and 538 AU/ml (<100), respectively. The patient did not have any clinical symptoms to suggest sicca syndrome (no dry eyes or mouth). TSH on admission was 0.60 (0.5–5.20 mcIU/ml) with repeat serial TSH remaining in normal limits. Clinically, she was never symptomatic with thyroiditis. Complement C4 was low at 7 mg/dl (12–43). Rheumatoid factor was 27 IU/ml (0–14). ANCA, SPEP, CCP, anti-Smith Ab, RNP Ab, and complement C3 were normal. Initial antiphospholipid screen (APS) was positive; however, repeat testing approximately 12 weeks later was negative. Initial APS enzyme-linked immunosorbent assay (ELISA) showed anti-cardiolipin Ab IgA < 9.5 (<12 APL), IgG 21.6 (<15 GPL), IgM 19.7 (<12.5 MPL), beta-2 glycoprotein 1 IgG 12.1 (<20 SUG), and beta-2 glycoprotein I IgM 24.5 (<20 SMU). Repeat APS panel was negative with all results at <9.5. DRVVT screen was 50 (0–52 seconds). The patient was determined to not have antiphospholipid syndrome due to lack of positive repeat APS Ab blood work. Infectious workup including VDRL, HIV, pericardial fluid Gram-stain, culture, AFB stain and culture, and virus culture was negative. Pericardial fluid cytology was negative for malignancy and revealed increased neutrophils and lymphocytes.

The patient was diagnosed with systemic lupus erythematosus and was started on intravenous (IV) methylprednisolone 100 mg for 3 days with transition to prednisone 40 mg daily, hydroxychloroquine 200 mg twice daily, and colchicine 0.6 mg twice daily. She was also treated with ibuprofen 400 mg every 6 hours and opioids for pain control. Over the next 48 hours, an additional 120 cc bloody fluid was drained after repositioning the pericardial drain, which was then successfully removed. In hospital day 3, troponin peaked at 3.09 ng/dl (0–0.05) and lupus myocarditis was considered. A cardiac MRI showed normal LV function and no evidence of myocarditis. However, it did reveal severe diffuse, circumferential pericardial contrast uptake involving both the visceral and parietal pericardium with trivial pericardial effusion. She continued to improve and was discharged after 8 days from the hospital with colchicine 0.6 mg twice daily, hydroxychloroquine 200 mg daily, and prednisone 40 mg daily. Colchicine was used to treat the patient for inflammatory pericarditis as imaging revealed inflammation, and she remained symptomatic despite evacuation of pericardial fluid.

Three weeks later, she presented with recurrent chest pain despite compliance with her medications. ECG showed new T-wave inversions in multiple leads and troponin peaked at 4 ng/dl (0–0.05). BNP was elevated at 742 pg/ml (0–100). A transesophageal echocardiogram showed an ejection fraction of 45% with mild-moderate mitral regurgitation. A cardiac MRI showed midmyocardial and epicardial hyperenhancement in the midlateral and inferolateral walls, suggestive of myocarditis. It also revealed persistent pericarditis similar to prior cardiac MRI but no pericardial effusion or constriction. Myocardial perfusion imaging showed fixed radiotracer defect in the mid-distal inferior and inferolateral walls concerning for myocardial scar. PET Myocardial Perfusion and Viability study showed resting hypoperfusion in the mid-inferior lateral region, which was matched on FDG suspected to be scar formation and flow-metabolic mismatch in the basal inferior and basal inferolateral regions, approximating 12% of the left ventricle. The myocardial scar was estimated to be 6% of the left ventricle myocardium. She was started on aspirin and carvedilol 3.125 mg twice daily. She was again treated with IV steroids and started on azathioprine 50 mg twice daily. Repeat anti-double-stranded DNA had decreased to 130 IU/ml (<100); however, complements C3 and C4 remained low at 76 mg/dl (80–200) and <6 mg/dl (12–43), respectively. Her symptoms improved, and she was discharged home after 6 days from the hospital.

Six weeks later, she presented to the hospital again with recurring chest pain that was associated with bilateral leg swelling, dyspnea with exertion, and orthopnea. BNP was markedly elevated at 1098 pg/ml (0–100). Transesophageal echocardiogram also revealed EF 35% with left ventricular global hypokinesis and moderate-severe mitral regurgitation. Infectious endocarditis was ruled out with serial blood cultures, and no vegetations were found on imaging. A third cardiac MRI was performed which showed a severely depressed ejection fraction 29% and midinferolateral wall akinesis with full thickness hyperenhancement. When compared to the prior MRI, it also showed progression of her myopericarditis.

Cardiac catheterization showed normal coronary arteries, ejection fraction 25%, global hypokinesis, and severe +4 mitral regurgitation with severely enlarged left atrium. Cardiovascular surgery was consulted regarding evaluation for mitral valve repair; however, recommendations were made to pursue surgery only if she were to fail maximum medical treatment. Given no recommendations for surgery, invasive myocardial biopsy was deferred as well. She was treated for acute decompensated congestive heart failure with IV furosemide, and later adequate diuresis was transitioned to oral furosemide 20 mg daily. She was also started on spironolactone 25 mg daily, carvedilol 6.25 mg twice daily, and lisinopril 5 mg daily.

Interestingly, a repeat anti-double-stranded DNA was normal at 83 IU/ml (<100); however, complement C4 remained low at 6 mg/dl (12–43). Given progression of her disease despite medication compliance, she was treated with 1 gram IV methylprednisolone for 3 days along with IVIG for 2 days. She was continued on hydroxychloroquine sulfate 200 mg twice daily and colchicine. Azathioprine was eventually discontinued and changed to mycophenolate mofetil 500 mg twice daily with plans to increase to 1000 mg twice daily.

She was monitored by serial echocardiograms which showed stabilization and mild improvement in her valve function. She was then discharged home after 12 days from the hospital. Repeat PET Myocardial Perfusion and Viability study performed 3 weeks later (and 4 months after initial presentation) showed similar findings to a prior study with active inflammation of the basal inferior, and basal inferior lateral regions were estimated to be 12% of the left ventricle myocardium. Myocardial scar/fibrosis was estimated to be 8% of the left ventricle myocardium. She was then started on cyclophosphamide with repeat echocardiogram showing improvement in ejection fraction to 36% and mild-moderate mitral regurgitation and complement levels improving. Fortunately, her most recent echocardiogram (2.5 years after initial diagnosis) reveals an EF of 55%, mild mitral regurgitation, and no hypokinesis appreciated. Her complement levels and anti-double-stranded DNA remain within normal range and no other manifestations of SLE. Unfortunately, due to prolonged, high-dose steroid use for over 1 year, she developed avascular necrosis of her bilateral femoral heads and condyles necessitating surgery on her bilateral knees and hip. Currently, her only immunosuppressive medication remains hydroxychloroquine.

3. Discussion

Our patient was very unusual because cardiac tamponade as a result of lupus-induced pericarditis was her initial presenting symptom of lupus and because her disease remained refractory and even progressed to myocarditis, resulting in severe mitral regurgitation and cardiomyopathy. In one retrospective study and literature review, 41 patients (out of 71 patients with SLE) were found to have tamponade. Patients with pericardial effusions who developed tamponade had a statistically significant ($P < 0.05$) lower C4 level at presentation as compared with patients who did not develop tamponade. This is consistent with our patient, who despite normalization of her anti-double-stranded DNA, continued to have consistently low C4 levels during her active disease. Decreased serum C4 levels, female sex, concurrent renal disease, haemolytic anemia, and pleurisy may all be potential predictors of tamponade in SLE patients with pericarditis and effusion [1].

Myocarditis has a varied clinical manifestation and can present with dyspnea, fever, orthopnea, chest pain, peripheral edema, or palpitations. The gold standard for confirmation of myocarditis is endomyocardial biopsy. However, the focal nature of myocarditis leads to significant sampling error with biopsy and, consequently, low sensitivity while also exposing the patient to the risk of complications including cardiac perforation and stroke [2]. In recent years, clinically overt myocarditis is uncommon, reported in only 7–10% of cases, probably as the consequence of the introduction of steroid therapy. Cardiac histological findings show small foci of fibrinoid necrosis with infiltrates of plasma cells and lymphocytes and small foci of myocardial fibrosis. Immunofluorescence studies demonstrate fine granular immune complexes and complement deposition in the walls and perivascular tissues of myocardial blood vessels, supporting the hypothesis that lupus myocarditis is an immune complex-mediated vascular phenomenon [3].

In one case series of lupus myocarditis, which looked at 24 patients, a bimodal age distribution was found. The data suggested that although patients with newly diagnosed SLE and lupus myocarditis are acutely ill at presentation, their prognosis is good with proper treatment. It also found that low left ventricular ejection fraction on presentation, which does not improve with treatment, is an indicator of poor prognosis. Eleven of the 22 patients had considerable valvular dysfunction on the initial echocardiogram with most (81%) having mitral regurgitation. The most likely cause in the majority of patients seems to be a functional change in the ventricular geometry, resulting in annular dilation [2] as was seen in our patient. In those patients who did not recover their systolic function, the valvular dysfunction persisted. Echocardiography was a useful investigation in monitoring the response to the therapy; however, because of the nonspecific findings, cardiac MRI is the diagnostic method of choice. Along with the aforementioned treatment recommendations, standard-of-care pharmacotherapy of patients with congestive heart failure is also recommended [2].

Monitoring active SLE disease is difficult and limited. Currently, there are scoring tools such as the British Isles Lupus Assessment Group (BILAG) index, the Systemic Lupus Activity Measure (SLAM) index, and Safety of Estrogens in Lupus National Assessment study-SLEDAI that attempt to measure disease activity and guide physicians on when to escalate treatment. However, these metrics often have administrative burden as well as other significant limitations. Traditional serum biomarkers can often reveal active disease and can help predict organ involvement. Unfortunately, they are not always accurate, and there are no clinical trials to date supporting routine use for monitoring disease activity. Therefore, in order to monitor active disease in our patient, we used a combination of clinical assessment, serum biomarkers, and imaging. A new promising lupus biomarker is the interferon signature characterized by the highly coordinated upregulation of type I IFN-inducible inflammatory cytokines, chemokines, and other genes whose expression levels are closely correlated with clinical and laboratory measures of SLE disease activity. This can lead to identification of patients at high risk for specific organ involvement and personalized, targeted treatment [4].

There are no standard guidelines for treating lupus myocarditis; most case reports have demonstrated a favorable response to pulse corticosteroids or cyclophosphamide along with supportive management [5]. IVIG is being increasingly used for the treatment of autoimmune diseases, including SLE, in an attempt to control severe manifestations unresponsive to other treatments. Perhaps, the most dramatic case report was a 20-year-old female with recent diagnosis of lupus (with active myositis treated with oral prednisone and azathioprine) who presented with acute myocarditis as evidenced by an ejection fraction of 15% and large pericardial effusion. Left and right cardiac catheterization was unremarkable, but she required intra-aortic balloon pump and soon developed cardiogenic shock. She subsequently arrested and received a pericardial window with biventricular assist devices. She was started on stress-dose steroids and IVIG with marked improvement, and within a week, her biventricular devices were removed. Within a month, her EF and creatine kinase had normalized [3].

There are no prospective controlled trials of IVIG in SLE, but many published case series have shown improvement of cutaneous, musculoskeletal, neuropsychiatric, serositic, haematological, vasculitic, and nephritic manifestations of SLE. There are few reports of lupus myocarditis treated with IVIG, but all have shown rapid improvement in the clinical and echocardiographic abnormalities [6]. The duration for treatment with IVIG is undetermined with ranges from 2 to 5 days. The standard dose used is 1 g/kg in most case reports. Although our patient did not show a significant improvement in her ejection fraction immediately, she clinically improved after treatment with IVIG and her active inflammation seemed to dissipate as evidenced by normalization of anti-dsDNA antibody levels and stabilization in her echocardiogram and valve dysfunction.

In more severe cases or in cardiac tamponade, a higher dose of corticosteroid is necessary, often given as an intravenous bolus (such as 1 gram of methylprednisolone daily for 3 days). In patients with recurrent pericarditis, chronic immunosuppression with methotrexate, azathioprine, or mycophenolate mofetil and the use of intravenous immunoglobulin may be beneficial [7]. In our case, the patient's underlying disease slowly progressed while on azathioprine. The overall disease progression was halted on mycophenolate mofetil, but the active inflammation was persistent in the myocardium. Only after receiving the cyclophosphamide therapy, the patient's underlying myocardium inflammation resolved and led to improvement in her ejection fraction and degree of mitral regurgitation.

In summary, while cardiac treatment modalities in SLE remain a challenge, patients who present with severe, life-threatening cardiac involvement justify the use of earlier and more aggressive immune therapy in order to achieve and maintain resolution of disease and improvement in ejection fraction.

Authors' Contributions

Nicole Marijanovich and Alexandra Halalau wrote the entire manuscript and approved the final version.

References

[1] E. Rosenbaum, E. Krebs, M. Cohen, A. Tiliakos, and C. T. Derk, "The spectrum of clinical manifestations, outcome and treatment of pericardial tamponade in patients with systemic lupus erythematosus: a retrospective study and literature review," *Lupus*, vol. 18, no. 7, pp. 608–612, 2009.

[2] G. M. Zawadowski, K. W. Klarich, K. G. Moder, W. D. Edwards, and L. T. Cooper Jr., "A contemporary case series of lupus myocarditis," *Lupus*, vol. 21, no. 13, pp. 1378–1384, 2012.

[3] A. Barnado and D. L. Kame, "Myocarditis successfully treated with intravenous immunoglobulin in a patient with systemic lupus erythematous and myositis," *American Journal of the Medical Sciences*, vol. 347, no. 3, pp. 256-257, 2014.

[4] M. F. Smith Jr., F. Hiepe, T. Dorner, and G. Bermester, "Biomarkers as tools for improved diagnostic and therapeutic monitoring in systemic lupus erythematosis," *Arthritis Research and Therapy*, vol. 11, no. 6, p. 255, 2009.

[5] V. Suri, S. Varma, K. Joshi, P. Malhotra, S. Kumari, and S. Jain, "Lupus myocarditis: marked improvement in cardiac function after intravenous immunoglobulin therapy," *Rheumatology International*, vol. 30, no. 11, pp. 1503–1505, 2010.

[6] D. Micheloud, M. Calderon, M. Caparros, and D. P. D'Cruz, "Intravenous immunoglobulin therapy in severe lupus myocarditis: good outcome in three patients," *Annals of the Rheumatic Diseases*, vol. 66, no. 7, pp. 986-987, 2007.

[7] A. Doria, L. Iaccarino, P. Sarzi-Puttini, F. Atzeni, M. Turriel, and M. Petri, "Cardiac involvement in systemic lupus erythematosus," *Lupus*, vol. 14, no. 9, pp. 683–686, 2005.

45

Concomitant Guillain Barre Syndrome and Transverse Myelitis as Initial Neuropsychiatric Manifestation in a Case of Lupus: A Diagnostic Quandary

Anshuman Srivastava,[1] Bijit Kumar Kundu,[2] and Diwakar Kumar Singh[1]

[1] *Department of Medicine, PGIMER and Dr. RML Hospital, New Delhi 110001, India*
[2] *Rheumatology Clinic, Department of Medicine, PGIMER and Dr. RML Hospital, New Delhi 110001, India*

Correspondence should be addressed to Bijit Kumar Kundu; bijit1973@gmail.com

Academic Editor: Mehmet Soy

Neuropsychiatric manifestations of systemic lupus erythematosus are varied. Presently nineteen in number, they are classified as whether affecting the central or the peripheral compartments of the nervous system. Its diagnosis however remains difficult, more so when two or more of the syndromes are found concomitantly in the same patient and when they occur in absence of the more classical rash, serositis, and haematological manifestations. We present a case of lupus where myelopathy as well as demyelination existed simultaneously as the initial neurologic manifestation.

1. Introduction

The neuropsychiatric manifestations of systemic lupus erythematosus (SLE), known commonly as neuropsychiatric SLE (NPSLE), include 19 different entities divided into central or peripheral affections which may be attributable directly to systemic lupus erythematosus (SLE) or associated with it in increasing frequencies. These do not correlate with systemic disease activity and can occur in combination. Transverse myelitis (TM) is a devastating manifestation, can occur at any time in the course of the disease, and involves small segments or the whole of the spinal cord anywhere from the medulla to the conus. Ascending paralysis similar to Guillain Barre Syndrome (GBS) has also been described. These are rare and along with chorea make up less than 3% of the cases of NPSLE, a fact which attests to the rarity of these manifestations. Compounding this rare scenario is the fact that the clinical distinction of demyelination and myelopathy can be difficult in the initial stages, both having overlapping features. Radiological and electrophysiological evidence can be incongruent to the clinical features as well as to each other, adding to the confusion already present. We present such a case where a 35-year-old female had features of both leading to diagnostic quandary.

2. Case Presentation

A 30-year-old lady presented with complaints of progressive ascending weakness of both lower limbs for a week for which a diagnosis of GBS was made elsewhere. After few days she also developed incontinence of urine and stools. A Magnetic Resonance Imaging (MRI) done then revealed myelitis of the spine at junction of the medulla and cervical spine. Owing to the diagnostic quandary, she was referred to our centre for further evaluation. Review of her history revealed a course consistent with the diagnosis of GBS but lack of any prodrome or viral illness prior to the onset of the weakness. Past history revealed occurrence of pain with minimal swelling affecting the small joints of hands, wrists, knees, and ankles, associated with Raynaud's phenomenon. These symptoms had been occurring for 2-3 months every winter for the last three years and always subsided with onset of summers. Only this time, the resolution of symptoms was not complete. She had been treated intermittently with nonsteroidal anti-inflammatory drugs (NSAIDs) and low dose corticosteroids by her general practitioner (GP). She had two healthy children, was a teetotaler, never suffered from tuberculosis, was not a known diabetic or hypertensive, and did not give any history of abortions. Family history was insignificant. General examination was unremarkable except for pallor. Central nervous system (CNS) examination revealed a conscious oriented lady with flaccid quadriparesis, areflexia, and unresponsive plantar reflexes. Cardiovascular, respiratory, and abdominal examinations were normal. Musculoskeletal examination revealed minimal to mild synovitis in few metacarpophalangeal (MCP) and interphalangeal (IP) joints of both hands and wrists. Laboratory investigations revealed haemoglobin (Hb) 9.2 g/dL, total leucocyte count (TLC) 7800/mm^3, total platelet count of 120000/mm^3, a normocytic normochromic blood picture, serum sodium (Na^+) 142 mEq/dL, serum potassium (K^+) of 4.6 mEq/dL, and normal liver and kidney function tests. Chest radiograph was reported to be normal. Serology for Human Immunodeficiency Viruses (HIV) types 1 and 2, Hepatitis B Virus Surface Antigen (HBsAg), Hepatitis C Virus (HCV), Herpes Simplex Virus (HSV) types 1 and 2, and Cytomegalovirus (CMV) was negative. Cerebrospinal fluid (CSF) analysis showed albuminocytological dissociation with sugar 85 mg/dL and proteins 110 mg/dL and no cells. MRI of brain and spinal cord reviewed showed hyperintensities in T2 weighted images in cervicomedullary junction (Figures 1 and 2). Nerve conduction study (NCS) showed pure motor involvement with increased distal latencies, decreased conduction velocities, normal amplitude, and absent F-waves with no affection of sensory nerves, features which in the background of rapidly progressive ascending areflexic quadriplegia suggested the diagnosis of the Acute Inflammatory Demyelinating Polyneuropathy (AIDP) subtype of GBS. Anti-Nuclear Antibody (ANA) was positive in 1 : 640 dilution and homogeneous in pattern by indirect immunofluorescence (IIF), and anti-smith antibody (anti-Sm) was positive with intensity of 65 by EUROLine scan. Levels of complement component C3 were low (76.2 mg/dL, normal 90–180 mg/dL) while component C4 levels were towards the lower limits of normal (10.5 mg/dL, normal 10–40 mg/dL). Direct Coombs test (DCT), rheumatoid factor (RF), and cyclic citrullinated peptide antibodies (anti-CCP) were negative. A provisional diagnosis of SLE with CNS involvement was kept in view of arthritis, CNS involvement, positive ANA, and low complements. Treatment was instituted immediately with intravenous methyl prednisolone 1 g once a day for three days followed by oral prednisolone at 1 mg/kg body weight daily, hydroxychloroquine 200 mg twice a day, and cyclophosphamide 750 mg infusion. Her neurologic status improved and a repeat neurological examination after 3 days showed improved power of 2/5 in both upper limbs. After two weeks her muscle power improved to 2/5 around hip joints and 3/5 around shoulders, elbows, knees, and ankle joints. Her bladder and bowel functions also improved and she could be decatheterised. Subsequent MRI screen of spine repeated after 3 weeks was normal.

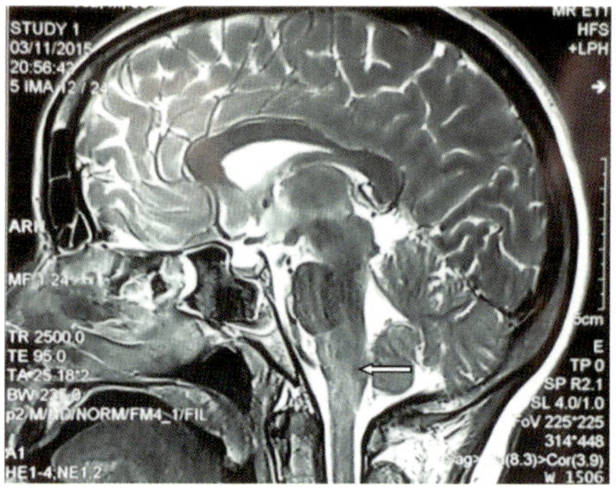

Figure 1: MRI of the brain in sagittal section showing hyperintensities at the cervicomedullary junction (white arrow).

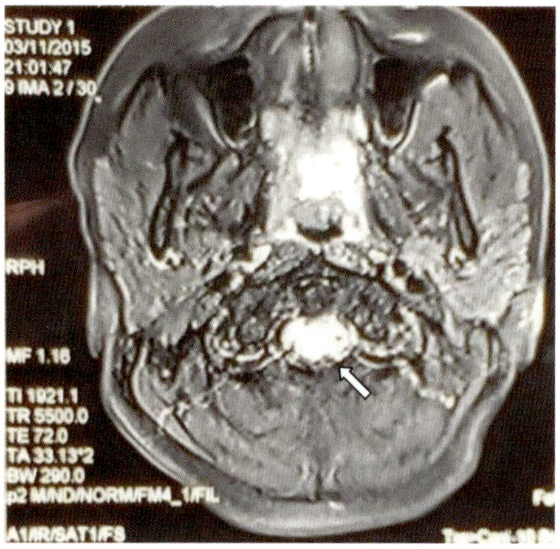

Figure 2: The same hyperintensity shown in the transverse section (white arrow).

The patient was put on monthly pulses of cyclophosphamide, and steroids were continued at 1 mg/kg body weight for 6 weeks and then tapered by 10% of the dose every two weeks. After 12 weeks, she had grade 4− (4 minus) muscle power around hips. Power around shoulders, elbows, wrists, knees, and ankles was grade 4. Grip was normal. She is able to carry out most of her activities of daily living.

3. Discussion

The prevalence as well as the prognosis of neuropsychiatric events in SLE is highly variable with almost a third being directly attributable to it. These have a negative effect on the health related quality of life [1]. The American College of Rheumatology (ACR) in 1999 defined 19 neuropsychiatric syndromes which occur in lupus. They can be classified into those affecting the central or the peripheral nervous systems [2] and are thought to be due to the effects of vascular abnormalities, different autoantibodies, and mediators of inflammation.

The 1997 ACR criteria included only seizures and organic brain syndrome (in absence of offending drugs or known metabolic derangements like uraemia, ketoacidosis, or electrolyte imbalance) in its criteria. The neurological manifestations of lupus in Systemic Lupus International Collaboration Clinics (SLICC) criteria include seizures, psychosis, mononeuritis multiplex (in the absence of other known causes such as primary vasculitis), myelitis, peripheral or cranial neuropathy (in the absence of other known causes such as primary vasculitis, infection, and diabetes mellitus), and acute confusional state (in the absence of other causes, including toxic/metabolic, uraemia, and drugs). The SLICC criteria containing many manifestations with less stringent timeframes aid in earlier diagnosis of NPSLE [3, 4].

Interestingly the commonest manifestations of NPSLE, namely, headache, psychosis, mood disorders, anxiety, and cognitive dysfunction, are the least specific. Still confounding the scenario is the fact that these syndromes have no correlation with disease activity and can occur at any stage of the disease, and in combination with other neurologic manifestations, thus making diagnosis difficult and liable to be missed and hence delaying treatment.

Among the rarer manifestations of SLE are an acute ascending demyelination akin to the classical Guillain Barre Syndrome (GBS) and transverse myelitis (TM) which are taught in medical schools. Though classical GBS and TM due to nonlupus causes are seen fairly commonly in medical school setting, those occurring as a result of lupus are seen in less than 3% of patients of lupus. However in lupus, TM is catastrophic, can occur at any time of the disease, and can involve small segments or entire spinal cord from medulla to conus. Though different syndromes in lupus are known to coexist or overlap, overlap of TM and GBS in the same patient of lupus could not be found in literature. However, coexistent TM and GBS have been reported in mycoplasma pneumonia in adolescents [5], in mumps [6], and after anti-Tumour Necrosis Factor (TNF) therapy [7].

GBS and TM can be difficult in absence of the classical rash of SLE to be attributed to as being due to SLE. Also watertight distinction between these two clinicopathologic entities may not be possible especially in the initial stages of manifestation because of overlapping clinical features and incongruence between clinical and radiological features. They are thus usually inferred to be due to causes other than SLE. Distinguishing even nonlupus TM and GBS assumes importance in view of the fact that GBS is usually treated with intravenous immunoglobulin (IVIg) or plasmapheresis, while steroids have no role. To elicit the cause of GBS and TM as SLE is of paramount importance because treatment of the same would include cytotoxic agent like cyclophosphamide and pulse steroids and because of the fact that, in spite of early diagnosis and treatment, only half of the patients show improvement [8].

Our patient had clinical findings suggestive of GBS with the nerve conduction study confirming the diagnosis. However MRI of brain and spine showed features of myelitis too. Retrospectively the whole clinical scenario could be explained by myelitis with spinal shock except for the gradual onset and the NCS findings. Thus our patient was a diagnostic dilemma with varied opinions and no unifying one till the diagnosis of NPSLE was made. Nonetheless immediate institution of pulse steroids and cytotoxic treatment led to improvement in the patient.

Test for anti-phospholipid antibodies (APLA) could not be done in our patient due to affordability issues and constitutes a limitation in our case. Anti-phospholipid syndromes (APS) either primary or secondary can be associated with various neurologic syndromes including transverse myelitis and GBS. The revised Sapporo or Sydney criteria [9] mandate fulfilment of at least one criteria clinical criterion, that is, vascular thrombosis or pregnancy related morbidity, and at least one laboratory criterion in order to make a diagnosis of APS. However our patient does not fulfil any of the two clinical criteria and thus APS could be presumed to be negative, albeit indirectly.

Behcet's disease (BD), sarcoidosis, vitamin B12 deficiency, vitamin D deficiency, and multiple sclerosis (MS) can share some of the clinical features of our case. However, they can be easily ruled out by detailed history, clinical examination, and basic investigations. BD can cause parenchymal lesions in brainstem as well as nonparenchymal lesions like aseptic meningitis, intracranial hypertension, cranial neuropathies or dural sinus thrombosis, arterial dissection, occlusion, and aneurysm [10], while sarcoidosis can cause cranial neuropathy, aseptic meningitis, mass lesions, encephalopathy, vasculopathy, seizures, hypothalamic-pituitary disorders, hydrocephalus, myelopathy, peripheral neuropathy, and myopathy and is usually suspected in a known case of sarcoidosis [11]. While absence of oral ulcers, a sine qua non for diagnosis of BD, along with high titre ANA in homogeneous pattern and albuminocytological dissociation in CSF rules out BD, the latter two along with no hilar lymphadenopathy on chest radiograph rule out sarcoidosis. Vitamin B12 deficiency can manifest as encephalopathy, myelopathy, peripheral neuropathy, and optic neuropathy. Reflexes are usually absent and weakness can be present [12]. However, the course is more prolonged, sensations are affected, and blood picture usually shows abnormalities like megaloblastic anaemia and hypersegmented neutrophils, features which were absent in our patient. Vitamin D deficiency can have proximal muscle weakness with normal sensations but can be easily distinguished by tender muscles, preserved reflexes, and normal CSF and NCS findings. Though MS presents in the same age group as our patient and is commoner in females, it is disseminated in time and space, spares the peripheral nervous system, and commonly affects the optic and sensory nerves, and associated systemic illness is not found, features which were absent in our patient [13].

It is our contention that, in any case of GBS and/or TM occurring singly or concomitantly, it is vital to keep the differential diagnosis of SLE especially in a lady of child bearing age even in the absence of any rash or other pointers to its diagnosis, more so if there is any incongruity between clinical, radiological, and electrophysiological findings. Sensitivity to and consideration of an autoimmune aetiology lead to prompt evaluation, early diagnosis, and early institution of treatment thus helping in improving prognosis.

Competing Interests

The authors declare that they have no competing interests.

References

[1] J. G. Hanly, "The nervous system and lupus," in *Systemic Lupus Erythematosus*, R. G. Lahita, Ed., pp. 727–746, Academic Press, Amsterdam, Netherlands, 5th edition, 2011.

[2] American College of Rheumatology Ad Hoc Committee on Neuropsychiatric Lupus Nomenclature, "The ACR nomenclature and case definitions for neuropsychiatric lupus syndromes," *Arthritis & Rheumatology*, vol. 42, no. 4, pp. 599–608, 1999.

[3] L. M. Amezcua-Guerra, V. Higuera-Ortiz, U. Arteaga-García, S. Gallegos-Nava, and C. Hübbe-Tena, "Performance of the 2012 Systemic Lupus International Collaborating Clinics and the 1997 American College of Rheumatology classification criteria for systemic lupus erythematosus in a real-life scenario," *Arthritis Care and Research*, vol. 67, no. 3, pp. 437–441, 2015.

[4] L. S. Ines, C. Silva, M. Galindo et al. et al., "Classification of systemic lupus erythematosus: systemic lupus international collaborating clinics versus american college of rheumatology criteria. A comparative study of 2,055 patients from a real-life, international systemic lupus erythematosus cohort," *Arthritis Care & Research*, vol. 67, no. 8, pp. 1180–1185, 2015.

[5] Y. Topcu, E. Bayram, P. Karaoglu, U. Yis, H. Guleryuz, and S. H. Kurul, "Coexistence of myositis, transverse myelitis, and Guillain Barré syndrome following *Mycoplasma pneumoniae* infection in an adolescent," *Journal of Pediatric Neurosciences*, vol. 8, no. 1, pp. 59–63, 2013.

[6] N. P. S. Bajaj, P. Rose, R. Clifford-Jones, and P. J. Hughes, "Acute transverse myelitis and Guillain-Barré overlap syndrome with serological evidence for mumps viraemia," *Acta Neurologica Scandinavica*, vol. 104, no. 4, pp. 239–242, 2001.

[7] S. Ugurlu, C. Saygin, D. Uzunaslan, K. Tascilar, B. Ince, and S. Saip, "Concomitant transverse myelitis and guillain-barre syndrome after adalimumab therapy in a case with ankylosing spondylitis," *Annals of the Rheumatic Diseases*, vol. 73, pp. 40–41, 2014.

[8] M. C. Hochberg, A. J. Silman, J. S. Smolen, M. E. Weinblatt, and M. H. Weisman, *Rheumatology*, Elsevier Mosby, Philadelphia, Pa, USA, 6th edition, 2015.

[9] S. Miyakis, M. D. Lockshin, T. Atsumi et al., "International consensus statement on an update of the classification criteria for definite antiphospholipid syndrome (APS)," *Journal of Thrombosis and Haemostasis*, vol. 4, no. 2, pp. 295–306, 2006.

[10] R. Shahien and A. Bowirat, "Neuro Behcet's disease: a report of 16 patients," *Journal of Neuropsychiatric Disease and Treatment*, vol. 6, pp. 219–225, 2010.

[11] A. Kumholz and B. J. Stern, "Neurologic manifestations of sarcoidosis," *Handbook of Clinical Neurology*, vol. 119, pp. 305–333, 2014.

[12] K. Scherer, "Neurologic manifestations of vitamin B_{12} deficiency," *The New England Journal of Medicine*, vol. 348, no. 22, p. 2208, 2003.

[13] S. L. Hauser and D. S. Goodin, "Multiple sclerosis and other demyelinating diseases," in *Harrison's Principles of Internal Medicine*, D. L. Casper, A. S. Fauci, S. L. Hauser, D. L. Longo, J. L. Jameson, and J. Loscalzo, Eds., pp. 2661–2674, McGraw Hill, New York, NY, USA, 19th edition, 2015.

Herpes Zoster Meningitis Complicating Combined Tocilizumab and Cyclosporine Therapy for Adult-Onset Still's Disease

Shinichiro Tsurukawa,[1] Nozomi Iwanaga,[1] Yasumori Izumi,[1] Atsunori Shirakawa,[2] Chieko Kawahara,[1] Tetsuo Shukuwa,[3] Miwako Inamoto,[4] Atsushi Kawakami,[5] and Kiyoshi Migita[1]

[1]*Department of Rheumatology, Clinical Research Center, NHO Nagasaki Medical Center, Kubara 2-1001-1, Omura 856-8562, Japan*
[2]*Department of Pharmacy, Clinical Research Center, NHO Nagasaki Medical Center, Kubara 2-1001-1, Omura 856-8562, Japan*
[3]*Department of Dermatology, Clinical Research Center, NHO Nagasaki Medical Center, Kubara 2-1001-1, Omura 856-8562, Japan*
[4]*Department of Ophthalmology, Clinical Research Center, NHO Nagasaki Medical Center, Kubara 2-1001-1, Omura 856-8562, Japan*
[5]*Department of Immunology and Rheumatology, Unit of Translational Medicine, Nagasaki University Graduate School of Biomedical Sciences, Sakamoto 1-7-1, Nagasaki 852-8501, Japan*

Correspondence should be addressed to Kiyoshi Migita; migita@nagasaki-mc.com

Academic Editor: Gregory J. Tsay

A 56-year-old female with refractory adult-onset Still's disease presented with ocular herpes zoster infection during TCZ treatment. After three days of acyclovir treatment (5 mg/kg), she developed a severe headache and high fever. Viral DNA isolation and cerebral spinal fluid abnormalities led to a herpes zoster meningitis diagnosis. Her meningitis was cured by high doses of intravenous acyclovir (10 mg/kg for 14 days). To our knowledge, this is the first report of meningeal herpes zoster infection in rheumatic diseases under TCZ treatment.

1. Introduction

Opportunistic viral infections are a well-recognized complication of biologics treatments for rheumatic diseases [1]. Cases of herpes zoster infections have been described in association with the immunosuppression induced by some rheumatic disease treatments [2]. Herpes zoster virus not only causes a primary infection (varicella/chickenpox) but also can be reactivated from a latent state, in which it is sequestered in the dorsal root ganglia [3]. A large prospective cohort of 3,266 rheumatoid arthritis (RA) patients on anti-TNF therapy found an increased risk of herpes zoster infection in RA patients, and the severity of many of these cases required hospitalization [4]. However, central nervous system herpes zoster viral infections have rarely been described in patients receiving TNF inhibitors [5], and, to our knowledge, there are no previous reports of herpes zoster meningitis associated with anti-IL-6 therapy. Here, we present the case of a 56-year-old female with adult onset Still's disease (AOSD) who developed herpes zoster meningitis while being treated with cyclosporin A, prednisolone, and an anti-IL-6 therapeutic, tocilizumab (TCZ).

2. Case Report

A 56-year-old female was referred to our hospital with a three-day history of left eye corneitis and a left frontal headache. She had been diagnosed with a systemic type of AOSD in 1999. Initial treatment with immunosuppressants (MTX and leflunomide) and biologics (TNF inhibitors and abatacept), which were combined with steroid treatments, had to be discontinued because of insufficient effects.

The patient had steroid-refractory AOSD; so, from 2010, she had been treated with TCZ (8 mg/kg in 4-week intervals) and cyclosporin A (200 ng/day) in addition to steroid therapy. The systemic manifestations of AOSD, such as spiking fever, skin rash, and hyperferritinemia, were controlled by these

Table 1: Laboratory findings.

Peripheral blood		Serological tests	
Red blood cells	$406 \times 10^4/\mu L$	C-reactive protein	<0.30 mg/dL
Hemoglobin	10.5 g/dL	Erythrocyte sedimentation rate	3.0 mm/hr
White blood cells	9600/μL	IgG	883 mg/dL (900–2000)
St	23.0%	Ferritin	613 ng/mL (10–85)
Seg	66.0%	C3	108 mg/dL (4–64)
Ly	6.0%	C4	24 mg/dL (17–45)
Mo	4.0%	CH50	42.7 U/mL (30–50)
AtyLy	1.0%	Anti-nuclear Ab	< ×40
Platelet	$12.1 \times 10^4/\mu L$	Anti-CCP Ab	<0.6 U/mL (<4.5)
Blood chemistry		β-D-glucan	(−)
Total protein	5.9 g/dL		
Albumin	3.9 g/dL	CSF	
Total bilirubin	0.6 mg/dL	Cell number	55/mm^3
Glutamic-oxaloacetic transaminase	176 IU/L (7–33)	Neutrophils	3%
Glutamic-pyruvic transaminase	181 IU/L (5–30)	Monocytes	97%
Lactate dehydrogenase	518 IU/L (260–480)		
Alkaline phosphatase	271 IU/L (80–250)	Protein	92 mg/dL
Creatinine kinase	21 IU/L (60–160)	Sugar	45 mg/dL
Total cholesterol	217 mg/dL	Cl	103 mEq/L
Blood urea nitrogen	10.8 mg/dL	Herpes zoster DNA (PCR method)	(+)
Creatinine	0.4 mg/dL		
Na	128 mEq/L		
K	3.5 mEq/L		
Cl	95 mEq/L		

Anti-CCP Ab, anti-cyclic citrullinated peptide antibody; CSF, cerebrospinal fluid; PCR, polymerase chain reaction.

treatments. A herpes zoster infection occurred five days after one of the TCZ infusions. At admission, the patient was afebrile and had a unilateral vesicular eruption with a well-defined dermatomal distribution involving the left ophthalmic verve area (trigeminal nerve V1) with corneal erosion but without visceral involvement. An acyclovir infusion treatment (5 mg/kg) was promptly started.

Three days after admission, the patient presented with high fever, severe headache, and vomiting. A detailed neurological examination demonstrated no focal motor or sensory deficits, and the cranial nerve test results were normal. A fundoscopy did not reveal any papilledema. Additionally, there was no nuchal rigidity, and both Brudzinski's sign and Kernig's sign were negative.

Laboratory studies revealed a peripheral white blood cell count of 9,600 cells/μL, with 77% neutrophils, 13% lymphocytes, and 5% monocytes. C-reactive protein was not detected, but the patient's liver transaminases and serum ferritin were slightly elevated (Table 1). A MRI examination of the patient's head was unremarkable. A lumbar puncture was performed, and the resulting cerebrospinal fluid (CSF) revealed an elevated protein level (92 mg/dL), decreased glucose level (45 mg/dL with a blood sugar level of 96 mg/dL), and a marked pleocytosis (55 cells/μL with 91% monocytes). While awaiting the results of a herpes zoster DNA detection test, we began treatment with a high dose of intravenous acyclovir (10 mg/kg) for 14 days based on a suspicion of herpes zoster meningitis. Later, a polymerase chain reaction assay of the CSF detected herpes zoster viral DNA, confirming our suspicions (Table 1). The patient's symptoms were improved by the high-dose acyclovir treatments, and she was discharged from the hospital after a total stay of 20 days. The elevated serum levels of transaminases and ferritin were also normalized by this therapy.

3. Discussion

To our knowledge, this is the first reported case of herpes zoster meningitis in an AOSD patient taking TCZ, and it highlights the risk of atypical and severe herpes zoster infection among immunosuppressed patients receiving biologics. In our case, the ophthalmic herpes zoster infection disseminated to a meningeal infection. As disseminated herpes zoster infections cause sequelae of the nervous system, early viral detection, antiviral therapy, and prevention strategies are particularly important for these patients [6].

The herpes zoster infection risk in rheumatic disease patients is high, and this risk appears to be increased in patients treated with biologics [2]. For example, in the SAMURAI study [7], the incidence of serious infections was 7.6% (0.6% herpes zoster) in the TCZ group versus 4.1% in the DMARDs group. Similarly, in the TOWARD study [8], the rate of serious infections per 100 patient-years was 5.9 (0.4% herpes zoster) in the TCZ group versus 4.7 in the control group. Likewise, the extension STREAM study [9] found a rate of serious infection of 5.7 per 100 patient-years and a rate of serious herpes infections of 1.1 events per 100 patient-years. The published rates of herpes zoster incidence during TCZ treatment are similar to those during treatment with anti-TNF inhibitors [4].

This case of herpes zoster meningitis in a patient with AOSD who was treated with TCZ must be considered within the context of herpes zoster in immunocompromised patients. In addition to the TCZ treatment, the patient was also treated with other immunosuppressive therapies, including cyclosporin A and steroids. Therefore, the herpes zoster infection risk attributable to the anti-IL-6 agent in this case is confounded by the immunosuppression caused by the combined treatment with prednisolone and cyclosporin A. Notably, other studies have also reported a higher risk for herpes zoster viral infection among patients receiving combination of immunosuppressive therapies. Specifically, glucocorticoid use had a significant association with herpes zoster, so it is likely that the usage of a moderate dose of glucocorticoid, in addition to cyclosporin A, could have contributed to the occurrence of herpes zoster meningitis seen in the present case.

Herpes zoster is caused by the reactivation of latent varicella zoster virus (VZV) maintained in the spinal dorsal root ganglia of the cranial nerves after primary infection. Virus replication following the primary infection depends upon several conditions, and protection from VZV reactivation from latency seems to depend on the VZV-specific T cell-mediated immunity that is elicited during the primary infection and declines with advancing age [10]. Meningoencephalitis, a rare manifestation of herpes zoster virus reactivation presumably caused by a centripetal spread of virus along the posterior root of the spinal cord, has been described in immunocompetent patients [11]. Other reports have demonstrated that IL-6 is required for an optimal immune response after ocular herpes simplex virus type 1 infection and is considered to contribute to resistance against herpesviruses [12].

Herpes zoster infections can be associated with subtle signs of aseptic meningitis, such as mild CSF mononuclear pleocytosis with a slight increase in protein, in up to 50% of patients [13], but this is rarely accompanied by virus isolation from the CSF. Therefore, when herpes zoster virus can be implicated in CNS infections in immunocompetent patients, investigations of the CSF are mandatory. For laboratory confirmation of herpes zoster virus, viral DNA detection by PCR, as was used in this case, is much more sensitive than virus culture, which has a low yield. Based on case reports and small series [14], a guideline from the Infectious Diseases Society of America suggests treating VZV encephalitis with intravenous acyclovir at 10–15 mg/kg every 8 hours for 10–14 days. Therefore, we treated the patient with 10 mg/kg for 14 days [15].

Immunization with a live attenuated vaccine reduces the risk of recurrent herpes zoster infection among immunocompetent individuals [16]. According to the American College of Rheumatology, however, the live herpes zoster vaccine is contraindicated in patients receiving immunosuppressive medications, such as biologic agents. Surprisingly [17], a recent study indicated that herpes zoster vaccination was not associated with a short-term increase in the herpes zoster incidence of Medicare beneficiaries with immune-mediated diseases, including those receiving biologics [18]. These data call into question the current recommendation of herpes zoster vaccine contraindication for patients receiving biologics. Therefore, further studies concerning the safety and effectiveness of herpes zoster vaccination among patients receiving biologics are needed.

In conclusion, this paper presents the first reported case of herpes zoster meningitis occurring opportunistically in association with TCZ therapy for AOSD. This case highlights the risk of severe, atypical opportunistic infections and the need for both early recognition of herpes zoster meningitis and aggressive management of this disease with antiviral therapy. It also draws attention to the potential cofounders of concomitant immunosuppression in the course of AOSD treatments, including TCZ.

Competing Interests

The authors declare that they have no competing interests.

References

[1] J. A. Singh, C. Cameron, S. Noorbaloochi et al., "Risk of serious infection in biological treatment of patients with rheumatoid arthritis: a systematic review and meta-analysis," *The Lancet*, vol. 386, no. 9990, pp. 258–265, 2015.

[2] H. Yun, F. Xie, E. Delzell et al., "Risks of herpes zoster in patients with rheumatoid arthritis according to biologic disease-modifying therapy," *Arthritis Care and Research*, vol. 67, no. 5, pp. 731–736, 2015.

[3] I. Steiner, "Human herpes viruses latent infection in the nervous system," *Immunological Reviews*, vol. 152, pp. 157–173, 1996.

[4] A. Strangfeld, J. Listing, P. Herzer et al., "Risk of herpes zoster in patients with rheumatoid arthritis treated with anti-TNF-α agents," *The Journal of the American Medical Association*, vol. 301, no. 7, pp. 737–744, 2009.

[5] C. Ma, B. Walters, and R. N. Fedorak, "Varicella zoster meningitis complicating combined anti-tumor necrosis factor and corticosteroid therapy in Crohn's disease," *World Journal of Gastroenterology*, vol. 19, no. 21, pp. 3347–3351, 2013.

[6] R. J. Whitley, "Therapeutic approaches to varicella-zoster virus infections," *Journal of Infectious Diseases*, vol. 166, no. 1, pp. S51–S57, 1992.

[7] N. Nishimoto, J. Hashimoto, N. Miyasaka et al., "Study of active controlled monotherapy used for rheumatoid arthritis, an IL-6 inhibitor (SAMURAI): evidence of clinical and radiographic benefit from an X-ray reader-blinded randomised controlled trial of tocilizumab," *Annals of the Rheumatic Diseases*, vol. 66, no. 9, pp. 1162–1167, 2007.

[8] M. C. Genovese, J. D. McKay, E. L. Nasonov et al., "Interleukin-6 receptor inhibition with tocilizumab reduces disease activity in rheumatoid arthritis with inadequate response to disease-modifying antirheumatic drugs: the tocilizumab in combination with traditional disease-modifying antirheumatic drug therapy study," *Arthritis and Rheumatism*, vol. 58, no. 10, pp. 2968–2980, 2008.

[9] N. Nishimoto, N. Miyasaka, K. Yamamoto, S. Kawai, T. Takeuchi, and J. Azuma, "Long-term safety and efficacy of tocilizumab, an anti-IL-6 receptor monoclonal antibody, in monotherapy, in patients with rheumatoid arthritis (the STREAM study): evidence of safety and efficacy in a 5-year extension study," *Annals of the Rheumatic Diseases*, vol. 68, no. 10, pp. 1580–1584, 2009.

[10] D. H. Gilden, B. K. Kleinschmidt-DeMasters, J. J. LaGuardia, R. Mahalingam, and R. J. Cohrs, "Neurologic complications of the reactivation of varicella-zoster virus," *New England Journal of Medicine*, vol. 342, no. 9, pp. 635–645, 2000.

[11] I. Steiner, P. G. Kennedy, and A. R. Pachner, "The neurotropic herpes viruses: herpes simplex and varicella-zoster," *Lancet Neurology*, vol. 6, no. 11, pp. 1015–1028, 2007.

[12] R. A. LeBlanc, L. Pesnicak, E. S. Cabral, M. Godleski, and S. E. Straus, "Lack of interleukin-6 (IL-6) enhances susceptibility to infection but does not alter latency or reactivation of herpes simplex virus type 1 in IL-6 knockout mice," *Journal of Virology*, vol. 73, no. 10, pp. 8145–8151, 1999.

[13] K. L. Roos, "Pearls and pitfalls in the diagnosis and management of central nervous system infectious diseases," *Seminars in Neurology*, vol. 18, no. 2, pp. 185–196, 1998.

[14] P. Cinque, S. Bossolasco, and A. Lundkvist, "Molecular analysis of cerebrospinal fluid in viral diseases of the central nervous system," *Journal of Clinical Virology*, vol. 26, no. 1, pp. 1–28, 2003.

[15] A. R. Tunkel, C. A. Glaser, K. C. Bloch et al., "The management of encephalitis: clinical practice guidelines by the Infectious Diseases Society of America," *Clinical Infectious Diseases*, vol. 47, no. 3, pp. 303–327, 2008.

[16] H. F. Tseng, M. Chi, N. Smith, S. M. Marcy, L. S. Sy, and S. J. Jacobsen, "Herpes zoster vaccine and the incidence of recurrent herpes zoster in an immunocompetent elderly population," *Journal of Infectious Diseases*, vol. 206, no. 2, pp. 190–196, 2012.

[17] S. Van Assen, N. Agmon-Levin, O. Elkayam et al., "EULAR recommendations for vaccination in adult patients with autoimmune inflammatory rheumatic diseases," *Annals of the Rheumatic Diseases*, vol. 70, no. 3, pp. 414–422, 2011.

[18] J. Zhang, F. Xie, E. Delzell et al., "Association between vaccination for herpes zoster and risk of herpes zoster infection among older patients with selected immune-mediated diseases," *The Journal of the American Medical Association*, vol. 308, no. 1, pp. 43–49, 2012.

Pneumatosis Intestinalis Associated with Juvenile Dermatomyositis

Takako Miyamae,[1,2] Naoko Ishiguro,[3] Maria Yonezawa,[4] Katsutoshi Tokushige,[4] and Hisashi Yamanaka[1]

[1] *Institute of Rheumatology, Tokyo Women's Medical University, No. 10-22, Kawadacho, Shinjuku-ku, Tokyo 162-0054, Japan*
[2] *Department of Pediatrics, Tokyo Women's Medical University, No. 8-1, Kawadacho, Shinjuku-ku, Tokyo 162-0054, Japan*
[3] *Department of Dermatology, Tokyo Women's Medical University, No. 8-1, Kawadacho, Shinjuku-ku, Tokyo 162-0054, Japan*
[4] *Institute of Gastroenterology, Tokyo Women's Medical University, No. 8-1, Kawadacho, Shinjuku-ku, Tokyo 162-0054, Japan*

Correspondence should be addressed to Takako Miyamae; tmiyamae@twmu.ac.jp

Academic Editor: Jamal Mikdashi

We herein report a case of pneumatosis intestinalis (PI), a condition characterized by the presence of gas within the wall of the digestive tract, associated with juvenile dermatomyositis (JDM). A 16-year-old girl, diagnosed with JDM at the age of 10, presented with abdominal pain and distention. She developed PI based on radiological findings that also included a dilated large intestine, extraluminal gas, and secondary diaphragmatic elevation. She was observed with medical therapy including bowel rest and hyperbaric oxygen therapy. However, she ultimately developed a strangulated obstruction 5 years after presentation with PI and large intestine resection and colostomy were performed emergently.

1. Introduction

Juvenile dermatomyositis (JDM) is an autoimmune vasculopathy of uncertain origin involving multiple organ systems. It is defined as chronic inflammation of the striated muscle and skin [1, 2]. Classic JDM presents with an insidious progression of malaise, fatigue, muscle weakness, fever, and a rash that may predate diagnosis by three to six months. In more than three-fourths of the children with JDM [3], the cutaneous abnormalities are pathognomonic of the disease at presentation. The most typical cutaneous manifestations are heliotrope discoloration of the upper eyelids and Gottron papules more frequently in young children. In cases with severe skin vasculopathy, cutaneous ulcers present in 5% to 10% of patients [4, 5].

Gastrointestinal manifestations may also be present as extra-muscular symptoms in JDM. Vasculopathy in the mucosa of the gastrointestinal tract with resulting tissue ischemia or an acute mesenteric infarction can occur [6].

Pneumatosis intestinalis (PI), first described in 1754, is a rare condition characterized by gas bubbles within the wall of the digestive tract. It has been associated with medical conditions including gastrointestinal and chronic pulmonary diseases [7]. However, it rarely occurs with autoimmune disorders. Among several PI cases associated with JDM, their gastrointestinal severity varies from benign to life-threatening causes [8]. We experienced a case of JDM complicated by PI eventually requiring a colostomy.

2. Case Presentation

In 1998, a girl presented with facial erythema and Gottron's papules at 10 years of age and visited the Department of Dermatology at Tokyo Women's Medical University. Muscle weakness and elevation of muscle-derived enzymes (creatine kinase 1105 IU/L, aldolase 30.9 IU/L, and myoglobin 470 ng/mL) developed during the following year. She was diagnosed as having JDM on clinical and pathological grounds after skin and muscle biopsy. Muscle biopsy revealed perivascular mononuclear inflammatory infiltrate, arterial wall thickening, and perifascicular atrophy. Anti-Jo-1 antibody was negative. Oral prednisolone (PSL, 60 mg/day,

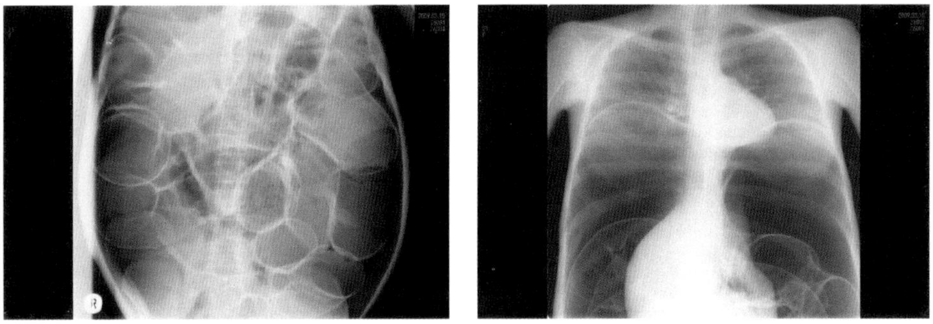

(a) (b)

FIGURE 1: Plain radiographs ((a) lateral view of the abdomen and (b) frontal view of the chest and abdomen) show extensive gas in the colon wall, a dominance of air in the abdominal cavity above the colon, and secondary diaphragmatic elevation.

2 mg/kg) alleviated the clinical symptoms and laboratory findings. Following a decrease in the dosage of PSL, myositis and skin erythema developed at age 14. The myositis remained stable whereas the skin rash intermittently progressed.

She presented with abdominal pain and severe distention when the dosage of PSL was decreased to 9 mg/day in 2004, at the age of 16. She was afebrile. Radiological examination demonstrated pneumatosis, a dilated large intestine, and dominance of air in the abdominal cavity suggesting the bowel-wall air above the colon (Figures 1(a) and 1(b)). She was not able to lie down on her back and developed respiratory distress because of the marked abdominal distention and secondary diaphragmatic elevation. She was diagnosed with PI and treated medically with bowel rest and hyperbaric oxygen therapy. She partially improved but abdominal pain and distention persisted, sometimes got a little better but then got worse again, and finally developed large bowel obstruction with strangulation in 2009 necessitating emergent large and small bowel resection with a double barrel colostomy. Further exploration revealed foci of necrosis with several perforations in both large and small intestines. Since the colostomy was performed, she was then receiving nutrition parenterally and has been free from abdominal pain with less distention without hyperbaric oxygen therapy during 6 years after the resection. Her steroids were changed from oral PSL to intravenous betamethasone at a dosage of 0.3 to 0.9 mg/day depending on skin manifestations but not on abdominal symptoms. In February 2015, anti-aminoacyl-tRNA synthetase antibodies were not detected and the patient was diagnosed with severe osteoporosis (% of young adult mean bone marrow density between lumbar vertebrae L2–L4: 53%), presumably caused by long term administration of betamethasone. She was then partially switched back to oral PSL. The dosage of PSL has been controlled based on gastrointestinal and skin manifestations and is currently maintained at 10 mg daily.

3. Discussion

We reported a case of PI associated with JDM eventually requiring large bowel resection and colostomy. PI is not a diagnosis but rather a physical or radiographic finding, usually as a result of a pathologic process. Impaired mucosal integrity, increased intraluminal pressure, bacterial flora, and intraluminal gas during illness all can lead to the presence of gas within the wall of the gastrointestinal tract [9].

Among autoimmune disorders, PI is commonly noted in systemic sclerosis but rarely associated with dermatomyositis or JDM. Previously, 8 cases of PI in JDM have been reported in the literature (Table 1). Two patients died of intestinal perforation and subsequent sepsis [10, 11]. The time required to normalization of gastrointestinal conditions varied from a week to over a year in those patients that survived. This patient had 5 years from the time of first manifestations of PI until the development of a strangulated obstruction and was never fully healthy during that time. Intestinal resection and colostomy were thought to be unavoidable.

In the JDM cases that developed PI, skin manifestations were more common than myositis. Two of the 8 cases had skin ulceration. The pathogenesis of PI in JDM is not clear. However, some authors have speculated that gastrointestinal ischemia secondary to vasculopathy could result in loss of integrity of the mucosa and bacterial production of gas with submucosal dissection of intraluminal gas [12]. The high frequency of skin manifestations and ulcers might suggest that skin vasculitis has a correlation with vasculopathy in the mucosa of the gastrointestinal tract. Interestingly, severity and prognosis of PI associated with JDM vary though the number of reported patients was small. Benign cases were diagnosed by routine X-ray finding without abdominal manifestations and resolved in natural course; however, there were fatal cases complicated with intestinal perforation, subsequent infection, and sepsis [Table 1]. The difference of the prognosis of PI is unclear but can be affected by severity of vessel vasculopathy, initial treatment, and myositis specific/associated antibodies.

Immunosuppressive treatments including glucocorticoids seemed to be effective in some of the reported cases and these were able to suppress the vasculopathy in the early phase of PI. In addition, they could help to cause the submucosal lymphoid tissue atrophy and subsequent dissection of air into the bowel wall that occurs. However, once peritonitis and sepsis occur, the problem is surgical. Considering the fact that

Table 1: Summary of reported cases of pneumatosis intestinalis associated with juvenile dermatomyositis.

	Onset age of PI	Period from JDM onset to PI onset	Treatment before PI onset	Manifestations of PI	Image findings and clinical diagnosis	Disease activity of JDM at PI onset	Clinical course of PI	Outcome
1 [13]	4.8, female	1 Y	GCs	Abdominal pain, diarrhea, constipation, and movable mass in the left lower quadrant	Cystoid gas collection in the mid transverse colon and splenic flexure	Calcinosis universalis was noted	Pneumatosis persisted for 25 months	Survived
2 [14]	8.5, female	3 Y	GCs, AZP, CY, and MTX	Abdominal pain and abdominal distention	Gas-filled hepatic flexure of colon and extraluminal gas	Refractory myositis and skin manifestations with disseminated subcutaneous calcification	Abdominal manifestations remitted during the next 10 days with PSL and MTX. Intramural gas persisted for four months	Survived
3 [15]	12, female	3 Y	None	Dysphagia	Cystoid gas collection	Noted myositis and dermatitis	Treated with oral GCs	Survived
4 [10]	8.5, female	1 Mo	GCs and MTX	Abdominal pain, vomiting, diarrhea, and fever	Perforation and peritonitis	Increased muscle weakness, rash, and rising muscle enzyme values recurred	Died 6 weeks after the development of PI owing to complications of perforations, peritonitis, and candida sepsis	Died
5 [11]	11, female	3 Mo	GCs and CY	Abdominal pain, bilious emesis, and fever	Extensive extraluminal gas collection in the right abdomen and flank. Peritonitis, retroperitoneal abscess, and duodenal perforation were found at laparotomy	Became bedridden because of progressive muscle weakness from JDM onset	Discharged 8.5 months after admission over multiple episodes of sepsis and 8 laparotomies	Survived
6 [11]	15, male	2 Y	GCs	Abdominal discomfort, pain, vomiting, fever, and hematemesis	Following appendicitis and appendectomy, PI occurred with duodenal perforation and peritonitis	Exacerbated muscle weakness two months previously	Died of perforation, sepsis and multiple organ failure on the 21st hospital day despite four laparotomies	Died
7 [12]	7, female	3 Mo	GCs and MTX	Abdominal pain	Intramural air in the ascending and transverse colon	Prominent skin rash and vascular ulcers in the axillar, minimal proximal muscle weakness	Treated with intravenous antibiotics and parental nutrition. Clinical improvement evident after a week	Survived
8 [8]	8, female	1 Mo	GCs, MTX, and mPSL pulse	Cough and abdominal distention	CT showed extensive PI in the large colon	Increased weakness and a vasculitic ulcer on upper eyelid and in the nare	Treated with intravenous antibiotics and a short period of bowel rest	Survived
Present case	16, female	6 Y	GCs	Abdominal pain and abdominal distention	Extensive gas-filled colon and extraluminal gas above colon	Intermittently worsened skin manifestations	Complicated with strangulated obstruction and large intestine resection and colostomy were performed	Survived

PI: pneumatosis intestinalis, JDM: juvenile dermatomyositis, Mo: month(s), Y: year(s), GCs: glucocorticoids, PSL: prednisolone, CY: cyclophosphamide, AZP: azathioprine, MTX: methotrexate, and mPSL: methylprednisolone.

most of the cases were reported before 2000, early diagnosis and timely initiation of immunosuppressive therapy may help to prevent vasculopathy and the development of PI. PI should be considered on the differential diagnosis in patients with JDM presenting with abdominal complaints, especially in patients with severe skin vasculitis.

Competing Interests

The authors declare that they have no competing interests.

References

[1] A. Bohan and J. B. Peter, "Polymyositis and dermatomyositis," *The New England Journal of Medicine*, vol. 292, no. 7, pp. 344–347, 1975.

[2] A. Bohan and J. B. Peter, "Polymyositis and dermatomyositis (second of two parts)," *The New England Journal of Medicine*, vol. 292, no. 8, pp. 403–407, 1975.

[3] L. G. Rider, C. B. Lindsley, and F. W. Miller, "Juvenile dermatomyositis," in *Textbook of Pediatric Rheumatology*, J. T. Cassidy and R. E. Petty, Eds., pp. 351–383, Elsevier Saunder, Philadelphia, Pa, USA, 7th edition, 2015.

[4] A. M. Huber, E. M. Dugan, P. A. Lachenbruch et al., "The cutaneous assessment tool: development and reliability in juvenile idiopathic inflammatory myopathy," *Rheumatology*, vol. 46, no. 10, pp. 1606–1611, 2007.

[5] N. Martin, P. Krol, S. Smith et al., "Comparison of children with onset of juvenile dermatomyositis symptoms before or after their fifth birthday in a UK and Ireland juvenile dermatomyositis cohort study," *Arthritis Care and Research*, vol. 64, no. 11, pp. 1665–1672, 2012.

[6] S. Inamdar, M. S. Slim, H. Bostwick, and L. Godine, "Treatment of duodenocutaneous fistula with somatostatin analog in a child with dermatomyositis," *Journal of Pediatric Gastroenterology and Nutrition*, vol. 10, no. 3, pp. 402–404, 1990.

[7] L. G. Koss, "Abdominal gas cysts (pneumatosiscystoidesintestinorumhominis): an analysis with a report of a case and acritical review of the literature," *Archives of Pathology*, vol. 53, no. 6, pp. 523–549, 1952.

[8] R. Berard, G. Chédeville, C. Saint-Martin, and R. Scuccimarri, "Benign pneumatosis intestinalis in a patient with juvenile dermatomyositis," *The Journal of Rheumatology*, vol. 37, no. 11, pp. 2442–2444, 2010.

[9] S. D. St Peter, M. A. Abbas, and K. A. Kelly, "The spectrum of pneumatosis intestinalis," *Archives of Surgery*, vol. 138, no. 1, pp. 68–75, 2003.

[10] T. J. Fischer, L. Cipel, and E. R. Stiehm, "Pneumatosis intestinalis associated with fatal childhood dermatomyositis," *Pediatrics*, vol. 61, no. 1, pp. 127–130, 1978.

[11] H. L. Magill, S. D. Hixson, G. Whitington, M. Igarashi, and A. Hannissian, "Duodenal perforation in childhood dermatomyositis," *Pediatric Radiology*, vol. 14, no. 1, pp. 28–30, 1984.

[12] J. C. Stefanski, A. K. Shetty, and A. Gedalia, "Abdominal pain in a girl with juvenile dermatomyositis," *Clinical Pediatrics*, vol. 37, no. 9, pp. 561–564, 1998.

[13] C. F. Mueller, R. Morehead, A. J. Alter, and W. Michener, "Pneumatosis intestinalis in collagen disorders," *The American Journal of Roentgenology, Radium Therapy, and Nuclear Medicine*, vol. 115, no. 2, pp. 300–305, 1972.

[14] M. A. Oliveros, J. J. Herbst, P. D. Lester, and F. A. Ziter, "Pneumatosis intestinalis in childhood dermatomyositis," *Pediatrics*, vol. 52, no. 5, pp. 711–712, 1973.

[15] E. M. Braunstein and S. J. White, "Pneumatosis intestinalis in dermatomyositis," *British Journal of Radiology*, vol. 53, no. 634, pp. 1011–1012, 1980.

ANA Negative Systemic Lupus Erythematosus Leading to CTEPH, TTP-Like Thrombocytopenia, and Skin Ulcers

Khalid Hamid Changal,[1] Fayaz Sofi,[2] Sheikh Shoaib Altaf,[3] Adnan Raina,[1] and Ab. Hameed Raina[1]

[1]*Internal Medicine, Sher-I-Kashmir Institute of Medical Sciences, Srinagar 190011, India*
[2]*Rheumatology and Internal Medicine, Sher-I-Kashmir Institute of Medical Sciences, Srinagar 190011, India*
[3]*Internal Medicine, Mercy Catholic Medical Center, Philadelphia, PA 19026, USA*

Correspondence should be addressed to Khalid Hamid Changal; khalidchangal@gmail.com

Academic Editor: Tsai-Ching Hsu

SLE affects almost every organ system, with differing degrees of severity. During its clinical course periods of flares may alternate with periods of remission culminating in disease and therapy related damage. We describe a case of ANA negative SLE with severe thrombocytopenia, cutaneous vasculitis, antiphospholipid antibody syndrome, and pulmonary artery hypertension. As there is no definitive cure for SLE the treatment lies in caring for the individual organ systems involved and simultaneously taking care of the patient as a whole.

1. Introduction

Systemic lupus erythematosus (SLE) is an autoimmune disorder that affects multiple organs. ANA (antinuclear antibody) negative SLE is a rare entity. The presentation in this case demonstrates how many organ systems can be affected in SLE and how complex the management is. Also it demonstrates that true ANA negative SLE does exist.

2. Case Presentation

The patient was a 26-year-old woman who had history of recurrent admissions for multiple problems. Despite being admitted multiple times she had not received a diagnosis for her recurrent admissions. Her first presentation was 2 years priorly. She had a right popliteal vein thrombosis for which she was put on treatment with warfarin. 5 months later, she suffered a massive pulmonary thromboembolism despite being on anticoagulation. Bed-side echocardiography had shown positive Mc Connell sign and she was thrombolysed with streptokinase. Warfarin was continued on discharge. Few months later she had an episode of hematemesis due to warfarin induced coagulopathy. Warfarin dose was adjusted. Few months later she was admitted again, this time with skin ulcers on posterior aspect of upper arms which were non-healing. The current admission was for recurrent skin ulcers (Figure 1) and breathlessness on exertion (functional classes II-III). In addition patient had generalized fatigue, malar rash, and photosensitivity. Hospital course was complicated with hematemesis. Esophagogastroduodenoscopy showed shallow erosions in stomach. Cardiovascular examination showed signs of right ventricular hypertrophy. A thorough evaluation was started. Hemogram showed anemia and thrombocytopenia. Platelet count was 20,000/micl. Peripheral blood film showed schistocytes and her serum lactate dehydrogenase was high. C-reactive protein was high. C3 levels were low. Other biochemical investigations were normal. Urinalysis was normal and there was no proteinuria. Chest X-ray showed increased cardiothoracic ratio and prominent left pulmonary conus (Figure 2). ANA and dsDNA were negative. ANA was tested using indirect immunofluorescence (IF-ANA) using HEp-2 cell substrates. dsDNA was tested using IF-ANA test using *Crithidia luciliae* as the substrate. Doppler ultrasound of lower limbs showed no evidence of DVT. An ultrasonogram of the abdomen showed congestive hepatosplenomegaly and mild ascites. Echocardiography

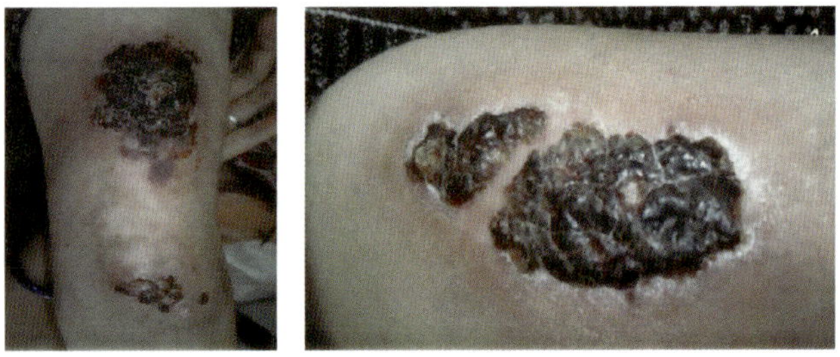

Figure 1: Pictures of the ulcers on the arms of the patient. Crustations have developed on the ulcers.

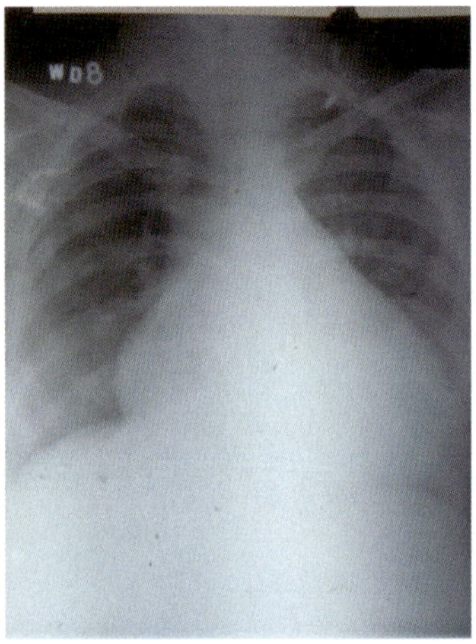

Figure 2: Chest X-ray showing increased cardiothoracic ratio and prominent left pulmonary conus.

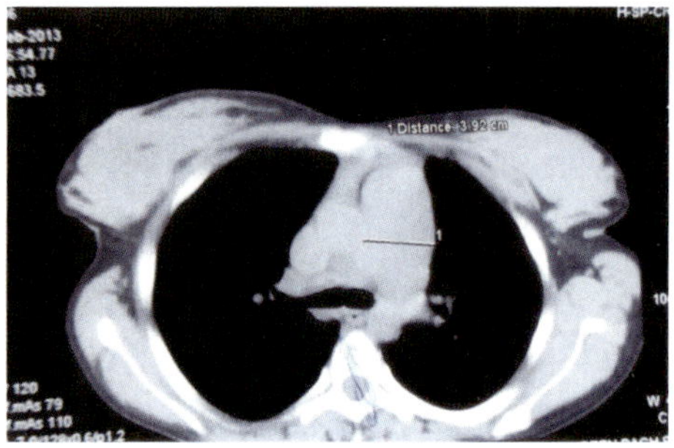

Figure 3: CT chest showing dilated pulmonary artery (marked by 1).

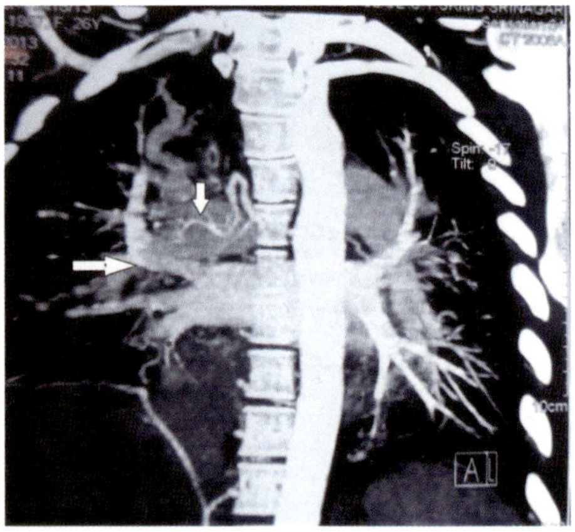

Figure 4: CT pulmonary angiography showing filling defects suggestive of thrombi in the pulmonary vessels (horizontal arrow). Pruning of pulmonary vessels is seen (asterisk). Also collateral vessels have started forming (vertical arrow).

showed normal left heart valves and function. Pulmonary artery was dilated. There were signs of severe pulmonary artery hypertension and severe tricuspid regurgitation. Investigations for APLA (antiphospholipid antibody) syndrome were ordered. Anti-Beta 2 glycoprotein antibody (anti β-2 gp Ab), lupus anticoagulant (LA), and anti-cardiolipin antibodies (ACL) were present. HRCT (high resolution computed tomography) of chest showed normal lung parenchyma but right ventricular and right atrial enlargement with signs of pulmonary artery hypertension (Figure 3). A CT pulmonary angiogram was done to evaluate the vasculature of lungs. The main pulmonary artery was dilated with a diameter of 3.6 cm. There were few filling defects in subsegmental branches of pulmonary artery involving left upper lobe. No thrombi could be found but the pulmonary vasculature showed peripheral pruning. These findings were suggestive of chronic thromboembolic pulmonary hypertension (Figure 4).

In view of the clinical features, thrombocytopenia, photosensitivity, and malar rash a primary diagnosis of SLE was made. Although ANA was negative a diagnosis of SLE can still be made as will be discussed in the discussion part. The cause for DVT and pulmonary embolism was attributed to secondary APLA (secondary to SLE) in view of DVT, ACL, LA, and Beta 2 gp Ab being present. The lab results were later reproduced more than 12 weeks apart. The recurrent skin ulcers were attributed to the cutaneous vasculitis secondary to SLE. The cause for pulmonary hypertension was chronic thromboembolic hypertension. Thrombocytopenia was due to SLE related thrombotic thrombocytopenic purpura (TTP) like pathology. As patient had multiple issues, the management was difficult. Critical thrombocytopenia was managed with pulse methylprednisolone for 5 days followed by oral steroids. Platelet count did not improve. Option of intravenous immunoglobulins was discussed with the patient but affordability was an issue. So patient was given oral azathioprine and dapsone. Platelet count started to improve. The treatment for PAH was medical as the patient was not a candidate for pulmonary thromboendarterectomy because the distal smaller vessels were involved. Second option was bosentan (affordability was again an issue). Patient was started on phosphodiesterase inhibitors (Tadalafil). Oxygen therapy was continued. Diuretics were rationalized. Anticoagulants were started once platelets improved. The skin ulcers started healing and improving while patient received pulse steroids for thrombocytopenia. Following up the patient few months later INR is stabilized within 2–2.5 without any bleeding episode. Latest platelet counts are 243,000/micl. Skin ulcers have cleared markedly with a little scared tissue. Patient still has functional class III symptoms.

3. Discussion

SLE is an autoimmune disease that is usually chronic but can present acutely too. Young women are usually affected, but it can occur in up to 20 percent of patients who are older than 50 years. SLE can manifest in any organ system and the pathology may vary from minor to life-threatening [1]. There can be a preclinical phase in which the patient may be apparently normal and tests positive for autoantibodies. This is followed by a clinically overt autoimmune phase in which the clinical phenotype of the disease starts to manifest. As the disease progresses there may be flares of active disease and remissions leading to cumulative damage of the organ systems affected [2]. This discussion is focused chiefly on the presentation features of the patient described.

SLE and Thrombocytopenia. Thrombocytopenia can be due to multiple reasons in SLE. The prevalence ranges from 7% to 30%. This is mostly due to peripheral destruction of platelets [3]. A TTP-like syndrome may occur in SLE as was present in our patient. There can be a microangiopathic hemolytic anemia with or without the other features of TTP like fever, thrombocytopenia, kidney involvement, and neurologic symptoms. Schistocytes in the peripheral blood smear and increased lactate dehydrogenase levels are strong pointers toward this disorder. In a patient with generalized lupus activity it is referred to as TTP-like syndrome. Immunosuppressive therapy is used for treatment. In the absence of generalized lupus activity it may be referred to as bonafide TTP. A similar syndrome can also occur in the presence of antiphospholipid antibodies [2]. Serum platelet-binding IgG and platelet-associated IgG have been found to be increased in SLE with thrombocytopenia. These antibodies can also be found in SLE patients who do not have thrombocytopenia thus making it not very specific [3–5]. Thrombocytopenia is an independent risk factor for increased mortality in SLE [6]. In a retrospective study of 632 patients with SLE it was found that thrombocytopenia is not directly associated with end organ damage and mortality but defines a subgroup of patients with higher morbidity and is thus a major complication of SLE, affecting overall prognosis [7]. Sultan et al. did a study that associated thrombocytopenia with disease activity in other organs [8]. Mild thrombocytopenia may require only observation. Corticosteroids are the treatment of choice for the initial management of more severe cases [9]. Treatment is considered if bleeding or severe bruising are present, or with platelet counts $<50 \times 109/L$ [10]. Azathioprine is introduced as a steroid-sparing agent [11]. Cyclosporine is also used but should be avoided in case of kidney disease [12]. Intravenous immunoglobulins (IVIG) can be very effective in some patients with lupus-associated thrombocytopenia. IVIG in SLE act by downregulation of autoantibody production, neutralization of pathogenic autoantibodies by anti-idiotypic antibodies, inhibition of complement-mediated damage, modulation of cytokine production, induction of apoptosis in lymphocytes and monocytes, and modulation of both B- and T-lymphocyte function [13, 14]. Relatively toxic drugs like cyclophosphamide may be used in severe thrombocytopenia refractory to other less toxic drugs [15]. Other drugs used include methotrexate, romiplostim, and mycophenolate mofetil. Rituximab and stem cell transplantation may be considered in refractory cases [16]. If treatment of thrombocytopenia with steroids or other drugs is unsuccessful, splenectomy may be considered [17]. The role of splenectomy has been controversial in SLE. One of the largest series of thrombocytopenic patients with SLE who have undergone splenectomy concluded that splenectomy should be considered safe and efficacious for thrombocytopenia associated with SLE [17]. However, one older study has suggested a poor outcome [18].

SLE and APLA. Antiphospholipid syndrome (APS) is an autoimmune disorder characterized by thromboembolic events or fetal deaths with the presence of antiphospholipid antibodies (APLAs) [19]. APLA can be primary or secondary. Secondary APS is most commonly associated with SLE. The prevalence of APLAs in SLE is reported to be 30% to 50% [20]. As the APLAs may be transiently positive, in order to be considered a part of APS it needs to be positive 12 weeks apart as per the Sapparo criteria. The lupus anticoagulant is an independent risk factor for acute myocardial infarction and ischemic stroke [21]. The treatment for thrombotic events and its prevention center on anticoagulation. The duration of treatment differs based on the patient characteristics and an individualized decision should be taken. Unprovoked thrombotic events, arterial events, or presence of APLA support prolonged anticoagulation.

SLE and Skin Ulcers. Kidney is the most common organ to be affected by SLE followed by skin [22]. The 3 major types of involvement of skin in SLE are chronic cutaneous lupus erythematosus (LE), subacute cutaneous LE, and systemic or acute cutaneous LE [23]. Cutaneous manifestations are varied and include malar rash, discoid LE (DLE), photosensitivity, mucosal DLE, subacute cutaneous lupus erythematosus, alopecia, lupus panniculitis/lupus profundus, lichenoid DLE, small vessel cutaneous leukocytoclastic vasculitis secondary to LE, secondary atrophie blanche, periungual telangiectasias, livedo reticularis, Raynaud's phenomenon, and bullous lesions (BSLE) [24]. Of these, the ones which can present as cutaneous ulcers include lupus profundus and cutaneous vasculitis. Lupus profundus presents as deep brawny indurations or subcutaneous nodule. The overlying skin may be erythematous, atrophic, and ulcerated and may leave a depressed scar. The most common sites of involvement are the lateral aspects of the arms and shoulders, thighs, buttocks, trunk, breast, face, and scalp. Cutaneous vasculitis presents in a number of morphological variants including ulcers. Other lesions which it can manifest by are punctate lesions, palpable purpura, urticaria, papules, erythematosus plaques or macules, and erythema with necrosis. The most common form of vasculitis is small vessel vasculitis.

SLE and ANA. ANA positivity is one of the criteria in the American College of Rheumatology's criteria for the classification of SLE which is primarily used as a research tool [23]. The description of ANA-negative lupus was first raised by Koller et al. in 1976. They described five patients who were

ANA-negative but had clinical features consistent with SLE [25]. Reports of ANA-negative SLE have decreased markedly in recent years probably because of the use of better substrates in ANA testing. Previously a variety of less efficient substrates were used like rat liver, mouse liver, human spleen, human prostate cell, and human granulocytes. The introduction of Hep-2 cells (a rapidly dividing human epithelial cell line) as a routine substrate for ANA determination has led to a well standardized assay with a marked increase in sensitivity [26]. Apart from antigen deficiency in the testing substrate other causes for ANA being negative in SLE include concurrent immunosuppressive treatment and persistent profound proteinuria with associated renal loss of immunoglobulins. ANA-negative lupus appeared to be a genuine and more common phenomenon a few decades ago. The current and latest evidence from the literature and experience in large centers suggests that true ANA-negative lupus is an extremely rare event [27]. In our case the substrate used for testing was Hep 2 cell based; the patient was not on immunosuppression when the testing was done and had no proteinuria. Also ANA has been repeated several months later and is negative. So our case represents a true ANA negative SLE.

SLE and Pulmonary Arterial Hypertension (PAH). The prevalence of PAH in SLE is around 0.5% to 17.5%. The pathophysiology of PAH may involve multiple mechanisms. It may be due to vasculitis, *in situ* thrombosis, or interstitial pulmonary fibrosis which increases pulmonary vascular resistance. PAH is defined as an increase in mean pulmonary arterial pressure ≥25 mmHg at rest, pulmonary artery wedge pressure, or left ventricular end diastolic pressure ≤15 mmHg and increased pulmonary vascular resistance [28, 29]. The various inflammatory and autoimmune mechanisms in SLE can lead to endothelial and smooth muscle proliferation causing damage to the pulmonary vasculature and leading to PAH. Studies have shown an imbalance between vasoconstrictors and vasodilators in the pulmonary vasculature. Vascular pathologic findings in patients with SLE associated PAH include plexiform lesions, muscular hypertrophy, and intimal proliferation [30]. Chronic thromboembolic pulmonary hypertension (CTEPH) is a pulmonary vascular disease due to chronic obstruction of major pulmonary arteries. It is one of the causes of pulmonary artery hypertension. Main features of CTEPH are a nonhomogeneous distribution of disease in segments of the pulmonary vascular tree and its association with venous thromboembolism [31]. In our case the PAH was chiefly caused by CTEPH but we feel that the underlying SLE also contributed independently to it.

References

[1] S. L. Gurevitz, J. A. Snyder, E. K. Wessel, J. Frey, and B. A. Williamson, "Systemic lupus erythematosus: a review of the disease and treatment options," *Consultant Pharmacist*, vol. 28, no. 2, pp. 110–121, 2013.

[2] G. Bertsias, R. Cervera, and D. T. Boumpas, "Systemic lupus erythematosus: pathogenesis and clinical features," in *EULAR Textbook of Rheumatic Diseases*, J. W. J. Bijlsma and E. Hachulla, Eds., pp. 476–505, BMJ Group, London, UK, 1st edition, 2012.

[3] S. E. Howe and D. M. Lynch, "Platelet antibody binding in systemic lupus erythematosus," *Journal of Rheumatology*, vol. 14, no. 3, pp. 482–486, 1987.

[4] F. Fabris, A. Casonato, M. L. Randi, G. Luzzatto, and A. Girolami, "Clinical significance of surface and internal pools of platelet-associated immunoglobulins in immune thrombocytopenia," *Scandinavian Journal of Haematology*, vol. 37, no. 3, pp. 215–220, 1986.

[5] M. Michel, V. Chanet, A. Dechartres et al., "The spectrum of Evans syndrome in adults: New insight into the disease based on the analysis of 68 cases," *Blood*, vol. 114, no. 15, pp. 3167–3172, 2009.

[6] C. C. Mok, K. W. Lee, C. T. K. Ho, C. S. Lau, and R. W. S. Wong, "A prospective study of survival and prognostic indicators of systemic lupus erythematosus in a southern Chinese population," *Rheumatology*, vol. 39, no. 4, pp. 399–406, 2000.

[7] P. D. Ziakas, S. Giannouli, E. Zintzaras, A. G. Tzioufas, and M. Voulgarelis, "Lupus thrombocytopenia: clinical implications and prognostic significance," *Annals of the Rheumatic Diseases*, vol. 64, no. 9, pp. 1366–1369, 2005.

[8] S. M. Sultan, S. Begum, and D. A. Isenberg, "Prevalence, patterns of disease and outcome in patients with systemic lupus erythematosus who develop severe haematological problems," *Rheumatology*, vol. 42, no. 2, pp. 230–234, 2003.

[9] P. D. Ziakas, J. G. Routsias, S. Giannouli, A. Tasidou, A. G. Tzioufas, and M. Voulgarelis, "Suspects in the tale of lupus-associated thrombocytopenia," *Clinical and Experimental Immunology*, vol. 145, no. 1, pp. 71–80, 2006.

[10] D. R. Budman and A. D. Steinberg, "Hematologic aspects of systemic lupus erythematosus. Current concepts," *Annals of Internal Medicine*, vol. 86, no. 2, pp. 220–229, 1977.

[11] M. Abu-Shakra and Y. Shoenfeld, "Azathioprine therapy for patients with systemic lupus erythematosus," *Lupus*, vol. 10, no. 3, pp. 152–153, 2001.

[12] B. Griffiths and P. Emery, "The treatment of lupus with cyclosporin A," *Lupus*, vol. 10, no. 3, pp. 165–170, 2001.

[13] Y. Levy, Y. Sherer, A. Ahmed et al., "A study of 20 SLE patients with intravenous immunoglobulin—clinical and serologic response," *Lupus*, vol. 8, no. 9, pp. 705–712, 1999.

[14] L. Rauova, J. Lukac, Y. Levy, J. Rovensky, and Y. Shoenfeld, "High-dose intravenous immunoglobulins for lupus nephritis—a salvage immunomodulation," *Lupus*, vol. 10, no. 3, pp. 209–213, 2001.

[15] D. T. Boumpas, S. Barez, J. H. Klippel, and J. E. Balow, "Intermittent cyclophosphamide for the treatment of autoimmune thrombocytopenia in systemic lupus erythematosus," *Annals of Internal Medicine*, vol. 112, no. 9, pp. 674–677, 1990.

[16] A. L. Hepburn, S. Narat, and J. C. Mason, "The management of peripheral blood cytopenias in systemic lupus erythematosus," *Rheumatology*, vol. 49, no. 12, pp. 2243–2254, 2010.

[17] Y. N. You, A. Tefferi, and D. M. Nagorney, "Outcome of splenectomy for thrombocytopenia associated with systemic lupus erythematosus," *Annals of Surgery*, vol. 240, no. 2, pp. 286–292, 2004.

[18] S. Hall, J. L. McCormick Jr., P. R. Greipp, C. J. Michet, and C. H. McKenna, "Splenectomy does not cure the thrombocytopenia of systemic lupus erythematosus," *Annals of Internal Medicine*, vol. 102, no. 3, pp. 325–328, 1985.

[19] W. A. Wilson, A. E. Gharavi, and J. C. Piette, "International classification criteria for antiphospholipid syndrome: synopsis of a post-conference workshop held at the Ninth International (Tours) aPL Symposium," *Lupus*, vol. 10, no. 7, pp. 457–460, 2001.

[20] M. T. McClain, M. R. Arbuckle, L. D. Heinlen et al., "The prevalence, onset, and clinical significance of antiphospholipid antibodies prior to diagnosis of systemic lupus erythematosus," *Arthritis and Rheumatism*, vol. 50, no. 4, pp. 1226–1232, 2004.

[21] C. C. Mok, C. S. Lau, and R. W. Wong, "Neuropsychiatric manifestations and their clinical associations in southern Chinese patients with systemic lupus erythematosus," *Journal of Rheumatology*, vol. 28, no. 4, pp. 766–771, 2001.

[22] G.-M. Deng and G. C. Tsokos, "Pathogenesis and targeted treatment of skin injury in SLE," *Nature Reviews Rheumatology*, vol. 11, no. 11, pp. 663–669, 2015.

[23] M. C. Hochberg, "Updating the American College of Rheumatology revised criteria for the classification of systemic lupus erythematosus," *Arthritis and Rheumatism*, vol. 40, no. 9, article 1725, 1997.

[24] L. Uva, D. Miguel, C. Pinheiro, J. P. Freitas, M. Marques Gomes, and P. Filipe, "Cutaneous manifestations of systemic lupus erythematosus," *Autoimmune Diseases*, vol. 2012, Article ID 834291, 15 pages, 2012.

[25] S. R. Koller, C. L. Johnston Jr., C. W. Moncure, and M. V. Waller, "Lupus erythematosus cell preparation, antinuclear factor incongruity. A review of diagnostic tests for systemic lupus erythematosus," *American Journal of Clinical Pathology*, vol. 66, no. 3, pp. 495–505, 1976.

[26] A. Kavanaugh, R. Tomar, J. Reveille, D. H. Solomon, and H. A. Homburger, "Guidelines for clinical use of the antinuclear antibody test and tests for specific autoantibodies to nuclear antigens. American College of Pathologists," *Archives of Pathology & Laboratory Medicine*, vol. 124, no. 1, pp. 71–81, 2000.

[27] L. S. Cross, A. Aslam, and S. A. Misbah, "Antinuclear antibody-negative lupus as a distinct diagnostic entity—does it no longer exist?" *Quarterly Journal of Medicine*, vol. 97, no. 5, pp. 303–308, 2004.

[28] V. V. McLaughlin, S. L. Archer, D. B. Badesch et al., "ACCF/AHA 2009 expert consensus document on pulmonary hypertension: a report of the American College of Cardiology Foundation task force on expert consensus documents and the American Heart Association developed in collaboration with the American College of Chest Physicians; American Thoracic Society, Inc.; and the Pulmonary Hypertension Association," *Journal of the American College of Cardiology*, vol. 53, no. 17, pp. 1573–1619, 2009.

[29] V. V. McLaughlin, S. L. Archer, D. B. Badesch et al., "ACCF/AHA 2009 expert consensus document on pulmonary hypertension: a report of the American College of Cardiology Foundation Task Force on Expert Consensus Documents and the American Heart Association: developed in collaboration with the American College of Chest Physicians, American Thoracic Society, Inc., and the Pulmonary Hypertension Association," *Circulation*, vol. 119, no. 16, pp. 2250–2294, 2009.

[30] A. Dhala, "Pulmonary arterial hypertension in systemic lupus erythematosus: current status and future direction," *Clinical and Developmental Immunology*, vol. 2012, Article ID 854941, 12 pages, 2012.

[31] I. M. Lang and M. Madani, "Update on chronic thromboembolic pulmonary hypertension," *Circulation*, vol. 130, no. 6, pp. 508–518, 2014.

Sarcoidosis: Is it a Possible Trigger of Inclusion Body Myositis?

Ali Zakaria, Issam Turk, Kenneth Leung, Ana Capatina-Rata, and Waseem Farra

Department of Internal Medicine, Division of Pulmonology, Division of Rheumatology, Providence-Providence Park Hospital, Michigan State University College of Human Medicine, Southfield, MI, USA

Correspondence should be addressed to Ali Zakaria; alizakaria86@hotmail.com

Academic Editor: Kuntal Chakravarty

Sarcoidosis is a multisystem disorder of unknown etiology, characterized pathologically by the presence of nonnecrotizing granulomatous inflammation in affected organs. Although skeletal muscle is involved in 50–80 percent of individuals with sarcoidosis, symptomatic myopathy has been shown to be a rare manifestation of the disease. Inclusion body myositis (IBM) is a rare acquired idiopathic inflammatory myopathy with the insidious onset of asymmetric and distal muscle weakness that characteristically involves the quadriceps, tibialis anterior, and forearm flexors. Moreover, dysphagia can be the presenting complaint in one-third of patients. Herein, we are presenting a case of 67-year-old African American female who presented with one-month history of new onset progressive dyspnea on exertion. She was diagnosed with stage IV sarcoidosis based on chest CT scan findings and transbronchial lung biopsy revealing nonnecrotizing granulomatous inflammation. Over the next three months after her diagnosis, she presented to the hospital with progressive dysphagia associated with asymmetrical distal muscle weakness. A quadriceps muscle biopsy revealed features consistent with inclusion body myositis. We are reporting this case as it may support the hypothesis of sarcoidosis being a trigger that possibly promotes the development of inclusion body myositis, leading to a very poor prognosis.

1. Introduction

Sarcoidosis is a multisystem disorder of unknown etiology, characterized pathologically by the presence of nonnecrotizing granulomatous inflammation in affected organs. Although skeletal muscle is involved in 50–80 percent of individuals with sarcoidosis, symptomatic myopathy has been shown to be a rare manifestation of the disease (0.5 to 2.5 percent of cases) [1]. Inclusion body myositis is a rare acquired idiopathic inflammatory myopathy with the insidious onset of asymmetric and distal muscle weakness that characteristically involves the quadriceps, tibialis anterior, and forearm flexors. Herein, we are reporting a case of a 62-year-old African American female with clinical and muscle biopsy findings consistent with sarcoidosis and inclusion body myositis.

2. Case Report

A 62-year-old African American female with a past medical history of hypertension presented to the emergency department of our hospital complaining of new onset dyspnea on exertion that had been progressively getting worse for the last month. Initial cardiac workup revealed elevated cardiac troponin T level with no electrocardiographic evidence of ischemic changes. Further evaluation with echocardiogram and coronary angiogram were negative for coronary artery disease. A chest computed tomography (CT) scan was performed and revealed increased bilateral interstitial lung markings with bilateral hilar and mediastinal lymphadenopathy most consistent with stage IV sarcoidosis (Figure 1). Bronchoscopy with transbronchial lung biopsy was performed and pathology revealed nonnecrotizing granulomatous inflammation (Figure 2). Her laboratory results were also supportive of the diagnosis as she had a calcium level of 10 mg/dL, 1,25-dihydroxy vitamin D level of 87 pg/mL (normal 20–79 pg/mL), angiotensin converting enzyme 98 unit/L (normal 8–52 unit/L), and a negative acid-fast bacilli, fungal, and viral tissue cultures. The patient refused the treatment with steroids and as such she was started on hydroxychloroquine 200 mg once daily and she was discharged in a stable condition.

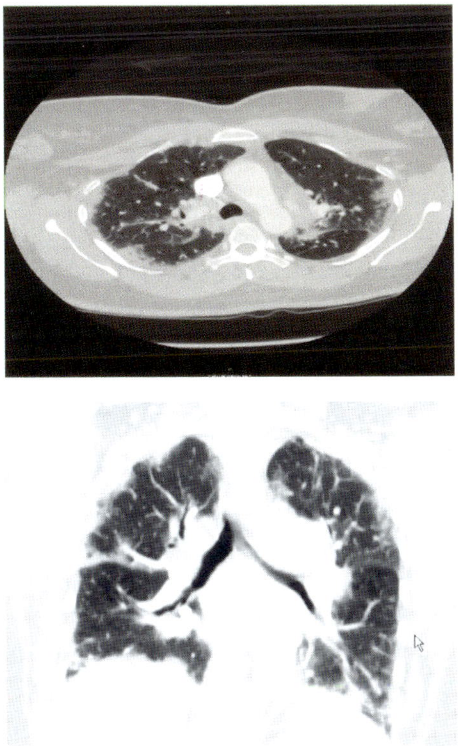

Figure 1: Chest computed tomography (CT) scan showing increased bilateral interstitial lung markings with bilateral hilar and mediastinal lymphadenopathy most consistent with stage IV sarcoidosis.

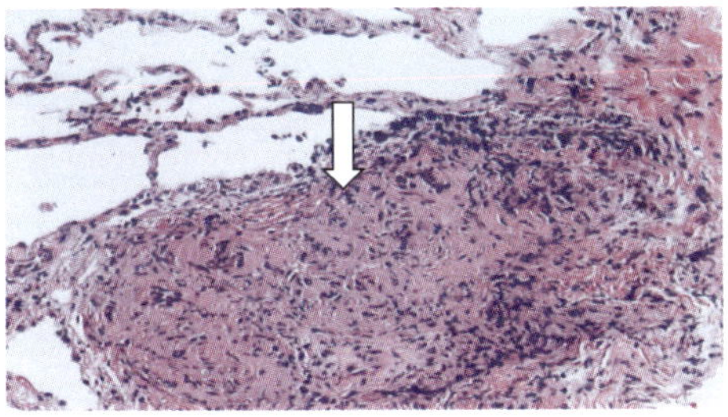

Figure 2: Transbronchial lung biopsy showing nonnecrotizing granulomatous inflammation with multinucleated giant cells (arrow).

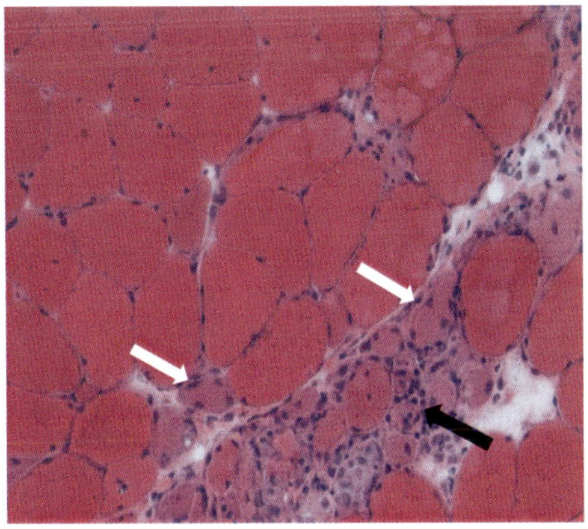

Figure 3: H & E stain of quadriceps muscle biopsy showing muscle atrophy (white arrows) and inflammatory cell infiltrate (black arrow).

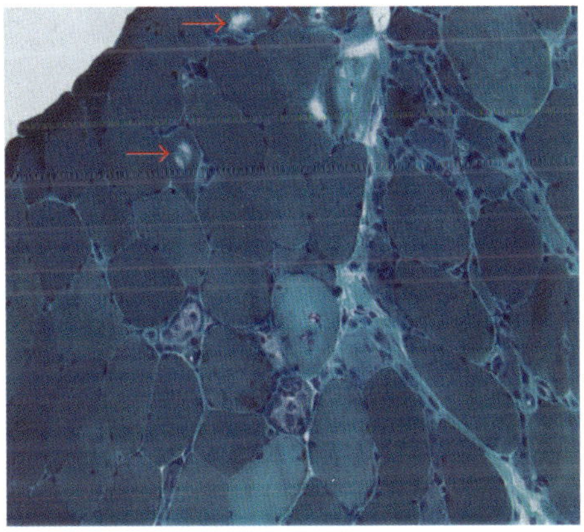

Figure 4: Gomori Trichrome stain of quadriceps muscle biopsy showing "rimmed vacuole" (red arrows) in a center of the myofiber, a classic feature of IBM.

Over the next three months after her diagnosis, her condition deteriorated. She presented to our clinic with progressive dysphagia associated with generalized muscle weakness as she was not able to rise up from sitting position and that impaired her activities of daily living. Her musculoskeletal exam revealed a normal hand grip bilaterally, right psoas strength 4/5, left psoas strength 4−/5, and bilateral deltoid strength 4/5. Her labs revealed an elevated troponin T and total creatine phosphokinase (CPK) of 11200 units/L, so she was readmitted to the hospital for further evaluation of possible sarcoid myopathy with cardiac involvement. Cardiac magnetic resonance image (CMR) revealed no myocardial enhancement to suggest an infiltrative myocardial disease. A quadriceps muscle biopsy was performed and histopathology showed basophilic atrophic nonnecrotic myofibers in clusters with rare rimmed vacuoles, enlarged reactive myonuclei, with endomysial and perivascular infiltrates of chronic inflammatory cells (Figures 3 and 4). Immunohistochemical staining revealed widespread increased sarcolemmal and sarcoplasmic staining for MHC class I antigen and strong staining of rare necrotic myofibers for MAC C5b-9. The thioflavin-S stain and the Mendell modification of the Congo red stain for amyloid were positive for fluorescently stained sarcoplasmic inclusions. A histopathologic picture is consistent with inclusion body myositis.

The dysphagia was further evaluated with videofluoroscopic swallowing study which revealed delayed and effortful swallow initiation, weak pharyngeal contraction, multiple swallows per bolus, and penetration and aspiration across barium consistencies given. Aspiration was both subepiglottic and transarytenoidal and occurred during the swallow as well as after swallow from pharyngeal residue, the patient was deemed at extremely high risk for aspiration, and a percutaneous endoscopic gastrostomy (PEG) tube was inserted.

The patient was started on methylprednisone 40 mg IV q12 hours and she was discharged from the hospital on taper dose of prednisone. During her two-week follow-up visit with her primary care physician as well as rheumatologist, her symptoms improved slightly, and her musculoskeletal exam revealed a right hand grip 3+/5, left hand grip 4+/5, right psoas 4−/5, left psoas 3+/5, and bilateral deltoid 4/5. She was started on methotrexate with a maintenance dose of prednisone. She was also evaluated by physical and occupational therapy with outpatient follow-up and home health care services.

3. Discussion

Sarcoidosis is a systemic granulomatous disease of unknown etiology, characterized by the formation of noncaseating granulomas. Musculoskeletal system involvement can be in the form of arthropathy, myopathy, bone lesions, and/or osteoporosis [2]. Symptomatic muscle disease is a rare manifestation of sarcoidosis, with three recognizable clinical patterns been described: insidious onset of proximal muscle weakness (the most common), acute myopathy with weakness and elevated muscle enzymes, and nodular myopathy (the least common) [3]. Although sarcoid myopathy in patients already diagnosed with sarcoidosis should be suspected among those with the insidious development of progressive proximal muscle weakness and abnormal laboratory findings, treating physicians should keep high index of suspicion for other etiologic causes of myopathy including and not limited to drug induced myopathy, granulomatosis with polyangiitis (Wegener's), polymyositis, dermatomyositis, and idiopathic inflammatory myopathy [4].

Inclusion body myositis (IBM) is a rare sporadic idiopathic inflammatory myopathy with a prevalence around 5–9 cases per million adults. The mean age of symptoms onset is 60 years old with male predominance [5, 6]. Several proposed diagnostic criteria for IBM have been published with the European Neuromuscular Centre (ENMC) 2013 criteria and a relatively new, simple, and clinically useful set of criteria has been proposed that has high sensitivity and specificity and it includes finger flexor or quadriceps weakness, endomysial inflammation, and invasion of nonnecrotic muscle fibers or rimmed vacuoles [7]. Given the relatively resistant nature of inclusion body myositis (IBM) to standard immunosuppressive therapy and the infrequent improvement in muscle strength most experts consider the goal of therapy to be prevention of further deterioration rather than improvement in strength [8, 9]. The prognosis of IBM is relatively poor as by 15 years most patients require assistance with basic daily activities, and some become wheelchair-bound or bedridden [10].

Although there is no apparent pathophysiological link; an association between sarcoid and inclusion body myositis was reported in 1986. However, very few cases have been reported thereafter [11–15]. The immunopathology of both diseases involves T-helper cells- (Th1-) mediated immunity [16], and some evidence suggests that muscle involvement in sarcoid may lead to the development of inclusion body myositis although a detailed understanding of the relationship between these two diseases is not yet fully known. It is important for the treating physicians to keep high index of suspicion for other etiologic causes of myopathy in patients who present with an unusual course of sarcoidosis or an uncommon pattern of muscle weakness, and a muscle biopsy should be considered as soon as possible if there is minimal response to the initial treatment of the disease.

4. Conclusion

Inclusion body myositis (IBM) is a rare sporadic idiopathic inflammatory myopathy. The association of IBM with sarcoidosis has been reported in very few cases. We are reporting this case as more research is needed to further elaborate on previously proposed theories of sarcoidosis being a trigger that possibly promotes the development of inclusion body myositis, leading to a very poor prognosis and/or inclusion body myositis (IBM) representing a common phenotypic endpoint of muscular sarcoidosis.

Acknowledgments

The authors would like to express their deepest appreciation to Dr. Juanita Evans and Dr. Steven Chin for their valuable expertise in providing and reading the histopathology slides.

References

[1] F. Fayad, F. Lioté, F. Berenbaum, P. Orcel, and T. Bardin, "Muscle involvement in sarcoidosis: a retrospective and followup studies," *Journal of Rheumatology*, vol. 33, no. 1, pp. 98–103, 2006.

[2] A. Abril and M. D. Cohen, "Rheumatologic manifestations of sarcoidosis," *Current Opinion in Rheumatology*, vol. 16, no. 1, pp. 51–55, 2004.

[3] A. Mathur and J. M. Kremer, "Immunopathology, musculoskeletal features, and treatment of sarcoidosis," *Current Opinion in Rheumatology*, vol. 5, no. 1, pp. 90–94, 1993.

[4] N. J. Simmonds and B. I. Hoffbrand, "Contracturing granulomatous myositis: a separate entity," *Journal of Neurology, Neurosurgery and Psychiatry*, vol. 53, no. 11, pp. 998–1000, 1990.

[5] M. Needham, A. Corbett, T. Day, F. Christiansen, V. Fabian, and F. L. Mastaglia, "Prevalence of sporadic inclusion body myositis and factors contributing to delayed diagnosis," *Journal of Clinical Neuroscience*, vol. 15, no. 12, pp. 1350–1353, 2008.

[6] M. M. Dimachkie and R. J. Barohn, "Inclusion body myositis," *Neurologic Clinics*, vol. 32, no. 3, pp. 629–646, 2014.

[7] T. E. Lloyd, A. L. Mammen, A. A. Amato, M. D. Weiss, M. Needham, and S. A. Greenberg, "Evaluation and construction of diagnostic criteria for inclusion body myositis," *Neurology*, vol. 83, no. 5, pp. 426–433, 2014.

[8] R. C. Griggs, "The current status of treatment for inclusion-body myositis," *Neurology*, vol. 66, no. 2, pp. S30–S32, 2006.

[9] R. L. Wortmann, "The dilemma of treating patients with inclusion body myositis," *Journal of Rheumatology*, vol. 19, no. 9, pp. 1327–1329, 1992.

[10] O. Benveniste, M. Guiguet, J. Freebody et al., "Long-term observational study of sporadic inclusion body myositis," *Brain*, vol. 134, no. 11, pp. 3176–3184, 2011.

[11] O. Sanmaneechai, A. Swenson, A. K. Gerke, S. A. Moore, and M. E. Shy, "Inclusion body myositis and sarcoid myopathy: coincidental occurrence or associated diseases," *Neuromuscular Disorders*, vol. 25, no. 4, pp. 297–300, 2015.

[12] S. Bouillot, M. Coquet, and X. Ferrer et al., "Inclusion body myositis associated with sacroidosis: a report of 3 cases," *Annales de Pathologie*, vol. 21, pp. 334–336, 2001.

[13] M. J. Danon, O. H. Perurena, S. Ronan, and J. R. Manaligod, "Inclusion body myositis associated with systemic sarcoidosis," *Canadian Journal of Neurological Sciences*, vol. 13, no. 4, pp. 334–336, 1986.

[14] S. Larue, T. Maisonobe, O. Benveniste et al., "Distal muscle involvement in granulomatous myositis can mimic inclusion body myositis," *Journal of Neurology, Neurosurgery and Psychiatry*, vol. 82, no. 6, pp. 674–677, 2011.

[15] G. Vattemi, P. Tonin, M. Marini et al., "Sarcoidosis and inclusion body myositis," *Rheumatology*, vol. 47, no. 9, pp. 1433–1435, 2008.

[16] B. De Paepe, K. De Keyzer, J.-J. Martin, and J. L. De Bleecker, "Alpha-chemokine receptors CXCR1-3 and their ligands in idiopathic inflammatory myopathies," *Acta Neuropathologica*, vol. 109, no. 6, pp. 576–582, 2005.

50

An Unusual Case of Systemic Lupus Erythematosus and Hemophagocytic Syndrome

Saika Sharmeen[1,2] and Nazia Hussain[2,3]

[1]*Department of Medicine, St. Luke's-Roosevelt Hospital Center, New York, NY 10025, USA*
[2]*Department of Medicine, Icahn School of Medicine at Mount Sinai, New York, NY 10025, USA*
[3]*Division of Rheumatology, Department of Medicine, St. Luke's-Roosevelt Hospital Center, New York, NY 10025, USA*

Correspondence should be addressed to Saika Sharmeen; ssharmeen@chpnet.org

Academic Editor: Shoichiro Ikuyama

Hemophagocytic syndrome (HS) or hemophagocytic lymphohistiocytosis (HLH) is an immune mediated phenomenon that can occur in the setting of an autoimmune disease, chronic immunosuppression, malignancy, or infection. It has been more commonly described in the pediatric population and less commonly in adults. We describe a case of a 52-year-old male who presented with a rash. He simultaneously met the Systemic Lupus International Collaborating Clinics (SLICC) criteria for the diagnosis of systemic lupus erythematosus (SLE) and the diagnostic criteria of HS as described in the hemophagocytic lymphohistiocytosis (HLH) 2004 trial. The bone marrow on autopsy showed the presence of abundant hemosiderophages with focal hemophagocytosis. SLE-associated HS might be underdiagnosed due to the overlap in clinical findings. This case represents the importance of prompt diagnosis and treatment of such a potentially fatal clinical syndrome.

1. Introduction

Systemic lupus erythematosus (SLE) is one of the collagen vascular diseases which may induce hemophagocytic syndrome (HS). The etiology of HS is essentially unknown but is thought to result from uncontrolled T lymphocyte activation that leads to macrophage activation and an increment of some cytokines such as tumor necrosis factor-α, interleukin-1 (IL-1), IL-6, IL-18, and interferon-γ [1]. Morphologically benign hemophagocytic histiocytes infiltrate the bone marrow and various organs, including the lymph nodes, liver, and spleen. Patients usually present with an acute febrile illness, which can sometimes become fulminant and lethal. Common manifestations include high fever, pancytopenia, hepatosplenomegaly, elevated liver enzymes, and high blood triglyceride and ferritin levels. Coagulopathy and central nervous system dysfunction often ensue, and less frequently the lungs and cardiac tissues are involved [2]. SLE in conjunction with HS is a rare presentation that has mainly been described in case reports and retrospective studies. It is a rare presentation in male patients and even more difficult to diagnose in a patient with history of alcohol abuse or cirrhosis where coagulopathy, elevated liver enzymes, and hepatosplenomegaly may also be expected. We demonstrate this difficulty in this case report of an African American male with history of alcohol abuse found to have SLE and HS. To our knowledge such a case in this demographic has never been reported.

2. Case

A 52-year-old African American male with past medical history only significant for alcohol abuse presented with four days of a pruritic rash. He was in his usual state of health until four days prior to admission when he noticed the rash. He could not remember if he first noticed it on his chest, abdomen, or legs. Over the next two days, it became more pruritic. He denied any shortness of breath or tongue swelling, as well as any constitutional symptoms including subjective fevers, night sweats, chills, or weight loss. He admitted to not seeing a primary care doctor in two years. He also denied any gait disturbance, gastrointestinal complaints, or urinary complaints but noted that his urine has been darker than usual. He endorsed daily alcohol use of about two to three beers daily but denied smoking or illicit drug use. He worked for the state and was working as of one day prior to admission. He admitted to recent travel in the northeast region. He denied taking any over-the-counter drugs or herbal medications.

Vitals at presentation were as follows: temp 98.9 degrees Fahrenheit, RR 16/min, HR 113–117/min, and BP 160/80 mmHg, saturating 100% on room air. On physical exam, skin exam was significant for nonblanching purpura on anterior calf bilaterally, pruritic nonblanching macules, and papules on chest, back, arms, abdomen, and petechial rash on his palms and soles bilaterally. The rash spared the groin area. Oral, ocular, and genital mucosa was clear. There was no skin tenderness. There was mild mucosal bleeding on lower lip. His eye exam showed scleral icterus. He also had lymphadenopathy on neck exam. He denied ever having a similar rash. On abdominal exam, he was found to have hepatosplenomegaly, with abdominal distention, and normoactive bowel sounds. There was no fluid shift. There was moderate pitting edema bilaterally but no clubbing or cyanosis. Neurologic exam was unremarkable at presentation.

Labs on presentation (Table 1) were significant for thrombocytopenia, hyponatremia, bilirubinemia, leukocytosis with left shift, normocytic anemia, and coagulopathy with elevated INR. His urine toxicology was negative. Urinalysis showed protein, moderate bilirubin, more than 182 RBC, 13 WBC, and trace leukocyte esterase. Urine sediment showed many RBCs with less than 50% dysmorphic cells but no obvious casts.

EKG showed sinus tachycardia 105 bpm, with left axis deviation. Chest X-ray was unremarkable. Computed tomography (CT) of abdomen and pelvis with contrast showed multiple hypodense hypovascular lesions scattered throughout the liver causing surface contour deformity with numerous subcentimeter periportal, periaortic splenic, and periesophageal lymph nodes. Spleen was notable for linear as well as rounded ill-defined hypodensities suggestive of splenic infarcts, abscess, or malignancy. The initial differential was broad including infectious etiology causing sepsis, or malignancy. Given the appearance of the rash as well as history of travel to northeast, the patient was started on doxycycline for suspicion of Rocky Mountain Spotted Fever and supportive management for his remaining findings.

Over the next few days of his hospital course he developed acute mental status change with CT head without contrast showing nonspecific left parietal/temporal scalp soft tissue swelling and no other pathologies. On hospital day 2 he was transferred to the medicine intensive care unit (ICU) for being febrile with T 101 degrees Fahrenheit, renal failure, hepatic dysfunction, and worsening coagulopathy. CT chest without contrast showed focal areas of ground glass attenuation right greater than left. These findings may represent in this clinical setting pulmonary hemorrhage as well as bilateral pleural effusions. All blood cultures, urine cultures, and all infectious workup were negative (Table 3). In the ICU he had a cardiac arrest requiring cardiac resuscitation and

Table 1: Lab values on presentation.

Variable	Lab values on admission	Reference range
Sodium	118	136–146 mmol/L
Potassium	4.9	3.5–5.1 mmol/L
Chloride	87	96–107 mmol/L
Carbon dioxide	23	22–30 mmol/L
Blood urea nitrogen	10	8–24 mmol/dL
Creatinine	0.89	0.66–1.25 mg/dL
Glucose	101	74–106 mg/dL
eGFR	90	>90
Calcium	7.7	8.4–10.3 mg/dL
Corrected calcium*	8.7	8.5–10.5 mg/dL
Protein, total	8.7	6.3–8.2 g/dL
Albumin	2.7	3.5–5 g/dL
Bilirubin, total	4.8	0.2–1.3 mg/dL
Bilirubin, direct	3.5	0.0–0.4 mg/dL
ALP	187	38–126 U/L
AST	366	15–46 U/L
ALT	66	13–69 U/L
WBC	14.3	3.4–11 k/μL
Hemoglobin	8.3	13.0–17 g/dL
Hct	27.7	38–51%
Platelet	72	150–450 k/μL
MCV	90.7	80–100 fL
Band	23	
Eosinophils (%)	2	0.0–0.6%
Neutrophil (%)	70	40–74%
Lymphocytes (%)	3	18–44%
Monocytes (%)	2	4.7–12.0%
Basophil (%)	0	0.1–1.4%
Partial thromboplastin time	51.3	22.5–35.5 secs
INR	3	0.9–1.1
PT	30.8	11.8–14.3 secs

*The normal albumin level defaults to 4 mg/dL standard units.

intubation, with return of spontaneous circulation. His hospital course was complicated with persistent fevers, gastrointestinal bleeding, acute kidney injury requiring hemodialysis, hypotension requiring pressor, and eventual acute respiratory distress syndrome with worsening liver failure. Later the lab results showed elevated ferritin level and LDH (Table 2). His rheumatologic workup (Table 3) revealed high titers of antidouble stranded DNA with low complement (C3/C4). Antinuclear antibody (ANA) was positive, antihistone antibodies (ab) negative, anti-Smith ab negative, antiribosomal P ab negative, antismooth muscle ab negative, and cardiolipin IgG/IgM moderately elevated. The patient was initially treated with broad spectrum antibiotics, despite negative cultures and infectious workup.

He received supportive management with packed red blood cell transfusion, fresh frozen plasma (FFP), and

Table 2: Additional labs.

Variable	Measurement	Reference range
DAT broad spectrum Coombs Ser (Direct Coombs)	Negative	Negative
GGT	100	12–58 U/L
Tryptase	4	2–10 ng/mL
Lipase	22	23–300 U/L
Uric acid	7.1	3.5–8.5 mg/dL
Lactic acid	7.4	0.7–2.1 mmol/L
Ammonia	42	9–30 μmol/L
Cryoglobulin	Negative	Negative
Creatine kinase	920	55–170 U/L
CRP, high sensitivity	10.4	Null
Sedimentation rate	100	0–13 mm/hr
LDH	2387	313–618 U/L
ADAMTS13 Activity	84	68–163% activity
G6PD	Adequate	Adequate
Haptoglobin, quant	22	30–200 mg/dL
Ferritin	700.7	22.0–322.0 ng/mL
Iron	41	49–181 μg/dL
Iron binding capacity, total (TIBC)	265	261–462 μg/dL
Thyroid stim. hormone	1	0.55–4.78 mIU/mL
Cortisol AM	16.54	4.0–22.0 μg/dL
Factor XI assay	66	50–150%
Factor X assay	66	50–150%
Factor II activity	64	70–150%
Factor VIII assay	279	50–150%
Factor VII assay	16	50–150%
Factor V assay	49	50–150%
Fibrinogen	123	225–483 mg/dL
D-dimer	13.29	<0.5 μg/mL

platelets. He was also treated with pulse dose steroids for 3 days and then intravenous (IV) Medrol 40 mg + 30 mg daily. He also received plasmapheresis followed by IV Cytoxan with mild initial improvement, but unfortunately his condition deteriorated and the patient passed away. The autopsy revealed marked diffuse intra-alveolar hemorrhage, pulmonary edema, cirrhotic liver with cholestasis, acute tubular necrosis, chronic pancreatitis, infarcted spleen, and evidence of esophageal varices in a patient with known chronic alcoholism. The bone marrow showed the presence of abundant hemosiderophages with focal hemophagocytosis, which added to the presence of fever, splenomegaly, skin rash, cytopenia, and increased ferritin which met the criteria for hemophagocytic lymphohistiocytosis.

3. Discussion

Our patient met 4 out of 17 (including at least one clinical criterion and one immunologic criterion) of the Systemic Lupus International Collaborating Clinics (SLICC) criteria

Table 3: Autoimmune and infectious workup.

Variable	Measurement	Reference range
ANA	Positive	Negative
ANA, quantitative	1:160	Negative
ANA, pattern	Speckled	Negative
ds DNA ab IgG Titer	300 or greater	0–29 IU/ML
C3	23	90–180 mg/dL
C4	3	10–40 mg/dL
Anti-Smith (Sm) interp.	Negative	Negative
SM-RNP antibodies interp.	Negative	Negative
SM-RNP ab interp.	Negative	Negative
Smith (ENA) ab, IgG	0.8	<16.00 EU/mL
SSA (Sjogren ab)	0.7	<16.00 EU/mL
SSB (Sjogren ab)	1	<16.00 EU/mL
Ribosomal P ab	<1.0	Negative
Smooth muscle ab	Negative	Negative
LKM 1 ab IgG	<20.0 U	Negative
GBM ab IgG	<1.0	<1.0 AI no antibody detected
Histone ab	1.2	<1.0 U negative
Cardiolipin ab IgM	24	Low to medium positive
Cardiolipin ab IgG	20	Indeterminate
β2-Glycoprotein I IgM	Negative	Negative
β2-Glycoprotein I IgA	9	Negative
ANCA vasculitides		
Proteinase 3 ab	<1.0	<1.0
Myeloperoxidase ab	<1.0	<1.0
Hep A ab, IgM	Nonreactive	Nonreactive
Hep A ab, total	Nonreactive	Nonreactive
Hep B sAg	Negative	Negative
Hep B Core ab, total	Reactive	Nonreactive
Hep BS ab	Reactive	Nonreactive
Hep C ab	Negative	Negative
HIV 1/2 ab screen, rapid	Nonreactive	Nonreactive
Cytomegalovirus, IgM	0.7	<0.9
Cytomegalovirus, Igg	Negative	Negative
EBV, DNA, QN, and PR-PCR	<200 COPIES/ML	Negative
Syphilis Screen Titer	Nonreactive	Nonreactive
Lyme Disease ab Screen	0.58	<0.91
RMSF IgM and IgG	Not detected	Not detected
B. Quintana IgM Scr	Negative	Negative
B. Quintana IgG Scr	Negative	Negative
B. Henselae ab IgG	Negative	Negative
Brucella IgG	0.16	<0.80 antibody not detected
Brucella IgM	0.07	<0.80 antibody not detected

TABLE 3: Continued.

Variable	Measurement	Reference range
AFB culture	Negative	Negative
Fungal culture	Negative	Negative
Viral culture	No virus isolated after 4 days	Negative
Gram stain	Few 2+ PMN no organisms	Negative
Bacterial culture	No growth	Negative

for the diagnosis of SLE [3]. Our patient's findings included thrombocytopenia and hemolytic anemia as two clinical criteria and positive anti-dsDNA ab and low complement (C3/C4) as immunologic criteria. Our patient also met the diagnostic criteria for HS as described in the hemophagocytic lymphohistiocytosis (HLH) 2004 trial.

He had a fever of 38.5°C for 7 days or more, splenomegaly, hemoglobin of 9 g/dL or less, platelets less than 100, hyperferritinemia, and hemophagocytosis in bone marrow [4]. Lambotte et al. described 8 cases where SLE was diagnosed simultaneously with HS pancytopenia with high ferritin level, uncommon in SLE, which is highly suggestive of HS [5]. Parodi et al. proposed preliminary diagnostic criteria for macrophage activation syndrome as a complication of juvenile SLE. The diagnostic criteria have a sensitivity and specificity of 92.1% and 90.9%, respectively, and an OR of 116.7% with a confidence interval between 21.9 and 621.6 at 95% confidence [6]. According to the diagnostic criteria proposed by Parodi et al., our patient met all clinical criteria including fever (>38°C), hepatomegaly (≥3 cm below the rib margin), splenomegaly (≥3 cm below the rib margin), hemorrhagic manifestations (purpura, easy bruising, or bleeding gums), and dysfunction of the central nervous system (irritability, disorientation, lethargy, headache, convulsions, or coma). He also met most of the laboratory criteria including cytopenia in 2 or more cell lines [4 leukocytes × 109/L, hemoglobin 90 g/L, or platelets 150 × 109, increased aspartate aminotransferase (>40 units/L), increased lactate dehydrogenase (>567 units/L), hypofibrinogenemia (fibrinogen <1.5 g/L), and hyperferritinemia (ferritin >500 μg/L)]. The histopathologic criteria were also met by evidence of hemophagocytic macrophages in bone marrow. For diagnosis, the simultaneous presence of at least one clinical criterion and at least 2 laboratory criteria is required.

HIV, cytomegalovirus, and Epstein-Barr virus are among the reported viral causes of HS [7, 8]. Although infections are a possible trigger for HS, our patient had an extensive infectious workup which was all shown to be negative (Table 2). Unfortunately, liver biopsy could not be done due to the coagulopathy. In addition, his disease continued to progress despite broad spectrum antibiotics and supportive treatment. His mild clinical improvement after pulse steroids and IV Cytoxan was in favor of the trigger for HS being autoimmune in etiology. This patient also received plasmapheresis without improvement. The presence of chronic alcoholism causing cirrhosis further complicated the diagnosis.

The current literature suggests that the goal of therapy for patients with HLH is to suppress life-threatening inflammation by destroying immune cells. The first treatment protocol for HLH (HLH-94) consists of induction therapy with weekly treatments of dexamethasone and etoposide (VP-16), followed by cyclosporine. Intrathecal methotrexate is given to those with central nervous system disease. After induction, patients who are recovering are weaned off therapy, while those who are not improving are continued on therapy as a bridge to allogeneic hematopoietic cell transplantation [9]. The newer HLH protocol initiated in 2004 (HLH-2004) differs from HLH-94 by earlier use of cyclosporine during the induction phase of treatment and adds hydrocortisone to intrathecal methotrexate. Treatment of secondary HLH is directed at control of the underlying condition. If unsuccessful, cytotoxic agents such as those in HLH-2004, steroids, intravenous γ-globulin, or targeted immune therapy have been used [10]. Steroids and other immunosuppressants including Rituximab have also been reported in successfully treating HS in the setting of SLE [11, 12]. Wong et al. reported an incidence of SLE-associated HS of 6 cases during a 3.5-year period among 250 SLE patients. They alluded to the fact that SLE-associated HS might be underdiagnosed due to the overlap in clinical findings [13]. Moreover, this case was even more difficult to diagnose because many of the findings that would be expected in a patient with alcoholic cirrhosis were also present in this patient.

4. Conclusion

In conclusion, a prompt diagnosis is essential for treating HS in the setting of SLE. Clinicians should raise a high index of suspicion in such a case.

References

[1] J. I. Henter, A. C. Horne, M. Arico, M. Egeler, A. H. Filipovich, and S. Imashuku, *Histiocyte Society Review HLH-2004: Diagnostic and Therapeutic Guidelines for Hemophagocytic Lymphohistiocytosis*, Wiley-Liss, Stockholm, Sweden, 2006.

[2] S. Fukaya, S. Yasuda, T. Hashimoto et al., "Clinical features of haemophagocytic syndrome in patients with systemic autoimmune diseases: analysis of 30 cases," *Rheumatology*, vol. 47, no. 11, pp. 1686–1691, 2008.

[3] M. Petri, A. M. Orbai, G. S. Alarcón et al., "Derivation and validation of the Systemic Lupus International Collaborating Clinics classification criteria for systemic lupus erythematosus," *Arthritis & Rheumatism*, vol. 64, no. 8, pp. 2677–2686, 2012.

[4] M. B. Jordan, C. E. Allen, S. Weitzman, A. H. Filipovich, and K. L. McClain, "How I treat hemophagocytic lymphohistiocytosis," *Blood*, vol. 118, no. 15, pp. 4041–4052, 2011.

[5] O. Lambotte, M. Khellaf, H. Harmouche et al., "Characteristics and long-term outcome of 15 episodes of systemic

lupus erythematosus-associated hemophagocytic syndrome," *Medicine*, vol. 85, no. 3, pp. 169–182, 2006.

[6] A. Parodi, S. Davì, A. B. Pringe et al., "Macrophage activation syndrome in juvenile systemic lupus erythematosus: a multinational multicenter study of thirty-eight patients," *Arthritis and Rheumatism*, vol. 60, no. 11, pp. 3388–3399, 2009.

[7] K. McClain, R. Gehrz, H. Grierson, D. Purtilo, and A. Filipovich, "Virus-associated histiocytic proliferations in children. Frequent association with Epstein-Barr virus and congenital or acquired immunodeficiencies," *The American Journal of Pediatric Hematology/Oncology*, vol. 10, no. 3, pp. 196–205, 1988.

[8] T.-L. Chen, W.-W. Wong, and T.-J. Chiou, "Hemophagocytic syndrome: an unusual manifestation of acute human immunodeficiency virus infection," *International Journal of Hematology*, vol. 78, no. 5, pp. 450–452, 2003.

[9] J.-I. Henter, A. Samuelsson-Horne, M. Aricò et al., "Treatment of hemophagocytic lymphohistiocytosis with HLH-94 immunochemotherapy and bone marrow transplantation," *Blood*, vol. 100, no. 7, pp. 2367–2373, 2002.

[10] M. P. Keith, C. Pitchford, and W. B. Bernstein, "Treatment of hemophagocytic lymphohistiocytosis with alemtuzumab in systemic lupus erythematosus," *Journal of Clinical Rheumatology*, vol. 18, no. 3, pp. 134–137, 2012.

[11] M. W. So, B. S. Koo, Y. J. Kim, Y.-G. Kim, C.-K. Lee, and B. Yoo, "Successful rituximab treatment of refractory hemophagocytic lymphohistiocytosis and autoimmune hemolytic anemia associated with systemic lupus erythematosus," *Modern Rheumatology*, vol. 24, no. 5, pp. 855–857, 2014.

[12] S. Kumakura and Y. Murakawa, "Clinical characteristics and treatment outcomes of autoimmune-associated hemophagocytic syndrome in adults," *Arthritis & Rheumatology*, vol. 66, no. 8, pp. 2297–2307, 2014.

[13] K.-F. Wong, P.-K. Hui, J. K. C. Chan, Y.-W. Chan, and S.-Y. Ha, "The acute lupus hemophagocytic syndrome," *Annals of Internal Medicine*, vol. 114, no. 5, pp. 387–390, 1991.

51

Pulmonary Sarcoidosis following Etanercept Treatment for Ankylosing Spondylitis

A. Majjad,[1] A. Bezza,[1] A. Biyi,[2] M. R. El Ochi,[3] and A. El Maghraoui[1]

[1]*Rheumatology Department, Mohammed V Military Academic Hospital, Faculty of Medicine and Pharmacy, Mohammed V University, Rabat, Morocco*
[2]*Nuclear Medicine Department, Mohammed V Military Academic Hospital, Faculty of Medicine and Pharmacy, Mohammed V University, Rabat, Morocco*
[3]*Anatomic Pathology Department, Mohammed V Military Academic Hospital, Faculty of Medicine and Pharmacy, Mohammed V University, Rabat, Morocco*

Correspondence should be addressed to A. Majjad; drmajjad@gmail.com

Academic Editor: Tsai-Ching Hsu

Antitumor necrosis factor therapies have revolutionized the treatment of some inflammatory diseases. However, the use of these agents is associated with the development of many paradoxical autoimmune diseases. Less well-recognized is the association with sarcoidosis. We report a 55-year-old female with long-standing ankylosing spondylitis who developed persistent dry cough and dyspnea while receiving etanercept therapy. High-resolution computed tomography scanning showed mediastinal lymphadenopathy and multiple nodules in both lung fields developed two months after the administration of etanercept. Lymph node biopsy was not practicable. Histopathological examination of minor salivary gland biopsy revealed noncaseating granulomata, and the serum angiotensin-converting enzyme was very elevated. All infectious studies were negative. Etanercept was discontinued plus a course of corticosteroids with a clinical improvement, and a follow-up high-resolution computed tomography scanning 4 months later showed evident regression of mediastinal lymph nodes and pulmonary nodules. Potential pathogenic mechanisms of this paradoxical effect of tumor necrosis factor-alpha blocking agents are discussed.

1. Background

Sarcoidosis is a rare granulomatous disease mainly affecting the lungs and lymph nodes. Its etiology remains unknown [1]. However, there are a small number of literatures possible that involve tumor necrosis factor-alpha blocking agents (anti-TNF-α), especially etanercept, in the development of pulmonary sarcoidosis [2]. Our case report supports possible relationship between etanercept therapy and the development of sarcoid-like granulomatosis.

2. Case Report

A 66-year-old female patient without medical history or professional exposures was diagnosed with ankylosing spondylitis 12 years ago. She had formerly responded to nonsteroidal inflammatory drugs. In 2006, she started treatment with infliximab, due to poor therapeutic response to various NSAIDs. After eight years of remission, the patient had repeated flares of ankylosing spondylitis symptoms with increased inflammatory back pain. In August 2015, due to persistent clinical activity with increased acute-phase reactant levels (C-reactive protein level of 16 mg/l), the treatment with etanercept at 25 mg twice weekly was started. Following national guidelines to exclude latent tuberculosis, mycobacterium tuberculosis research in sputum and interferon-gamma test were negative and a chest radiograph was normal. Two months after etanercept therapy onset, the patient developed persistent dry cough and dyspnea without fever or night

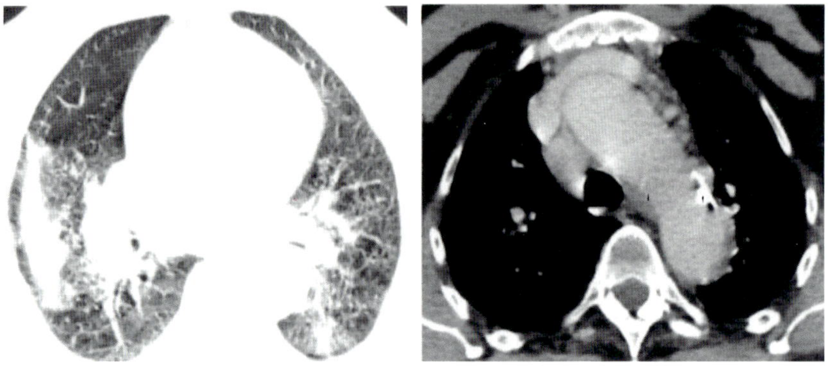

Figure 1

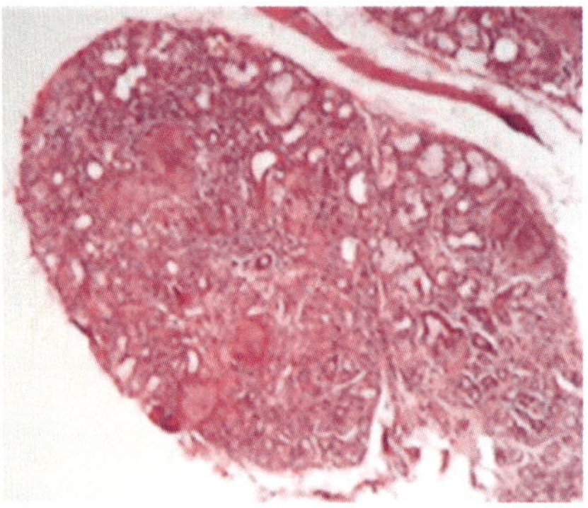

Figure 2

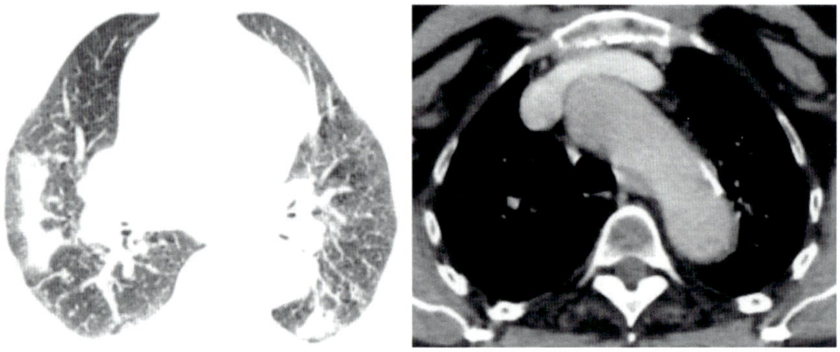

Figure 3

sweating. Physical examination was unremarkable apart from tachypnea and severe spinal stiffness. High-resolution computed tomography (HRCT) scanning showed mediastinal lymphadenopathy and multiple nodules in both lung fields (Figure 1). Echocardiography was normal. The blood analysis demonstrated ESR 35 mm/h, CRP 14 mg/l, and normal renal and hepatic function tests. Sputum culture and polymerase chain reaction and interferon-gamma release assays were negative. Viral serology (human immunodeficiency virus, hepatitis B virus, and hepatitis C virus) and syphilis serology were negative. Serum angiotensin-converting enzyme was very elevated at 147 UI/ml (reference range 8–52 UI/ml). Calcemia and calciuria tests were normal. The pulmonary function test showed restrictive ventilatory alteration. It was not possible to perform neither bronchoscopy nor thoracoscopy because of respiratory failure and severe ankylosis of the cervical spine. Histopathological examination of minor salivary gland biopsy revealed a chronic granulomatous sialadenitis without caseous necrosis (Figure 2). Diseases showing similar histologic changes were excluded, and a diagnosis of sarcoidosis was made. Etanercept was discontinued plus a course of corticosteroids with 40 mg/day of prednisone for two months. An evident improvement of cough and dyspnea was seen. Follow-up HRCT 4 months later showed regression of mediastinal lymph nodes and pulmonary nodules (Figure 3).

3. Discussion

Sarcoidosis is a multisystem disorder characterized by the accumulation of lymphocytes, mononuclear phagocytes, and noncaseating granulomas in involved tissues. Etiology of sarcoidosis is still not identified. The role of viral, bacterial, and parasitic infections is not clearly determined. The role of some drugs and environmental exposure are still considered [3]. Due to unknown causes, active macrophages and lymphocytes are accumulated in this or that organ and produce increased number of interleukins, TNF-α. The TNF-α is the key cytokine that participates in the formation of granulomas in sarcoidosis [3, 4].

At present, there are five anti-TNF-α agents currently available: four monoclonal antibodies (infliximab, adalimumab, golimumab, and certolizumab) and a soluble TNF-α receptor fusion protein (etanercept) [5]. Anti-TNF-α agents, especially infliximab and sometimes adalimumab, are effective in refractory sarcoidosis [6, 7]. However, there have been a few cases of sarcoidosis occurring during anti-TNF-α therapy. In a recent review of literature published on January 2016, SimJae Kyeom et al. found 59 cases of sarcoidosis occurring during anti-TNF-α therapy in the medical literature. Thirty-seven (61.6%) occurred after etanercept, 13 (21.6%) after adalimumab, and 9 (15%) after infliximab. In this study, twenty-eight had rheumatoid arthritis. The lung and/or lymph node were the most commonly affected organs (64%), followed by the skin (37%) and the eye (15%). Prognosis seems to be favorable since 52 of 59 cases displayed a partial or complete resolution after anti-TNF-α withdrawal with or without steroids [2].

The pathogenesis of sarcoidosis induced by anti-TNF-α remains unclear. However, some potential hypotheses have been proposed. Mainly followed hypothesis is that sarcoidosis is of an infectious origin favored by an immunosuppressant effect of anti-TNF-α, especially with some microorganisms that are implicated in the development of sarcoidosis (*Propionibacterium acnes* and *Propionibacterium granulosum*) [8]. Another hypothesis is that the disease is an immunological disorder, with an imbalance in Th17 lymphocytes and Treg lymphocytes, favoring Th17 and formation of granulomas via the increased expression of IL17 and TNF-α. Currently, there are many reports supporting this latter hypothesis [9–11]. Indeed, more than 60% of the reported cases occurred with etanercept. There are two hypotheses that may explain this greater association: on one hand, the difference in pharmacological proprieties between the synthesized anti-TNF-α receptor and monoclonal antibodies: the antibodies neutralize both soluble and membrane forms of TNF-α, whereas etanercept neutralizes just the soluble form. This partial inhibition permits the redistribution of TNF-α in areas of elevated concentration such as the lungs and lymph nodes [11]. On the other hand, several studies suggest that monoclonal antibodies, in contrast to etanercept, inhibit the expression of IL17 and INF-gamma, cytokines strongly involved in granuloma formation [12]. Taking into account that it is not the only case of sarcoidosis developed with the anti-TNF therapy, the pathogenesis of granulomas under the effect of the therapy needs to be studied. Besides, it is possible that similar complications of anti-TNF therapy may be developed in carriers of HLA-A1, B8, and B13 antigens as it is known that those antigens are met more frequently in sarcoidosis patients compared to the general population [13]. In summary, it is important for clinicians to be aware of this rare complication of anti-TNF therapy. Sarcoidosis granulomas may be formed not only in the intrathoracic lymphatic nodes, lungs, and salivary glands but in other organs too (liver, spleen, eyes, heart, skin, etc.). If the biopsy of the affected organ is difficult, minor salivary gland biopsy may be an excellent alternative and help in diagnosis [11, 13].

4. Conclusion

Pulmonary sarcoidosis is an uncommon effect of anti-TNF therapy. The pathogenic mechanism is unclear. Minor salivary gland biopsy may help in diagnosis. The management requires discontinuing anti-TNF plus a course of steroids.

Consent

Written informed consent was obtained from the patient for publication of this case report.

Acknowledgments

The authors thank the patient and her family.

References

[1] N. Unterstell, A. L. Bressan, L. A. Serpa, and A. C. Gripp, "Systemic sarcoidosis induced by etanercept: first Brazilian case report," *Anais Brasileiros de Dermatologia*, vol. 88, no. 6, pp. 197–199, 2013.

[2] J. K. Sim, S. Y. Lee, J. J. Shim, and K. H. Kang, "Pulmonary sarcoidosis induced by adalimumab: a case report and literature review," *Yonsei Medical Journal*, vol. 57, no. 1, pp. 272-273, 2016.

[3] J. Müller-Quernheim, A. Prasse, and G. Zissel, "Pathogenesis of sarcoidosis," *La Presse Médicale*, vol. 41, no. 6, pp. e275–e287, 2012.

[4] N. W. Lukacs, S. W. Chensue, R. M. Strieter, K. Warmington, and S. L. Kunkel, "Inflammatory granuloma formation is mediated by TNF-alpha-inducible intercellular adhesion molecule-1," *Journal of Immunology*, vol. 152, no. 12, pp. 5883–5889, 1994.

[5] A. Mounach and A. El Maghraoui, "Efficacy and safety of adalimumab in ankylosing spondylitis," *Open Access Rheumatology*, vol. 6, pp. 83–90, 2014.

[6] R. P. Baughman, M. Drent, M. Kavuru et al., "Infliximab therapy in patients with chronic sarcoidosis and pulmonary involvement," *American Journal of Respiratory and Critical Care Medicine*, vol. 174, no. 7, pp. 795–802, 2006.

[7] N. J. Sweiss, I. Noth, M. Mirsaeidi et al., "Efficacy results of a 52-week trial of adalimumab in the treatment of refractory sarcoidosis," *Sarcoidosis, Vasculitis, and Diffuse Lung Diseases*, vol. 31, no. 1, pp. 46–54, 2014.

[8] Y. Eishi, M. Suga, I. Ishige et al., "Quantitative analysis of mycobacterial and propionibacterial DNA in lymph nodes of Japanese and European patients with sarcoidosis," *Journal of Clinical Microbiology*, vol. 40, no. 1, pp. 198–204, 2002.

[9] D. E. Furst, R. Wallis, M. Broder, and D. O. Beenhouwer, "Tumor necrosis factor antagonists: different kinetics and/or mechanisms of action may explain differences in the risk for developing granulomatous infection," *Seminars in Arthritis and Rheumatism*, vol. 36, no. 3, pp. 159–167, 2006.

[10] C. Prior and P. L. Haslam, "Increased levels of serum interferon-gamma in pulmonary sarcoidosis and relationship with response to corticosteroid therapy," *American Review of Respiratory Disease*, vol. 143, no. 1, pp. 53–60, 1991.

[11] C. Vigne, F. Coury, Y. Pacheco, and J. Tebib, "AB0452 sarcoidosis: an underestimated and potentially dramatic side effect of anti-TNF-α," *Annals of the Rheumatic Diseases*, vol. 71, no. 3, p. 663, 2013.

[12] É. Toussirot, "Sarcoïdose induite par les anti-TNFα," Commentaires à propos l'article de Vigne C et al. (Joint Bone Spine 2013; 80: 104–107)," *Revue du Rhumatisme*, vol. 80, no. 6, pp. 631-632, 2013.

[13] K. Bellil, I. Chelly, G. I. Ben et al., "Salivary gland biopsy: experience of La Rabta Hospital's pathology department," *La Tunisie Medicale*, vol. 85, no. 1, pp. 64–66, 2007.

52

Combination Immunosuppressive Therapy Including Rituximab for Epstein-Barr Virus-Associated Hemophagocytic Lymphohistiocytosis in Adult-Onset Still's Disease

Eva Johanna Schäfer,[1] Wolfram Jung,[1] and Peter Korsten[2]

[1]*Department of Hematology and Oncology, University Medical Center Göttingen, Göttingen, Germany*
[2]*Department of Nephrology and Rheumatology, University Medical Center Göttingen, Göttingen, Germany*

Correspondence should be addressed to Peter Korsten; peter.korsten@med.uni-goettingen.de

Academic Editor: Gregory J. Tsay

Hemophagocytic lymphopcytosis (HLH) is a life-threatening condition. It can occur either as primary form with genetic defects or secondary to other conditions, such as hematological or autoimmune diseases. Certain triggering factors can predispose individuals to the development of HLH. We report the case of a 25-year-old male patient who was diagnosed with HLH in the context of adult-onset Still's disease (AOSD) during a primary infection with Epstein-Barr virus (EBV). During therapy with anakinra and dexamethasone, he was still symptomatic with high-spiking fevers, arthralgia, and sore throat. His laboratory values showed high levels of ferritin and C-reactive protein. His condition improved after the addition of rituximab and cyclosporine to his immunosuppressive regimen with prednisolone and anakinra. This combination therapy led to a sustained clinical and serological remission of his condition. While rituximab has been used successfully for HLH in the context of EBV-associated lymphoma, its use in autoimmune diseases is uncommon. We hypothesize that the development of HLH was triggered by a primary EBV infection and that rituximab led to elimination of EBV-infected B-cells, while cyclosporine ameliorated the cytokine excess. We therefore propose that this combination immunosuppressive therapy might be successfully used in HLH occurring in the context of autoimmune diseases.

1. Introduction

Hemophagocytic lymphohistiocytosis (HLH) is a potentially life-threatening condition characterized by excessive macrophage activity and cytokine production resulting in multiorgan failure [1, 2]. Primary HLH occurs in children with HLH-associated genetic defects or a family history of HLH, while secondary HLH develops after exposure to immunological trigger factors of underlying infections, autoimmune diseases, or malignancies [3]. In the setting of rheumatic conditions, HLH is also termed macrophage activation syndrome (MAS) and occurs most frequently in patients with systemic juvenile idiopathic arthritis (sJIA), adult-onset Still's disease (AOSD), and systemic lupus erythematosus (SLE) [4].

2. Case Presentation

We report the case of a 25-year-old man who had been diagnosed with AOSD five years before admission. His condition had been successfully controlled with 100 mg/d of anakinra and 5 mg/d of prednisolone. Previous attempts to reduce his immunosuppressive therapy had failed due to frequent relapses with severe arthritis and episodes of high-spiking fevers. His family history was negative for autoimmune diseases or inherited diseases.

On admission to another hospital, he presented with high fever, sore throat, and arthralgia. Laboratory tests revealed kidney and liver failure and he was transferred to the intensive care unit with suspected sepsis. His prior immunosuppressive treatment with prednisolone and anakinra was stopped and empiric antibiotic therapy was initiated. During the diagnostic process, anemia, thrombocytopenia, highly elevated ferritin levels, C-reactive protein levels, hypertriglyceridemia, hypofibrinogenemia, elevated soluble interleukin- (IL-) 2 receptor, and splenomegaly were detected. A bone marrow biopsy was performed and hemophagocytosis was demonstrated. The clinical picture was compatible with HLH/MAS according to current classification criteria, which have been developed for HLH in the context of sJIA [5]. Chemotherapy with etoposide and dexamethasone according to the HLH-94 protocol [6] was started and the patient was transferred to our hospital in slightly improved condition.

After one week, the patient deteriorated again with high fever, pancytopenia, and high levels of inflammatory markers. Physical examination on admission to our hospital was remarkable for cervical lymphadenopathy and severe tonsillopharyngitis. Computed abdominal tomography revealed hepatosplenomegaly as well as cervical and mesenteric lymphadenopathy. Chemotherapy was stopped because neutropenic fever developed and the patient appeared septic. Second-line empirical antibiotic therapy was started and dexamethasone reduced to 20 mg/d. Microbiological testing revealed a primary Epstein-Barr virus (EBV) infection with positive anti-EBV-VCA-IgM antibodies and viral load of 10^4 copies/mL as determined by polymerase chain reaction.

We initiated treatment with rituximab once a week at a dose of 375 mg/m^2 and achieved virus suppression after three cycles with undetectable copy numbers. Anakinra was reinstituted for AOSD and dexamethasone therapy continued at a dose of 8 mg/d. Blood count normalized and symptoms improved significantly, but quotidian fever and high levels of inflammatory values persisted. Addition of cyclosporine resulted in further clinical improvement of the patient and normalization of abnormal laboratory values. The patient course and the respective treatments are depicted in Figure 1.

3. Discussion

Early diagnosis of HLH in rheumatologic patients is essential to improve survival, because mortality rates ranging from 8% to 60% have been reported in the literature depending on the setting and population studied [7–11]. In general, higher mortality rates have been reported in patients with HLH secondary to underlying hematological malignancies.

The diagnosis of HLH/MAS is often delayed because of possible differential diagnoses. These include conditions that can present with similar clinical presentations and laboratory abnormalities, most importantly sepsis or systemic inflammatory response syndromes. Ferritin levels, however, are usually markedly higher in HLH patients and deemed a highly characteristic feature of HLH by most experts, which led to its recognition as mandatory criterion in the recently developed classification criteria [5]. Nevertheless, it has been argued that fever or ferritin levels can be lower in patients receiving anti-IL-1 (such as canakinumab) or anti-IL-6 therapies (such as tocilizumab) [12, 13]. Other diseases which should be excluded are infectious hepatitis, visceral leishmaniasis, brucellosis, familial hyperlipidemia, and flares of underlying conditions, notably sJIA and SLE [5, 14].

In our patient, infectious hepatitis was excluded by negative serologic testing. Visceral leishmaniasis (also termed kala-azar), which is a protozoan infection transmitted by the bite of the sand fly, can have a similar presentation. The disease is not endemic in Germany and it was very unlikely with a negative travel history of the patient to an endemic area. Brucellosis, a zoonotic disease caused by various species of *Brucella* organisms, is endemic in Germany and can present with a wide array of clinical symptoms similar to those of HLH [15]. Infection can occur by contact to domestic or wild animals including cattle, sheep, goats, or wild boars [15], making occupational exposure the most important risk factor. It has also occurred in laboratory workers exposed during routine analyses [16]. Serologic testing for brucellosis was also negative in our patient.

Recently, the so-called "HScore" has been developed for the diagnosis of reactive HLH [17]. Of note, use of different cut-off values of the HScore might be necessary in patients with underlying rheumatic conditions [18]. EBV-related HLH secondary to hematological malignancies has been successfully treated with rituximab-containing regimens, the rationale being depletion of EBV-infected B-cells [19]. In a recent case report, the use of rituximab in conjunction with chemotherapy according to the HLH-2004 protocol was unsuccessful [20]. The patient in this report also presented with a sepsis-like syndrome and was tested positive for EBV. There was, however, no underlying rheumatic condition.

In our case, on the contrary, the HLH-94 protocol was started and then terminated because of suspected sepsis. A combination immunosuppressive therapy including dexamethasone, anakinra, rituximab, and cyclosporine was necessary to achieve clinical and laboratory remission. We hypothesize that the EBV infection was the trigger for the secondary HLH in our case and led to a severe flare of the underlying AOSD. This sequence of events is probable in our view, because the clinical symptoms during the primary EBV infection (lymphadenopathy and hepatosplenomegaly) were different compared to his previous flares and rapidly disappeared upon virus suppression. By contrast, the high-spiking fevers, arthralgia, and high serological inflammatory activity persisted, which was similar to previous documented flares of his AOSD.

In conclusion, suppression of the triggering factor (EBV infection) was likely achieved with rituximab, but the severe AOSD flare and subsequent cytokine release, which occurred afterwards, required a more T-cell specific immunosuppression (i.e., cyclosporine) to be controlled. A similar approach was recently reported in a young male patient who developed secondary HLH associated with EBV with SLE as underlying autoimmune disorder [21]. We are not aware of any previous reports of rituximab-containing regimens in the treatment of EBV-related HLH in the context of AOSD and therefore propose that this combination therapy might be successfully applied in this population.

Additional Points

(i) Secondary HLH may be triggered by primary viral infections, such as Epstein-Barr virus. (ii) EBV-associated

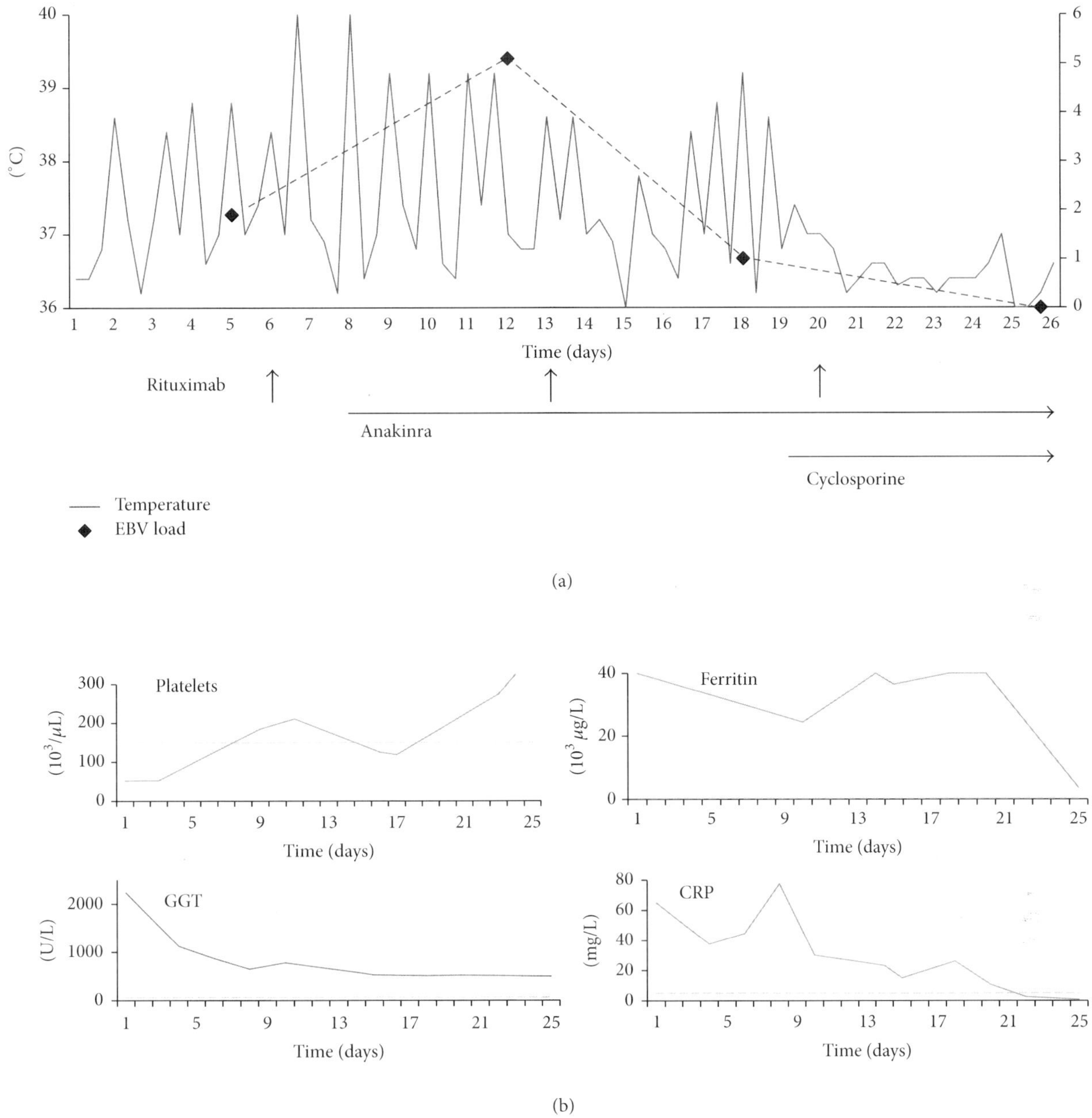

Figure 1: Clinical response in relation to treatment with rituximab, anakinra, and cyclosporine. (a) Fever curve and treatment overview. Body temperature was taken twice a day via an infrared ear thermometer. Rituximab was started on day 6 at a dose of 375 mg/m^2 and repeated once a week indicated by an arrow until virus suppression was achieved after the third infusion. Anakinra was started on day 8 at a dose of 100 mg daily and cyclosporine on day 19 at a dose of 200 mg daily (blood level aiming at 100 μg/L). (b) Correlating laboratory parameters over time. Dotted lines indicate the respective upper reference ranges. CRP: C-reactive protein; EBV: Epstein-Barr virus; GGT: gamma-glutamyltransferase.

HLH in the context of autoimmune diseases may be treated successfully using a combination immunosuppressive therapy including rituximab.

Competing Interests

The authors declare that there are no competing interests regarding the publication of this paper.

Authors' Contributions

Eva Johanna Schäfer and Peter Korsten collected the data and wrote the manuscript. Eva Johanna Schäfer, Wolfram Jung, and Peter Korsten analyzed and interpreted the data and treated the patient. Wolfram Jung revised the manuscript critically. All authors approved the final version of the manuscript for publication.

Acknowledgments

The authors acknowledge the support by the Open Access Publication Funds of the Göttingen University.

References

[1] G. Janka, "Familial and acquired hemophagocytic lymphohistiocytosis," *Annual Review of Medicine*, vol. 63, no. 1, pp. 233–246, 2012.

[2] G. S. Schulert and A. A. Grom, "Pathogenesis of macrophage activation syndrome and potential for cytokine- directed therapies," *Annual Review of Medicine*, vol. 66, no. 1, pp. 145–159, 2015.

[3] B. E. Favara, A. C. Feller, M. Pauli et al., "Contemporary classification of histiocytic disorders. The WHO Committee on Histiocytic/Reticulum Cell Proliferations. Reclassification Working Group of the Histiocyte Society," *Medical and Pediatric Oncology*, vol. 29, no. 3, pp. 157–166, 1997.

[4] S. Sawhney, P. Woo, and K. J. Murray, "Macrophage activation syndrome: a potentially fatal complication of rheumatic disorders," *Archives of Disease in Childhood*, vol. 85, no. 5, pp. 421–426, 2001.

[5] A. Ravelli, F. Minoia, S. Davì et al., "2016 classification criteria for macrophage activation syndrome complicating systemic juvenile idiopathic arthritis," *Annals of the Rheumatic Diseases*, vol. 75, no. 3, pp. 481–489, 2016.

[6] J.-I. Henter, M. Arico, R. M. Egeler et al., "HLH-94: a treatment protocol for hemophagocytic lymphohistiocytosis," *Medical and Pediatric Oncology*, vol. 28, no. 5, pp. 342–347, 1997.

[7] K. Kaito, M. Kobayashi, T. Katayama et al., "Prognostic factors of hemophagocytic syndrome in adults: analysis of 34 cases," *European Journal of Haematology*, vol. 59, no. 4, pp. 247–253, 1997.

[8] F. Minoia, S. Davì, A. Horne et al., "Clinical features, treatment, and outcome of macrophage activation syndrome complicating systemic juvenile idiopathic arthritis: a multinational, multicenter study of 362 patients," *Arthritis and Rheumatology*, vol. 66, no. 11, pp. 3160–3169, 2014.

[9] R. Dhote, J. Simon, T. Papo et al., "Reactive hemophagocytic syndrome in adult systemic disease: report of twenty-six cases and literature review," *Arthritis Care and Research*, vol. 49, no. 5, pp. 633–639, 2003.

[10] A. A. Grom, "Macrophage activation syndrome and reactive hemophagocytic lymphohistiocytosis: the same entities?" *Current Opinion in Rheumatology*, vol. 15, no. 5, pp. 587–590, 2003.

[11] S. Rivière, L. Galicier, P. Coppo et al., "Reactive hemophagocytic syndrome in adults: a retrospective analysis of 162 patients," *The American Journal of Medicine*, vol. 127, no. 11, pp. 1118–1125, 2014.

[12] A. A. Grom, N. T. Ilowite, V. Pascual et al., "Rate and clinical presentation of macrophage activation syndrome in patients with systemic juvenile idiopathic arthritis treated with canakinumab," *Arthritis and Rheumatology*, vol. 68, no. 1, pp. 218–228, 2016.

[13] M. Shimizu, Y. Nakagishi, K. Kasai et al., "Tocilizumab masks the clinical symptoms of systemic juvenile idiopathic arthritis-associated macrophage activation syndrome: the diagnostic significance of interleukin-18 and interleukin-6," *Cytokine*, vol. 58, no. 2, pp. 287–294, 2012.

[14] A. Ravelli, *Macrophage Activation Syndrome Differential Diagnoses*, 2016, http://emedicine.medscape.com/article/1380671-differential.

[15] E. M. Galińska and J. Zagórski, "Brucellosis in humans—etiology, diagnostics, clinical forms," *Annals of Agricultural and Environmental Medicine*, vol. 20, no. 2, pp. 233–238, 2013.

[16] R. M. Traxler, M. W. Lehman, E. A. Bosserman et al., "A literature review of laboratory-acquired brucellosis," *Journal of Clinical Microbiology*, vol. 51, no. 9, pp. 3055–3062, 2013.

[17] L. Fardet, L. Galicier, O. Lambotte et al., "Development and validation of the hscore, a score for the diagnosis of reactive hemophagocytic syndrome," *Arthritis and Rheumatology*, vol. 66, no. 9, pp. 2613–2620, 2014.

[18] E. D. Batu, A. Erden, E. Seyhoğlu et al., "Assessment of the HScore for reactive haemophagocytic syndrome in patients with rheumatic diseases," *Scandinavian Journal of Rheumatology*, 2016.

[19] D. Chellapandian, R. Das, K. Zelley et al., "Treatment of Epstein Barr virus-induced haemophagocytic lymphohistiocytosis with rituximab-containing chemo-immunotherapeutic regimens," *British Journal of Haematology*, vol. 162, no. 3, pp. 376–382, 2013.

[20] T. Y. Shaw and M. Schivo, "Weathering a cytokine storm: a case of EBV-induced hemophagocytic lymphohistiocytosis," *Journal of Investigative Medicine High Impact Case Reports*, vol. 4, no. 2, 2016.

[21] A. Rudinskaya, M. Shao, and R. G. Lahita, "A young male with more than lupus," *Lupus*, vol. 25, no. 13, pp. 1491–1496, 2016.

A Case of Familial Mediterranean Fever with Extensive Lymphadenopathy and Complex Heterozygous Genotype Presenting

Jawad Al-Khafaji,[1] **Fran Ganz-Lord**,[2] **Venkata Rajesh Konjeti**,[1] **and Aaron D. Viny**[3]

[1]*Department of Medicine, Virginia Commonwealth University Health System, Richmond, VA 23298, USA*
[2]*CareMount Medical, Chappaqua, NY 10514, USA*
[3]*Human Oncology & Pathogenesis Program, Memorial Sloan Kettering Cancer Center, New York, NY 10065, USA*

Correspondence should be addressed to Jawad Al-Khafaji; jawad.al-khafaji@vcuhealth.org

Academic Editor: Mehmet Soy

Familial Mediterranean fever (FMF) is an inherited disease caused by loss of function mutations in the *MEFV* gene encoding pyrin, a negative regulator of interleukin-1. The disease is characterized by recurrent fever and self-limited attacks of joint, chest, and abdominal pain but lymphadenopathy is an infrequent manifestation. While mesenteric lymphadenopathy has been described in several cases in the literature; hilar, paratracheal, axillary, pelvic, and retroperitoneal lymphadenopathy are extremely rare and have been reported separately in very few individuals. In this report, we present a patient with late-onset FMF with extensive lymphadenopathy in all of the aforementioned anatomic regions. Genetic analysis identified three heterozygous pyrin mutations in a patient with no affected family members. Genetic investigation of the patient's mother identified a novel carrier haplotype E148Q/P369S. The proband also inherited the previously described and rare A744S mutation previously not thought to be a disease-defining lesion. This unique compound heterozygous genotype resulted in a novel genotype-phenotype association producing an atypical clinical presentation of FMF that fits within the pattern of several case reports of late-onset disease with respect to clinical course and therapeutic response.

1. Introduction

Familial Mediterranean fever (FMF) is an inherited autonomous inflammatory disease predominantly affecting people of Mediterranean descent, including Sephardic Jews, Turks, Armenians, and Arabs [1]. The disease is hallmarked by three clinical sequelae [1–3]: (1) self-limited, recurrent episodes of fever (lasting 2–4 days), (2) inflammation of the peritoneal, pleural, pericardial, and synovial membranes and skin, leading to chest and abdominal pain, arthralgias, and erysipelas-like erythema, and (3) systemic AA amyloidosis that leads to nephropathy if left untreated. About 60% of patients with FMF experience their first attack before the age of 10, 90% before reaching 20 years, and nearly all present before age 40 [1, 4]. Late-onset FMF is defined as diagnosis above 40 years of age, which is a rare occurrence, affecting about only 0.5% of FMF patients [4].

The disease has been linked to mutations within the gene *MEFV* on chromosome 16 which encodes pyrin, a protein found almost exclusively in mature granulocytes and is a regulator of interleukin-1- (IL-1-) mediated inflammation [5]. Loss-of-function mutations within the pyrin/marenostrin protein complex are believed to cause dysregulation of IL-1 inflammatory response either by a functional mutation in pyrin or increased sensitivity of pyrin to cleavage by caspace-1 [6, 7]. Originally discovered serendipitously, colchicine has become the mainstay of therapy, ameliorating both the inflammatory response as well as resultant amyloid deposition [8]. While the precise mechanism remains incompletely understood, it is likely that colchicine exerts its effect through impairing inflammatory cell activity through conformational changes to microtubules, and new evidence also implicates transcriptional suppression of inflammatory proteins [9, 10].

The genetic basis for the disease has been well described in the last two decades. Founder mutations have been identified at amino acid positions 680, 694, and 726, all within exon 10, leading to alterations of the C-terminus and comprise the majority (86–93%) of cases. Subsequently, several nonfounder mutations have been found in exons 2, 5, and 10 within well-described haplotypes [11].

In this report, we present a case of a late-onset FMF (age 42 years) with a unique phenotype manifesting with retroperitoneal paraaortic, paratracheal, hilar, pelvic, and axillary lymphadenopathy in the setting of a complex heterozygous genotype implicating A744S as a new disease modifying locus.

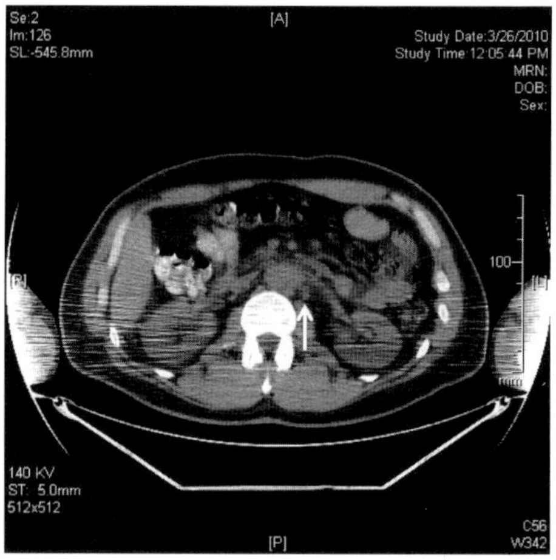

FIGURE 1: CT image of periaortic lymphadenopathy.

2. Case Presentation

A 42-year-old man of Armenian descent was admitted to the internal medicine service complaining of intermittent fever and night sweats for one month. The fevers continued for >36 hours, peaked at 40°C, and were associated with diffuse myalgias, rigors, and diaphoresis. He also reported drenching night sweats and a 20 lb. weight loss over the previous month. He does not smoke and drinks alcohol sparingly. His past medical history and family history were unremarkable. His review of systems was otherwise unremarkable. He is married with two children and works at a petroleum tank farm with exposure to benzenes and industrial solvents. His physical exam upon admission was significant for fever of 39.1°C, marked diaphoresis, tenderness to palpation in the lower extremities bilaterally, blanching maculopapular rash on the legs bilaterally and left forearm, and subcentimeter mobile, nontender inguinal lymph nodes bilaterally. Myalgias and fevers continued throughout the hospital stay. His myalgias were only moderately relieved by the aggressive use of opiates and NSAIDs. The patient continued to complain of the same symptoms throughout his hospital stay during which he was evaluated for fever of unknown origin.

Laboratory evaluation was significant for ESR 66 mm/hr, C-reactive protein 10.79 mg/L, creatinine kinase 34 U/L, and lactate dehydrogenase 117 U/L. His complete blood count, liver, kidney and thyroid function tests were all within normal limits, as were his serum electrolytes, iron studies, uric acid, amylase, proteins, and immunoglobulins. Serial blood, urine, and sputum cultures, including mycobacterium, were negative. Serologic testing was negative for HIV, EBV, CMV, HBV, HCV, and Syphilis. A PPD was also negative. His EKG, chest X-ray, and abdominal sonography were normal. Testing for the following autoimmune factors was negative: ANA, anti-dsDNA, RF, anti-smith, anti-RNP, anti-SSA, anti-SSB, and CCP.

A malignancy work-up included bone marrow examination. Core biopsy, aspirate, flow cytometry, molecular pathology, immunohistochemistry, and cultures (for tuberculosis, bacteria, and fungi) were all unrevealing. Flow cytometry of peripheral blood was normal, no atypical cells were identified by peripheral smear, and there was no M-spike detected in serum or urine. Whole body PET/CT scan showed hypermetabolic retroperitoneal enlarged lymph nodes in the left paraaortic region at the level of the renal vessels (largest 1.7 × 2.5 cm) and minimally active lymph nodes in the following regions: right axillary region (1.8 cm), right lower paratracheal region (1.5 cm), right upper lung (8 mm), retrocaval, common iliac, internal iliac and obturator regions bilaterally and left external iliac (all subcentimeter), and the inguinal region bilaterally (largest 1.2 cm).

CT-guided aspiration biopsy of the retroperitoneal periaortic lymph node (Figure 1) showed atypical lymphoid proliferation of small lymphocytes, which were polyclonal by flow cytometric analysis. Surgical consultation was requested for an excisional biopsy of the periaortic lymph node; however, this was deferred due to unacceptable risk related to anatomical location of the node.

The patient was given the presumptive diagnosis of a low-grade lymphoproliferative disorder and in addition to careful expectant management, an empiric trial of prednisone was started despite the risk of losing diagnostic lymph node architecture. The patient was discharged and had outpatient follow-up one week later. Over the next several weeks, the patient noted a subjective improvement in his symptoms. However, attempts to taper the prednisone dose resulted in a relapse of fevers and myalgias.

Although very atypical in presentation, the diagnosis of familial Mediterranean fever was considered given the robust response to steroids and his Armenian descent. Genetic studies were performed and an empiric trial of colchicine 0.6 mg daily was also initiated. The patient reported a near immediate relief of symptoms and was then able to be tapered off of prednisone completely. One month later, the *MEFV* genetic results were returned, which confirmed the diagnosis. His genetic tests were significant for a complex heterozygous genotype with the three mutations: E148Q, P369S, and A744S. The patient's mother was also genotyped to determine allelic distribution and risk of inheritance. The patient's mother's test was significant for heterozygosity at

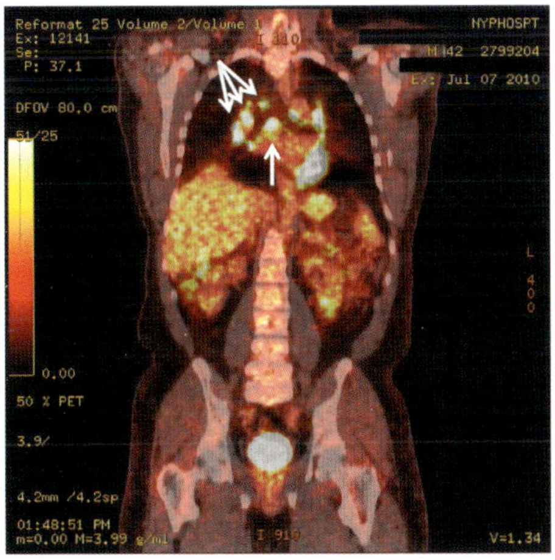

Figure 2: Positron emission tomography imaging of mediastinal lymphadenopathy.

the A744S locus. The patient's father was not willing to undergo genetic counseling or testing but denies any symptoms that might be attributed to FMF. Thus, the father's presumed haplotype E148Q/P369S is likely not sufficient to produce any symptoms or clinical phenotype.

Three months later, a follow-up PET scan was performed to evaluate the patient's previously identified lymphadenopathy (Figure 2). The study revealed near resolution previous paraaortic lymph node and resolved axillary and pelvic lymphadenopathy. However, new extensive hypermetabolic mediastinal and hilar lymphadenopathy were identified, revealing new right upper paratracheal node (1.7 cm), enlarging right lower paratracheal node (1.6 cm), subcarinal node (2.7 cm), and bilateral hypermetabolic hilar lymphadenopathy. At this point, several core needle biopsies of the subcarinal and peritracheal lymph nodes were performed under CT-guidance. Pathologic examination showed nonspecific reactive heterogeneous population of lymphocytes and was negative for granulomatous and amyloidal disease. Molecular pathology, immunohistochemistry, and flow cytometry were unremarkable.

Despite these findings, the patient continued to do well and remained symptom-free on colchicine.

3. Discussion

In this report, we describe a unique presentation of an Armenian man with familial Mediterranean fever with extensive lymphadenopathy in the hilum, mesentery, and retroperitoneal regions with a novel complex heterozygous genotype. His genetics implicate A744S as a phenotype defining mutation in conjunction with the E148Q/P369S haplotype.

MEFV gene defects in FMF have been well described with mutations clustering at the C-terminus and presumed to affect interactions with regulatory molecules such as 14-3-3 [12]. Other *MEFV* gene mutations found to correlate with disease cluster in the splice junction between exon 1–3 [13, 14]. More than 317 mutations have been identified [15]. The most frequent of which include M694V, M694I, M680I,

Table 1: Review of literature of lymphadenopathy in familial Mediterranean fever.

Anatomical region	Number of cases	Reference
Abdominal	13	[25, 27–29, 31, 32]
Retroperitoneal†	5	[25–28]
Thoracic (hilar and paratracheal)†	2	[25]
Peripheral (cervical and axillary)	2	[25, 30]
Pelvic/inguinal†	0	—

†Anatomic region where lymphadenopathy was identified in the current report.

and V726A [12]. These mutations are associated with a younger age of onset, a variable response to colchicine, and the complications of amyloidosis and renal failure [11, 16, 17]. The distribution, prevalence, and penetrance of FMF mutations seem to have implications in disease severity and age of onset. Although disease most often presents before 20 years of age, onset of the disease after the fourth decade has been reported in only 0.5% of FMF patient population and most had milder disease [4, 18–21]. These patients uniformly had absence of the prototypical M694V mutation, and a favorable response to colchicine was noted in all patients with late-onset FMF compared with other patient populations of younger ages [4]. This suggests that the specific genotype-phenotype association in FMF has a spectrum likely reflecting the capacity of each mutation to maintain varying functional capacity. The heterozygous nature of these mutations predicts a dominant negative effect, with one wild type copy of *MEFV* unable to suppress IL-1 sufficiently.

Therefore, a compound heterozygous genotype with two unaffected parents, as seen in this patient, may reflect limited functional effects of E148Q/P369S and A744S in isolation, but sufficiently reduced function in combination. The former two mutations have been well studied and have been linked to a milder disease phenotype but independently do not cause a disease phenotype [4, 20, 22, 23]. The third mutation is a rare mutation described in the literature but is by itself not particularly associated with any serious disease manifestations [24]. This patient presented with FMF after age 40 and had extensive lymph node involvement. Both of these are rare features but may reflect the slow smoldering nature of this particular genotype, permissive of nodal disease.

When present, lymphadenopathy is most commonly found in the abdomen involving primarily the mesenteric region [25–29]. Retroperitoneal lymphadenopathy has only been reported in 4 patients with FMF [25 28]. Peripheral lymphadenopathy has been reported in only two cases [25, 30]. Paratracheal and hilar lymphadenopathy have each been reported in only one case report [25]. These FMF patient cases with lymphadenopathy that are reported in the literature are summarized in Table 1. When reported, biopsy of these lymph nodes uniformly showed nonspecific lymphoid hyperplasia [25, 26, 30, 31]. In this patient, biopsies of paraaortic, hilar, and paratracheal lymph nodes also showed nonspecific reactive lymphocytes, without infectious or malignant stigmata, and are similar to what has been described elsewhere [25, 26, 30, 31]. The significance of lymphadenopathy in FMF is not well understood, and the clinical significance of their locations is also yet to be studied. Whether they correlate to the disease process (i.e., evolution, severity, and prognosis) is unclear.

This patient has multiple rare findings for FMF. His extensive lymphadenopathy adds to the extremely rare cases reported in the literature of hilar, para-tracheal lymphadenopathy, axillary, and retroperitoneal lymphadenopathy. The age of onset of this patient's FMF illness also adds to the very few cases of late-onset FMF patients. Furthermore, his remarkable complex heterozygous genotype has two-fold impact. First, it establishes a functional consequence of A744S, a rare *MEFV* mutation previously not linked to disease and second, it strengthens the dogma of nonfounder pyrin mutations producing a distinct clinical and prognostic disease.

References

[1] E. Sohar, J. Gafni, M. Pras, and H. Heller, "Familial Mediterranean fever. A survey of 470 cases and review of the literature," *American Journal of Medicine*, vol. 43, no. 2, pp. 227–253, 1967.

[2] M. Bektas, I. Soykan, D. Goren et al., "A rare cause of ascites: familial Mediterranean fever," *Turkish Journal of Gastroenterology*, vol. 19, no. 1, pp. 64–68, 2008.

[3] A. M. Ozel, L. Demirturk, Y. Yazgan et al., "Familial Mediterranean fever. A review of the disease and clinical and laboratory findings in 105 patients," *Digestive and Liver Disease*, vol. 32, no. 6, pp. 504–509, 2000.

[4] N. Tamir, P. Langevitz, D. Zemer et al., "Late-onset familial Mediterranean fever (FMF): a subset with distinct clinical, demographic, and molecular genetic characteristics," *American Journal of Medical Genetics*, vol. 87, no. 1, pp. 30–35, 1999.

[5] M. Lidar and A. Livneh, "Familial Mediterranean fever: clinical, molecular and management advancements," *Netherlands Journal of Medicine*, vol. 65, no. 9, pp. 318–324, 2007.

[6] J. J. Chae, G. Wood, K. Richard et al., "The familial Mediterranean fever protein, pyrin, is cleaved by caspase-1 and activates NF-kappaB through its N-terminal fragment," *Blood*, vol. 112, no. 5, pp. 1794–1803, 2008.

[7] S. Ozen, H. M. Hoffman, J. Frenkel, and D. Kastner, "Familial Mediterranean fever (FMF) and beyond: a new horizon. Fourth international congress on the systemic autoinflammatory diseases held in Bethesda, USA, 6–10 November 2005," *Annals of the Rheumatic Diseases*, vol. 65, no. 7, pp. 961–964, 2006.

[8] S. E. Goldfinger, "Colchicine for familial Mediterranean fever," *New England Journal of Medicine*, vol. 287, no. 25, p. 1302, 1972.

[9] E. Ben-Chetrit, S. Bergmann, and R. Sood, "Mechanism of the anti-inflammatory effect of colchicine in rheumatic diseases: a possible new outlook through microarray analysis," *Rheumatology*, vol. 45, no. 3, pp. 274–282, 2006.

[10] D. Rigante, I. La Torraca, L. Avallone, A. L. Pugliese, S. Gaspari, and A. Stabile, "The pharmacologic basis of treatment with colchicine in children with familial Mediterranean fever," *European Review for Medical and Pharmacological Sciences*, vol. 10, no. 4, pp. 173–178, 2006.

[11] A. Bernot, C. da Silva, J. L. Petit et al., "Non-founder mutations in the MEFV gene establish this gene as the cause of familial Mediterranean fever (FMF)," *Human Molecular Genetics*, vol. 7, no. 8, pp. 1317–1325, 1998.

[12] M. Medlej-Hashim, J. Loiselet, G. Lefranc, and A. Megarbane, "Familial Mediterranean fever (FMF): from diagnosis to treatment," *Sante*, vol. 14, no. 4, pp. 261–266, 2004.

[13] S. Papin, P. Duquesnoy, C. Cazeneuve et al., "Alternative splicing at the MEFV locus involved in familial Mediterranean fever regulates translocation of the marenostrin/pyrin protein to the nucleus," *Human Molecular Genetics*, vol. 9, no. 20, pp. 3001–3009, 2000.

[14] I. Touitou, "The spectrum of familial Mediterranean fever (FMF) mutations," *European Journal of Human Genetics*, vol. 9, no. 7, pp. 473–483, 2001.

[15] D. Kishida, M. Yazaki, A. Nakamura et al., "One novel and two uncommon *MEFV* mutations in Japanese patients with familial Mediterranean fever: a clinicogenetic study," *Rheumatology International*, vol. 38, no. 1, pp. 105–110, 2017.

[16] R. Gershoni-Baruch, M. Shinawi, K. Leah, K. Badarnah, and R. Brik, "Familial Mediterranean fever: prevalence, penetrance and genetic drift," *European Journal of Human Genetics*, vol. 9, no. 8, pp. 634–637, 2001.

[17] E. Yilmaz, S. Ozen, B. Balci et al., "Mutation frequency of familial Mediterranean fever and evidence for a high carrier rate in the Turkish population," *European Journal of Human Genetics*, vol. 9, no. 7, pp. 553–555, 2001.

[18] The International FMF Consortium, "Ancient missense mutations in a new member of the RoRet gene family are likely to cause familial Mediterranean fever," *Cell*, vol. 90, no. 4, pp. 797–807, 1997.

[19] A. Livneh, P. Langevitz, Y. Shinar et al., "MEFV mutation analysis in patients suffering from amyloidosis of familial Mediterranean fever," *Amyloid*, vol. 6, no. 1, pp. 1–6, 1999.

[20] M. Rozenbaum and I. Rosner, "The clinical features of familial Mediterranean fever of elderly onset," *Clinical and Experimental Rheumatology*, vol. 12, no. 3, pp. 347-348, 1994.

[21] Y. Shinar, A. Livneh, P. Langevitz et al., "Genotype-phenotype assessment of common genotypes among patients with familial Mediterranean fever," *Journal of Rheumatology*, vol. 27, no. 7, pp. 1703–1707, 2000.

[22] D. Marek-Yagel, I. Bar-Joseph, E. Pras, and Y. Berkun, "Is E148Q a benign polymorphism or a disease-causing mutation?," *Journal of Rheumatology*, vol. 36, no. 10, p. 2372, 2009.

[23] T. Sarkisian, H. Ajrapetyan, and G. Shahsuvaryan, "Molecular study of FMF patients in Armenia," *Current Drug Target–Inflammation & Allergy*, vol. 4, no. 1, pp. 113–116, 2005.

[24] I. Aksentijevich, Y. Torosyan, J. Samuels et al., "Mutation and haplotype studies of familial Mediterranean fever reveal new ancestral relationships and evidence for a high carrier frequency with reduced penetrance in the Ashkenazi Jewish population," *American Journal of Human Genetics*, vol. 64, no. 4, pp. 949–962, 1999.

[25] S. Siegal, "Familial paroxysmal polyserositis. analysis of fifty cases," *American Journal of Medicine*, vol. 36, no. 6, pp. 893–918, 1964.

[26] D. Rimon, Y. Meir, and L. Cohen, "Retroperitoneal lymphadenopathy in familial Mediterranean fever," *Postgraduate Medical Journal*, vol. 65, no. 768, pp. 776–778, 1989.

[27] R. Zissin, V. Rathaus, G. Gayer, M. Shapiro-Feinberg, and M. Hertz, "CT findings in patients with familial Mediterranean fever during an acute abdominal attack," *British Journal of Radiology*, vol. 76, no. 901, pp. 22–25, 2003.

[28] D. Aharoni, N. Hiller, and I. Hadas-Halpern, "Familial Mediterranean fever: abdominal imaging findings in 139 patients and review of the literature," *Abdominal Imaging*, vol. 25, no. 3, pp. 297–300, 2000.

[29] G. E. Ishak, N. J. Khoury, G. A. Birjawi, Y. R. El-Zein, L. N. Naffaa, and M. C. Haddad, "Imaging findings of familial Mediterranean fever," *Clinical Imaging*, vol. 30, no. 3, pp. 153–159, 2006.

[30] A. D. Schwabe and R. S. Peters, "Familial Mediterranean fever in armenians. Analysis of 100 cases," *Medicine*, vol. 53, no. 6, pp. 453–462, 1974.

[31] H. A. Reimann, J. Moadie, S. Semerdjian, and P. F. Sahyoun, "Periodic peritonitis; heredity and pathology: report of seventy-two cases," *Journal of the American Medical Association*, vol. 154, no. 15, pp. 1254–1259, 1954.

[32] M. Wikstrom, A. Wolf, D. Birk, and H. J. Brambs, "Abdominal CT in familial Mediterranean fever: a case report," *Abdominal Imaging*, vol. 23, no. 2, pp. 147–149, 1998.

Development of Eosinophilic Fasciitis during Infliximab Therapy for Psoriatic Arthritis

Richard Hariman,[1] Payal Patel,[1] Jennifer Strouse,[1] Michael P. Collins,[2] and Ann Rosenthal[1]

[1] *Division of Rheumatology, Department of Medicine, Medical College of Wisconsin, 9200 W. Wisconsin Avenue, Milwaukee, WI 53226, USA*
[2] *Department of Neurology, Medical College of Wisconsin, 9200 W. Wisconsin Avenue, Milwaukee, WI 53226, USA*

Correspondence should be addressed to Richard Hariman; rhariman@mcw.edu

Academic Editor: Mario Salazar-Paramo

Eosinophilic fasciitis (EF) is a rare disorder involving chronic inflammation of the fascia and connective tissue surrounding muscles, nerves, and blood vessels. While its pathogenesis is not entirely understood, this disorder is thought to be autoimmune or allergic in nature. We present here a case of a 59-year-old male who developed peripheral eosinophilia and subsequent eosinophilic fasciitis during treatment with infliximab. To our knowledge, eosinophilic fasciitis has not been previously described in patients during treatment with an inhibitor of tumor necrosis factor α.

1. Introduction

Eosinophilic fasciitis is a rare disorder involving chronic inflammation of fascia and connective tissue surrounding muscles, nerves, and blood vessels [1]. We report a case of eosinophilic fasciitis in a 59-year-old male patient undergoing treatment with infliximab for psoriatic arthritis. Infliximab infusion triggered eosinophilic fasciitis three months after his medication dose was increased from 3 mg/kg to 5 mg/kg. To our knowledge, eosinophilic fasciitis has not been described in patients during therapy with a tumor necrosis factor-α (TNF-α) inhibitor.

2. Case Description

Mr. E was a 59-year-old former mechanic and current smoker with psoriatic arthritis who presented to the hospital with a 2-month history of worsening lower extremity swelling, arthralgias of his hands and feet, and new onset of muscle pain. He had a 20-year history of poorly controlled psoriasis and had developed psoriatic arthritis about 3 years prior to admission. He had been treated with methotrexate, azathioprine, etanercept, adalimumab, and golimumab without success due to either poor clinical response or infectious complications largely related to cellulitis from large open skin lesions. For the past 9 months, he had been taking infliximab 3 mg/kg IV infusion every 6 weeks along with erythromycin for prophylaxis against infections with an initial good response for both his skin and joint disease. When his synovitis recurred four months prior to admission, the infliximab dose was increased to 5 mg/kg every 6 weeks. The patient reported initial improvement in his joint and skin symptoms with this dose adjustment. However, over the several weeks prior to admission, he noted increasing muscle pain, stiffness, swelling in his legs, and weight gain.

He denied fevers, weakness, or recent acute respiratory or gastrointestinal illness but did note some night sweats. Past medical history was notable for depression and COPD. Review of systems was otherwise negative. Family history was notable for a poorly characterized autoimmune disease in a grandmother.

Medications on admission were citalopram 40 mg daily, infliximab 5 mg/kg every 6 weeks, naproxen 220 mg BID, hydrocodone/acetaminophen 7.5 mg/325 mg every 6 hours as needed, tramadol 50 mg every 6 hours as needed, folic acid 1 mg daily, fluocinonide 0.05% cream topically for psoriasis, erythromycin 250 mg BID for infection prophylaxis, and topical clotrimazole.

His vital signs at the time of admission were a temperature of 98.2 F, pulse of 87, respiratory rate of 16, blood pressure

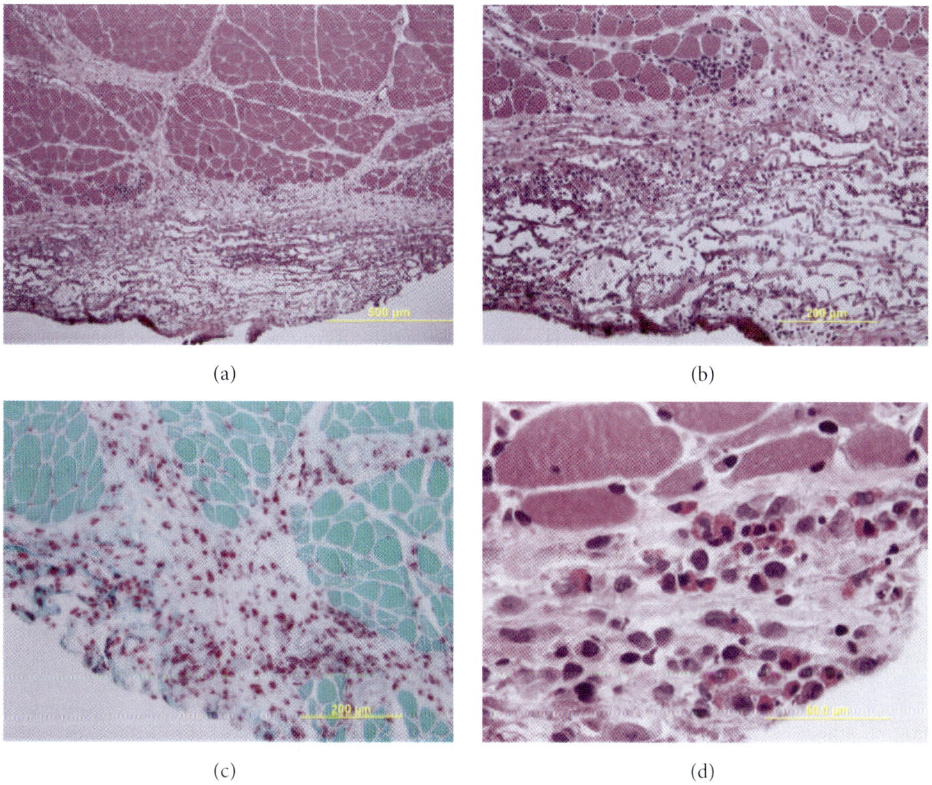

FIGURE 1: Deltoid muscle biopsy. (a) Low power view showing marked thickening and edema of epimysium and, to lesser extent, perimysium accompanied by diffuse chronic inflammation (H&E stain). There is only minor focal involvement of underlying endomysium. Muscle fascicles are relatively spared. (b) Higher power view of epimysium demonstrating noncohesive chronic inflammation and rarefaction/necrosis of connective tissue (H&E stain). A single necrotic fiber undergoing phagocytosis is observed in the adjacent fascicle. (c) Infiltrates are composed primarily of histiocytes, highlighted as red-staining cells in this preparation (acid phosphatase stain). (d) High power view of more focal collection of eosinophils within the epimysium (H&E stain).

of 133/73, and oxygen level of 95% on room air. His weight was 63.4 kg which was 7 kg greater than his previous recorded weight 6 months ago. He had mild synovitis of the second and third metacarpophalangeal joints of his left hand. Both wrists were tender to palpation. He also had new leg edema bilaterally with diffuse muscle tenderness to palpation. His legs were warm and erythematous. Muscle strength in upper and lower extremities modestly decreased due to pain in all extremities proximally and distally. Scattered small psoriatic lesions were noted over his bilateral knees, distal legs, and dorsal feet.

Laboratory studies revealed creatinine kinase level of 22 U/L (normal 39–308 U/L) and an aldolase level which was mildly elevated at 11 U/L (normal < 8 U/L). He had a peripheral eosinophilia with eosinophils accounting for up to 30% of his white blood cells. During the hospital stay, his absolute eosinophil count varied between 700 and 2200/μL. He had developed new, mild, normocytic anemia with hemoglobin of 12.0 g/dL and mean corpuscular volume of 94.8 fL. Previous hemoglobin 1 month priorly was 13.8 g/dL. Erythrocyte sedimentation rate was 36 mm/h (normal 0–15) and C-reactive protein was 78.7 (normal 0–10).

Dermatology, rheumatology, and hematology services were consulted. The differential diagnosis included DRESS syndrome (drug rash with eosinophilia and systemic symptoms), malignancy, hypereosinophilic syndrome, inflammatory myopathy, and eosinophilic fasciitis. DRESS syndrome was felt to be unlikely due to the absence of liver involvement. The patient improved with supportive care and outpatient workup was arranged.

The patient underwent a bone marrow biopsy to evaluate hypereosinophilic syndrome. The biopsy showed hypercellular marrow with marked eosinophilia, but no other significant abnormal cell populations were noted. A scheduled infliximab infusion was performed 2 weeks after hospitalization but had to be stopped due to the development of urticaria during the infusion. A CT scan of the chest, abdomen, and pelvis revealed no evidence of malignancy. The patient underwent an EMG of his right upper extremity to evaluate inflammatory myopathy which showed no definite evidence of a myopathic process. Because of the elevated aldolase level which subsequently increased to 14.3 U/L 3 weeks later, a muscle biopsy of the left deltoid muscle was performed. The biopsy showed diffuse thickening and edema of the epimysium and, to a lesser extent, perimysium, accompanied by a chronic, polymorphic inflammatory infiltrate and foci of fibrinoid necrosis of the involved fibrous connective tissue (Figures 1(a) and 1(b)). The inflammatory cells included

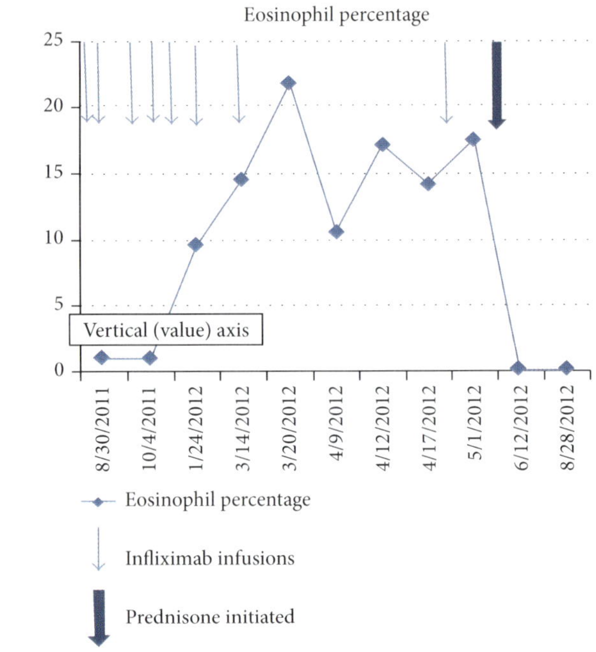

Figure 2: Peripheral eosinophil counts. This graph shows the eosinophil percentage as a function of time. The thin arrows denote the dates of infliximab infusions. The thick arrow shows the initiation of steroid treatment.

histiocytes, lymphocytes, focally prevalent eosinophils, and scattered plasma cells (Figures 1(c) and 1(d)).

These aggregates only rarely infiltrated into the adjacent endomysium. The muscle fibers themselves were relatively spared, with only rare necrotic fibers in perifascicular areas abutting the interstitial inflammation (Figure 1(b)). The findings were indicative of eosinophilic fasciitis. Infliximab was then discontinued and he was started on 60 mg prednisone daily with excellent resolution of his symptoms. Within 24 hours of initiation of prednisone, his muscle pains significantly diminished. Three weeks after initiation of steroid treatment, his edema had resolved, and his eosinophilia normalized.

3. Discussion

We describe a patient who developed biopsy-confirmed eosinophilic fasciitis (EF) on infliximab. Peripheral eosinophilia and typical skin changes occurred after his infliximab dose was increased from 3 mg/kg dose to 5 mg/kg and preceded the development of EF (Figure 2). The pathogenesis of EF is not fully understood, although autoimmune and allergic pathways are thought to be involved. Vigorous exercise, *Borrelia* infection, and malignancy have been associated with EF, although our patient did not have any of these conditions.

The diagnosis of EF is established by clinical, laboratory, and histological findings [1]. Universally accepted international diagnostic criteria are lacking. Clinical manifestations of EF include painful swelling with progressive circumferential induration and thickening of the subcutaneous fat, dermis, and fascia, a finding typically seen in the extremities. All of these features were noted in our patient. The trunk area can also be affected, while the face, fingers, and feet are usually spared. Peripheral eosinophilia may occur in up to 60% of patients. One can also see elevated gamma globulin levels in some cases. Histologically, a full-thickness wedge tissue biopsy of the clinically affected area will show inflammation of the lower subcutis and deep fascia, occasionally extending into the underlying muscle. Muscle biopsy findings in our patient showed inflammation within the perimysial septa and overlying epimysial connective tissue, as is typical of this condition. In a study performed by Wasserman et al., increased eosinophilic chemotactic activity was noted in patients with EF suggesting that elevated peripheral eosinophil activity may have a direct role in this disease process [2].

It seems counterintuitive that a TNF-α inhibitor such as infliximab would induce EF. TNF-α is a potent chemotactic agent for eosinophils [3] and downregulates eosinophil apoptosis [4]. Several previous cases of eosinophilia have been noted with TNF-α inhibitors. Adalimumab was linked with a case of eosinophilic myocarditis [5]. Infliximab has been implicated in a case of eosinophilic cellulitis known as Wells' Syndrome [6], a syndrome of recurrent granulomatous dermatitis with eosinophilia. Infliximab and other TNF-α inhibitors can induce autoimmune syndromes such as systemic lupus erythematous [7]. While the mechanisms of these effects are unclear, off-target effects of these drugs or repercussions of antibody formation against these foreign proteins may explain this association.

In regard to treatment, corticosteroids remain the standard therapy for EF, although some patients may improve spontaneously with time. In the setting of malignancy, treating the underlying malignancy is the key to treatment of EF. Other immunologic steroid-sparing medications such as methotrexate, azathioprine, cyclosporine, and rituximab have been tried successfully in the treatment of EF [8]. Interestingly, Khanna et al. reported 3 patients with steroid-resistant EF who improved with addition of infliximab at 3 mg/kg every 8 weeks [9].

In conclusion, we report a case of a 59-year-old male who developed peripheral eosinophilia and subsequent eosinophilic fasciitis during treatment with infliximab for psoriatic arthritis. To our knowledge, this is the first reported case of eosinophilic fasciitis developing from tumor necrosis factor-α inhibitors. The mechanism of the development of eosinophilic fasciitis from these medications is unknown, but the description of other eosinophilic syndromes with TNF-α inhibitors suggests a possible etiologic link that warrants further study.

Competing Interests

The authors declare that they have no competing interests.

References

[1] I. Pinal-Fernandez, A. Selva-O'Callaghan, and J. M. Grau, "Diagnosis and classification of eosinophilic fasciitis," *Autoimmunity Reviews*, vol. 13, no. 4-5, pp. 379–382, 2014.

[2] S. I. Wasserman, J. R. Seibold, T. A. Medsger Jr., and G. P. Rodnan, "Serum eosinophilotactic activity in eosinophilic fasciitis," *Arthritis and Rheumatism*, vol. 25, no. 11, pp. 1352–1356, 1982.

[3] A. E. El-Shazly, V. Moonen, M. Mawet et al., "IFN-γ and TNF-α potentiate prostaglandin D2-induced human eosinophil chemotaxis through up-regulation of CRTH2 surface receptor," *International Immunopharmacology*, vol. 11, no. 11, pp. 1864–1870, 2011.

[4] H. Kankaanranta, P. Ilmarinen, X. Zhang et al., "Tumour necrosis factor-α regulates human eosinophil apoptosis via ligation of TNF-receptor 1 and balance between NF-κB and AP-1," *PLoS ONE*, vol. 9, no. 2, Article ID e90298, 2014.

[5] R. Adamson, Y. Yazici, E. S. Katz, S. G. Greisman, and D. Steiger, "Fatal acute necrotizing eosinophilic myocarditis temporally related to use of adalimumab in a patient with relapsing polychondritis," *Journal of Clinical Rheumatology*, vol. 19, no. 7, pp. 386–389, 2013.

[6] N. Tugnet, A. Youssef, and A. J. Whallett, "Wells' syndrome (eosinophilic cellulitis) secondary to infliximab," *Rheumatology*, vol. 51, no. 1, pp. 195–196, 2012.

[7] N. Shakoor, M. Michalska, C. A. Harris, and J. A. Block, "Drug-induced systemic lupus erythematosus associated with etanercept therapy," *The Lancet*, vol. 359, no. 9306, pp. 579–580, 2002.

[8] D. Lebeaux, C. Francés, S. Barete et al., "Eosinophilic fasciitis (Shulman disease): new insights into the therapeutic management from a series of 34 patients," *Rheumatology*, vol. 51, no. 3, pp. 557–561, 2012.

[9] D. Khanna, H. Agrawal, and P. J. Clements, "Infliximab may be effective in the treatment of steroid-resistant eosinophilic fasciitis: report of three cases," *Rheumatology*, vol. 49, no. 6, Article ID keq062, pp. 1184–1188, 2010.

Permissions

All chapters in this book were first published in CRR, by Hindawi Publishing Corporation; hereby published with permission under the Creative Commons Attribution License or equivalent. Every chapter published in this book has been scrutinized by our experts. Their significance has been extensively debated. The topics covered herein carry significant findings which will fuel the growth of the discipline. They may even be implemented as practical applications or may be referred to as a beginning point for another development.

The contributors of this book come from diverse backgrounds, making this book a truly international effort. This book will bring forth new frontiers with its revolutionizing research information and detailed analysis of the nascent developments around the world.

We would like to thank all the contributing authors for lending their expertise to make the book truly unique. They have played a crucial role in the development of this book. Without their invaluable contributions this book wouldn't have been possible. They have made vital efforts to compile up to date information on the varied aspects of this subject to make this book a valuable addition to the collection of many professionals and students.

This book was conceptualized with the vision of imparting up-to-date information and advanced data in this field. To ensure the same, a matchless editorial board was set up. Every individual on the board went through rigorous rounds of assessment to prove their worth. After which they invested a large part of their time researching and compiling the most relevant data for our readers.

The editorial board has been involved in producing this book since its inception. They have spent rigorous hours researching and exploring the diverse topics which have resulted in the successful publishing of this book. They have passed on their knowledge of decades through this book. To expedite this challenging task, the publisher supported the team at every step. A small team of assistant editors was also appointed to further simplify the editing procedure and attain best results for the readers.

Apart from the editorial board, the designing team has also invested a significant amount of their time in understanding the subject and creating the most relevant covers. They scrutinized every image to scout for the most suitable representation of the subject and create an appropriate cover for the book.

The publishing team has been an ardent support to the editorial, designing and production team. Their endless efforts to recruit the best for this project, has resulted in the accomplishment of this book. They are a veteran in the field of academics and their pool of knowledge is as vast as their experience in printing. Their expertise and guidance has proved useful at every step. Their uncompromising quality standards have made this book an exceptional effort. Their encouragement from time to time has been an inspiration for everyone.

The publisher and the editorial board hope that this book will prove to be a valuable piece of knowledge for researchers, students, practitioners and scholars across the globe.

List of Contributors

Fabiola Caracseghi and Consuelo Modesto
Pediatric Rheumatology Department, Vall d'Hebron University Hospital, P. Vall d'Hebron 119-129, 08035 Barcelona, Spain

Jaume Izquierdo-Blasco and Manuel Roig-Quilis
Pediatric Neurology Department, Vall d'Hebron University Hospital, P. Vall d'Hebron 119-129, 08035 Barcelona, Spain

Angel Sanchez-Montanez
Pediatric Radiology Department, Vall d'Hebron University Hospital, P. Vall d'Hebron 119-129, 08035 Barcelona, Spain

Susana Melendo-Perez
Pediatric Emergency Department, Vall d'Hebron University Hospital, P. Vall d'Hebron 119-129, 08035 Barcelona, Spain

Michael A. Hunt, Jeanie R. Zabukovec, Sue Peters, Courtney L. Pollock, Meghan A. Linsdell and Lara A. Boyd
Department of Physical Therapy, University of British Columbia, Vancouver, BC, Canada V6T 1Z3

Taro Masuda, Yasumori Izumi, Hayato Takeshita, Chieko Kawahara,Yoshika Tsuji, Nozomi Iwanaga and Kiyosi Migita
Departments of General Internal Medicine and Rheumatology, Nagasaki Medical Center, Kubara 2-1001-1, Omura, Nagasaki 856-8562, Japan

Hirokazu Kurohama and Masahiro Ito
Department of Pathology, Nagasaki Medical Center, Kubara 2-1001-1, Omura, Nagasaki 856-8562, Japan

Miwako Inamoto
Department of Ophthalmology, Nagasaki Medical Center, Kubara 2-1001-1, Omura, Nagasaki 856-8562, Japan

Keiichi Kase
Department of Otolaryngology, Nagasaki Medical Center, Kubara 2-1001-1, Omura, Nagasaki 856-8562, Japan

Atsushi Kawakami
Department of Rheumatology, Nagasaki University Hospital, Sakamoto 1-7-1, Nagasaki 852-8501, Japan

Syuichi Koarada, Yoshinobu Nakao, Yukiko Tokuda, Yukihide Ono, Satoko Tashiro, Akihito Maruyama, Nobuyuki Ono, Akihide Ohta and Yoshifumi Tada
Division of Rheumatology, Faculty of Medicine, Saga University, 5-1-1 Nabeshima, Saga 849-8501, Japan

Masahiko Tsuboi
Nagasaki Medical Hospital of Rheumatology, 1-21 Aburaya-machi, Nagasaki 850-0832, Japan

Mitsunori Komine
Tsuruta Rehabilitation Clinic, 174-8 Ogi-Ushizu, Saga 849-0305, Japan

Muhammet Cinar, Sedat Yilmaz, Ismail Simsek, Hakan Erdem, Salih Pay and Ayhan Dinc
Division of Rheumatology, Gulhane Military Medical Academy School of Medicine, 06018 Etlik, Ankara, Turkey

Hatice Tugba Sanal
Department of Radiology, Gulhane Military Medical Academy School of Medicine, 06018 Etlik, Ankara, Turkey

E. Roos, S. J. M. Breugem, G. R. Schaap and J. A.M. Bramer
Department of Orthopedic Surgery, Academic Medical Center, 1100DD Amsterdam, Netherlands

M. Maas
Department of Radiology, Academic Medical Center, Amsterdam, Netherlands

Talal Hilal
Department of Internal Medicine, University of Kentucky College of Medicine, Charles T Wethington Building 304B,900 South Limestone Street, Lexington, KY 40536, USA

Eiko Saito, Shinji Sato, Shinichi Nogi, Noriko Sasaki, Naofumi Chinen, Kiri Honda, Takayuki Wakabayashi, Chiho Yamada and Yasuo Suzuki
Division of Rheumatology, Department of Internal Medicine, Tokai University School of Medicine, 142 Shimokasuya, Isehara 160-8582, Japan

Naoya Nakamura
Department of Pathology, Tokai University School of Medicine, 142 Shimokasuya, Isehara 160-8582, Japan

Valéria Valim, Roberta Hora Rocha, Roberta Barcelos Couto, Thaysa Simões Paixão and Érica Vieira Serrano
Department of Internal Medicine, Universidade Federal do Espirito Santo, Marechal Campos Avenue 1355,29040-715 Vitoria, ES, Brazil

Lu Wang and Maria M. Picken
Department of Pathology and Laboratory Medicine, Loyola University Medical Center, 2160 S 1st Avenue, Maywood, IL 60153, USA

Crystal Rose, Paul Mellen and George Branam
Department of Pathology, Ball Memorial Hospital, Indiana University Health, 2401WUniversity Avenue, Muncie, IN 47303, USA

Fawad Aslam and Elizabeth B. Russell
Division of Rheumatology, Department of Internal Medicine, University of Arkansas for Medical Sciences, Little Rock, AR 72205, USA
Division of Rheumatology, Department of Internal Medicine, John L. McClellan Memorial Veterans Hospital, Little Rock, AR 72205, USA

Firas Bannout
Division of Rheumatology, Department of Internal Medicine, John L. McClellan Memorial Veterans Hospital, Little Rock, AR 72205, USA
Department of Neurology, University of Arkansas for Medical Sciences, Little Rock, AR 72205, USA

L. Watson
Department of Paediatric Nephrology, Institute of Child Health, Alder Hey Children's NHS Foundation Trust Hospital, Eaton Road, Liverpool L12 2AP, UK

P. Brogan
Department of Paediatric Rheumatology, Great Ormond Street NHS Hospital, LondonWC1N 3JH, UK

I. Peart
Department of Paediatric Cardiology, Alder Hey Children's NHS Foundation Trust Hospital, Eaton Road, Liverpool L12 2AP, UK

C. Landes and N. Barnes
Department of Paediatric Radiology, Alder Hey Children's NHS Foundation Trust Hospital, Eaton Road, Liverpool L12 2AP, UK

G. Cleary
Department of Paediatric Rheumatology, Alder Hey Children's NHS Foundation Trust Hospital, Eaton Road, Liverpool L12 2AP, UK

Yu Zuo, Michelle Foshat, You-wen Qian, Brent Kelly, Brock Harper and Bernard Karnath
Department of Internal Medicine, University of Texas Medical Branch, 301 University Boulevard, Galveston, TX 77555, USA

Valérie Huyge and Serge Goldman
Department of Nuclear Medicine, Hôpital Erasme, Université Libre de Bruxelles (ULB), 1070 Brussels, Belgium

Muhammad S. Soyfoo
Department of Rheumatology, Hôpital Erasme, Université Libre de Bruxelles (ULB), 1070 Brussels, Belgium

Marta Baleva
Department of Clinical Immunology, University Hospital Alexandrovska, Sofia, Bulgaria

Krasimir Nikolov
Department of Dermatology and Venereology, Medical University, 9002 Varna, Bulgaria

Emil Manov, Anastas Stoikov and Rebhat Shabani
Department of Internal Medicine II, University Hospital Alexandrovska, Sofia, Bulgaria

Lyubomir Dourmishev
Department of Dermatology and Venereology, University Hospital Alexandrovska, Sofia, Bulgaria

Milena Nikolova
Department of Nephrology, University Hospital Alexandrovska, Sofia, Bulgaria

Raya Saba, Shawn G. Kwatra, Bishwas Upadhyay, Aibek E. Mirrakhimov and Farah N. Khan
Department of Internal Medicine, Saint Joseph Hospital, 2900 N. Lake Shore, Chicago, IL 60657, USA

Mariangelí Arroyo-Ávila, Ruth M. Fred-Jiménez and Luis M. Vilá
Division of Rheumatology, Department of Medicine, University of Puerto Rico, Medical Sciences Campus, San Juan, PR 00936, USA

Jose R. Zaragoza, Natalia Vernon, and Gisoo Ghaffari
Division of Allergy and Immunology, Penn State Hershey Allergy, Asthma and Immunology, 500 University Drive, UPC II, Suite 1300, Hershey, PA 17033, USA

Naoshi Nishina, Yuko Kaneko, Masataka Kuwana, Hironari Hanaoka, Hideto Kameda and Tsutomu Takeuchi
Division of Rheumatology, Department of Internal Medicine, School of Medicine, Keio University, 35 Shinanomachi Shinjuku-ku, Tokyo 160-8582, Japan

Shuji Mikami
Division of Diagnostic Pathology, Keio University Hospital, Tokyo 160-8582, Japan

Yasuo Iwata
Iwata Orthopedics and Rheumatology Clinic, No. 13-5, 1A Nakasuji 8-Chome, Takarazuka, Hyogo 665-9874, Japan

Basheer Tashtoush, Roya Memarpour and Jose Ramirez
Department of Pulmonary and Critical Care Medicine, Cleveland Clinic Florida, 2950 Cleveland Clinic Boulevard, Weston, FL 33331, USA

Yasmin Johnston
Department of Clinical Pathology, Cleveland Clinic Florida, 2950 Cleveland Clinic Boulevard,Weston, FL 33331, USA

Howard Van Gelder, Kim M. Wu, Philip J. Clements and Robert I. Morris
UCLA-Olive View Rheumatology Program, Division of Rheumatology, Olive View-UCLA Medical Center, 14445 Olive View Drive, 2B182, Sylmar, CA 91342, USA

Andrew L. Wong and Emil R. Heinze
UCLA-Olive View Rheumatology Program, Division of Rheumatology, Olive View-UCLA Medical Center, 14445 Olive View Drive, 2B182, Sylmar, CA 91342, USA
UCLA-Olive View Internal Medicine Program, Department of Medicine, Olive View-UCLA Medical Center, 14445 Olive View Drive, 2B182, Sylmar, CA 91342, USA

Nayiri Gharibian and Dharmi B. Patel
UCLA-Olive View Internal Medicine Program, Department of Medicine, Olive View-UCLA Medical Center, 14445 Olive View Drive, 2B182, Sylmar, CA 91342, USA

Mohammad E. Naffaa, Alexander P. Rozin Alexandra Balbir-Gurman and Yolanda Braun-Moscovici
The B. Shine Rheumatology Unit, Rambam Health Care Campus, 31096 Haifa, Israel
Rappaport Faculty of Medicine, Technion-Israel Institute of Technology, 31096 Haifa, Israel

Netanel Horowitz
Rappaport Faculty of Medicine, Technion-Israel Institute of Technology, 31096 Haifa, Israel
Hematology Institute, Rambam Health Care Campus, 31096 Haifa, Israel

Ofer Ben-Itzhak
Rappaport Faculty of Medicine, Technion-Israel Institute of Technology, 31096 Haifa, Israel
Pathology Institute, Rambam Health Care Campus, 31096 Haifa, Israel

Vahid Ziaee
Department of Pediatrics, Tehran University of Medical Sciences, Tehran, Iran
Pediatric Rheumatology Research Group, Rheumatology Research Center, Tehran University of Medical Sciences, Tehran, Iran
Division of Pediatric Rheumatology, Children's Medical Center, Pediatrics Center of Excellence, Tehran 14194, Iran

Mohammad Hassan Moradinejad
Department of Pediatrics, Tehran University of Medical Sciences, Tehran, Iran
Division of Pediatric Rheumatology, Children's Medical Center, Pediatrics Center of Excellence, Tehran 14194, Iran
Growth and Development Research Center, Tehran University of Medical Sciences, Tehran, Iran

Reyhaneh Bayat
Growth and Development Research Center, Tehran University of Medical Sciences, Tehran, Iran

Franchesca Cruz-Pérez, Salvador Vilá, Grissel Ríos, and Luis M. Vilá
Division of Rheumatology, Department of Medicine, University of Puerto Rico Medical Sciences Campus, San Juan, PR, USA

Elena Tsitsami and Charis Papadopoulou
Pediatric Rheumatology Unit, 1st Department of Pediatrics, Children's Hospital "Aghia Sophia", University of Athens, 115 27 Athens, Greece

Matthaios Speletas
Department of Immunology and Histocompatibility, School of Medicine, University of Thessaly, 411 10 Biopolis, Larissa, Greece

NurGen Düzgün, Orhan Küçük Gahin and Askin Ates
Department of Internal Medicine-Rheumatology, Ankara University, Faculty of Medicine, Akademik Yerleşke, Sıhhıye, 06100 Ankara, Turkey

Kayhan Çetin Atasoy, Ayse Erden and Seda Kaynak Fahap
Department of Radiology, Ankara University, Faculty of Medicine, Akademik Yerles¸ke, Sıhhıye, 06100 Ankara, Turkey

Canan Togay Isikay
Department of Neurology, Ankara University, Faculty of Medicine, Akademik Yerles¸ke, Sıhhıye, 06100 Ankara, Turkey

Demet Menekse Gerede
Department of Cardiology, Ankara University, Faculty of Medicine, Akademik Yerles¸ke, Sıhhıye, 06100 Ankara, Turkey

Muhammed Arif ibis
Department of Internal Medicine, Ankara University, Faculty of Medicine, Akademik Yerles¸ke, Sıhhıye, 06100 Ankara, Turkey

Hisashi Yamanaka
1Institute of Rheumatology, Tokyo Women's Medical University, 10-22 Kawada-cho, Shinjuku-ku, Tokyo 162-0054, Japan

Takako Miyamae, Yumi Tani and Takayuki Kishi
Institute of Rheumatology, Tokyo Women's Medical University, 10-22 Kawada-cho, Shinjuku-ku, Tokyo 162-0054, Japan
Department of Pediatrics, Tokyo Women's Medical University, 8-1 Kawada-cho, Shinjuku-ku, Tokyo 162-8666, Japan

Takuma Hara and Aki Hanaya
Department of Pediatrics, Tokyo Women's Medical University, 8-1 Kawada-cho, Shinjuku-ku, Tokyo 162-8666, Japan

Shanti Virupannavar and Heather Laird-Fick
Internal Medicine, Michigan State University, 138 Service Road, A225 Clinical Center, East Lansing, MI 48825, USA

Anthony Brandau
Internal Medicine and Hematology/Oncology, McLaren of Greater Lansing, 401West Greenlawn Avenue, Lansing, MI 48910, USA

Carla Guggenheim
Internal Medicine and Rheumatology, Michigan State University, 138 Service Road, A225 Clinical Center, East Lansing, MI 48825, USA

Fernando Gonzalez-Ibarra, Sahar Eivaz-Mohammadi, Shiri Surapaneni and Mazhar Elamir
Department of Internal Medicine, Mount Sinai School of Medicine, Jersey City Medical Center, 355 Grand Street, Jersey City, NJ 07302, USA

Hazem Alsaadi
Department of Internal Medicine, Jersey City Medical Center, St. George's University School of Medicine, Jersey City, NJ 07302, USA

Amer K. Syed
Laureate National Institute of Medicine, Jersey City Medical Center, 355 Grand Street, Jersey City, NJ 07302, USA

Simon Badin
Department of Hematology, Mount Sinai School of Medicine, Jersey City Medical Center, Jersey City, NJ 07302, USA

Valentin Marian
Department of Rheumatology, Mount Sinai School of Medicine, Jersey City Medical Center, Jersey City, NJ 07302, USA

Yoshio Nagayama and Akihide Nampei
Department of Orthopaedic Surgery, Osaka Rosai Hospital, 1179-3 Nagasonecho, Kita-ku, Sakai 591-8025, Japan

Naoki Matsushiro
Department of Otolaryngology, Osaka Police Hospital, 10-31 Kitayamacho, Tennoji-ku, Osaka 543-0035, Japan

Hideo Hashimoto
Rinku Hashimoto Rheumatology Orthopaedics, 1 Rinku Orai kita, Izumisano, Osaka 598-0048, Japan

Kenrin Shi
Department of Orthopaedic Surgery, Osaka University Graduate School of Medicine, 2-2 Yamadaoka, Suita, Osaka, Japan

Yahia Z. Imam
General Medicine Division, Department of Medicine, Hamad Medical Corporation, Doha, Qatar

Issa Mattar
General Medicine Division, Department of Medicine, Hamad Medical Corporation, Doha, Qatar

Weill Cornell Medical School, Hamad Medical Corporation, Doha, Qatar

Housam Aldeen Sarakbi
Rheumatology Division, Department of Medicine, Hamad Medical Corporation, Doha, Qatar
Weill Cornell Medical School, Hamad Medical Corporation, Doha, Qatar

Nagui Abdelwahab
Department of Radiology, Faculty of Medicine, Cairo University, Giza, Egypt

Richard A. Lau, Ramandeep Bains and Philip J. Clements
1UCLA-Olive View Rheumatology Program, Division of Rheumatology, Olive View-UCLA Medical Center, 14445 Olive View Drive,2B182, Sylmar, CA 91342, USA

Emil R. Heinze and Andrew L. Wong
UCLA-Olive View Rheumatology Program, Division of Rheumatology, Olive View-UCLA Medical Center, 14445 Olive View Drive, 2B182, Sylmar, CA 91342, USA
UCLA-Olive View Internal Medicine Program, Department of Medicine, Olive View-UCLA Medical Center, 14445 Olive View Drive,2B182, Sylmar, CA 91342, USA

Duminda Suraweera and Jane Ma
UCLA-Olive View Internal Medicine Program, Department of Medicine, Olive View-UCLA Medical Center, 14445 Olive View Drive,2B182, Sylmar, CA 91342, USA

Rajesh Gopalarathinam
Department of Internal Medicine, Allegheny General Hospital, 320 E. North Avenue, Pittsburgh, PA 15212, USA

Eric Orlowsky
Department of Rheumatology, Allegheny General Hospital, 320 E. North Avenue, Pittsburgh, PA 15212, USA

Ramesh Kesavalu
Department of Rheumatology, Lakeside Community Healthcare Medical Group, 1500 S. Central Avenue No. 200,Glendale, CA 91204, USA

Sreeteja Yelaminchili
Department of Internal Medicine, Capital Health Regional Medical Center, 750 Brunswick Avenue, Trenton, NJ 08638, USA

Champa Nataraja
Barwon Health, Bellerine Street, Geelong, VIC 3220, Australia

Hedley Griffith
Barwon Health, Bellerine Street, Geelong, VIC 3220, Australia
Barwon Rheumatology Service, 156 Bellerine Street, Geelong, VIC 3220, Australia

Ozan Volkan Yurdakul, Okan Küçükakkaş and Aylin Rezvani
Department of Physical Medicine and Rehabilitation, Bezmialem Foundation University, Istanbul, Turkey

Abdulkerim Furkan Tamer
Department of Nephrology, Gaziosmanpasa Taksim Training and Research Hospital, Istanbul, Turkey

Tracy M. Frech
Division of Rheumatology, Department of Internal Medicine, University of Utah School of Medicine, 4B200 30 N. 1900 E., Salt Lake City, UT 84132, USA

Kathleen Boynton and Kathryn Peterson
Division of Gastroenterology, Department of Internal Medicine, University of Utah, 50 N Medical Drive, Salt Lake City, UT 84132, USA

Erinn Downs-Kelly
Department of Anatomic Pathology, University of Utah, 50 N Medical Drive, Salt Lake City, UT 84132, USA

Bryan Jones
Department of Ophthalmology, University of Utah, 50 N Medical Drive, Salt Lake City, UT 84132, USA

John D. Kriesel
Division of Infectious Diseases, Department of Internal Medicine, University of Utah, 50 N Medical Drive, Salt Lake City, UT 84132, USA

Devin Malik and Sheela Tejwani
Department of Hematology Oncology, Henry Ford Hospital, 2799 W. Grand Blvd., Detroit, MI 48202, USA

Richa Handa
Department of Internal Medicine, Henry Ford Allegiance Health, 205 N. East Ave., Jackson, MI 49201, USA

Andrew Petraszko
Department of Radiology, Henry Ford Hospital, 2799 W. Grand Blvd., Detroit, MI 48202, USA

Hussein Halabi and Israa Mulla
King Faisal Specialist Hospital and Research Center, Jeddah 21499, Saudi Arabia

M. Colaci, D. Giuggioli, C. Vacchi and C. Ferri
Rheumatology Unit, Azienda Ospedaliero-Universitaria Policlinico di Modena, University of Modena and Reggio Emilia, Modena, Italy

Koichiro Takahashi, Hironori Sadamatsu, Shinsuke Ogusu, Kazutoshi Komiya, Tomomi Nakamura, Shinya Kimura and Naoko Sueoka-Aragane
Division of Hematology, Respiratory Medicine and Oncology, Department of Internal Medicine, Faculty of Medicine, Saga University, 5-1-1 Nabeshima, Saga 849-8501, Japan

Aneeta R. Kiran, Richard A. Lau, Kim M. Wu and Philip J. Clements
UCLA-Olive View Rheumatology Program, Division of Rheumatology, Olive View-UCLA Medical Center,14445 Olive View Drive, No. 2B182, Sylmar, CA 91342, USA

Andrew L. Wong and Emil R. Heinze
UCLA-Olive View Internal Medicine Program, Department of Medicine, Olive View-UCLA Medical Center,14445 Olive View Drive, No. 2B182, Sylmar, CA 91342, USA

Yanal Alnimer, Suresh Subedi, Thair Dawood and Ghassan Bachuwa
Internal Medicine Department, Hurley Medical Center, Flint, MI, USA

Nicole Marijanovich
Internal Medicine Department, Beaumont Hospital, Royal Oak, MI, USA
9 North Beaumont Hospital, Royal Oak, MI, USA
Oakland University William Beaumont School of Medicine, Rochester, MI, USA

Alexandra Halalau
Internal Medicine Department, Beaumont Hospital, Royal Oak, MI, USA
Oakland University William Beaumont School of Medicine, Rochester, MI, USA
General Internal Medicine Division, Beaumont Hospital, Royal Oak, MI, USA

Anshuman Srivastava and Diwakar Kumar Singh
Department of Medicine, PGIMER and Dr. RML Hospital, New Delhi 110001, India

Bijit Kumar Kundu
Rheumatology Clinic, Department of Medicine, PGIMER and Dr. RML Hospital, New Delhi 110001, India

Shinichiro Tsurukawa, Nozomi Iwanaga, Yasumori Izumi, Chieko Kawahara and Kiyoshi Migita
Department of Rheumatology, Clinical Research Center, NHO Nagasaki Medical Center, Kubara 2-1001-1, Omura 856-8562, Japan

Atsunori Shirakawa
Department of Pharmacy, Clinical Research Center, NHO Nagasaki Medical Center, Kubara 2-1001-1, Omura 856-8562, Japan

Tetsuo Shukuwa
Department of Dermatology, Clinical Research Center, NHO Nagasaki Medical Center, Kubara 2-1001-1, Omura 856-8562, Japan

Miwako Inamoto
Department of Ophthalmology, Clinical Research Center, NHO Nagasaki Medical Center, Kubara 2-1001-1, Omura 856-8562, Japan

Atsushi Kawakami
Department of Immunology and Rheumatology, Unit of Translational Medicine, Nagasaki University Graduate School of Biomedical Sciences, Sakamoto 1-7-1, Nagasaki 852-8501, Japan

Hisashi Yamanaka
Institute of Rheumatology, TokyoWomen'sMedical University,No. 10-22, Kawadacho, Shinjuku-ku, Tokyo 162-0054, Japan

Takako Miyamae
Institute of Rheumatology, TokyoWomen'sMedical University,No. 10-22, Kawadacho, Shinjuku-ku, Tokyo 162-0054, Japan
Department of Pediatrics, TokyoWomen's Medical University, No. 8-1, Kawadacho, Shinjuku-ku, Tokyo 162-0054, Japan

Naoko Ishiguro
Department of Dermatology, TokyoWomen's Medical University, No. 8-1, Kawadacho, Shinjuku-ku, Tokyo 162-0054, Japan

Maria Yonezawa and Katsutoshi Tokushige
Institute of Gastroenterology, TokyoWomen's Medical University, No. 8-1, Kawadacho, Shinjuku-ku, Tokyo 162-0054, Japan

Khalid Hamid Changal, Adnan Raina and Ab. Hameed Raina
Internal Medicine, Sher-I-Kashmir Institute of Medical Sciences, Srinagar 190011, India

Fayaz Sofi
Rheumatology and Internal Medicine, Sher-I-Kashmir Institute of Medical Sciences, Srinagar 190011, India

Sheikh Shoaib Altaf
Internal Medicine, Mercy Catholic Medical Center, Philadelphia, PA 19026, USA

Ali Zakaria, Issam Turk, Kenneth Leung, Ana Capatina-Rata and Waseem Farra
Department of Internal Medicine, Division of Pulmonology, Division of Rheumatology, Providence-Providence Park Hospital, Michigan State University College of Human Medicine, Southfield, MI, USA

Saika Sharmeen
Department of Medicine, St. Luke's-Roosevelt Hospital Center, New York, NY 10025, USA
Department of Medicine, Icahn School of Medicine at Mount Sinai, New York, NY 10025, USA

Nazia Hussain
Department of Medicine, Icahn School of Medicine at Mount Sinai, New York, NY 10025, USA
Division of Rheumatology, Department of Medicine, St. Luke's-Roosevelt Hospital Center, New York, NY 10025, USA

A. Majjad, A. Bezza and A. El Maghraoui
Rheumatology Department, Mohammed V Military Academic Hospital, Faculty of Medicine and Pharmacy, Mohammed V University, Rabat, Morocco

A. Biyi
Nuclear Medicine Department, Mohammed V Military Academic Hospital, Faculty of Medicine and Pharmacy, Mohammed V University, Rabat, Morocco

M. R. El Ochi
Anatomic Pathology Department, Mohammed V Military Academic Hospital, Faculty of Medicine and Pharmacy, Mohammed V University, Rabat, Morocco

Eva Johanna Schäfer and Wolfram Jung
Department of Hematology and Oncology, University Medical Center Göttingen, Göttingen, Germany

Peter Korsten
Department of Nephrology and Rheumatology, University Medical Center G¨ottingen, G¨ottingen, Germany

Jawad Al-Khafaji and Venkata Rajesh Konjeti
Department of Medicine, Virginia Commonwealth University Health System, Richmond, VA 23298, USA

Fran Ganz-Lord
CareMount Medical, Chappaqua, NY 10514, USA

Aaron D. Viny
Human Oncology and Pathogenesis Program, Memorial Sloan Kettering Cancer Center, New York, NY 10065, USA

Richard Hariman, Payal Patel, Jennifer Strouse and Ann Rosenthal
Division of Rheumatology, Department of Medicine, Medical College of Wisconsin, 9200W.Wisconsin Avenue, Milwaukee, WI 53226, USA

Michael P. Collins
Department of Neurology, Medical College of Wisconsin, 9200W.Wisconsin Avenue, Milwaukee, WI 53226, USA

Index